Model-Informed Precision Dosing

Model-Informed Precision Dosing

Editors

Jonás Samuel Pérez-Blanco
José Martínez Lanao

MDPI • Basel • Beijing • Wuhan • Barcelona • Belgrade • Manchester • Tokyo • Cluj • Tianjin

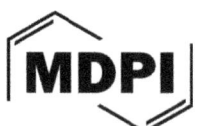

Editors
Jonás Samuel Pérez-Blanco
University of Salamanca
Salamanca
Spain

José Martínez Lanao
University of Salamanca
Salamanca
Spain

Editorial Office
MDPI
St. Alban-Anlage 66
4052 Basel, Switzerland

This is a reprint of articles from the Special Issue published online in the open access journal *Pharmaceutics* (ISSN 1999-4923) (available at: https://www.mdpi.com/journal/pharmaceutics/special_issues/model).

For citation purposes, cite each article independently as indicated on the article page online and as indicated below:

LastName, A.A.; LastName, B.B.; LastName, C.C. Article Title. *Journal Name* **Year**, *Volume Number*, Page Range.

ISBN 978-3-0365-6896-6 (Hbk)
ISBN 978-3-0365-6897-3 (PDF)

© 2023 by the authors. Articles in this book are Open Access and distributed under the Creative Commons Attribution (CC BY) license, which allows users to download, copy and build upon published articles, as long as the author and publisher are properly credited, which ensures maximum dissemination and a wider impact of our publications.

The book as a whole is distributed by MDPI under the terms and conditions of the Creative Commons license CC BY-NC-ND.

Contents

About the Editors ix

Jonás Samuel Pérez-Blanco and José M. Lanao
Model-Informed Precision Dosing (MIPD)
Reprinted from: *Pharmaceutics* **2022**, *14*, 2731, doi:10.3390/pharmaceutics14122731 1

Heleen Gastmans, Erwin Dreesen, Sebastian G. Wicha, Nada Dia, Ellen Spreuwers, Annabel Dompas, et al.
Systematic Comparison of Hospital-Wide Standard and Model-Based Therapeutic Drug Monitoring of Vancomycin in Adults
Reprinted from: *Pharmaceutics* **2022**, *14*, 1459, doi:10.3390/pharmaceutics14071459 5

Vanesa Escudero-Ortiz, Vanessa Domínguez-Leñero, Ana Catalán-Latorre, Joseba Rebollo-Liceaga and Manuel Sureda
Relevance of Therapeutic Drug Monitoring of Tyrosine Kinase Inhibitors in Routine Clinical Practice: A Pilot Study
Reprinted from: *Pharmaceutics* **2022**, *14*, 1216, doi:10.3390/pharmaceutics14061216 19

Paulo Teixeira-da-Silva, Jonás Samuel Pérez-Blanco, Dolores Santos-Buelga, María José Otero and María José García
Population Pharmacokinetics of Valproic Acid in Pediatric and Adult Caucasian Patients
Reprinted from: *Pharmaceutics* **2022**, *14*, 811, doi:10.3390/pharmaceutics14040811 39

Laurynas Mockeliunas, Lina Keutzer, Marieke G. G. Sturkenboom, Mathieu S. Bolhuis, Lotte M. G. Hulskotte, Onno W. Akkerman and Ulrika S. H. Simonsson
Model-Informed Precision Dosing of Linezolid in Patients with Drug-Resistant Tuberculosis
Reprinted from: *Pharmaceutics* **2022**, *14*, 753, doi:10.3390/pharmaceutics14040753 51

Cyril Leven, Anne Coste and Camille Mané
Free and Open-Source Posologyr Software for Bayesian Dose Individualization: An Extensive Validation on Simulated Data
Reprinted from: *Pharmaceutics* **2022**, *14*, 442, doi:10.3390/pharmaceutics14020442 67

Woojin Jung, Heeyoon Jung, Ngoc-Anh Thi Vu, Gwan-Young Kim, Gyoung-Won Kim, Jung-woo Chae, et al.
Model-Based Equivalent Dose Optimization to Develop New Donepezil Patch Formulation
Reprinted from: *Pharmaceutics* **2022**, *14*, 244, doi:10.3390/pharmaceutics14020244 81

Femke de Velde, Brenda C. M. de Winter, Michael N. Neely, Jan Strojil, Walter M. Yamada, Stephan Harbarth, et al.
Parametric and Nonparametric Population Pharmacokinetic Models to Assess Probability of Target Attainment of Imipenem Concentrations in Critically Ill Patients
Reprinted from: *Pharmaceutics* **2021**, *13*, 2170, doi:10.3390/pharmaceutics13122170 91

Ferdinand Anton Weinelt, Miriam Songa Stegemann, Anja Theloe, Frieder Pfäfflin, Stephan Achterberg, Lisa Schmitt, et al.
Development of a Model-Informed Dosing Tool to Optimise Initial Antibiotic Dosing—A Translational Example for Intensive Care Units
Reprinted from: *Pharmaceutics* **2021**, *13*, 2128, doi:10.3390/pharmaceutics13122128 107

Ana Valero, Alicia Rodríguez-Gascón, Arantxa Isla, Helena Barrasa, Ester del Barrio-Tofiño, Antonio Oliver, et al.
Pseudomonas aeruginosa Susceptibility in Spain: Antimicrobial Activity and Resistance Suppression Evaluation by PK/PD Analysis
Reprinted from: *Pharmaceutics* **2021**, *13*, 1899, doi:10.3390/pharmaceutics13111899 121

Dong-Hwan Lee, Hyoung-Soo Kim, Sunghoon Park, Hwan-il Kim, Sun-Hee Lee and Yong-Kyun Kim
Population Pharmacokinetics of Meropenem in Critically Ill Korean Patients and Effects of Extracorporeal Membrane Oxygenation
Reprinted from: *Pharmaceutics* **2021**, *13*, 1861, doi:10.3390/pharmaceutics13111861 139

Unai Caballero, Elena Eraso, Javier Pemán, Guillermo Quindós, Valvanera Vozmediano, Stephan Schmidt and Nerea Jauregizar
In Vitro Pharmacokinetic/Pharmacodynamic Modelling and Simulation of Amphotericin B against *Candida auris*
Reprinted from: *Pharmaceutics* **2021**, *13*, 1767, doi:10.3390/pharmaceutics13111767 155

Alexandre Le Marouille, Emma Petit, Courèche Kaderbhaï, Isabelle Desmoulins, Audrey Hennequin, Didier Mayeur, et al.
Pharmacokinetic/Pharmacodynamic Model of Neutropenia in Real-Life Palbociclib-Treated Patients
Reprinted from: *Pharmaceutics* **2021**, *13*, 1708, doi:10.3390/pharmaceutics13101708 167

Rodrigo Alonso, Ainara Rodríguez-Achaerandio, Amaia Aguirre-Quiñonero, Aitor Artetxe, Ilargi Martínez-Ballesteros, Alicia Rodríguez-Gascón, et al.
Molecular Epidemiology, Antimicrobial Surveillance, and PK/PD Analysis to Guide the Treatment of *Neisseria gonorrhoeae* Infections
Reprinted from: *Pharmaceutics* **2021**, *13*, 1699, doi:10.3390/pharmaceutics13101699 181

Idoia Bilbao-Meseguer, Helena Barrasa, Eduardo Asín-Prieto, Ana Alarcia-Lacalle, Alicia Rodríguez-Gascón, Javier Maynar, et al.
Population Pharmacokinetics of Levetiracetam and Dosing Evaluation in Critically Ill Patients with Normal or Augmented Renal Function
Reprinted from: *Pharmaceutics* **2021**, *13*, 1690, doi:10.3390/pharmaceutics13101690 197

Ruben Faelens, Zhigang Wang, Thomas Bouillon, Paul Declerck, Marc Ferrante, Séverine Vermeire and Erwin Dreesen
Model-Informed Precision Dosing during Infliximab Induction Therapy Reduces Variability in Exposure and Endoscopic Improvement between Patients with Ulcerative Colitis
Reprinted from: *Pharmaceutics* **2021**, *13*, 1623, doi:10.3390/pharmaceutics13101623 211

Jurij Aguiar Zdovc, Jurij Hanžel, Tina Kurent, Nejc Sever, Matic Koželj, Nataša Smrekar, et al.
Ustekinumab Dosing Individualization in Crohn's Disease Guided by a Population Pharmacokinetic–Pharmacodynamic Model
Reprinted from: *Pharmaceutics* **2021**, *13*, 1587, doi:10.3390/pharmaceutics13101587 223

Christina Schräpel, Lukas Kovar, Dominik Selzer, Ute Hofmann, Florian Tran, Walter Reinisch, et al.
External Model Performance Evaluation of Twelve Infliximab Population Pharmacokinetic Models in Patients with Inflammatory Bowel Disease
Reprinted from: *Pharmaceutics* **2021**, *13*, 1368, doi:10.3390/pharmaceutics13091368 239

**Silvia Marquez-Megias, Amelia Ramon-Lopez, Patricio Más-Serrano,
Marcos Diaz-Gonzalez, Maria Remedios Candela-Boix and Ricardo Nalda-Molina**
Evaluation of the Predictive Performance of Population Pharmacokinetic Models of
Adalimumab in Patients with Inflammatory Bowel Disease
Reprinted from: *Pharmaceutics* **2021**, *13*, 1244, doi:10.3390/pharmaceutics13081244 . . . . **261**

**Martin Šíma, Danica Michaličková, Pavel Ryšánek, Petra Cihlářová, Martin Kuchař,
Daniela Lžičařová, et al.**
No Time Dependence of Ciprofloxacin Pharmacokinetics in Critically Ill Adults: Comparison
of Individual and Population Analyses
Reprinted from: *Pharmaceutics* **2021**, *13*, 1156, doi:10.3390/pharmaceutics13081156 . . . . **275**

**Francisco José Toja-Camba, Nerea Gesto-Antelo, Olalla Maroñas, Eduardo Echarri Arrieta,
Irene Zarra-Ferro, Miguel González-Barcia, et al.**
Review of Pharmacokinetics and Pharmacogenetics in Atypical Long-Acting
Injectable Antipsychotics
Reprinted from: *Pharmaceutics* **2021**, *13*, 935, doi:10.3390/pharmaceutics13070935 . . . . **289**

About the Editors

Jonás Samuel Pérez Blanco

Jonás Samuel Pérez Blanco is a research scientist currently working as assistant professor in pharmacokinetics at the University of Salamanca (Spain). His PhD and postdoctoral research in pharmacometrics at Janssen Pharmaceutica (Johnson & Johnson) allowed him to have a strong bacground in PK, PKPD and Exposure-Response modeling & simulations with NONMEM and R in different therapeutic areas such as Oncology, Central Nervous System (CNS) and Infectious Diseases and Vaccinology (IDV). He has da wide expertise in clinical trials, pharmacometrics, clinical pharmacology, late drug development of small molecules, analitycal methods (UHPLC), virtual training (second life) and teaching in academia (Pharmacy & Master degree, TDM and HPLC courses).

José Martínez Lanao

Professor of Pharmacy and Pharmaceutical Technology. University of Salamanca. Head of the Research group of Experimental and Clinical pharmacokinetics in the Institute of Biomedical Research of Salamanca (IBSAL) and Head of Pharmaceutical R & D Laboratory. of the University of Salamanca. He is an International expert in experimental and clinical pharmacokinetics, population pharmacokinetics, therapeutic drug monitoring (TDM), modeling and simulation and drug delivery and has published numerous articles in indexed journals and book chapters and supervised many PhD theses in this field. He is a member of the editorial board of different international journals.

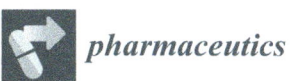

Editorial

Model-Informed Precision Dosing (MIPD)

Jonás Samuel Pérez-Blanco [1,2,*] and José M. Lanao [1,2]

[1] Area of Pharmacy and Pharmaceutical Technology, Department of Pharmaceutical Sciences, University of Salamanca, 37007 Salamanca, Spain
[2] The Institute for Biomedical Research of Salamanca (IBSAL), 37007 Salamanca, Spain
* Correspondence: jsperez@usal.es

Model-informed precision dosing (MIPD) is an advanced quantitative approach focusing on individualized dosage optimization, integrating complex mathematical and statistical models of drugs and disease combined with individual demographic and clinical patient characteristics. MIPD has been highlighted as a current and useful tool for drug dosage optimization in drug development processes and clinical practice.

This Special Issue focuses on new MIPD strategies and methodologies to optimize drug dosage in specific populations. A total of twenty manuscripts, nineteen research articles and one review article, are published in this Special Issue.

Population pharmacokinetics (popPK) and dose optimization in different types of patients constitutes a useful working tool within the framework of the MIPD approach. Population pharmacokinetic models are of essential in the selection of doses of a wide variety of drugs and especially drugs with a narrow therapeutic margin in special populations, such as pediatric patients, critically ill patients, etc.

In this Special Issue, a total of eleven manuscripts on popPK and the dosage of various drugs are presented, addressing antibiotics, including linelozid, meropenem, imipenem and ciprofloxacin, in special populations such as critically ill patients. Other popPK studies included in this Special Issue focus on different drugs, such as valproic acid in pediatric and adult Caucasian patients, donezepil administered in patch formulations, levetiracetam in critically ill patients with normal or augmented renal function, and monoclonal antibodies such as infliximab or adalimumab for anti-TNF therapy in patients with inflammatory bowel disease.

One of the manuscripts focuses on building a popPK model to establish MIPD algorithm to optimize the dosing of linezolid in patients with multidrug and extensively drug-resistant tuberculosis and propose three sampling occasions to derive an individualized dose that results in effective and safe dosage regimens [1].

Considering the therapeutic importance of the use of antibiotics in patient populations with great inter- and intra-individual variability, this Special Issue includes MIPD-based dosing strategies for antibiotics, such as meropenem, imipenem and ciprofloxacin, for patients in intensive care units. Based on a popPK model of meropenem for critically ill adult patients using probability target attainment (PTA), prolonged infusion or a high-dosage regimen of meropenem is proposed, particularly when treating critically ill patients with increased renal clearance or those infected with pathogens with decreased in vitro susceptibility. This study also concludes that extracorporeal membrane oxygenation (ECMO) use does not affect meropenem PK in critically ill patients [2].

A tabular precision dosing tool for the initial therapy of meropenem, integrating hospital-specific pathogen susceptibility and based on popPK in intensive care units, was developed [3]. Parametric and non-parametric popPK models were also optimized for the dosage of imipenem in critically ill patients, which is appropriate for individuals with high glomerular filtration rates (eGFRs), but insufficient for low eGFRs [4].

In another comparative study, an individual and popPK analysis of ciprofloxacin in critically ill patients in the first 36 h of treatment was performed. No differences were

Citation: Pérez-Blanco, J.S.; Lanao, J.M. Model-Informed Precision Dosing (MIPD). *Pharmaceutics* **2022**, *14*, 2731. https://doi.org/10.3390/pharmaceutics14122731

Received: 25 November 2022
Accepted: 2 December 2022
Published: 6 December 2022

Publisher's Note: MDPI stays neutral with regard to jurisdictional claims in published maps and institutional affiliations.

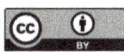

Copyright: © 2022 by the authors. Licensee MDPI, Basel, Switzerland. This article is an open access article distributed under the terms and conditions of the Creative Commons Attribution (CC BY) license (https://creativecommons.org/licenses/by/4.0/).

reported between ciprofloxacin pharmacokinetic parameters between early and late phases of treatment, and creatinine clearance was identified as a covariate of ciprofloxacin pharmacokinetics [5]. In this same type of population, a study on the population pharmacokinetics of the antiepileptic levetiracetam in critically ill patients with normal or augmented renal function was carried out, proposing specific dosing schemes for this kind of population [6].

The good predictability of a popPK model of valproic acid was found based on the characterization of the valproic acid apparent clearance (CL/F) in pediatric and adult Caucasian patients. The popPK model demonstrates the influence of co-administration with carbamazepine, phenytoin, and phenobarbital on the pharmacokinetics of valproic acid [7].

A two-compartmental popPK model of the antipsychotic donezepil with two transit compartments was used for the characterization of this drug after the administration of transdermal patches in comparison with the oral route of administration, establishing dose equivalence between both routes of administration [8]. Additionally, and in the therapeutic group of antipsychotics, a review on the PK and pharmacogenetic data regarding the three major long-acting injectable (LAI) atypical antipsychotics, risperidone, paliperidone, and aripiprazole, is included in this Special Issue. The main conclusions of this review are the role of CYP2D6 in the PK of LAI aripiprazole and common aspects in the popPK models developed for these drugs, such as the influence of body weight, administration site, and needle characteristics. The manuscript also suggests that the combination of pharmacogenetics and PK leads to individualized dosing antipsychotic therapy [9].

This Special Issue also includes three papers on popPK and the dosing of two monoclonal antibodies, infliximab and adalimumab in patients with gastrointestinal tract diseases, such as ulcerative colitis and Crohn's disease.

The predictive performance of twelve different published infliximab popPK models for inflammatory bowel disease patients was evaluated. Two of the models were suggested to have the best predictive performance and may be used as MIPD approaches for infliximab therapy in this kind of population [10]. A similar manuscript allows the best predictive performance for two Adalimumab popPK models to be established [11].

Different dosing strategies have been tested in comparison to standard dosing for increasing infliximab exposure during induction therapy in patients with ulcerative colitis. A dose of 10 mg/kg improves the probability of endoscopic improvement together with dose adaptation based on the interindividual variability of the patients [12].

In addition, this Special Issue includes several studies on pharmacokinetic/pharmacodynamic models (PK/PD). Focusing on applications in the field of infectious diseases, three manuscripts of this type are included. The anti-pseudomonal activity of different antibiotics against *P. aeruginosa* was evaluated using a PK/PD analysis with three different PK/PD indices based on the probability of target attainment (PTA). According to the results of this study, the most active antibacterial against *P. aeruginosa* was ceftazidime/avibactam, followed by ceftolozane/tazobactam and colistin [13]. In the same way, PK/PD analysis was used as a tool to optimize the treatment of *Neisseria gonorrhoeae* infections. The conclusions of this study suggest that ceftriaxone and oral cefixime are good candidates for treating gonorrhea [14].

A semi-mechanistic pharmacokinetic/pharmacodynamic (PK/PD) modelling and simulation approach was tested to evaluate the activity of Amphotericin B against *Candida auris* in vitro. The model includes two fungal stages consisting of a drug-susceptible fungal subpopulation and a drug-resistant subpopulation. In addition, a modified Emax sigmoidal model better describes this drug effect [15].

Neutropenia is usually associated with palbociclib toxicity in patients with breast cancer who are treated with this drug. A PK/PD model of five compartments, including a blood compartment, stem cell compartment and three transit compartments, was used to evaluate the relationship between plasma concentrations of palbociclib and absolute neutrophile count. According to the results, palbociclib < 100 μg/L can limit the risk of grade 4 neutropenia [16].

The dosing individualization of ustekimab in Crohn's disease was based on a semi-mechanistic popPK/PD model composed of a two-compartment PK model linked to an indirect response model. This model allows individualized treatments with ustekimab in patients with Crohn´s disease [17].

Bayesian algorithms are a fundamental element of the MIPD framework because they can be used to forecast individualized dosing to obtain target therapeutic concentrations in patients enrolled in therapeutic drug monitoring (TDM) programs. In this Special Issue, several papers focus on this objective.

Bayesian software is an important tool in hospitals for the routine dosage individualization of a wide spectrum of drugs in different patient populations undergoing TDM programs. Posologyr is an open-source R package developed for Bayesian individual parameter estimation and dose individualization with different drugs. The performance of this computer program was tested against NONMEM for maximum a posteriori (MAP) points estimates and against Monolix for the estimation of full posterior distributions of individual parameters in a wide variety of models [18].

In this Special Issue, two articles focused on Bayesian forecasting for dosage adaptation following TDM. One of these addresses the predictive performance in vancomycin TDM testing five different model-based approaches and suggests the potential benefit of model-based vancomycin dosing in adult patients compared with the standard TDM [19]. The other contribution focuses on the use of the routine TDM of tyrosine kinase inhibitors (TKI), such as erlotinib, imatinib, lapatinib and sorafenib in cancer therapy. The results of the study demonstrate the high inter- and intra-individual variability in the PK behavior of this type of drug, as well as the utility of routine TDM to optimize doses and assess adherence, as well as interactions with food and other drugs [20].

In summary, this Special Issue demonstrates the rise of the MIPD as a powerful tool in the field of precision medicine for the optimization of treatments, with direct implications in increasing the safety and efficacy of pharmacological treatments.

Funding: This research received no external funding.

Conflicts of Interest: The authors declare no conflict of interest.

References

1. Mockeliunas, L.; Keutzer, L.; Sturkenboom, M.G.G.; Bolhuis, M.S.; Hulskotte, L.M.G.; Akkerman, O.W.; Simonsson, U.S.H. Model-Informed Precision Dosing of Linezolid in Patients with Drug-Resistant Tuberculosis. *Pharmaceutics* **2022**, *14*, 753. [CrossRef] [PubMed]
2. Lee, D.H.; Kim, H.S.; Park, S.; Kim, H.I.; Lee, S.H.; Kim, Y.K. Population Pharmacokinetics of Meropenem in Critically Ill Korean Patients and Effects of Extracorporeal Membrane Oxygenation. *Pharmaceutics* **2021**, *13*, 1861. [CrossRef] [PubMed]
3. Weinelt, F.A.; Stegemann, M.S.; Theloe, A.; Pfäfflin, F.; Achterberg, S.; Schmitt, L.; Huisinga, W.; Michelet, R.; Hennig, S.; Kloft, C. Development of a Model-Informed Dosing Tool to Optimise Initial Antibiotic Dosing-A Translational Example for Intensive Care Units. *Pharmaceutics* **2021**, *13*, 2128. [CrossRef] [PubMed]
4. de Velde, F.; de Winter, B.C.M.; Neely, M.N.; Strojil, J.; Yamada, W.M.; Harbarth, S.; Huttner, A.; van Gelder, T.; Koch, B.C.P.; Muller, A.E.; et al. Parametric and Nonparametric Population Pharmacokinetic Models to Assess Probability of Target Attaiment of Imipenem Concentrations in Critically Ill Patients. *Pharmaceutics* **2021**, *13*, 2170. [CrossRef] [PubMed]
5. Šíma, M.; Michaličková, D.; Ryšánek, P.; Cihlářová, P.; Kuchař, M.; Lžičařová, D.; Beroušek, J.; Hartinger, J.M.; Vymazal, T.; Slanař, O. No Time Dependence of Ciprofloxacin Pharmacokinetics in Critically Ill Adults: Comparison of Individual and Population Analyses. *Pharmaceutics* **2021**, *13*, 1156. [CrossRef] [PubMed]
6. Bilbao-Meseguer, I.; Barrasa, H.; Asín-Prieto, E.; Alarcia-Lacalle, A.; Rodríguez-Gascón, A.; Maynar, J.; Sánchez-Izquierdo, J.Á.; Balziskueta, G.; Griffith, M.S.; Quilez Trasobares, N.; et al. Population Pharmacokinetics of Levetiracetam and Dosing Evaluation in Critically Ill Patients with Normal or Augmented Renal Function. *Pharmaceutics* **2021**, *13*, 1690. [CrossRef] [PubMed]
7. Teixeira-da-Silva, P.; Pérez-Blanco, J.S.; Santos-Buelga, D.; Otero, M.J. García Population Pharmacokinetics of Valproic Acid in Pediatric and Adult Caucasian Patients. *Pharmaceutics* **2022**, *14*, 811. [CrossRef] [PubMed]
8. Jung, W.; Jung, H.; Vu, N.T.; Kim, G.Y.; Kim, G.W.; Chae, J.W.; Kim, T.; Yun, H.Y. Model-Based Equivalent Dose Optimization to Develop New Donepezil Patch Formulation. *Pharmaceutics* **2022**, *14*, 244. [CrossRef] [PubMed]
9. Toja-Camba, F.J.; Gesto-Antelo, N.; Maroñas, O.; Echarri Arrieta, E.; Zarra-Ferro, I.; González-Barcia, M.; Bandín-Vilar, E.; Mangas Sanjuan, V.; Facal, F.; Arrojo Romero, M.; et al. Review of Pharmacokinetics and Pharmacogenetics in Atypical Long-Acting Injectable Antipsychotics. *Pharmaceutics* **2021**, *13*, 935. [CrossRef] [PubMed]

10. Schräpel, C.; Kovar, L.; Selzer, D.; Hofmann, U.; Tran, F.; Reinisch, W.; Schwab, M.; Lehr, T. External Model Performance Evaluation of Twelve Infliximab Population Pharmacokinetic Models in Patients with Inflammatory Bowel Disease. *Pharmaceutics* **2021**, *13*, 1368. [CrossRef] [PubMed]
11. Marquez-Megias, S.; Ramon-Lopez, A.; Más-Serrano, P.; Diaz-Gonzalez, M.; Candela-Boix, M.R.; Nalda-Molina, R. Evaluation of the Predictive Performance of Population Pharmacokinetic Models of Adalimumab in Patients with Inflammatory Bowel Disease. *Pharmaceutics* **2021**, *13*, 1244. [CrossRef] [PubMed]
12. Faelens, R.; Wang, Z.; Bouillon, T.; Declerck, P.; Ferrante, M.; Vermeire, S.; Dreesen, E. Model-Informed Precision Dosing during Infliximab Induction Therapy Reduces Variability in Exposure and Endoscopic Improvement between Patients with Ulcerative Colitis. *Pharmaceutics* **2021**, *13*, 1623. [CrossRef] [PubMed]
13. Valero, A.; Rodríguez-Gascón, A.; Isla, A.; Barrasa, H.; Del Barrio-Tofiño, E.; Oliver, A.; Canut, A.; Solinís, M.Á. *Pseudomonas aeruginosa* Susceptibility in Spain: Antimicrobial Activity and Resistance Suppression Evaluation by PK/PD Analysis. *Pharmaceutics* **2021**, *13*, 1899. [CrossRef] [PubMed]
14. Alonso, R.; Rodríguez-Achaerandio, A.; Aguirre-Quiñonero, A.; Artetxe, A.; Martínez-Ballesteros, I.; Rodríguez-Gascón, A.; Garaizar, J.; Canut, A. Molecular Epidemiology, Antimicrobial Surveillance, and PK/PD Analysis to Guide the Treatment of *Neisseria gonorrhoeae* Infections. *Pharmaceutics* **2021**, *13*, 1699. [CrossRef] [PubMed]
15. Caballero, U.; Eraso, E.; Pemán, J.; Quindós, G.; Vozmediano, V.; Schmidt, S.; Jauregizar, N. In Vitro Pharmacokinetic/Pharmacodynamic Modelling and Simulation of Amphotericin B against *Candida auris*. *Pharmaceutics* **2021**, *13*, 1767. [CrossRef] [PubMed]
16. Marouille, A.L.; Petit, E.; Kaderbhaï, C.; Desmoulins, I.; Hennequin, A.; Mayeur, D.; Fumet, J.D.; Ladoire, S.; Tharin, Z.; Ayati, S.; et al. Pharmacokinetic/Pharmacodynamic Model of Neutropenia in Real-Life Palbociclib-Treated Patients. *Pharmaceutics* **2021**, *13*, 1708. [CrossRef] [PubMed]
17. Aguiar Zdovc, J.; Hanžel, J.; Kurent, T.; Sever, N.; Koželj, M.; Smrekar, N.; Novak, G.; Štabuc, B.; Dreesen, E.; Thomas, D.; et al. Ustekinumab Dosing Individualization in Crohn's Disease Guided by a Population Pharmacokinetic-Pharmacodynamic Model. *Pharmaceutics* **2021**, *13*, 1587. [CrossRef] [PubMed]
18. Leven, C.; Coste, A.; Mane, C. Free and Open-Source Posologyr Software for Bayesian Dose Individualization: An Extensive Validation on Simulated Data. *Pharmaceutics* **2022**, *14*, 442. [CrossRef] [PubMed]
19. Gastmans, H.; Dreesen, E.; Wicha, S.G.; Dia, N.; Spreuwers, E.; Dompas, A.; Allegaert, K.; Desmet, S.; Lagrou, K.; Peetermans, W.E.; et al. Systematic Comparison of Hospital-Wide Standard and Model-Based Therapeutic Drug Monitoring of Vancomycin in Adults. *Pharmaceutics* **2022**, *14*, 1459. [CrossRef] [PubMed]
20. Escudero-Ortiz, V.; Domínguez-Leñero, V.; Catalán-Latorre, A.; Rebollo-Liceaga, J.; Sureda, M. Relevance of Therapeutic Drug Monitoring of Tyrosine Kinase Inhibitors in Routine Clinical Practice: A Pilot Study. *Pharmaceutics* **2022**, *14*, 1216. [CrossRef] [PubMed]

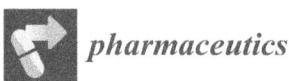

Article

Systematic Comparison of Hospital-Wide Standard and Model-Based Therapeutic Drug Monitoring of Vancomycin in Adults

Heleen Gastmans [1,†], Erwin Dreesen [2,†], Sebastian G. Wicha [3], Nada Dia [2], Ellen Spreuwers [1], Annabel Dompas [4], Karel Allegaert [2,5,6], Stefanie Desmet [7,8], Katrien Lagrou [7,8], Willy E. Peetermans [9,10], Yves Debaveye [11], Isabel Spriet [1,2,‡] and Matthias Gijsen [1,2,*,‡]

1. Pharmacy Department, UZ Leuven, 3000 Leuven, Belgium; heleen.gastmans@uzleuven.be (H.G.); ellen.spreuwers@uzleuven.be (E.S.); isabel.spriet@uzleuven.be (I.S.)
2. Clinical Pharmacology and Pharmacotherapy, Department of Pharmaceutical and Pharmacological Sciences, KU Leuven, 3000 Leuven, Belgium; erwin.dreesen@kuleuven.be (E.D.); nada.dia@kuleuven.be (N.D.); karel.allegaert@kuleuven.be (K.A.)
3. Department of Clinical Pharmacy, Institute of Pharmacy, University of Hamburg, 20146 Hamburg, Germany; sebastian.wicha@uni-hamburg.de
4. Department of Information Technology, University Hospitals Leuven, 3000 Leuven, Belgium; annabel.dompas@uzleuven.be
5. Department of Development and Regeneration, KU Leuven, 3000 Leuven, Belgium
6. Department of Hospital Pharmacy, Erasmus MC University Medical Center, 3015 GD Rotterdam, The Netherlands
7. Laboratory of Clinical Bacteriology and Mycology, Department of Microbiology, Immunology and Transplantation, KU Leuven, 3000 Leuven, Belgium; stefanie.desmet@uzleuven.be (S.D.); katrien.lagrou@uzleuven.be (K.L.)
8. Department of Laboratory Medicine, UZ Leuven, 3000 Leuven, Belgium
9. Laboratory of Clinical Infectious and Inflammatory Disease, Department of Microbiology, Immunology and Transplantation, KU Leuven, 3000 Leuven, Belgium; willy.peetermans@uzleuven.be
10. Department of General Internal Medicine, UZ Leuven, 3000 Leuven, Belgium
11. Laboratory for Intensive Care Medicine, Department of Cellular and Molecular Medicine, KU Leuven, 3000 Leuven, Belgium; yves.debaveye@uzleuven.be
* Correspondence: matthias.gijsen@uzleuven.be; Tel.: +32-16-340087
† Shared first authors.
‡ Shared last author.

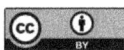

Abstract: We aimed to evaluate the predictive performance and predicted doses of a single-model approach or several multi-model approaches compared with the standard therapeutic drug monitoring (TDM)-based vancomycin dosing. We performed a hospital-wide monocentric retrospective study in adult patients treated with either intermittent or continuous vancomycin infusions. Each patient provided two randomly selected pairs of two consecutive vancomycin concentrations. A web-based precision dosing software, TDMx, was used to evaluate the model-based approaches. In total, 154 patients contributed 308 pairs. With standard TDM-based dosing, only 48.1% (148/308) of all of the second concentrations were within the therapeutic range. Across the model-based approaches we investigated, the mean relative bias and relative root mean square error varied from −5.36% to 3.18% and from 24.8% to 28.1%, respectively. The model averaging approach according to the squared prediction errors showed an acceptable bias and was the most precise. According to this approach, the median (interquartile range) differences between the model-predicted and prescribed doses, expressed as mg every 12 h, were 113 [−69; 427] mg, −70 [−208; 120], mg and 40 [−84; 197] mg in the case of subtherapeutic, supratherapeutic, and therapeutic exposure at the second concentration, respectively. These dose differences, along with poor target attainment, suggest a large window of opportunity for the model-based TDM compared with the standard TDM-based vancomycin dosing. Implementation studies of model-based TDM in routine care are warranted.

Keywords: vancomycin; therapeutic drug monitoring; population pharmacokinetics; precision dosing; predictive performance; model averaging; model selection; Bayesian forecasting

1. Introduction

Vancomycin is a glycopeptide antibiotic, administered intravenously to treat severe infections due to Gram-positive bacteria. Vancomycin is widely used across different patient populations [1]. Considering its relatively narrow therapeutic range, plasma concentrations are usually monitored during therapy, and therapeutic drug monitoring (TDM) is ubiquitously applied to guide vancomycin dosing [2,3].

Until recently, most institutions used concentrations obtained during intermittent (trough concentration, C_{trough}) or continuous infusion to guide vancomycin dosing as was recommended in the first consensus guideline for the TDM of vancomycin in 2009 [3]. In the 2020 update of this guideline, the ratio of the area under the concentration–time curve over 24 h to the minimum inhibitory concentration (AUC/MIC) was recommended over the use of vancomycin concentrations to guide the treatment of serious infections caused by methicillin-resistant *Staphylococcus aureus* [2]. Despite this recommendation, the pharmacokinetic/pharmacodynamic (PK/PD) index of interest that should be used to guide vancomycin dosing is still under debate [4–7]. Some argue that the evidence for using AUC/MIC-based TDM over the monitoring of vancomycin concentrations is inconclusive and that it is too early to justify the increased resource use associated with AUC/MIC monitoring [4,6,8]. As a result, there has not been a universal application of AUC/MIC-based TDM of vancomycin to date, and single vancomycin concentrations are still regularly used to guide dosing.

Irrespective of the PK/PD index, evidence reveals that many patients still experience vancomycin exposure outside of the therapeutic range with standard TDM-based strategies, associated with either reduced efficacy or increased toxicity [9,10]. Therefore, Bayesian forecasting has been proposed to provide standardized and accurate dose adaptations following the TDM of vancomycin [2,10]. Bayesian forecasting relies on the combination of previously developed pharmacokinetic population (pop) PK models and patient information, such as plasma concentrations, previous dosing information, and patient characteristics. The individually generated PK estimates then allow the prediction of future exposure according to specific dosing adaptations. This whole process is commonly referred to as model-informed precision dosing (MIPD) [11].

Currently, several dosing software modules offer vancomycin MIPD [11]. However, the accuracy of model-based dosing recommendations depends on the PopPK model used [12]. Several studies illustrated that it is particularly challenging to select one appropriate PopPK model of vancomycin for use in real-world clinical practice [13,14]. Recently, Uster et al. suggested two multi-model approaches—a model selection algorithm (MSA) and a model averaging algorithm (MAA)—that might address this important challenge and stimulate the integration of model-based vancomycin dosing in clinical practice [15].

Therefore, in this study, we aimed to evaluate the predictive performance and the predicted doses of a single-model approach and several multi-model approaches based on seven vancomycin models for the Bayesian forecasting of vancomycin dosing compared with the standard TDM-based dosing in a hospital-wide setting for both intermittent and continuous infusion regimens in adults.

2. Materials and Methods

2.1. Study Design, Patients, and Data Collection

This study was designed as a retrospective, monocentric, and hospital-wide evaluation study in adults. The study was approved by the Ethics Committee Research UZ/KU Leuven (S65213).

All adult patients admitted to any ward at the University Hospitals Leuven between January 2019 and January 2021 and treated with either intermittent or continuous vancomycin infusion were eligible for inclusion. To cover a hospital-wide adult patient population, both patients admitted to the intensive care unit (ICU) wards and non-ICU wards were included. Patients were excluded if they did not provide a minimum of three vancomycin plasma concentrations measured consecutively during one treatment course. Patients with two consecutive concentrations measured after >72 h were also excluded.

Demographic, clinical, and laboratory data were collected from the patients' medical files. For each patient, two randomly selected pairs of two consecutive vancomycin plasma concentrations were selected by a 'Research Randomizer' tool [16] as illustrated in Figure 1. For each pair of two consecutive plasma concentrations, the vancomycin dosing information was collected from the first vancomycin dose until the time of the second vancomycin concentration.

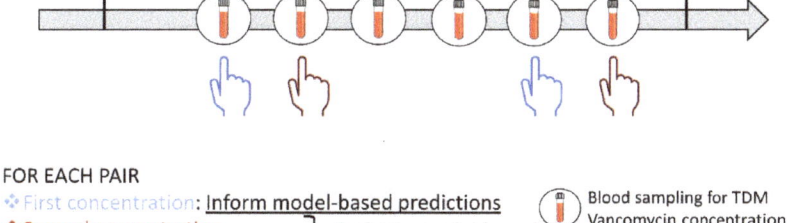

Figure 1. Schematic representation of the inclusion of two pairs of two consecutive vancomycin concentrations using a random example as illustration. The first concentration of each pair was used to inform the model-based predictions. The second concentration was blinded from the models and was used to evaluate the performance of the model-based prediction. The model-predicted dose after the first concentration was used to evaluate the model-based doses compared with the standard TDM-based doses.

2.2. Bayesian Forecasting

A free web-based MIPD software, TDMx [17], was used to evaluate the model-based vancomycin concentrations and doses. Five different model-based approaches were evaluated. First, a single-model approach using the Goti model [18] was evaluated. The Goti model was developed using a large and heterogeneous set of hospitalized patients. This specific model was selected as it was demonstrated to be the most suitable single model to drive model-based vancomycin dosing in both hospitalized non-ICU patients [14] and ICU patients [13]. Next, two automated multi-model algorithms were also evaluated, i.e., the MSA and the MAA [15]. Both algorithms were recently developed and validated in a heterogeneous population and integrated into TDMx. In TDMx, MSA and MAA predictions are based on seven vancomycin PopPK models [18–24]. These seven PopPK models were developed in distinct populations covering a broad hospital setting, including hospitalized, critically ill, extremely obese, dialysis, sepsis, trauma, and post-cardiac surgery patients. Therefore, these vancomycin models were considered representative of the hospital-wide adult patient population investigated in our study. The characteristics of these vancomycin models were reported in detail previously [15]. All models included at least creatinine clearance or serum creatinine and total body weight as covariates. All of the covariates included in the seven vancomycin models were collected except for the Simplified Acute Physiology Score (SAPS) score, which is not collected at our institution.

Both multi-model approaches used all of the available models simultaneously to provide predictions. The prediction of the MSA was the prediction of the best-fitting model for an individual patient based on the goodness-of-fit of each model to the previous vancomycin concentration (i.e., how well did the model predict the previous vancomycin concentration). Similarly, the MAA considered the same previously collected data. However, instead of selecting the best-fitting model, the prediction of the MAA was based on the weighted predictions of all of the PopPK models. The MSA and MAA both required a criterion to quantify the individual model's fit and to attribute the final weighting schemes.

Two different criteria to assess the models' fit metrics were evaluated: the objective function value (OFV) and the squared prediction errors (SSE). These weighting schemes were described in detail previously [15]. The MSA and MAA were evaluated according to these two weighting schemes. As such, we evaluated five different model-based approaches in this study: the Goti model, the MSA with weighting according to the OFV (MSA_{OFV}) or the SSE (MSA_{SSE}), and the MAA with weighting according to the OFV (MAA_{OFV}) or the SSE (MAA_{SSE}).

2.3. Evaluation of the Model-Based Approaches

For each of the five above-mentioned model-based approaches, we evaluated the predictive performance regarding the vancomycin model-based predictions. Subsequently, the model-based approach with the best predictive performance was used to evaluate the model-based vancomycin doses compared with the standard TDM-based doses. Additionally, a sensitivity analysis was performed using the model-based approach with the worst predictive performance to evaluate the robustness of the model-predicted doses across the different model-based approaches.

Initially, the first vancomycin concentration of each pair was used to inform the model-based predictions as illustrated in Figure 1. The second vancomycin concentration was then used to evaluate the predictive performance of the model-based dosing by comparing the model-based predicted concentration with the observed vancomycin concentration. The model-predicted concentration was based on patient characteristics, previously administered doses (up to the second plasma concentration), and the previous and most recent vancomycin concentration.

The bias, relative bias (rBias), and relative root mean square error (rRMSE) were calculated to compare the individually predicted and observed second vancomycin concentration of each pair.

$$\text{Bias} = \frac{1}{n} \times \sum_{1}^{i} (predicted_i - observed_i) \quad (1)$$

$$\text{rBias} = \frac{1}{n} \times \sum_{1}^{i} \left(\frac{predicted_i - observed_i}{observed_i} \right) \times 100\% \quad (2)$$

$$\text{rRMSE} = \sqrt{\frac{1}{n} \times \sum_{1}^{i} \frac{(predicted_i - observed_i)^2}{(observed_i)^2}} \times 100\% \quad (3)$$

where n is the total number of second vancomycin concentrations.

The predictive performance was considered acceptable if the mean bias was $\leq \pm 2$ mg/L for concentrations below 20 mg/L or if the rBias was $\leq \pm 10\%$ for concentrations of 20 mg/L and higher, thereby meeting the analytical quality requirements of the Royal College of Pathologists of Australasia applied at our institution. The 95% confidence intervals of the mean (relative) bias also included 0. Additionally, an rRMSE as low as possible was aimed for.

At an individual level (i.e., for each pair separately), the acceptable bias was also evaluated according to the above-mentioned criteria. The performance was considered acceptable if the bias was $\leq \pm 2$ mg/L for concentrations below 20 mg/L or if the rBias was $\leq \pm 10\%$ for concentrations of 20 mg/L and higher. The classification accuracy was also evaluated; it was defined as no change in exposure category (i.e., subtherapeutic, supratherapeutic, or therapeutic) between the predicted vancomycin concentration and the observed concentration. Therapeutic exposure was defined as vancomycin concentrations between 12.5–17.5 mg/L or 20–25 mg/L depending on intermittent or continuous infusion, respectively.

Next, the prescribed doses were compared with the model-based doses predicted to reach the target concentration of 15 mg/L and 22.5 mg/L according to the local hospital's guidelines for intermittent and continuous infusion, respectively. In clinical practice, it is common to prescribe a dose that is considered to reach therapeutic exposure at steady state. In contrast, model-based dosing aims to attain therapeutic exposure as soon as possible, i.e., at the next dosing interval. Therefore, the model-based doses were predicted as the first two doses to be administered after the first concentration of each pair. The prescribed dose in clinical practice was compared with the model-predicted second dose—which was a steady-state dose—since the model-predicted first dose was often not representative of the steady-state dose. All model-predicted and prescribed doses were normalized to a twice-daily dosing regimen, i.e., doses were expressed as dose every 12 h (q12h).

The absolute differences were calculated and evaluated graphically by comparing observed versus individually predicted vancomycin concentrations. Additionally, the correlation between the model-predicted and prescribed doses was evaluated using the intraclass correlation coefficient (ICC), which is an index of agreement between two measurements [25]. The ICC values were reported according to the best practices for reporting ICC parameters [26]. The subgroup analyses were performed to investigate the dose differences according to the vancomycin exposure at the second concentration (i.e., subtherapeutic, supratherapeutic, or therapeutic exposure).

2.4. Statistics

Statistical and graphical analyses of the data were performed using IBM SPSS Statistics 27 and R (version 4.0.0, R Core Team, Vienna, Austria). The figures were constructed in Microsoft PowerPoint (version 2203, Microsoft 365 MSO, Washington, DC, USA) and R (version 4.0.0, R Core Team, Vienna, Austria). The data were reported as count and percentage or median and interquartile range (IQR) as appropriate. A Wilcoxon signed-rank test was performed to evaluate the differences between vancomycin concentrations in patients receiving intermittent or continuous infusions separately since different targets were aimed for in both groups. The statistical significance was defined using a two-sided p-value ≤ 0.05. In line with previous studies, we aimed to collect data from 150 patients to represent the adult hospital-wide population that received vancomycin at the University Hospitals Leuven. To further increase the sample size, two pairs of vancomycin concentrations were collected for each patient. As such, we considered data from 150 patients, corresponding to 300 pairs of two consecutive vancomycin concentrations, appropriate for performing a robust evaluation of the predictive performance and predicted doses of model-based vancomycin dosing.

3. Results

3.1. Clinical Data

In total, 616 vancomycin concentrations were collected from 154 patients. Each patient contributed four vancomycin concentrations (i.e., two pairs of two consecutive concentrations per patient). As shown in Table 1, both ICU and non-ICU patients receiving intermittent and continuous infusion therapy were included. The median [IQR] age was 63 [53; 72] years old. The reasons for hospital admission and vancomycin therapy were diverse, as illustrated in Table 1. On the day of the first vancomycin concentration, renal replacement therapy was present in 23 (7.5%) of all pairs.

Table 1. Patient characteristics.

Per Patient			
	All (n = 154)	Intermittent (n = 95)	Continuous (n = 59)
Male, n (%)	103 (66.9)	68 (71.6)	35 (59.3)
Caucasian, n (%)/Afro-American, n (%)	149 (96.8)/5 (3.2)	90 (94.7)/5 (5.3)	59 (100)
Age (years), median [IQR]	63 [53; 72]	63 [55; 74]	60 [49; 68]
Weight (kg), median [IQR]	76 [64; 94]	77 [63; 95]	74 [65; 94]
Diabetes mellitus (type I, type II, and corticosteroid-induced), n (%)	43 (27.9)	32 (33.7)	11 (16.8)
Intensive care unit, n (%)	60 (39)	30 (31.6)	30 (50.8)
In-hospital mortality, n (%)	43 (27.9)	17 (17.3)	26 (44.1)
Reason for Hospital Admission (n = 154)			
Surgical, n (%)	54 (35.1)	45 (47.4)	9 (15.3)
Medical, n (%)	44 (28.6)	23 (24.2)	21 (35.6)
Emergency, n (%)	51 (33.1)	26 (27.4)	25 (42.4)
Others, n (%)	5 (3.2)	1 (1.1)	4 (6.8)
Focus of the Infection (n = 154)			
Respiratory, n (%)	21 (13.6)	10 (10.5)	11 (18.6)
Gastrointestinal, n (%)	7 (4.5)	5 (5.3)	2 (3.4)
Endocarditis, n (%)	6 (3.9)	3 (3.2)	3 (5.1)
Urinary, n (%)	3 (1.9)	3 (3.2)	0 (0)
Skin and soft tissue, n (%)	19 (12.3)	16 16.8)	3 (5.1)
Bone and joint, n (%)	24 (15.6)	20 (21.1)	4 (6.8)
Catheter-related, n (%)	18 (11.7)	9 (9.5)	9 (15.3)
Abdominal, n (%)	15 (9.7)	9 (9.5)	6 (10.2)
Postoperative, n (%)	10 (6.5)	7 (7.4)	3 (5.1)
Neutropenic fever, n (%)	25 (16.2)	8 (8.4)	17 (28.8)
Other, n (%)	6 (3.9)	5 (5.3)	1 (1.7)
Clinical and Biochemical Data on the Day of the First Vancomycin Concentration Measurement			
	All (n = 308)	Intermittent (n = 190)	Continuous (n = 118)
Serum creatinine (mg/dL), median [IQR]	0.83 [0.64; 1.22]	0.82 [0.61; 1.17]	0.84 [0.67; 1.34]
eGFR CKD-EPI (mL/min/1.73 m^2), median [IQR]	87 [59; 104]	86 [61; 102]	88 [54.5; 107]
eCrCl CG (mL/min), median [IQR]	93 [58; 132]	90.2 [60; 132]	98 [51; 129]
Serum albumin (g/L) [a], median [IQR], n	31.2 [27.8; 34.6], 175	30.5 [26.8; 34.3], 62	31.9 [29; 34; 8], 113
Serum urea nitrogen (mg/dL), median [IQR]	31 [21; 55]	28 [20; 45]	39 [24; 77]
SOFA score [b], median [IQR], n	11 [7; 15], 120	8 [5; 12], 60	15 [11; 18], 60
Intermittent hemodialysis, n (%)	3 (1.0)	0 (0)	3 (2.5)
Intermittent peritoneal dialysis, n (%)	2 (0.6)	2 (1.1)	0 (0)
Continuous veno-venous hemofiltration, n (%)	18 (5.8)	5 (2.6)	13 (11)
Use of furosemide, n (%)	45 (14.6)	30 (15.8)	15 (12.7)

eCrCl CG: estimated creatinine clearance according to the Cockcroft–Gault equation; eGFR CKD-EPI: estimated glomerular filtration ratio according to the Chronic Kidney Disease Epidemiology Collaboration equation; IQR: interquartile range; n: count; SOFA: sequential organ failure assessment. [a] If available; [b] If ICU patient.

Among the first vancomycin concentrations of each pair, 45.1% were within the therapeutic range, with 31.2% and 23.7% of the concentrations being subtherapeutic and supratherapeutic, respectively. Following the standard TDM-based dose optimization, 48.1% of the second vancomycin concentrations of each pair were in the therapeutic range. The proportion of the subtherapeutic concentrations decreased to 21.4%, in contrast with the proportion of the supratherapeutic concentrations, which increased to 30.5% (Table 2).

As shown in Table 2, the median vancomycin concentration was 15 mg/L and 21.3 mg/L in the first sample of each pair and increased significantly to 15.7 mg/L and

22.1 mg/L in the second sample in patients receiving intermittent (p = 0.004) and continuous infusions (p = 0.0003), respectively.

Table 2. Vancomycin concentrations (two pairs per patient) during intermittent (trough) and continuous infusion.

Vancomycin trough Concentrations during Intermittent Infusion (n = 190).	
First concentration (mg/L), median [IQR]	15.0 [12; 17.7]
Second concentration (mg/L), median [IQR]	15.7 [13.7; 18.3]
Vancomycin Concentrations during Continuous Infusion (n = 118)	
First concentration (mg/L), median [IQR]	21.3 [17.4; 23.5]
Second concentration (mg/L), median [IQR]	22.1 [19.3; 25;5]
Exposure at Second Concentration (n = 308)	
Therapeutic exposure [a], n (%)	148 (48.1)
Supratherapeutic exposure [b], n (%)	94 (30.5)
Subtherapeutic exposure [c], n (%)	66 (21.4)

[a] 12.5–17.5 mg/L (intermittent) and 20–25 mg/L (continuous); [b] >17.5 mg/L (intermittent) and >25 mg/L (continuous); [c] <12.5 mg/L (intermittent) and <20 mg/L (continuous).

3.2. Evaluation of the Model-Based Approaches

3.2.1. Predictive Performance

Across the five model-based approaches investigated in our study, the mean bias in the overall population ranged from −1.53 mg/L to −0.11 mg/L. Depending on the model-based approach, the mean rBias ranged from −5.36% to 3.18% in the overall population, and 95% confidence intervals were all within ±10% as illustrated in Figure 2. However, the 95% confidence intervals did not include 0 for the MSA$_{OFV}$ approach. The rRMSE was ≤28.1% for all model-based approaches (Figure 2). The goodness-of-fit plots showed a clinically acceptable fit of the predicted concentrations with the observed concentrations across all five model-based approaches, as illustrated in Figure 3. At the individual level, acceptable rBias was found in 38–46.4% of all predicted concentrations (Supplementary Table S1). The classification accuracy was 47.7–55.5%, depending on the model-based approach.

The analyses in the subpopulations are shown in Table S2. The performance remained similar or even better in non-ICU patients or patients receiving the intermittent vancomycin infusion. However, in ICU patients or patients receiving the continuous vancomycin infusion, the performance decreased slightly. In these patients, only the Goti model showed 95% confidence intervals of the mean rBias, including 0. Additionally, for two of the multi-model-based approaches (i.e., MSA$_{OFV}$ and MAA$_{OFV}$), the 95% confidence intervals exceeded ± 10%.

3.2.2. Model-Predicted Vancomycin Doses Compared with Standard TDM-Based Doses

Based on the predictive performance, we selected the MAA$_{SSE}$ approach as the model-based approach with the best predictive performance (defined as a combination of the lowest overall rBias and rRMSE). The dose differences were calculated with the doses predicted according to the MAA$_{SSE}$ approach. The median differences between the second (i.e., steady-state) model-predicted dose q12h and the prescribed (i.e., standard TDM-based) dose q12h were 113 [−69; 427] mg, −70 [−208; 120] mg, and 40 [−84; 197] mg in the case of subtherapeutic, supratherapeutic, and therapeutic exposure at the time of the second vancomycin concentration, respectively. These differences are depicted in Figure 4, together with the differences between the first model-predicted dose and the prescribed dose. The differences with the first model-predicted dose were substantially larger than that of the second model-predicted dose.

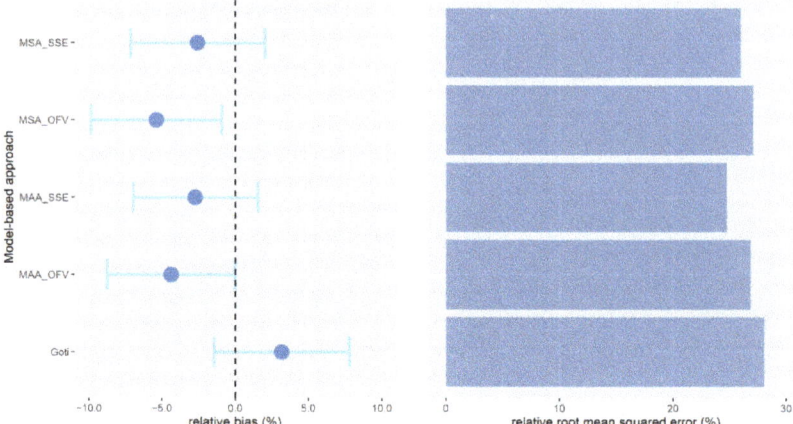

Figure 2. Overall relative bias and relative root mean square error of the predicted versus the observed second vancomycin concentration of each pair for the five model-based approaches investigated (i.e., the model selection algorithm [MSA] and the model averaging algorithm [MAA], according to the objective function value [OFV] and the squared prediction errors [SSE], and the single-model approach according to the Goti model). The blue dots represent the mean relative bias, and the blue error bars represent the 95% confidence intervals.

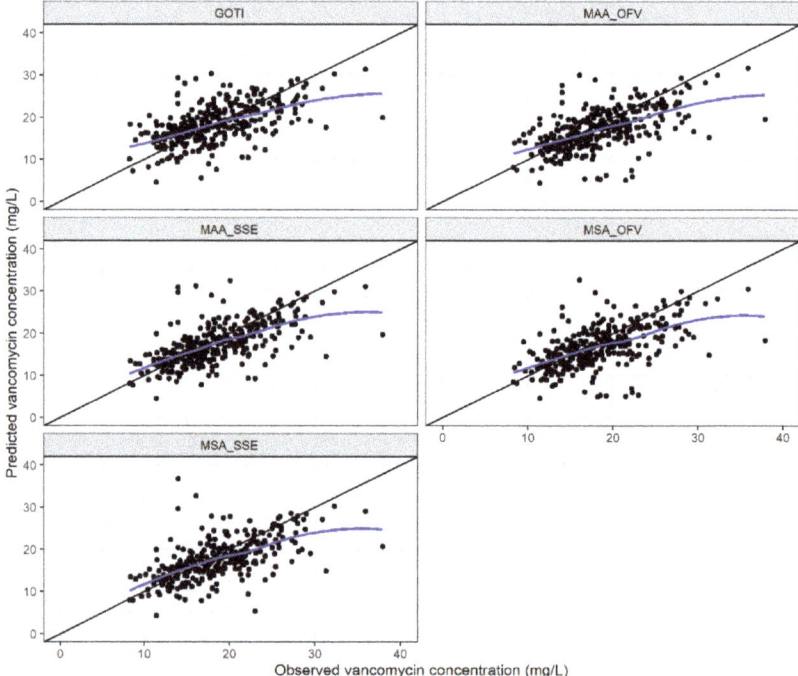

Figure 3. Goodness-of-fit plots of the predicted versus observed second vancomycin concentration of each pair for the five model-based approaches (i.e., the model selection algorithm [MSA] and the model averaging algorithm [MAA], according to the objective function value [OFV] and the squared prediction errors [SSE], and the single-model approach according to the Goti model). The blue line represents the local polynomial regression fit. The line of identity represents a perfect model fit.

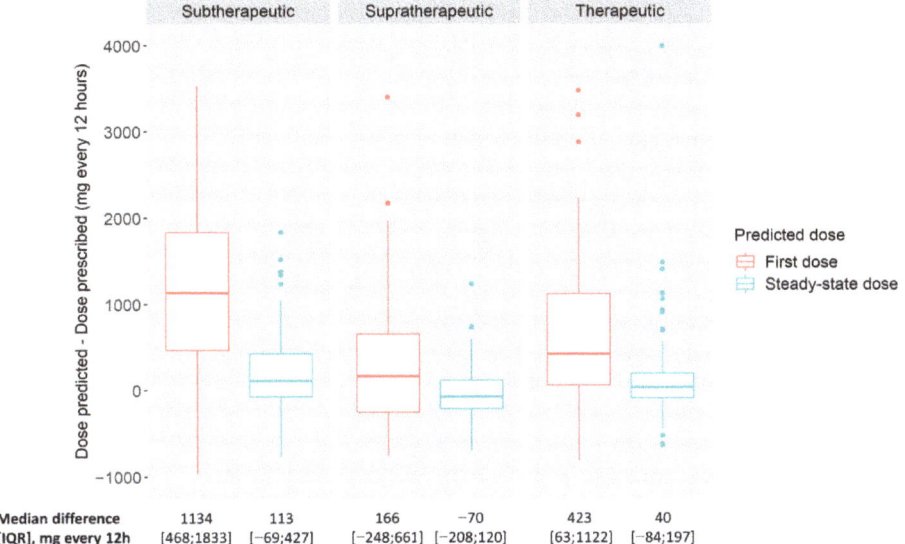

Figure 4. Boxplots of the difference between the vancomycin doses predicted by the MAA$_{SSE}$ approach and the prescribed vancomycin doses, including the median (interquartile range) difference. The doses were normalized to a twice-daily dosing regimen, i.e., the doses were expressed as dose q12h. The differences were shown in three groups depending on the exposure at the time of the second vancomycin concentration of each pair (i.e., subtherapeutic, supratherapeutic, or therapeutic). The vancomycin doses were predicted based on the first vancomycin concentration of each pair of concentrations. The red and blue boxplots represent the dose differences based on the first and second dose predicted to reach therapeutic exposure, respectively. The therapeutic exposure was defined as concentrations between 12.5–17.5 mg/L or between 20–25 mg/L for intermittent or continuous infusion, respectively.

Overall, the ICC showed a moderate correlation between the second model-predicted dose and the prescribed dose (0.656). The correlation remained moderate in the case of the subtherapeutic and therapeutic vancomycin concentrations, as illustrated by an ICC of 0.665 and 0.596, respectively. In the case of the supratherapeutic vancomycin concentrations, the ICC showed a good correlation (0.821).

For the sensitivity analysis, the MSA$_{OFV}$ approach was selected as the approach with the worst performance as this was the only model-based approach that did not show an overall mean rBias, including 0 in its 95% confidence intervals. As shown in , similar differences between the second model-predicted dose q12h and the prescribed dose q12h were observed with the MSA$_{OFV}$ compared with the dose differences calculated with the MAA$_{SSE}$ approach.

4. Discussion

In our study, we investigated TDM-based vancomycin dose optimization in a broad and diverse population of hospitalized adult patients receiving either intermittent or continuous vancomycin infusions. We demonstrated that a single-model approach or multi-model approach performs well, as illustrated by the acceptable predictive performance. Moreover, the model-based vancomycin dose predictions suggest a potential for increased therapeutic exposure compared with the standard TDM-based dosing.

A great deal of vancomycin PopPK models have been developed in both specific and general adult patient populations [13,14,27]. However, it remains challenging to select and implement the right model to guide the vancomycin dosing for an individual patient. Many models have failed to show good predictive performance outside the population they were developed in [13,14,27]. In our study, we showed that the Goti model, as well as different multi-model approaches, performs acceptably well in a broad set of hospitalized patients. The Goti model [18] as single-model approach is probably the simplest model-based approach and covers many of the standard hospitalized patients. Interestingly, we observed that the MAA$_{SSE}$ approach showed slightly better performance. A potential explanation might be that the multi-model approach performs better in specific patient populations for which the Goti model is not suitable. It should be noted that we only used the most recent previous vancomycin concentration to inform the TDM-based dose optimization. Multiple previous concentrations were deemed unnecessary. This agreed with recent studies demonstrating that performance metrics were superior [27], or similar [14], when based on the most recent vancomycin concentration compared with a higher number of previous concentrations.

Recently, Heus and co-workers [27] found that the Okada [28] and Colin [29] PopPK models performed best in a set of non-ICU patients treated with continuous infusion vancomycin. They also found the multi-model approaches investigated in this study performed similarly well as these single models. Noteworthy, in their study, the Goti model showed overall high imprecision and overpredicted the observed vancomycin concentrations. Heus et al. related this discrepancy to the difference in the mode of administration and potential variation in assay methods for vancomycin and serum creatinine concentration. In the future, the performance of the multi-model approaches in the population investigated in our study might be further improved by including the Okada and Colin models. Still, in our study including both intermittent and continuous infusion, the Goti model performed well. Our results are in accordance with previous studies that found the Goti model to perform acceptably well with similar rBias and rRMSE in patients receiving intermittent or continuous infusions of vancomycin [13,14]. Interestingly, these studies also included dialysis patients, as in our study (23/308), whereas that of Heus and co-workers [27] excluded dialysis patients. We also performed subanalyses to identify potential subpopulations in which specific model-based approaches performed differently. Whereas the predictive performance remained similar in non-ICU patients or patients receiving an intermittent vancomycin infusion, the performance decreased slightly in ICU patients or patients receiving a continuous infusion. Nevertheless, the overall predictive performance was acceptable in the total population for four out of the five model-based approaches (Supplementary Table S1). In the future, the specific subpopulations in which the model-based approaches perform worse should be further expanded on. The benefit of including additional models in the multi-model approaches may also be investigated in order to make model-based vancomycin dosing even more widely applicable.

Although the acceptable performance at an individual level was only found in 38–46.4% of all predicted concentrations, the classification accuracy was higher (47.7–55.5%). It should be noted that we defined stricter criteria for acceptable performance than those of previous studies (i.e., rBias ± 10% versus rBias ± 20% [13–15] or 2.5 mg/L [27]). Using an rBias ± 20%, an acceptable bias was attained in 60.1–69.5% of all predicted concentrations, which overestimated the classification accuracy. Eventually, the MAA$_{SSE}$ approach was selected to perform dose predictions, as overall it was the least biased and most precise approach. Moreover, the MAA$_{SSE}$ approach showed good performance at an individual level and good classification accuracy compared with the other approaches.

Even though the vancomycin concentrations increased significantly after the standard TDM-based dose optimization, less than 50% of all second concentrations still showed therapeutic exposure (i.e., 48.1%). This agreed with a recent study revealing poor target attainment in adults with real-life standard TDM-based vancomycin dosing [10].

In our study, the model-predicted doses show only moderate to good correlation with prescribed doses. This finding illustrates a large opportunity for improvement in therapeutic exposure during vancomycin therapy that might be addressed with model-based TDM. The model-predicted doses suggest a potential increase in therapeutic exposure as suggested by the differences with the prescribed dose (Figure 4). In patients with subtherapeutic vancomycin exposure after the standard TDM-based dose optimization, the predicted doses are mostly larger than the prescribed doses. Hence, if the predicted doses had been administered to those patients, the subtherapeutic exposure may have been avoided in a substantial proportion of these patients. On the other hand, the lower doses were most frequently predicted in patients with supratherapeutic exposure after the standard TDM-based dose optimization. Therefore, less supratherapeutic exposure may also be expected from model-based dosing. Considering a dose modification of 125 mg or more as clinically relevant, the model-based vancomycin dosing would most frequently lead to a dose increase or a dose reduction in patients with a subtherapeutic or supratherapeutic second vancomycin concentration, respectively (Supplementary Table S3). In patients with a therapeutic second vancomycin concentration, the doses remained mostly unchanged. These findings were also confirmed in the sensitivity analysis when using the model-based approach with the worst predictive performance, i.e., the MSA_{OFV} approach. This finding strongly suggests that this is a benefit of the model-based vancomycin dosing compared with that of the standard TDM-based dosing.

It should be noted that the dose differences were calculated with the second model-predicted dose after the first TDM measurement. When using MIPD, the user should be aware that model-based predictions aim for direct target attainment, often resulting in relatively low or high doses immediately after a TDM measurement. In contrast, the subsequent (i.e., second) dose will be more reflective of the steady-state dose required to keep the exposure at the predefined target. This finding was confirmed by the large dose differences observed when comparing the first model-predicted dose with the prescribed dose (Figure 4). We opted to compare with the second model-based dose, as most often in clinical practice the clinicians will adapt the vancomycin dose to the new steady-state dose they believe is adequate for reaching the target exposure.

This study has several strengths. First, we intentionally performed our study in a broad and heterogeneous set of adult patients, hence increasing its external generalizability. Second, we evaluated both single and multi-model approaches. Third, we performed a comprehensive evaluation of the model-based approaches using goodness-of-fit plots, predictive performance, classification accuracy, and sensitivity analysis. Moreover, whereas previous studies only evaluated the predictive performance [13–15,27], we also evaluated model-predicted doses in relation to the exposure. Notwithstanding, several limitations to our study should also be taken into account. First, we need to acknowledge the limitations inherent to the retrospective and monocentric design of our study. Therefore, the findings may not necessarily be extrapolated to other centers, and prospective validation is needed. When prospectively validating model-based vancomycin dosing, one should be cautious of those patients for which predicted exposure is substantially over- or underestimated (i.e., inacceptable rBias at the individual level). These might represent patients with erroneous sampling or specific patients not appropriately covered by the included PopPK models. Second, we only included a subset of all available vancomycin PopPK models. We did not include the Okada [28] and Colin [29] models, which were recently found to perform the best in continuous-infusion vancomycin patients without dialysis [27]. Nevertheless, our analysis showed good overall predictive performance. Third, it should be noted that we did not include children, although children may also benefit from a similar model-based approach [10,29]. Fourth, our sample size of 154 patients is rather limited. However, our sample size is within the range of previous studies investigating the predictive performance of vancomycin model-based approaches. Interestingly, we performed an interim analysis—after inclusion of the first 65 patients—that showed results similar to the final results, hence supporting the robustness of our results [30]. Finally, we did not consider AUC/MIC targets as these are not commonly used at our institution and were therefore not available.

In conclusion, our study confirmed the predictive performance and illustrated the potential benefit of model-based vancomycin dosing compared with the standard TDM-based dosing in a broad and heterogeneous population. The Goti model, as well as most of the multi-model approaches, showed good overall performance. The MAA$_{SSE}$ approach showed the best overall performance. Using this approach, the clinically relevant differences and moderate correlation between the model-based and prescribed dosing, along with the poor target attainment with the standard TDM-based dosing, suggested a large window of opportunity for the model-based TDM to increase therapeutic exposure. Implementation studies—preferably prospectively—of the model-based TDM in routine care are warranted.

Supplementary Materials: The following supporting information can be downloaded at: https://www.mdpi.com/article/10.3390/pharmaceutics14071459/s1, Supplementary Table S1: Acceptable performance and classification accuracy across the five model-based approaches; Supplementary Table S2: Relative bias and relative root mean square error of the five model-based approaches; Supplementary Table S3: Clinically relevant differences between model-predicted and prescribed vancomycin doses; Supplementary Figure S1: Boxplots of the difference between vancomycin doses predicted by the MSA$_{OFV}$ approach and prescribed vancomycin doses.

Author Contributions: Conceptualization, E.D., I.S., and M.G.; methodology, H.G., E.D., S.G.W., I.S. and M.G.; software, S.G.W. and A.D.; validation, E.D., K.A., I.S. and M.G.; formal analysis, H.G., E.D., S.G.W., I.S. and M.G.; investigation, H.G., S.G.W., N.D., E.S. and M.G.; resources, E.D., S.G.W., K.A. and I.S.; data curation, E.D., S.G.W., N.D., A.D. and M.G.; writing—original draft preparation, H.G., E.D., I.S. and M.G.; writing—review and editing, S.G.W., N.D., E.S., A.D., K.A., S.D., K.L., W.E.P. and Y.D.; visualization, H.G., S.G.W. and M.G.; supervision, E.D., S.D., K.L., W.E.P., Y.D., I.S. and M.G.; project administration, H.G. and M.G.; funding acquisition, E.D., K.A., I.S. and M.G. All authors have read and agreed to the published version of the manuscript.

Funding: M.G. is a postdoctoral research fellow at KU Leuven (file number PDMT2/21/077). The funders had no role in study design, data collection and interpretation, or the decision to submit the work for publication.

Institutional Review Board Statement: This study was conducted in accordance with the Declaration of Helsinki and approved by the Ethics Committee Research UZ/KU Leuven (S65213; March 24 2021).

Informed Consent Statement: Patient consent was waived due to the retrospective nature of this study.

Data Availability Statement: The data are contained within the article and supplementary material. Additional data are available upon reasonable request.

Conflicts of Interest: S.G.W. is the developer of the TDMx software.

References

1. Rybak, M.J. The pharmacokinetic and pharmacodynamic properties of vancomycin. *Clin. Infect. Dis.* **2006**, *42* (Suppl. 1), S35–S39. [CrossRef] [PubMed]
2. Rybak, M.J.; Le, J.; Lodise, T.P.; Levine, D.P.; Bradley, J.S.; Liu, C.; Mueller, B.A.; Pai, M.P.; Wong-Beringer, A.; Rotschafer, J.C.; et al. Therapeutic monitoring of vancomycin for serious methicillin-resistant *Staphylococcus aureus* infections: A revised consensus guideline and review by the American Society of Health-System Pharmacists, the Infectious Diseases Society of America, the Pediatric Infectious Diseases Society, and the Society of Infectious Diseases Pharmacists. *Am. J. Health Syst. Pharm.* **2020**, *77*, 835–864. [CrossRef] [PubMed]
3. Rybak, M.; Lomaestro, B.; Rotschafer, J.C.; Moellering, R., Jr.; Craig, W.; Billeter, M.; Dalovisio, J.R.; Levine, D.P. Therapeutic monitoring of vancomycin in adult patients: A consensus review of the American Society of Health-System Pharmacists, the Infectious Diseases Society of America, and the Society of Infectious Diseases Pharmacists. *Am. J. Health Syst. Pharm.* **2009**, *66*, 82–98. [CrossRef]
4. Dalton, B.R.; Dersch-Mills, D.; Langevin, A.; Sabuda, D.; Rennert-May, E.; Greiner, T. Appropriateness of basing vancomycin dosing on area under the concentration-time curve. *Am. J. Health. Syst. Pharm.* **2019**, *76*, 1718–1721. [CrossRef]
5. Wright, W.F.; Jorgensen, S.C.J.; Spellberg, B. Heaping the Pelion of Vancomycin on the Ossa of Methicillin-resistant *Staphylococcus aureus*: Back to Basics in Clinical Care and Guidelines. *Clin. Infect. Dis.* **2021**, *72*, e682–e684. [CrossRef]
6. Dalton, B.R.; Rajakumar, I.; Langevin, A.; Ondro, C.; Sabuda, D.; Griener, T.P.; Dersch-Mills, D.; Rennert-May, E. Vancomycin area under the curve to minimum inhibitory concentration ratio predicting clinical outcome: A systematic review and meta-analysis with pooled sensitivity and specificity. *Clin. Microbiol. Infect.* **2020**, *26*, 436–446. [CrossRef] [PubMed]

7. Tsutsuura, M.; Moriyama, H.; Kojima, N.; Mizukami, Y.; Tashiro, S.; Osa, S.; Enoki, Y.; Taguchi, K.; Oda, K.; Fujii, S.; et al. The monitoring of vancomycin: A systematic review and meta-analyses of area under the concentration-time curve-guided dosing and trough-guided dosing. *BMC Infect. Dis.* **2021**, *21*, 153. [CrossRef]
8. Stewart, J.J.; Jorgensen, S.C.; Dresser, L.; Lau, T.T.; Gin, A.; Thirion, D.J.; Nishi, C.; Dalton, B. A Canadian perspective on the revised 2020 ASHP–IDSA–PIDS–SIDP guidelines for vancomycin AUC-based therapeutic drug monitoring for serious MRSA infections. *Off. J. Assoc. Med. Microbiol. Infect. Dis. Can.* **2021**, *6*, 3–9. [CrossRef]
9. Stocker, S.L.; Carland, J.E.; Reuter, S.E.; Stacy, A.E.; Schaffer, A.L.; Stefani, M.; Lau, C.; Kirubakaran, R.; Yang, J.J.; Shen, C.F.J.; et al. Evaluation of a Pilot Vancomycin Precision Dosing Advisory Service on Target Exposure Attainment Using an Interrupted Time Series Analysis. *Clin. Pharmacol. Ther.* **2021**, *109*, 212–221. [CrossRef]
10. Van Der Heggen, T.; Buyle, F.M.; Claus, B.; Somers, A.; Schelstraete, P.; De Paepe, P.; Vanhaesebrouck, S.; De Cock, P. Vancomycin dosing and therapeutic drug monitoring practices: Guidelines versus real-life. *Int. J. Clin. Pharm.* **2021**, *43*, 1394–1403. [CrossRef]
11. Kantasiripitak, W.; Van Daele, R.; Gijsen, M.; Ferrante, M.; Spriet, I.; Dreesen, E. Software Tools for Model-Informed Precision Dosing: How Well Do They Satisfy the Needs? *Front. Pharmacol.* **2020**, *11*, 620. [CrossRef] [PubMed]
12. Turner, R.B.; Kojiro, K.; Shephard, E.A.; Won, R.; Chang, E.; Chan, D.; Elbarbry, F. Review and Validation of Bayesian Dose-Optimizing Software and Equations for Calculation of the Vancomycin Area under the Curve in Critically Ill Patients. *Pharmacotherapy* **2018**, *38*, 1174–1183. [CrossRef] [PubMed]
13. Cunio, C.B.; Uster, D.W.; Carland, J.E.; Buscher, H.; Liu, Z.; Brett, J.; Stefani, M.; Jones, G.R.D.; Day, R.O.; Wicha, S.G.; et al. Towards precision dosing of vancomycin in critically ill patients: An evaluation of the predictive performance of pharmacometric models in ICU patients. *Clin. Microbiol. Infect.* **2020**, *27*, 783-e7. [CrossRef]
14. Broeker, A.; Nardecchia, M.; Klinker, K.P.; Derendorf, H.; Day, R.O.; Marriott, D.J.; Carland, J.E.; Stocker, S.L.; Wicha, S.G. Towards precision dosing of vancomycin: A systematic evaluation of pharmacometric models for Bayesian forecasting. *Clin. Microbiol. Infect.* **2019**, *25*, e1281–e1286. [CrossRef] [PubMed]
15. Uster, D.W.; Stocker, S.L.; Carland, J.E.; Brett, J.; Marriott, D.J.E.; Day, R.O.; Wicha, S.G. A Model Averaging/Selection Approach Improves the Predictive Performance of Model-Informed Precision Dosing: Vancomycin as a Case Study. *Clin. Pharmacol. Ther.* **2021**, *109*, 175–183. [CrossRef]
16. Available online: https://www.randomizer.org/ (accessed on 17 March 2022).
17. Wicha, S.G.; Kees, M.G.; Solms, A.; Minichmayr, I.K.; Kratzer, A.; Kloft, C. TDMx: A novel web-based open-access support tool for optimising antimicrobial dosing regimens in clinical routine. *Int. J. Antimicrob. Agents* **2015**, *45*, 442–444. [CrossRef]
18. Goti, V.; Chaturvedula, A.; Fossler, M.J.; Mok, S.; Jacob, J.T. Hospitalized Patients with and without Hemodialysis Have Markedly Different Vancomycin Pharmacokinetics: A Population Pharmacokinetic Model-Based Analysis. *Ther. Drug Monit.* **2018**, *40*, 212–221. [CrossRef]
19. Adane, E.D.; Herald, M.; Koura, F. Pharmacokinetics of vancomycin in extremely obese patients with suspected or confirmed *Staphylococcus aureus* infections. *Pharmacotherapy* **2015**, *35*, 127–139. [CrossRef]
20. Mangin, O.; Urien, S.; Mainardi, J.L.; Fagon, J.Y.; Faisy, C. Vancomycin pharmacokinetic and pharmacodynamic models for critically ill patients with post-sternotomy mediastinitis. *Clin. Pharmacokinet.* **2014**, *53*, 849–861. [CrossRef]
21. Medellín-Garibay, S.E.; Ortiz-Martín, B.; Rueda-Naharro, A.; García, B.; Romano-Moreno, S.; Barcia, E. Pharmacokinetics of vancomycin and dosing recommendations for trauma patients. *J. Antimicrob. Chemother.* **2016**, *71*, 471–479. [CrossRef]
22. Revilla, N.; Martín-Suárez, A.; Pérez, M.P.; González, F.M.; Fernández de Gatta Mdel, M. Vancomycin dosing assessment in intensive care unit patients based on a population pharmacokinetic/pharmacodynamic simulation. *Br. J. Clin. Pharmacol.* **2010**, *70*, 201–212. [CrossRef] [PubMed]
23. Roberts, J.A.; Taccone, F.S.; Udy, A.A.; Vincent, J.L.; Jacobs, F.; Lipman, J. Vancomycin dosing in critically ill patients: Robust methods for improved continuous-infusion regimens. *Antimicrob. Agents Chemother.* **2011**, *55*, 2704–2709. [CrossRef] [PubMed]
24. Thomson, A.H.; Staatz, C.E.; Tobin, C.M.; Gall, M.; Lovering, A.M. Development and evaluation of vancomycin dosage guidelines designed to achieve new target concentrations. *J. Antimicrob. Chemother.* **2009**, *63*, 1050–1057. [CrossRef]
25. Watson, P.F.; Petrie, A. Method agreement analysis: A review of correct methodology. *Theriogenology* **2010**, *73*, 1167–1179. [CrossRef] [PubMed]
26. Koo, T.K.; Li, M.Y. A Guideline of Selecting and Reporting Intraclass Correlation Coefficients for Reliability Research. *J. Chiropr. Med.* **2016**, *15*, 155–163. [CrossRef] [PubMed]
27. Heus, A.; Uster, D.W.; Grootaert, V.; Vermeulen, N.; Somers, A.; In't Veld, D.H.; Wicha, S.G.; De Cock, P.A. Model-informed precision dosing of vancomycin via continuous infusion: A clinical fit-for-purpose evaluation of published PK models. *Int. J. Antimicrob. Agents* **2022**, *59*, 106579. [CrossRef]
28. Okada, A.; Kariya, M.; Irie, K.; Okada, Y.; Hiramoto, N.; Hashimoto, H.; Kajioka, R.; Maruyama, C.; Kasai, H.; Hamori, M.; et al. Population Pharmacokinetics of Vancomycin in Patients Undergoing Allogeneic Hematopoietic Stem-Cell Transplantation. *J. Clin. Pharmacol.* **2018**, *58*, 1140–1149. [CrossRef]
29. Colin, P.J.; Allegaert, K.; Thomson, A.H.; Touw, D.J.; Dolton, M.; de Hoog, M.; Roberts, J.A.; Adane, E.D.; Yamamoto, M.; Santos-Buelga, D.; et al. Vancomycin Pharmacokinetics Throughout Life: Results from a Pooled Population Analysis and Evaluation of Current Dosing Recommendations. *Clin. Pharmacokinet.* **2019**, *58*, 767–780. [CrossRef]
30. Gastmans, H.; Dreesen, E.; Dia, N.; Desmet, S.; Lagrou, K.; Peetermans, W. Model-based TDM of vancomycin: A retrospective comparison with routine TDM-based dosing. In *Oral Presentation at the European Congress of Clinical Microbiology and Infectious Diseases*; Abstract/Presentation Number: 1258/O00302; ESCMID Library: Lisbon, Portugal, May 2022.

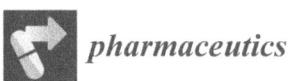 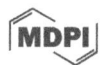

Article

Relevance of Therapeutic Drug Monitoring of Tyrosine Kinase Inhibitors in Routine Clinical Practice: A Pilot Study

Vanesa Escudero-Ortiz [1,2], Vanessa Domínguez-Leñero [3], Ana Catalán-Latorre [1], Joseba Rebollo-Liceaga [1] and Manuel Sureda [1,*]

[1] Plataforma de Oncología, Hospital Quirónsalud Torrevieja, 03184 Torrevieja, Spain; vanesa.escudero@quironsalud.es (V.E.-O.); ana.catalan@quironsalud.es (A.C.-L.); joseba.rebollo@quironsalud.es (J.R.-L.)
[2] Pharmacy and Clinical Nutrition Group, Universidad CEU Cardenal Herrera, 03203 Elche, Spain
[3] Servicio de Farmacia, Hospital Universitario Morales Meseguer, 30008 Murcia, Spain; vanedole80@hotmail.com
* Correspondence: manuel.sureda@quironsalud.es

Abstract: Introduction: The main goal of treatment in cancer patients is to achieve the highest therapeutic effectiveness with the least iatrogenic toxicity. Tyrosine kinase inhibitors (TKIs) are anticancer oral agents, usually administered at fixed doses, which present high inter- and intra-individual variability due to their pharmacokinetic characteristics. Therapeutic drug monitoring (TDM) can be used to optimize the use of several types of medication. Objective: We evaluated the use of TDM of TKIs in routine clinical practice through studying the variability in exposure to erlotinib, imatinib, lapatinib, and sorafenib and dose adjustment. Materials and methods: We conducted a retrospective analytical study involving patients who received treatment with TKIs, guided by TDM and with subsequent recommendation of dose adjustment. The quantification of the plasma levels of the different drugs was performed using high-performance liquid chromatography (HPLC). The Clinical Research Ethics Committee of the Hospital Quirónsalud Torrevieja approved this study. Results: The inter-individual variability in the first cycle and in the last monitored cycle was 46.2% and 44.0% for erlotinib, 48.9 and 50.8% for imatinib, 60.7% and 56.0% for lapatinib and 89.7% and 72.5% for sorafenib. Relationships between exposure and baseline characteristics for erlotinib, imatinib, lapatinib and sorafenib were not statistically significant for any of the variables evaluated (weight, height, body surface area (BSA), age and sex). Relationships between height ($p = 0.021$) and BSA ($p = 0.022$) were statistically significant for sorafenib. No significant relationships were observed between C_{trough} and progression-free survival (PFS) or overall survival (OS) for any drug, except in the case of sunitinib (correlation between C_{trough} and PFS $p = 0.023$) in the exposure–efficacy analysis. Conclusions: Erlotinib, imatinib, lapatinib and sorafenib show large inter-individual variability in exposure. TDM entails a significant improvement in exposure and enables more effective and safe use of TKIs in routine clinical practice.

Keywords: therapeutic drug monitoring; tyrosine kinase inhibitors; cancer; personalized medicine

Citation: Escudero-Ortiz, V.; Domínguez-Leñero, V.; Catalán-Latorre, A.; Rebollo-Liceaga, J.; Sureda, M. Relevance of Therapeutic Drug Monitoring of Tyrosine Kinase Inhibitors in Routine Clinical Practice: A Pilot Study. *Pharmaceutics* **2022**, *14*, 1216. https://doi.org/10.3390/pharmaceutics14061216

Academic Editors: José Martínez Lanao and Jonás Samuel Pérez-Blanco

Received: 24 March 2022
Accepted: 6 June 2022
Published: 8 June 2022

Publisher's Note: MDPI stays neutral with regard to jurisdictional claims in published maps and institutional affiliations.

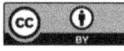

Copyright: © 2022 by the authors. Licensee MDPI, Basel, Switzerland. This article is an open access article distributed under the terms and conditions of the Creative Commons Attribution (CC BY) license (https://creativecommons.org/licenses/by/4.0/).

1. Introduction

The main goal of pharmacologic treatment in cancer patients is to achieve the highest therapeutic effectiveness with the least iatrogenic toxicity. However, the dosage regimens to achieve this goal can differ considerably from patient to patient. In routine clinical practice, the standardized dosage regimens of the drugs administered are very satisfactory in some patients but may show minimal efficacy or even generate adverse reactions in others [1].

Pharmacokinetic studies the relationship between the dosage regimens used and the corresponding time course of drug and/or metabolite concentrations in the body [2]. The inherent variability in pharmacokinetic processes constitutes one of the main causes of the different clinical responses observed in individual patients.

TDM is the clinical practice of measuring specific drugs at designated intervals to maintain a constant concentration in a patient's bloodstream, thereby optimizing individual dosage regimens [3]. Drugs typically considered good candidates for TDM were those with a narrow therapeutic window and a clear correlation between exposure and clinical response as antibiotics, antiretrovirals, antiarrhythmics, anticonvulsants, immunosuppressants or antineoplastics.

TKIs are a type of enzyme inhibitor that specifically block the action of one or more tyrosine kinases [4], involving processes such as cell proliferation and survival, transcription, angiogenesis and progression to metastasis. Other effects are mediated by the interaction with therapeutic targets such as epidermal growth factor receptor (EGFR), ATP-binding cassette (ABC) transporters, vascular endothelial growth factor receptor (VEGFR), human epidermal growth factor receptor 2 (HER2), platelet-derived growth factor receptor (PDGFR) or stem cell factor receptor (c-KIT) [5]. TKIs cause fewer non-specific toxicities than standard chemotherapy due to their high affinity for specific molecular mutations of tumor cells [6,7] and can be used both as monotherapy and in combination.

TKIs are usually given at a fixed dose and taken via the oral route. Fixed-dose therapies present a wide range of plasma concentrations, with inter-individual variability in trough concentrations (C_{trough}) of up to 23 fold [8]. In the case of subtherapeutic exposure, selection of resistant cell clones can be favored, or the agent inadequately considered non-active. Overexposure can cause undesirable toxicities [9].

Although oral administration implies theoretical advantages to both patients and the health system, evidence suggests that adherence to oral cancer therapies is far from optimal [10–15]. Several studies have examined adherence to imatinib treatment in patients with gastrointestinal stromal tumor (GIST) or chronic myeloid leukemia (CML), showing high rates of non-compliance [11,12,16], which can result in a low C_{trough} of imatinib [17]. In patients with CML treated for several years, poor adherence may be the most important cause of not reaching adequate molecular responses [18]. Food–drug interactions and gastrointestinal surgery are other areas of concern. High-fat meals can increase the area under the plasma concentration–time curve (AUC) of nilotinib by up to 80% [19] and that of lapatinib by more than 3 fold [20]. Pazopanib exposure in terms of AUC is doubled when administered with food compared to when administered in the fasted state [21]. Saturation of gastrointestinal absorption has been described for nilotinib at doses greater than 400 mg [22]; and for sorafenib at doses greater than 800 mg [23]. For pazopanib, due to solubility limitations in the digestive tract, a dose higher than 800 mg does not translate into an increase in plasma AUC [24]. Imatinib concentrations were significantly lower in patients undergoing gastrectomy [25,26], possibly due to decreased gastrointestinal transit time or lack of gastric acid secretion [26].

Regarding distribution process, most TKIs are substrates for membrane efflux transporters (e.g., ABCB1 and ABCG2) or uptake transporters (e.g., SLC22A1) [27–31] and present a high affinity for plasma proteins (e.g., 1-acid glycoprotein [AGP] and albumin), with only the free fraction of the drug (corresponding to a small percentage of total plasma levels) exerting any therapeutic action [32,33]. Other emerging parameters to consider are body composition and muscle mass [34,35].

Pharmacogenetics causes part of the high inter-individual variability observed to date in the metabolism of TKIs [8]. TKIs are primarily metabolized by CYP3A4, with a secondary role for other CYP enzymes [27]. Interactions among drugs can explain why the metabolic genotype does not accurately reflect the phenotype and limit the application of pharmacogenomic methods [36]. For all these reasons, dose adjustment is highly recommended for TKIs [37]. Finally, some TKIs have active metabolites for which variations in the enzymes responsible for metabolism translate into variations in plasma concentrations [8].

Most patients with advanced cancer acquire genetically based mechanisms of therapeutic resistance as the disease progresses [38]. Recent advances in high-throughput gene expression profiling enable the identification of differentially expressed genes involved in processes such as drug sensitivity and resistance, signaling pathways relevant to cancer biology, and tumor therapeutic targets in a semi-quantitative and rapid manner. Therefore, it is of interest to explore not only mutations in the genome, but also the expression of multiple genes capable of predicting the outcome of a drug in the clinical setting [39,40].

In general, there is a relationship between the concentration of the drug in plasma and the response and toxicity of the drug. TDM relies on the hypothesis that the concentration of a drug in the blood reflects the concentration at the site of action much better than the administered dose and constitutes a valid tool to complement pharmacogenomic techniques [41,42].

At present, there are more than 30 TKIs available for the treatment of several hematologic and solid tumors. Pharmacokinetic parameters obtained through TDM may be an important biomarker to optimize treatment [43]. Currently, there are numerous ongoing studies of TKIs, usually with highly selected patients. Data on real-world populations are necessary due to widespread use in very different clinical conditions.

The Plataforma de Oncología of Hospital Quirónsalud Torrevieja implemented TDM of TKIs in 2010. Since then, many cases of drug–drug interactions, drug–food interactions, and underdosing or overexposure to the drug at standard doses were detected. The results were analyzed with the aim of evaluating variability in real-world populations and assessing the effectiveness of TDM of TKIs in the routine clinical practice.

2. Materials and Methods

2.1. Patients

Patients were included in the present study if erlotinib, imatinib, lapatinib or sorafenib was part of their cancer drug therapy in the period 2016–2020. Selection criteria were not previously defined in this study, because the patient cohort should reflect a real-world cohort.

Patients' medical records were reviewed with the aim of studying all possible factors related to the patient and the medication that may influence the evolution of the plasma concentrations of TKIs. Sociodemographic and anthropometric, pharmacological treatment, clinical, toxicity and therapeutic drug monitoring data were collected. Treatment response was determined according to the RECIST.13. Adverse events were recorded by grade according to the Common Terminology Criteria for Adverse Events version 3.0 (CTCAE v 3.0) [44].

This study was reviewed and approved by the Clinical Research Ethics Committee of the Hospital Quirónsalud Torrevieja and conducted according to Good Clinical Practice guidelines and the Declaration of Helsinki. Patients received information about this study and provided written informed consent.

2.2. Treatment and Blood Sampling

Patients included in this study received drugs at doses previously established by their doctors, according to data sheet indications and clinical judgment. In all cases, drug dose was prescribed before the patient enrolled onto this study and was not affected by this study prior to enrollment.

Monitoring was carried out in all cases after at least fifteen days from the start of treatment, when the plasma levels of the drug were considered at steady state. Blood samples were extracted just before ingestion of the tablet/s and at different times after ingestion. The drug was administered in the fasted state and patients were told they could eat food after the second blood sample was drawn. Sampling times, which are defined for each drug in Table 1, were selected based on the optimal sampling theory and pharmacokinetic models previously published in the scientific literature [45–48]. Blood samples were extracted into tubes with lithium heparin as an anticoagulant and immediately protected from light with aluminum foil. The total blood volume extracted was between 4 and 5 mL for each sample. All samples were centrifuged after extraction at 3500 r.p.m. for 10 min at room temperature and the plasma obtained was frozen at $-80\ ^\circ$C until bioanalysis.

Table 1. Blood sampling times for monitored TKIs.

Drug	Sampling Times
Erlotinib	
Imatinib	Before drug administration and then at 1, 2, 4 and 6 h after drug administration
Lapatinib	
Sorafenib	Before drug administration and then at 1, 3, 6 and 8 h after drug administration

Bioanalysis was carried out using high-performance liquid chromatography (HPLC) coupled with ultraviolet (UV) detection. All the techniques used for the quantification of erlotinib, imatinib, lapatinib and sorafenib were previously validated in the Personalized Pharmacotherapy Unit of Hospital Quirónsalud Torrevieja according to the Guidelines of the Food and Drug Administration (FDA) [49] and the European Medicines Agency (EMA) [50], in terms of linearity, precision, accuracy, selectivity, specificity and performance.

2.2.1. Erlotinib

As the stationary phase, an Ultrabase® C_{18} chromatographic column, 4.6 mm in diameter by 150 mm in length, made of stainless steel and filled with a C_{18} reversed-phase siliceous substrate with a particle size of 5 µm, was used. A mixture of 40% of 0.02 M ammonium acetate, pH = 7, and 60% acetonitrile: methanol at a ratio of 70:30 (v/v) was used as the mobile phase. The linearity of the technique included a concentration range of 0.05–7.5 µg/mL. The limit of quantification was 0.5 µg/mL. Solid–liquid extraction was used and the analysis time was 9 min.

2.2.2. Imatinib

The stationary phase used was an Ultrabase® C_{18} chromatographic column, 4.6 mm in diameter by 150 mm in length, made of stainless steel and filled with a C_{18} reversed-phase siliceous substrate with a particle size of 5 µm. The mobile phase used was a 40% mixture of 0.02 M ammonium acetate, pH = 7, and 60% acetonitrile: methanol at a ratio of 70:30 (v/v). The linearity of the technique included a concentration range of 0.05–5 µg/mL. The limit of quantification was 0.5 µg/mL. Solid–liquid extraction was used and the analysis time was 10 min.

2.2.3. Lapatinib

The stationary phase used was a Kromasil® C_{18} chromatographic column, 4.6 mm in diameter by 150 mm in length, made of stainless steel and filled with a C_{18} reversed-phase siliceous substrate with a particle size of 5 µm. The mobile phase used was a mixture of acetonitrile and 0.02 M ammonium acetate, pH = 3.5, at a ratio of 53:47 (v/v). The linearity of the technique included a concentration range of 0.02–10 µg/mL. The limit of quantification was 0.2 µg/mL. Liquid–liquid extraction was used and the analysis time was 12 min [51].

2.2.4. Sorafenib

The stationary phase used was a Kromasil® C_{18} chromatographic column, 4.6 mm in diameter by 150 mm in length, made of stainless steel and filled with a C_{18} reversed-phase siliceous substrate with a particle size of 5 µm. The mobile phase used was a mixture of acetonitrile and 0.02 M ammonium acetate, pH = 3.5, at a ratio of 53:47 (v/v). The linearity of the technique included a concentration range of 0.1–20 µg/mL. The limit of quantification was 0.1 µg/mL. Liquid–liquid extraction was used and the analysis time was 12 min [52].

2.3. Pharmacokinetic Analysis

2.3.1. Erlotinib

The pharmacokinetic analysis of erlotinib, like that of imatinib, lapatinib and sorafenib, was performed with the NONMEM VII version 2.0 software (ICON, Hanover, MD, USA) using the POSTHOC option [53]. The program was compiled with the DIGITAL Visual Fortran version 6.6C program. The graphics were made with the S-Plus 6.1 Professional Edition program for Windows (Insightful, Seattle, WA, USA). A one-compartment pharmacokinetic model with first-order absorption and elimination kinetics was selected to describe erlotinib plasma concentrations, as performed previously by other authors [45]. The fixed-effect parameters estimated by the model were V (volume of distribution, L), CL (plasma clearance, L/h) and K_a (absorption constant). The model included plasma ALT concentration and age as covariates in CL, and weight in V.

2.3.2. Imatinib

To describe the plasma concentrations of imatinib, a one-compartment pharmacokinetic model with zero-order absorption and first-order elimination kinetics was selected, as performed previously by other authors [46]. The model was parameterized in terms of D1 (zero-order absorption duration), V and CL, and included the plasma concentration of α 1-acid glycoprotein as a covariate in CL.

2.3.3. Lapatinib

In the case of lapatinib, a one-compartment pharmacokinetic model with first-order absorption and elimination kinetics was selected, as performed previously by other authors [47]. The fixed-effect parameters estimated by the model were V, CL and K_a. The model included plasma ALT concentration and age as covariates in CL, and weight in V.

2.3.4. Sorafenib

Sorafenib plasma concentrations were described using a one-compartment pharmacokinetic model previously used by Jain L et al. to describe the pharmacokinetics of sorafenib [48]. The model uses 4 absorption transit compartments, enterohepatic circulation, and first-order elimination kinetics.

2.4. Statistical Methods

The statistical analysis was carried out with the SPSS software (version 20.0 for Windows®, Chicago, IL, USA). All data were stored in the database and filtered through distributions of unknown values for every variable and through distributions to detect uncommon values. Two-sided significance tests were used in the analyses performed, considering a probability of error α ($p < 0.05$) as significant.

For the descriptive analysis of the data, the categorical variables were expressed as a percentage, while the continuous variables were expressed as the mean (standard deviation (SD)). To describe the normality in the distribution of continuous variables, the distribution profile of the values of each variable was evaluated through histograms and trend lines, in addition to performing the Kolmogorov–Smirnov test. To validate the assumption of homogeneity of variances, Levene's test was used.

A linear regression model with an established Pearson's correlation coefficient (r) between continuous variables was used for the analytical treatment of the data.

To compare the mean values of continuous variables in different events, Student's *t*-test was used for those variables with a normal distribution and the Mann–Whitney U test was used for those that did not follow a normal distribution.

To compare the variation in categorical variables (rash, diarrhea, fatigue, abdominal pain, hypertension, and mucositis) between the first and the last monitored cycle, the non-parametric chi-square test was performed.

To assess the relationship between treatments protocols and disease progression or mortality, a Kaplan–Meier survival curve was plotted.

3. Results

3.1. Patients

The plasma levels of erlotinib, lapatinib, imatinib or sorafenib were monitored in 58 patients (57% women and 43% men) receiving 141 cycles of each drug (mean 2.4 cycles/patient, range 1–12) for dose individualization. A summary of all baseline characteristics of patients is shown in Table 2.

Table 2. Baseline characteristics.

Baseline Characteristics	Treatment			
	Erlotinib	Lapatinib	Imatinib	Sorafenib
Number of Patients in Treatment	22	16	9	11
Number of total cycles monitored	55	35	22	29
Cycles monitored by patient (n, %)				
1 cycle	8 (38.1)	9 (56.3)	3 (33.3)	7 (63.6)
2 cycles	6 (28.6)	4 (25.0)	2 (22.2)	1 (9.1)
3 cycles	3 (13.6)	2 (12.5)	2 (22.2)	1 (9.1)
4 cycles	2 (9.5)	–	1 (11.1)	1 (9.1)
>5 cycles	3 (14.3)	1 (6.3)	1 (11.1)	1 (9.1)
Gender (n. %)				
Male	14 (63.6)	4 (25.0)	3 (33.3)	4 (36.4)
Female	8 (36.4)	12 (75.0)	6 (66.7)	7 (63.6)
Age (mean (SD). years)	63.0 (12.3)	54.5 (12.6)	50.8 (16.4)	57.1 (15.6)
Weight (mean (SD). Kg)	80.2 (14.6)	69.7 (11.0)	78.50 (18.2)	71.2 (13.3)
Size (mean (SD). cm)	169.7 (9.3)	163.8 (8.4)	168 (11.5)	166.6 (12.2)
Body surface area (mean (SD). m^2)	1.9 (0.2)	1.7 (0.1)	1.87 (0.3)	1.8 (0.2)
Metastasis (number of patients. %)	19 (86.4)	15 (93.8)	5 (55.6)	9 (81.8)
Previous lines of treatment (range)	1.64 (0–7)	2.4 (1–6)	0.56 (0–2)	1.91 (0–5)

n: number of patients. SD: standard deviation.

A total of 710 plasma samples (307 for erlotinib, 137 for lapatinib, 114 for imatinib and 152 for sorafenib) were analyzed according to sampling times detailed in Table 1. We observed large interpatient variability for all drugs, as shown in Figure 1.

The mean interpatient variability in dose-normalized plasma concentrations in the first monitored cycle, expressed as a coefficient of variation (CV, %), was 46.2%, 60.7%, 48.9% and 89.7%, for erlotinib, lapatinib, imatinib and sorafenib, respectively. After TDM and dose adjustments, the mean interpatient variability in dose-normalized plasma concentrations in the last monitored cycle was 44%, 56%, 50.8% and 75.5%, respectively.

No significant effect of body weight, age, height or BSA on TKI plasma concentrations was observed, except for a negative correlation between height ($r = -0.4$, $p = 0.021$) and BSA ($r = -0.4$, $p = 0.022$) versus plasma concentrations of sorafenib. A non-significant increase in the C_{trough} of drugs was observed in women vs. men.

3.1.1. Erlotinib

In 21 of the monitored cycles (38.2%), the recommendation was to increase the prescribed dose. A total of 5 of the 22 patients included in this study required a mean dose increase of 46.6% in the last monitored cycle compared to the first one. In 30 of the monitored cycles (54.5%), the recommendation was to maintain the current dose since the concentrations were within the therapeutic target interval. In two of the cycles (3.6%), it was recommended to decrease the dose, with a dose reduction of 24.9% in the last monitored cycle with respect to the first one in 2 patients. In addition, in two of the monitored cycles (3.6%), it was recommended to suspend administration of the drug.

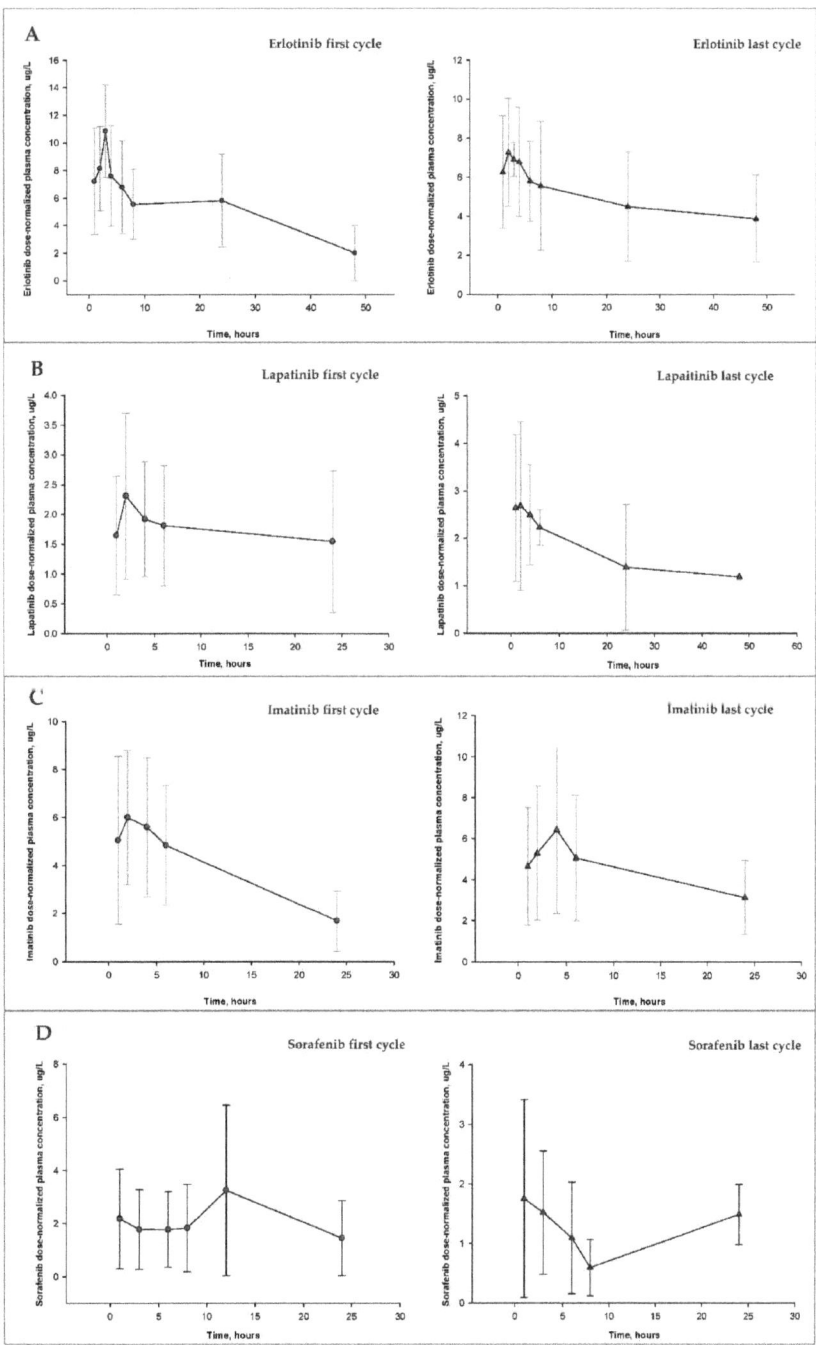

Figure 1. Dose-normalized plasma concentration profiles after administration of drug to patients receiving the dose of erlotinib (**A**), lapatinib (**B**), imatinib (**C**) or sorafenib (**D**) in the first or last monitored cycle. The symbols (circles and triangles) represent the mean dose-normalized plasma concentrations of patients at different times. The error bar for each point represents the standard deviation for each mean.

3.1.2. Imatinib

In seven of the monitored cycles (31.8%), the recommendation was to increase the prescribed dose since the concentrations were below the target therapeutic range—this meant a mean dose increase of 77.7% in the last monitored cycle compared to the dose administered in the first one for 3 of the 9 patients included. In 15 of the monitored cycles (68.2%), the recommendation was to maintain the current dose since the concentrations were within the therapeutic range. There were no recommendations to reduce the dose of imatinib, since no concentrations were found above the target level.

3.1.3. Lapatinib

In five of the monitored cycles (14.3%), the recommendation was to increase the prescribed dose—this meant a mean increase of 175% in the last monitored cycle with respect to the first one for 2 of the 16 patients included. In 24 of the monitored cycles (68.6%), the recommendation was to maintain the current dose since the concentrations were within the therapeutic range. In three of the cycles (8.6%), it was recommended to reduce the initial dose for concentrations above the therapeutic range, with a dose reduction of 62.5% of the dose administered in the last cycle with respect to the first one in 2 of the patients included. In three of the monitored cycles (8.6%), the recommendation was to suppress the drug.

3.1.4. Sorafenib

In five of the monitored cycles (17.2%), the recommendation was to increase the prescribed dose since the concentrations were below the therapeutic range, with a mean increase of 200% in the last compared to the first one in 2 of the 11 patients included. In 21 of the monitored cycles (72.4%), the recommendation was to maintain the current dose. In two of the cycles (6.9%), it was recommended to decrease the initial dose since concentrations were above the therapeutic range, with a reduction of 50% of the dose in the last one with respect to that in the first one in 1 patient. In one cycle (3.4%), it was recommended to suspend administration of the drug.

3.2. Response and Survival

Table 3 shows the survival data in terms of PFS and OS. The maximum follow-up period was 100 months for erlotinib, 176 months for imatinib, 105 months for lapatinib, and 62 months for sorafenib.

Table 3. Survival analysis.

Drug	Progression-Free Survival (Months)			Overall Survival (Months)		
	Median	SE	CI 95%	Median	SE	CI 95%
Erlotinib	8	4.7	0.0–17.1	32	31.6	0.0–93.9
Imatinib	28	11.9	4.6–54.4	90	29.9	31.3–148.0
Lapatinib	8	3.0	2.1–13.9	46	18.9	9.0–83.0
Sorafenib	9	3.4	2.3–15.6	9	5.1	0.1–19.1

SE: Standard error. CI 95%: 95% confidence interval.

No significant relationship between PFS and C_{trough} ($p > 0.203$ in all cases) or between OS and C_{trough} ($p > 0.251$ in all cases) was observed for none of the TKIs under study.

3.3. The Exposure–Toxicity Relationship

A total of 33 of the patients included in the present study developed toxicity at the start of treatment: 9 erlotinib patients (45.4%), 5 imatinib patients (55.5%), 12 lapatinib patients (75%), and 7 sorafenib patients (63.3%). The toxicity incidence data for each drug are detailed in Table 4.

Table 4. Incidence of toxicity.

Characteristic	Erlotinib		Imatinib		Lapatinib		Sorafenib	
Patients with toxicity [n. (%)]		9 (45.4)		5 (55.5)		12 (75.0)		7 (63.3)
Toxicity [n. (%)]	RI G1	9 (45.4)	Anemia G2	2 (22.2)	RI G1	6 (37.5)	Abdominal pain	2 (18.2)
	Skin rash G1	5 (22.7)	RI G1	2 (22.2)	Anemia G1	3 (18.7)	IR G1	2 (18.2)
	Anemia G1	4 (18.1)	Fatigue G1	1 (11.1)	Diarrhea G1	2 (12.5)	Anemia G1	2 (18.2)
	RI G2	4 (18.1)	Anemia G1	1 (11.1)	Pain	2 (12.5)	Diarrea G2	1 (9.1)
	Skin rash G2	3 (13.6)	RI G2	1 (11.1)	Anemia G2	2 (12.5)	Anemia G2	1 (9.1)
	Skin rash G3	3 (13.6)			Neutr. G3	2 (12.5)	Thromb. G1	1 (9.1)
	Diarrhea G2	3 (13.6)			RI G2	2 (12.5)		
	Fatigue G2	2 (9.1)			Skin rash G1	1 (6.2)		
	Anemia G2	2 (9.1)			Skin rash G3	1 (6.2)		
	Mucositis G3	1 (4.5)			Diarrhea G2	1 (6.2)		
	Thromb. G3	1 (4.5)			Diarrhea G3	1 (6.2)		
					Mucositis G3	1 (6.2)		
					Anemia G3	1 (6.2)		

n: number of patients. G: grade. RI: renal insufficiency. Thromb.: trombopenia. Neutr.: neutropenia.

Patients were classified into four groups to assess the toxicities developed based on exposure to each of the drugs: (1) patients with drug concentrations below the target level and without toxicities, (2) patients with drug concentrations below the target level and with toxicities, (3) patients with drug concentrations above the target level and without toxicities and (4) patients with drug concentrations above the target level and with toxicities. The distribution of patients according to the four groups described above is shown in Figure 2.

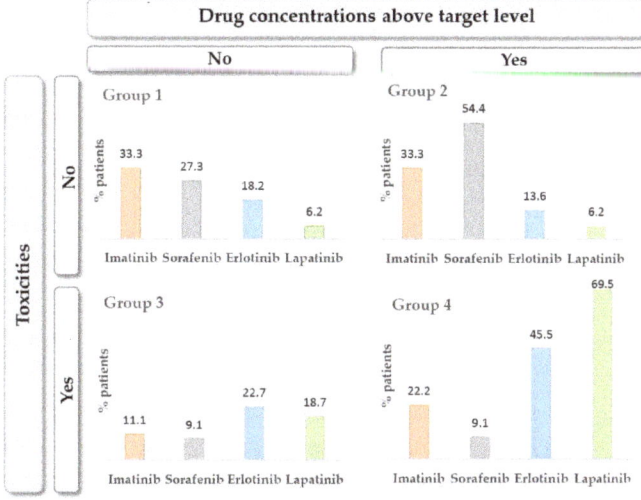

Figure 2. Groups of patients according to exposure to the drugs under study.

4. Discussion

TDM aims to maximize the therapeutic effectiveness of pharmacologic treatments while reducing the iatrogenic toxicity produced by them. TDM was typically considered advantageous for drugs with a large inter-individual variability in exposure with relatively low intra-individual variation, a significant exposure–efficacy relationship, a narrow therapeutic window, and availability of a validated bioanalytical assay [22]. It has been postulated recently that this could also represent a useful tool to individualize dosing and optimize treatment using drugs with a wide therapeutic window and high cost [54–56].

TKIs are drugs with a narrow therapeutic window and high cost which are commonly administered at fixed doses. Even though TKIs present high variability in their pharmacokinetics, which translates into high inter- and intra-individual variability in drug exposure as stated above [57,58], the standard dose described in the corresponding data sheet of the drugs is administered to all candidate patients, resulting in unpredictable plasma concentrations [27]. Clinical trials do not identify all real-world scenarios because frail patients, those on specific diets, variable dosage intervals, or concomitant polimedication are systematically excluded from them. Post-marketing studies detect or better describe different side effects that can decrease adherence to the treatment, reducing the efficacy of these drugs. TDM can improve tolerability and subsequently adherence [59].

Oral cancer therapies have theoretical advantages, both for patients and the healthcare system, but not without drawbacks. Adverse effects increase therapeutic non-compliance and symptoms of anxiety and depression. These, in turn, cause loss of control of the disease, higher costs due to increased and longer admissions in the hospital, and loss of quality of life. TDM, in this context, enables identification inadequate dosing, adapting the dose to the individual needs of the patient and avoiding abandonment of therapy due to toxicity or futility and unjustified changes in therapy caused by low plasma levels of the drug [59].

The present evaluation has been performed on adult real-world patients, with no inclusion or exclusion criteria other than an expected efficacy of the TKI in their clinical situation. They presented high variability in terms of tumor type, disease stage, pre-treatment, duration of treatment, etc. In this population, the variability in drug exposure can be much greater than in clinical trials and the response to treatment, both in terms of efficacy and toxicity, reflects it. This enabled the detection of personalized influences of different factors on exposure, response, and toxicity of TKI treatments and highlighted the benefit of TDM in routine clinical practice.

4.1. Erlotinib

In the case of erlotinib, data on underdosed patients found in the present study differed from those obtained by Lankheet et al. [60], who used a plasma concentration of 500 mg/L as the therapeutic target [61] and found that 11.1% of patients had plasma concentrations below the target, a percentage of underdosed patients that is clearly lower than that reported here. In this study, all the patients included had a diagnosis of lung cancer, so this lower percentage of underdosed patients may be due to lower interpatient variability.

The data sheet of erlotinib [62] recommend a dose of 150 mg/day for adult patients with non-small-cell lung cancer (NSCLC) and 100 mg/day for those with pancreatic cancer. In the present study, patients started with standard doses, but five of them received higher doses in the last cycle because they could not otherwise reach therapeutic levels within the optimal range. Erlotinib dose adjustment is only recommended in the data sheet when co-administered with CYP3A4 inhibitors or inducers, CYP1A2 inhibitors, or in smokers, but, as shown, dose adjustments based on TDM are necessary in other situations.

No effect of weight, height, BSA, age or sex on the plasma C_{trough} was detected in the present study, as was the case in the patients studied by Lankheet et al. [60] and other population studies involving 1859 NSCLC patients [63], 291 NSCLC patients [62], 80 NSCLC patients [64] and 204 pancreatic cancer patients [62].

A direct relationship between exposure to erlotinib and observed clinical response must be proven [65]. Some authors describe a statistically significant correlation between exposure and efficacy [66,67], while others only point to a non-statistically significant trend or relationship between both parameters [68,69]. The preclinical study carried out by Hidalgo et al. [61] suggested that a target C_{trough} greater than 500 mg/L in humans would be adequate for the inhibition of EGFR receptors, so this target concentration was adopted for later studies.

In the present study, PFS is similar (8 months) to previously published results, whereas OS is greater (32 months). Motoshima et al. found PFS and OS of 6.3 months and 16.9 months, respectively, in 26 NSCLC patients [67]. The differences observed may be due to the smaller number of patients recruited in this study, their complexity and underlying pathogenesis, and the follow-up time.

No statistically significant relationship was found between dose-normalized C_{trough} and PFS ($p = 0.630$) or OS ($p = 0.593$). Similarly, Tiseo et al., in their study of 56 patients with NSCLC, found no significant relationship between a $C_{trough} \geq 4.6$ nmol/mL or greater skin toxicity (patients with greater skin toxicity had better results from treatment) with an improvement in OS ($p = 0.351$) or PFS ($p = 0.127$) [66]. In a phase II study involving 16 NSCLC patients, C_{trough} was measured on days 2 and 8 of treatment. The ratio of C_{trough} on day 8 to C_{trough} on day 2 represented the accumulation of erlotinib over time. A high ratio was related to a low metabolism of erlotinib and therefore higher exposure, and correlated positively with PFS ($p = 0.004$) but not with OS [67]. Another study of patients with HNSC evaluated three ranges of samples depending on the time elapsed after taking the drug—in 42 patients, the C_{trough} was between 20 and 25 h after the dose; in 77 patients, C_{max} was between 2 and 5 h post dose; in 47 patients, the concentration was stated for between 5 and 10 h post dose. The median concentration between 5 and 10 h post dose for erlotinib predicted better OS ($p = 0.021$) [68].

The main analytical parameters related to toxicity (hemoglobin, hematocrit, neutrophils, leukocytes, platelets, creatinine, bilirubin, GOT, GPT and alkaline phosphatase), showed no significant differences in the first monitored cycle with respect to the last, as with the defined toxicities themselves (fatigue, diarrhea, abdominal pain, hypertension, mucositis, anemia, neutropenia, thrombocytopenia, and renal insufficiency (RI)). Most of the grade 3 toxicities described were in the first monitored cycle (rash, mucositis and thrombocytopenia), before carrying out TDM and dose adjustment, compared to the last monitored cycle (13, 6% vs. 7.1%, 4.5% vs. 0%, and 4.5% vs. 0%, respectively). Grade 2 skin rash was the only relevant toxicity observed in a higher percentage of patients in the last monitored cycle (13.6% in the first monitored cycle vs. 14.3% in the last). This may be due to the relationship between the skin rash produced by erlotinib and tumor response, for which the rash is a potential marker of activity [68–71]. Development of cutaneous rash has been related to drug exposure and clinical benefit with erlotinib. Soulieres et al. [68] reported higher OS in patients who developed a grade ≥ 2 skin rash ($p = 0.045$, $n = 115$). In addition, the C_{trough} in this group of patients was higher, although not statistically significant, than the C_{trough} in patients with a rash grade lower than 2 (1097–1126 mg/L vs. 803 mg/L, $p = 0.49$).

No significant relationship was found between the different degrees of skin rash and C_{trough} (rash G1 $p = 0.870$, rash G2 $p = 0.746$ and rash G3 $p = 0.374$) in the present study. In a phase II study of 57 NSCLC patients, the OS of patients with grade 2 rash was 19.6 months, the OS of patients grade 1 rash was 8.5 months and the OS of patients without rash was 1.5 months [72]. Other groups reported similar results [66–69]. Despite some studies showing a relationship between pharmacokinetic parameters and efficacy, and between toxicity and treatment efficacy, pharmacokinetic parameters did not correlate with toxicity in all cases [66–68]. This indicates that the skin rash is not simply a reflection of exposure to erlotinib, in accordance with the results in this study. The largest study to determine this relationship was carried out in 339 NSCLC patients, demonstrating a relationship between AUC_{0-24} and C_{max} with the appearance of rash. However, the correlation was not considered relevant, as there was a large overlap in AUC_{0-24} and C_{max} between patients with and without toxicity [63].

The only significant correlation between the analytical parameters collected and C_{trough} was an inversely proportional relationship with alkaline phosphatase ($p = 0.025$). There are studies that show a relationship between the pharmacokinetic parameters of erlotinib and liver function, although none of them relates it with plasma concentrations [63]. These results led to the recommendation of dose adjustment of erlotinib in hepatic insufficiency.

The relationship between C_{trough} and grade 1 RI was the only statistically significant ($p > 0.013$) relationship between C_{trough} and a toxicity (fatigue, diarrhea, abdominal pain, hypertension, mucositis, anemia and thrombocytopenia). It was not considered clinically relevant, since the 10 patients who presented with grade 1 RI already presented with this at the beginning of this study, in the first monitored cycle. In the literature, we have not found studies showing a relationship between RI and C_{trough}, although it seems logical to think that, since only 9% of a single dose is eliminated in the urine [73], there is no relationship between renal function and the pharmacokinetic parameters of erlotinib.

4.2. Imatinib

Imatinib showed large variability both in the first and in the last monitored cycle (mean CV first cycle 48.91% vs. mean CV last cycle 50.84%). In different populations, the pharmacokinetic analysis revealed that weight, age, sex, diagnosis, AGP, albumin, granulocytes, white series, hemoglobin and gastrectomy might be factors that explain the variability between patients, but they have not been considered significant for dose adjustments [26,28,33]. As with other TKIs, this variation can be explained by the oral route, whether the drug is administered with food, presystemic metabolism at the intestinal level, membrane transporters, binding to plasma proteins or hepatic metabolism through cytochrome CYP3A4 and CYP3A5. In addition, therapeutic compliance can vary between patients or even in the same patient [2,27]. Patients included in the present study show variability in drug exposure comparable to that observed in other studies [60].

All imatinib dose adjustments made following TDM indications were to increase the dose. In 31.8% of cycles, plasma concentrations were below the established 50% population prediction interval. Dose adjustment in these patients led to a mean increase of 77.7% in the last monitored cycle compared to the first. There are studies confirming the fact that after 8 months of treatment with imatinib, exposure to the drug decreases due to the induction of liver enzymes [60,74].

As detailed in the data sheet of imatinib [75], the recommended dose for adult patients ranges from 100 to 800 mg/day, depending on the indication. Although the patients included started with the standard dose, three of them had to receive higher doses because they did not reach therapeutic levels with the initial doses. Dose adjustment is only recommended in the data sheet when co-administered with inhibitors or inducers of CYP3A4, with liver dysfunction or RI [75]. As evidenced in this study, dose adjustments based on TDM are necessary in additional situations where optimal therapeutic levels are not reached if the patient's condition allows it.

No significant relationship was observed between dose-normalized plasma C_{trough} in every cycle and PFS and OS. Other authors found that patients with lower exposure to imatinib showed a lower overall rate of benefit (complete response + partial response + stable disease), suggesting that a determinate level of C_{trough} is necessary to maintain the response in patients with GIST [76]. Another prospective study demonstrated a decrease of approximately 30% in C_{trough} after 3 months of treatment [74]. Therefore, it would be advisable to repeat TDM after 3 months of treatment. Widmer et al. demonstrated the relevance of achieving adequate levels of imatinib to maintain therapeutic responses in a study of 38 patients with GIST [33]. This work also suggested that sustained exposure is associated with a better response, more than total exposure to the drug. In the present study, no relationship was found between C_{trough} and PFS or OS, probably due to the low number of patients recruited.

No significant differences were found in the analytical parameters or defined toxicities in the first monitored cycle with respect to the last. Grade 2 toxicities observed, specifically grade 2 anemia, were in the first cycle, before TDM and dose adjustment, compared to the last (22.2% vs. 16.7%), except grade 2 RI (11.1% vs. 33.3%). Chronic RI is described in the data sheet as an adverse reaction of unknown frequency for imatinib [75]. There was no significant correlation between the analytical parameters and C_{trough}, except for hemoglobin and hematocrit, where a significant and inversely proportional relationship with C_{trough} was observed. Other authors reported a direct relationship between C_{trough} and analytical alterations or some toxic manifestations, probably related to longer treatment or higher casuistry [77,78].

4.3. Lapatinib

Patients treated with lapatinib in this study had different tumors: breast cancer, GIST, pancreas, colon, esophagus, etc. Due to this heterogeneity, the dosage in the monitored treatment cycles varied between 125 mg/day in some patients and 1250 mg/day. There is no similar study in the literature on a real-world population for comparison.

Large variability was observed in the dose-normalized plasma concentrations at different sampling times, both in the first cycle and in the last (mean CV first cycle: 60.7% vs. average CV last cycle: 56.0%), in concordance with other TKIs previously analyzed. Interpatient variability in lapatinib exposure found in the literature shows data for C_{trough} and an AUC of 55–97% and 42–117%, respectively [20,79–82], consistent with that obtained in the present study. Regarding variability in intra-patient exposure, EPAR data for lapatinib show a CV of AUC between 30% and 36% on average in healthy subjects. There are no other studies in which variability has been measured. Therefore, patients included in this study show interpatient variability in drug exposure comparable to the few studies available in the literature. As other authors have shown for other TKIs, this variability may be influenced by patients' adherence to treatment, concomitant medication or previous lines of treatment received, etc. [60].

As detailed in the data sheet of lapatinib [79], the recommended dose in adult patients with HER2-positive breast cancer is 750 to 1500 mg/day, depending on the concomitant medication administered. Dose adjustment is only recommended when cardiac events, diarrhea or other grade 2 toxicities occur. In the case of severe hepatic insufficiency, it is recommended to suspend treatment and not restart it. In the present study, 7 of the 16 patients treated began at a reduced dose for impaired liver function. Only in 2 of the patients who started at a reduced dose was it necessary to increase the dose for inadequate plasma levels. In the remaining 5 patients with a reduced dose, optimal levels within the 50% population prediction interval were observed. In patients with impaired liver function, TDM enabled the quantification of drug exposure and subsequent satisfactory dose adjustment.

In situations other than impaired liver function in which optimal therapeutic levels are not reached or when they are reached with doses lower than the standard, as long as the patient's condition allows it, dose adjustments based on TDM are necessary. Even so, based on the data available in the literature, the individualization of the dose of lapatinib with TDM based solely on a target dose is not recommended because they are studies carried out in a very limited and heterogeneous population [57,58].

In the present study, no significant relationship was observed between dose-normalized plasma C_{trough} at each monitored cycle and PFS or OS. A clear exposure–efficacy relationship for lapatinib has not been identified in the literature. Lapatinib was found to be well tolerated at doses ranging from 175 to 1800 mg once daily or 500 to 900 mg twice daily [81]. In a phase I trial, it was found that most patients who responded to lapatinib had a C_{trough} ranging from 300 to 600 mg/L (n = 67 patients with metastatic solid tumors) [81]. However, the results are difficult to interpret as response data are limited and the population is highly heterogeneous.

The analytical parameters related to toxicity in the first monitored cycle with respect to the last showed no significant differences, as with the defined toxicities themselves. The most serious side effects observed, at grade 2 and grade 3, were mostly in the first cycle (rash, diarrhea, mucositis, anemia and neutropenia), before performing TDM and dose adjustment, compared to the last monitored cycle. It is remarkable in the case of lapatinib that toxicities were detected in 25 cases in the first monitored cycle, while toxicities were only detected in 5 cases after performing TDM. TDM of lapatinib reduced toxicity events presented by the study population by 80%, very important in an otherwise useful drug with a high degree of therapeutic withdrawal due to toxicity.

GOT and GPT were the only analytical parameters that correlated with C_{trough}, showing a directly proportional relationship. These data are consistent with those found in the literature. Higher systemic exposure to lapatinib was previously described in patients with severe liver failure, with a mean AUC of lapatinib increased by more than 60% and a 3-fold higher $t_{1/2}$ than that observed in patients with normal liver function [79,80]. No relationship was found between fatigue, rash, diarrhea, abdominal pain, hypertension, mucositis or thrombocytopenia and C_{trough} ($p > 0.093$). Other studies described similar results, with diarrhea directly and positively related to dose ($p < 0.03$) but not to C_{trough}. This fact suggests that diarrhea is caused by a local effect of the drug on the intestinal epithelium [81,82].

4.4. Sorafenib

Due to the different origin of the tumors treated with sorafenib (liver, breast, oral cavity, etc.), the dosage guidelines varied from 200 mg/day in some patients to 600 mg/8 h in other cases. There is no study in the literature that includes a similar real-world population with TDM data for comparison with that shown here.

The large variability observed in dose-normalized plasma concentrations at different sampling times in previous TKIs analyzed was also observed in the case of sorafenib (mean CV first cycle: 89.7% vs. mean CV last cycle: 72.5%). In addition to other already mentioned factors, sorafenib intake is recommended outside of meals or with a moderate or low-fat meal due to the influence of food in pharmacokinetics. It also presents pre-systemic metabolism at the intestinal level. The variability in exposure between patients found in the literature shows data for C_{trough}, AUC and apparent oral Cl of 25–104%, 12–117% and 13–80%, respectively [83–86]. Therefore, the variability in drug exposure in patients included in this study is comparable to that observed in other previously published studies.

The data sheet of sorafenib recommend a dose of 400 mg twice daily for adult patients with hepatocellular carcinoma, renal cell carcinoma or differentiated thyroid carcinoma [83]. In the present study, only two patients started at the standard doses, while nine of the patients started at a reduced dose, either because it was administered in combination with chemotherapy, due to their age (78-year-old patient), as a result of cumulative toxicity, or because they were in a bad clinical condition. One of the patients who started at a reduced dose required an increase from 400 mg/day to higher than 1800 mg/day (350%) to reach levels within the therapeutic range. Another patient required a 50% reduction from 400 mg/day due to levels above the population prediction interval. (Sorafenib dose adjustment is recommended in the data sheet only to manage possible toxicities or with co-administration of neomycin or other antibiotics that cause ecological alterations in the gastrointestinal microflora and may lead to decreased bioavailability or if the drug is administered with inducers of metabolic enzymes. As has been observed in this study, it is necessary to make dose adjustments based on TDM in situations other than suggested if the patient's condition allows it.

The correlation analysis of height and BSA with plasma C_{trough} shows a positive relationship in both cases ($p = 0.021$ and $p = 0.022$, respectively). No studies assessing the clinical significance of this relationship were found.

In the present study, no significant relationship was observed between dose-normalized plasma C_{trough} at every monitored cycle and PFS ($p = 0.940$) or OS ($p = 0.909$). A clear relationship between exposure and efficacy has not been established at present for sorafenib, with some studies showing a relationship [87,88] and others not doing so [27].

The difference between the first and last cycles monitored was significant only for hemoglobin ($p = 0.031$) and hematocrit ($p = 0.031$) when hematological parameters were analyzed according to exposure to sorafenib. The most remarkable toxicities observed were anemia and grade 3 neutropenia, which mainly occurred in the last cycle (50% and 25%, respectively), that is, after performing TDM and dose adjustment. Hematological toxicities such as anemia or neutropenia are described as frequent in the data sheet of sorafenib after continued administration of the drug, even at levels within the therapeutic range [83]. The correlation study performed between C_{trough} and the different analytical parameters or toxic manifestations show statistically significant results for platelets ($r = -0.483$, $p = 0.043$), GPT ($r = -0.478$, $p = 0.045$) and alkaline phosphatase ($r = -0.746$, $p = 0.001$). Most of the studies which relate exposure and toxicity to sorafenib use AUC as a pharmacokinetic parameter [34,87,89], so they are not comparable to the present study. Fukudo et al. showed that C_{trough} at steady state correlates with grade 2 hand–foot syndrome ($p = 0.0045$) and hypertension ($p = 0.0453$). Although the toxicities they described were not the same as those related in the present work, an exposure–toxicity relationship was shown in both studies [88].

In the study by subgroups of the toxicities for each TKI evaluated, patients in group 1 (patients with concentrations below therapeutic levels and no toxicities) and group 4 (patients with levels above the therapeutic range and toxicities), the results are similar to those reported in the literature for erlotinib and imatinib [60]. The authors conclude that 65.7% of the patients treated with erlotinib and 47.3% of those treated with imatinib would benefit most from TDM as a tool to improve the exposure–efficacy and exposure–toxicity relationships. These percentages were slightly different from ours (63.7% and 55.5%, respectively), but significant enough to consider performing TDM. A total of 75.9% and 36.4% of lapatinib and sorafenib patients, respectively, would benefit most from TDM. There is no similar study in the literature to compare these results.

5. Conclusions

Erlotinib, imatinib, lapatinib and sorafenib show high inter-individual and intra-individual variability in exposure. A similar scenario might be anticipated for other TKIs.

TDM of TKIs adds remarkable value to routine clinical practice. TDM enables assessment of underdosing, lack of adherence to treatment and changes in exposure due to interaction with food or other drugs. TDM-guided dose corrections result in a significant improvement in exposure and enable more effective and safe use of TKIs, avoiding the ineffectiveness and toxicity of these drugs in certain patients and clinical situations, as has been the current practice with other medications (antibiotics, digoxin, anticonvulsants, etc.).

Author Contributions: Data curation, V.E.-O., V.D.-L., A.C.-L. and M.S.; Formal analysis, V.E.-O., V.D.-L., A.C.-L. and J.R.-L.; Investigation, V.E.-O., V.D.-L., A.C.-L., J.R.-L. and M.S.; Methodology, V.E.-O., V.D.-L.; Supervision, V.E.-O. and M.S.; Validation, M.S.; Visualization, V.E.-O.; Writing—original draft, V.E.-O., V.D.-L. and M.S.; Writing—review & editing, V.E.-O., V.D.-L., A.C.-L., J.R.-L. and M.S. All authors have read and agreed to the published version of the manuscript.

Funding: This research was partially founded by Fundación TEDECA, which also covered APC.

Institutional Review Board Statement: This study was reviewed and approved by the Clinical Research Ethics Committee of the Hospital Quirónsalud Torrevieja and conducted according to Good Clinical Practice guidelines and the Declaration of Helsinki.

Informed Consent Statement: All the patients included in this study provided written informed consent.

Data Availability Statement: Data are available upon reasonable request.

Conflicts of Interest: The authors declare no conflict of interest.

References

1. Holford, N.H.; Sheiner, L.B. Kinetics of pharmacologic response. *Pharmacol. Ther.* **1982**, *16*, 143–166. [CrossRef]
2. Sheiner, L.B.; Beal, S.; Rosenberg, B.; Marathe, V.V. Forecasting individual pharmacokinetics. *Clin. Pharmacol. Ther.* **1979**, *26*, 294–305. [CrossRef] [PubMed]
3. Kang, J.S.; Lee, M.H. Overview of therapeutic drug monitoring. *Korean J. Intern. Med.* **2009**, *24*, 1–10. [CrossRef] [PubMed]
4. Zhao, Y.; Thomas, H.D.; Batey, M.A.; Cowell, I.G.; Richardson, C.J.; Griffin, R.J.; Calvert, A.H.; Newell, D.R.; Smith, G.C.; Curtin, N.J. Preclinical evaluation of a potent novel DNA-dependent protein kinase inhibitor NU7441. *Cancer Res.* **2006**, *66*, 5354–5362. [CrossRef]
5. Giamas, G.; Man, Y.L.; Hirner, H.; Bischof, J.; Kramer, K.; Khan, K.; Ahmed, S.S.; Stebbing, J.; Knippschild, U. Kinases as targets in the treatment of solid tumors. *Cell. Signal.* **2010**, *22*, 984–1002. [CrossRef]
6. Cohen, P. Protein kinases—the major drug targets of the twenty-first century? *Nat. Rev. Drug Discov.* **2002**, *1*, 309–315. [CrossRef]
7. Zhang, J.; Yang, P.L.; Gray, N.S. Targeting cancer with small molecule kinase inhibitors. *Nat. Rev. Cancer* **2009**, *9*, 28–39. [CrossRef]

8. Gao, B.; Yeap, S.; Clements, A.; Balakrishnar, B.; Wong, M.; Gurney, H. Evidence for therapeutic drug monitoring of targeted anticancer therapies. *J. Clin. Oncol.* **2012**, *30*, 4017–4025. [CrossRef]
9. von Mehren, M.; Widmer, N. Correlations between imatinib pharmacokinetics, pharmacodynamics, adherence, and clinical response in advanced metastatic gastrointestinal stromal tumor (GIST): An emerging role for drug blood level testing? *Cancer Treat. Rev.* **2011**, *37*, 291–299. [CrossRef]
10. Wood, L. A review on adherence management in patients on oral cancer therapies. *Eur. J. Oncol. Nurs.* **2012**, *16*, 432–438. [CrossRef]
11. Tsang, J.; Rudychev, I.; Pescatore, S.L. Prescription compliance and persistency in chronic myelogenous leukemia (CML) and gastrointestinal stromal tumor (GIST) patients (pts) on imatinib (IM). *J. Clin. Oncol.* **2006**, *24*, 6119. [CrossRef]
12. Feng, W.; Henk, H.; Thomas, S.; Baladi, J.; Hatfield, A.; Goldberg, G.A. Compliance and persistency with imatinib. *J. Clin. Oncol.* **2006**, *24*, 6038. [CrossRef]
13. Levine, A.M.; Richardson, J.L.; Marks, G.; Chan, K.; Graham, J.; Selser, J.N.; Kishbaugh, C.; Shelton, D.R.; Johnson, C.A. Compliance with oral drug therapy in patients with hematologic malignancy. *J. Clin. Oncol.* **1987**, *5*, 1469–1476. [CrossRef] [PubMed]
14. Gater, A.; Heron, L.; Abetz-Webb, L.; Coombs, J.; Simmons, J.; Guilhot, F.; Rea, D. Adherence to oral tyrosine kinase inhibitor therapies in chronic myeloid leukemia. *Leuk. Res.* **2012**, *36*, 817–825. [CrossRef]
15. Jabbour, E.J.; Kantarjian, H.; Eliasson, L.; Cornelison, A.M.; Marin, D. Patient adherence to tyrosine kinase inhibitor therapy in chronic myeloid leukemia. *Am. J. Hematol.* **2012**, *87*, 687–691. [CrossRef]
16. de Almeida, M.H.; Pagnano, K.B.; Vigorito, A.C.; Lorand-Metze, I.; de Souza, C.A. Adherence to tyrosine kinase inhibitor therapy for chronic myeloid leukemia: A Brazilian single-center cohort. *Acta Haematol.* **2013**, *130*, 16–22. [CrossRef]
17. Bui, B.N.; Italiano, A.; Miranova, A.; Bouchet, S.; Molimard, M. Trough imatinib plasma levels in patients treated for advanced gastrointestinal stromal tumors evidence of large interpatient variations under treatment with standard doses. *J. Clin. Oncol.* **2008**, *26*, 10564. [CrossRef]
18. Marin, D.; Bazeos, A.; Mahon, F.X.; Eliasson, L.; Milojkovic, D.; Bua, M.; Apperley, J.F.; Szydlo, R.; Desai, R.; Kozlowski, K.; et al. Adherence is the critical factor for achieving molecular responses in patients with chronic myeloid leukemia who achieve complete cytogenetic responses on imatinib. *J. Clin. Oncol.* **2010**, *28*, 2381–2388. [CrossRef]
19. Tanaka, C.; Yin, O.Q.; Sethuraman, V.; Smith, T.; Wang, X.; Grouss, K.; Kantarjian, H.; Giles, F.; Ottmann, O.G.; Galitz, L.; et al. Clinical pharmacokinetics of the BCR-ABL tyrosine kinase inhibitor nilotinib. *Clin. Pharmacol. Ther.* **2010**, *87*, 197–203. [CrossRef]
20. Koch, K.M.; Reddy, N.J.; Cohen, R.B.; Lewis, N.L.; Whitehead, B.; Mackay, K.; Stead, A.; Beelen, A.P.; Lewis, L.D. Effects of food on the relative bioavailability of lapatinib in cancer patients. *J. Clin. Oncol.* **2009**, *27*, 1191–1196. [CrossRef]
21. Heath, E.I.; Chiorean, E.G.; Sweeney, C.J.; Hodge, J.P.; Lager, J.J.; Forman, K.; Malburg, L.; Arumugham, T.; Dar, M.M.; Suttle, A.B.; et al. A phase I study of the pharmacokinetic and safety profiles of oral pazopanib with a high-fat or low-fat meal in patients with advanced solid tumors. *Clin. Pharmacol. Ther.* **2010**, *88*, 818–823. [CrossRef]
22. Kantarjian, H.; Giles, F.; Wunderle, L.; Bhalla, K.; O'Brien, S.; Wassmann, B.; Tanaka, C.; Manley, P.; Rae, P.; Mietlowski, W.; et al. Nilotinib in imatinib-resistant CML and Philadelphia chromosome-positive ALL. *N. Engl. J. Med.* **2006**, *354*, 2542–2551. [CrossRef] [PubMed]
23. Hornecker, M.; Blanchet, B.; Billemont, B.; Sassi, H.; Ropert, S.; Taieb, F.; Mir, O.; Abbas, H.; Harcouet, L.; Coriat, R.; et al. Saturable absorption of sorafenib in patients with solid tumors: A population model. *Investig. New Drugs.* **2012**, *30*, 1991–2000. [CrossRef] [PubMed]
24. Hurwitz, H.I.; Dowlati, A.; Saini, S.; Savage, S.; Suttle, A.B.; Gibson, D.M.; Hodge, J.P.; Merkle, E.M.; Pandite, L. Phase I trial of pazopanib in patients with advanced cancer. *Clin. Cancer Res.* **2009**, *15*, 4220–4227. [CrossRef] [PubMed]
25. Pavlovsky, C.; Egorin, M.J.; Shah, D.D.; Beumer, J.H.; Rogel, S.; Pavlovsky, S. Imatinib mesylate pharmacokinetics before and after sleeve gastrectomy in a morbidly obese patient with chronic myeloid leukemia. *Pharmacotherapy* **2009**, *29*, 1152–1156. [CrossRef] [PubMed]
26. Yoo, C.; Ryu, M.H.; Kang, B.W.; Yoon, S.K.; Ryoo, B.Y.; Chang, H.M.; Lee, J.L.; Beck, M.Y.; Kim, T.W.; Kang, Y.K. Cross-sectional study of imatinib plasma trough levels in patients with advanced gastrointestinal stromal tumors: Impact of gastrointestinal resection on exposure to imatinib. *J. Clin. Oncol.* **2010**, *28*, 1554–1559. [CrossRef]
27. van Erp, N.P.; Gelderblom, H.; Guchelaar, H.J. Clinical pharmacokinetics of tyrosine kinase inhibitors. *Cancer Treat. Rev.* **2009**, *35*, 692–706. [CrossRef]
28. Petain, A.; Kattygnarath, D.; Azard, J.; Chatelut, E.; Delbaldo, C.; Geoerger, B.; Barrois, M.; Séronie-Vivien, S.; LeCesne, A.; Vassal, G. Innovative Therapies with Children with Cancer European consortium. Population pharmacokinetics and pharmacogenetics of imatinib in children and adults. *Clin. Cancer Res.* **2008**, *14*, 7102–7109. [CrossRef]
29. Tang, S.C.; Lagas, J.S.; Lankheet, N.A.; Poller, B.; Hillebrand, M.J.; Rosing, H.; Beijnen, J.H.; Schinkel, A.H. Brain accumulation of sunitinib is restricted by P-glycoprotein (ABCB1) and breast cancer resistance protein (ABCG2) and can be enhanced by oral elacridar and sunitinib coadministration. *Int. J. Cancer* **2012**, *130*, 223–233. [CrossRef]
30. Bazeos, A.; Marin, D.; Reid, A.G.; Gerrard, G.; Milojkovic, D.; May, P.C.; de Lavallade, H.; Garland, P.; Rezvani, K.; Apperley, J.F.; et al. hOCT1 transcript levels and single nucleotide polymorphisms as predictive factors for response to imatinib in chronic myeloid leukemia. *Leukemia* **2010**, *24*, 1243–1245. [CrossRef]

31. White, D.L.; Saunders, V.A.; Dang, P.; Engler, J.; Venables, A.; Zrim, S.; Zannettino, A.; Lynch, K.; Manley, P.W.; Hughes, T. Most CML patients who have a suboptimal response to imatinib have low OCT-1 activity: Higher doses of imatinib may overcome the negative impact of low OCT-1 activity. *Blood* **2007**, *110*, 4064–4072. [CrossRef]
32. Widmer, N.; Decosterd, L.A.; Leyvraz, S.; Duchosal, M.A.; Rosselet, A.; Debiec-Rychter, M.; Csajka, C.; Biollaz, J.; Buclin, T. Relationship of imatinib-free plasma levels and target genotype with efficacy and tolerability. *Br. J. Cancer* **2008**, *98*, 1633–1640. [CrossRef]
33. Widmer, N.; Decosterd, L.A.; Csajka, C.; Leyvraz, S.; Duchosal, M.A.; Rosselet, A.; Rochat, B.; Eap, C.B.; Henry, H.; Biollaz, J.; et al. Population pharmacokinetics of imatinib and the role of alpha-acid glycoprotein. *Br. J. Clin. Pharmacol.* **2006**, *62*, 97–112. [CrossRef]
34. Mir, O.; Coriat, R.; Blanchet, B.; Durand, J.P.; Boudou-Rouquette, P.; Michels, J.; Ropert, S.; Vidal, M.; Pol, S.; Chaussade, S.; et al. Sarcopenia predicts early dose-limiting toxicities and pharmacokinetics of sorafenib in patients with hepatocellular carcinoma. *PLoS ONE* **2012**, *7*, e37563. [CrossRef]
35. Antoun, S.; Baracos, V.E.; Birdsell, L.; Escudier, B.; Sawyer, M.B. Low body mass index and sarcopenia associated with dose-limiting toxicity of sorafenib in patients with renal cell carcinoma. *Ann. Oncol.* **2010**, *21*, 1594–1598. [CrossRef]
36. Thomas-Schoemann, A.; Blanchet, B.; Bardin, C.; Noé, G.; Boudou-Rouquette, P.; Vidal, M.; Goldwasser, F. Drug interactions with solid tumour-targeted therapies. *Crit. Rev. Oncol. Hematol.* **2014**, *89*, 179–196. [CrossRef]
37. Haouala, A.; Zanolari, B.; Rochat, B.; Montemurro, M.; Zaman, K.; Duchosal, M.A.; Ris, H.B.; Leyvraz, S.; Widmer, N.; Decosterd, L.A. Therapeutic Drug Monitoring of the new targeted anticancer agents imatinib, nilotinib, dasatinib, sunitinib, sorafenib and lapatinib by LC tandem mass spectrometry. *J. Chromatogr. B Analyt. Technol. Biomed. Life Sci.* **2009**, *877*, 1982–1996. [CrossRef]
38. de Castro, D.G.; Clarke, P.A.; Al-Lazikani, B.; Workman, P. Personalized cancer medicine: Molecular diagnostics, predictive biomarkers, and drug resistance. *Clin. Pharmacol. Ther.* **2013**, *93*, 252–259. [CrossRef]
39. Von Hoff, D.D.; Stephenson, J.J., Jr.; Rosen, P.; Loesch, D.M.; Borad, M.J.; Anthony, S.; Jameson, G.; Brown, S.; Cantafio, N.; Richards, D.A.; et al. Pilot study using molecular profiling of patients' tumors to find potential targets and select treatments for their refractory cancers. *J. Clin. Oncol.* **2010**, *28*, 4877–4883. [CrossRef]
40. Rebollo, J.; Sureda, M.; Martinez, E.M.; Fernández-Morejón, F.J.; Farré, J.; Muñoz, V.; Fernández-Latorre, F.; Manzano, R.G.; Brugarolas, A. Gene Expression Profiling of Tumors From Heavily Pretreated Patients With Metastatic Cancer for the Selection of Therapy: A Pilot Study. *Am. J. Clin. Oncol.* **2017**, *40*, 140–145. [CrossRef]
41. Chatelut, A.C.; Quaranta, S.; Ciccolini, J.; Lacarelle, B. Applications cliniques, limites et perspectives des analyses pharmacogénétiques et pharmacocinétiques des traitements anticancéreux [Clinical application, limits and perspectives of pharmacogenetic and pharmacokinetic analysis of anticancer drugs]. *Ann. Biol. Clin.* **2014**, *72*, 527–542. [CrossRef]
42. Gervasini, G.; Benítez, J.; Carrillo, J.A. Pharmacogenetic testing and therapeutic drug monitoring are complementary tools for optimal individualization of drug therapy. *Eur. J. Clin. Pharmacol.* **2010**, *66*, 755–774. [CrossRef]
43. Verheijen, R.B.; Yu, H.; Schellens, J.H.M.; Beijnen, J.H.; Steeghs, N.; Huitema, A.D.R. Practical Recommendations for Therapeutic Drug Monitoring of Kinase Inhibitors in Oncology. *Clin. Pharmacol. Ther.* **2017**, *102*, 765–776. [CrossRef]
44. *Common Terminology Criteria for Adverse Events (CTCAE)*; Version 5; US Department of Health and Human Services, National Institutes of Health, National Cancer Institute: Washington, DC, USA, 2017.
45. Thomas, F.; Rochaix, P.; White-Koning, M.; Hennebelle, I.; Sarini, J.; Benlyazid, A.; Malard, L.; Lefebvre, J.L.; Chatelut, E.; Delord, J.P. Population pharmacokinetics of erlotinib and its pharmacokinetic/pharmacodynamic relationships in head and neck squamous cell carcinoma. *Eur. J. Cancer* **2009**, *45*, 2316–2323. [CrossRef]
46. Schmidli, H.; Peng, B.; Riviere, G.J.; Capdeville, R.; Hensley, M.; Gathmann, I.; Bolton, A.E.; Racine-Poon, A.; IRIS Study Group. Population pharmacokinetics of imatinib mesylate in patients with chronic-phase chronic myeloid leukaemia: Results of a phase III study. *Br. J. Clin. Pharmacol.* **2005**, *60*, 35–44. [CrossRef]
47. Rezai, K.; Urien, S.; Isambert, N.; Roche, H.; Dieras, V.; Berille, J.; Bonneterre, J.; Brain, E.; Lokiec, F. Pharmacokinetic evaluation of the vinorelbine-lapatinib combination in the treatment of breast cancer patients. *Cancer Chemother. Pharmacol.* **2011**, *68*, 1529–1536. [CrossRef]
48. Jain, L.; Woo, S.; Gardner, E.R.; Dahut, W.L.; Kohn, E.C.; Kummar, S.; Mould, D.R.; Giaccone, G.; Yarchoan, R.; Venitz, J.; et al. Population pharmacokinetic analysis of sorafenib in patients with solid tumours. *Br. J. Clin. Pharmacol.* **2011**, *72*, 294–305. [CrossRef]
49. Guidance for Industry. Bioanalytical Method Validation. U.S. Department of Health and Human Services. Food and Drug Administration Center for Drug Evaluation and Research (CDER). Available online: http://www.fda.gov/downloads/Drugs/GuidanceComplianceRegulatoryInformation/Guidances/ucm070107.pdf (accessed on 1 August 2018).
50. Validation of Analytical Procedures: Text and Methodology. Ich Topic Q2 (R1). CPMP/ICH/381/95-ICH Q2 (R1). Available online: http://www.ich.org/products/guidelines/quality/quality-single/article/validation-of-analyticalprocedures-text-and-methodology.html (accessed on 1 August 2018).
51. Escudero-Ortiz, V.; Pérez-Ruixo, J.J.; Valenzuela, B. Development and validation of a high-performance liquid chromatography ultraviolet method for lapatinib quantification in human plasma. *Ther. Drug Monit.* **2013**, *35*, 796–802. [CrossRef]
52. Escudero-Ortiz, V.; Pérez-Ruixo, J.J.; Valenzuela, B. Development and validation of an HPLC-UV method for sorafenib quantification in human plasma and application to patients with cancer in routine clinical practice. *Ther. Drug Monit.* **2014**, *36*, 317–325. [CrossRef]

53. Beal, S.L.; Sheiner, L.B.; Boeckman, A.J. (Eds.) *NONMEN Users Guides (1989–2006)*; ICON Development Solutions: Ellicott, MA, USA, 1989.
54. Sureda, M.; Calvo, E.; Mata, J.J.; Escudero-Ortiz, V.; Martinez-Navarro, E.; Catalán, A.; Rebollo, J. Dosage of anti-PD-1 monoclonal antibodies: A cardinal open question. *Clin. Transl. Oncol.* **2021**, *23*, 1511–1519. [CrossRef]
55. Sureda, M.; Mata, J.J.; Catalán, A.; Escudero, V.; Martínez-Navarro, E.; Rebollo, J. Therapeutic drug monitoring of nivolumab in routine clinical practice. A pilot study. *Farm. Hosp.* **2020**, *44*, 81–86. [CrossRef] [PubMed]
56. Chatelut, E.; Hendrikx, J.J.M.A.; Martin, J.; Ciccolini, J.; Moes, D.J.A.R. Unraveling the complexity of therapeutic drug monitoring for monoclonal antibody therapies to individualize dose in oncology. *Pharmacol. Res. Perspect.* **2021**, *9*, e00757. [CrossRef]
57. de Wit, D.; Guchelaar, H.-J.; den Hartigh, J.; Gelderblom, H.; van Erp, N.P. Individualized dosing of tyrosine kinase inhibitors: Are we there yet? *Drug Discov. Today* **2015**, *20*, 18–36. [CrossRef]
58. Yu, H.; Steeghs, N.; Nijenhuis, C.M.; Schellens, J.H.; Beijnen, J.H.; Huitema, A.D. Practical guidelines for therapeutic drug monitoring of anticancer tyrosine kinase inhibitors: Focus on the pharmacokinetic targets. *Clin. Pharmacokinet.* **2014**, *53*, 305–325. [CrossRef]
59. Lucas, C.J.; Martin, J.H. Pharmacokinetic-Guided Dosing of New Oral Cancer Agents. *J. Clin. Pharmacol.* **2017**, *57* (Suppl. S10), 78–98. [CrossRef]
60. Lankheet, N.A.; Knapen, L.M.; Schellens, J.H.; Beijnen, J.H.; Steeghs, N.; Huitema, A.D. Plasma concentrations of tyrosine kinase inhibitors imatinib, erlotinib, and sunitinib in routine clinical outpatient cancer care. *Ther. Drug Monit.* **2014**, *36*, 326–334. [CrossRef]
61. Hidalgo, M.; Siu, L.L.; Nemunaitis, J.; Rizzo, J.; Hammond, L.A.; Takimoto, C.; Eckhardt, S.G.; Tolcher, A.; Britten, C.D.; Denis, L.; et al. Phase I and pharmacologic study of OSI-774, an epidermal growth factor receptor tyrosine kinase inhibitor, in patients with advanced solid malignancies. *J. Clin. Oncol.* **2001**, *19*, 3267–3279. [CrossRef]
62. Erlotinib Summary of Product Characteristics. Available online: https://www.ema.europa.eu/en/documents/product-information/tarceva-epar-product-information_en.pdf (accessed on 15 June 2018).
63. Lu, J.F.; Eppler, S.M.; Wolf, J.; Hamilton, M.; Rakhit, A.; Bruno, R.; Lum, B.L. Clinical pharmacokinetics of erlotinib in patients with solid tumors and exposure-safety relationship in patients with non-small cell lung cancer. *Clin. Pharmacol. Ther.* **2006**, *80*, 136–145. [CrossRef]
64. Rudin, C.M.; Liu, W.; Desai, A.; Karrison, T.; Jiang, X.; Janisch, L.; Das, S.; Ramirez, J.; Poonkuzhali, B.; Schuetz, E.; et al. Pharmacogenomic and pharmacokinetic determinants of erlotinib toxicity. *J. Clin. Oncol.* **2008**, *26*, 1119–1127. [CrossRef]
65. Catalán-Latorre, A.; Sureda, M.; Brugarolas-Masllorens, A.; Escudero-Ortiz, V. Therapeutic Drug Monitoring of Erlotinib in Non-Small Cell Lung Carcinoma: A Case Study. *Ther. Drug Monit.* **2021**, *43*, 447–450. [CrossRef]
66. Tiseo, M.; Andreoli, R.; Gelsomino, F.; Mozzoni, P.; Azzoni, C.; Bartolotti, M.; Bortesi, B.; Goldoni, M.; Silini, E.M.; De Palma, G.; et al. Correlation between erlotinib pharmacokinetics, cutaneous toxicity and clinical outcomes in patients with advanced non-small cell lung cancer (NSCLC). *Lung Cancer* **2014**, *83*, 265–271. [CrossRef] [PubMed]
67. Motoshima, K.; Nakamura, Y.; Sano, K.; Ikegami, Y.; Ikeda, T.; Mizoguchi, K.; Takemoto, S.; Fukuda, M.; Nagashima, S.; Iida, T.; et al. Phase II trial of erlotinib in patients with advanced non-small-cell lung cancer harboring epidermal growth factor receptor mutations: Additive analysis of pharmacokinetics. *Cancer Chemother. Pharmacol.* **2013**, *72*, 1299–1304. [CrossRef] [PubMed]
68. Soulieres, D.; Senzer, N.N.; Vokes, E.E.; Hidalgo, M.; Agarwala, S.S.; Siu, L.L. Multicenter phase II study of erlotinib, an oral epidermal growth factor receptor tyrosine kinase inhibitor, in patients with recurrent or metastatic squamous cell cancer of the head and neck. *J. Clin. Oncol.* **2004**, *22*, 77–85. [CrossRef] [PubMed]
69. Wacker, B.; Nagrani, T.; Weinberg, J.; Witt, K.; Clark, G.; Cagnoni, P.J. Correlation between development of rash and efficacy in patients treated with the epidermal growth factor receptor tyrosine kinase inhibitor erlotinib in two large phase III studies. *Clin. Cancer Res.* **2007**, *13*, 3913–3921. [CrossRef] [PubMed]
70. Steffens, M.; Paul, T.; Hichert, V.; Scholl, C.; von Mallek, D.; Stelzer, C.; Sörgel, F.; Reiser, B.; Schumann, C.; Rüdiger, S.; et al. Dosing to rash?—The role of erlotinib metabolic ratio from patient serum in the search of predictive biomarkers for EGFR inhibitor-mediated skin rash. *Eur. J. Cancer* **2016**, *55*, 131–139. [CrossRef] [PubMed]
71. Mita, A.C.; Papadopoulos, K.; de Jonge, M.J.; Schwartz, G.; Verweij, J.; Mita, M.M.; Ricart, A.; Chu, Q.S.; Tolcher, A.W.; Wood, L.; et al. Erlotinib 'dosing-to-rash': A phase II intrapatient dose escalation and pharmacologic study of erlotinib in previously treated advanced non-small cell lung cancer. *Br. J. Cancer* **2011**, *105*, 938–944. [CrossRef]
72. Pérez-Soler, R.; Chachoua, A.; Hammond, L.A.; Rowinsky, E.K.; Huberman, M.; Karp, D.; Rigas, J.; Clark, G.M.; Santabárbara, P.; Bonomi, P. Determinants of tumor response and survival with erlotinib in patients with non—small-cell lung cancer. *J. Clin. Oncol.* **2004**, *22*, 3238–3247. [CrossRef]
73. Ling, J.; Johnson, K.A.; Miao, Z.; Rakhit, A.; Pantze, M.P.; Hamilton, M.; Lum, B.L.; Prakash, C. Metabolism and excretion of erlotinib, a small molecule inhibitor of epidermal growth factor receptor tyrosine kinase, in healthy male volunteers. *Drug Metab. Dispos.* **2006**, *34*, 420–426. [CrossRef]
74. Eechoute, K.; Fransson, M.N.; Reyners, A.K.; de Jong, F.A.; Sparreboom, A.; van der Graaf, W.T.; Friberg, L.E.; Schiavon, G.; Wiemer, E.A.; Verweij, J.; et al. A long-term prospective population pharmacokinetic study on imatinib plasma concentrations in GIST patients. *Clin. Cancer Res.* **2012**, *18*, 5780–5787. [CrossRef]
75. Lyseng-Williamson, K.; Jarvis, B. Imatinib. *Drugs* **2001**, *61*, 1765–1774; discussion 1775–1776. [CrossRef]

76. Demetri, G.D.; Wang, Y.; Wehrle, E.; Racine, A.; Nikolova, Z.; Blanke, C.D.; Joensuu, H.; von Mehren, M. Imatinib plasma levels are correlated with clinical benefit in patients with unresectable/metastatic gastrointestinal stromal tumors. *J. Clin. Oncol.* **2009**, *27*, 3141–3147. [CrossRef] [PubMed]
77. Larson, R.A.; Druker, B.J.; Guilhot, F.; O'Brien, S.G.; Riviere, G.J.; Krahnke, T.; Gathmann, I.; Wang, Y.; IRIS (International Randomized Interferon vs STI571) Study Group. Imatinib pharmacokinetics and its correlation with response and safety in chronic-phase chronic myeloid leukemia: A subanalysis of the IRIS study. *Blood* **2008**, *111*, 4022–4028. [CrossRef] [PubMed]
78. Guilhot, F.; Hughes, T.P.; Cortes, J.; Druker, B.J.; Baccarani, M.; Gathmann, I.; Hayes, M.; Granvil, C.; Wang, Y. Plasma exposure of imatinib and its correlation with clinical response in the Tyrosine Kinase Inhibitor Optimization and Selectivity Trial. *Haematologica* **2012**, *97*, 731–738. [CrossRef] [PubMed]
79. Lapatinib Summary of Product Characteristics. Available online: https://www.ema.europa.eu/en/documents/product-information/tyverb-epar-product-information_en.pdf (accessed on 15 June 2018).
80. Midgley, R.S.; Kerr, D.J.; Flaherty, K.T.; Stevenson, J.P.; Pratap, S.E.; Koch, K.M.; Smith, D.A.; Versola, M.; Fleming, R.A.; Ward, C.; et al. A phase I and pharmacokinetic study of lapatinib in combination with infusional 5-fluorouracil, leucovorin and irinotecan. *Ann. Oncol.* **2007**, *18*, 2025–2029. [CrossRef]
81. Burris, H.A., 3rd; Hurwitz, H.I.; Dees, E.C.; Dowlati, A.; Blackwell, K.L.; O'Neil, B.; Marcom, P.K.; Ellis, M.J.; Overmoyer, B.; Jones, S.F.; et al. Phase I safety, pharmacokinetics, and clinical activity study of lapatinib (GW572016), a reversible dual inhibitor of epidermal growth factor receptor tyrosine kinases, in heavily pretreated patients with metastatic carcinomas. *J. Clin. Oncol.* **2005**, *23*, 5305–5313. [CrossRef]
82. Nakagawa, K.; Minami, H.; Kanezaki, M.; Mukaiyama, A.; Minamide, Y.; Uejima, H.; Kurata, T.; Nogami, T.; Kawada, K.; Mukai, H.; et al. Phase I dose-escalation and pharmacokinetic trial of lapatinib (GW572016), a selective oral dual inhibitor of ErbB-1 and -2 tyrosine kinases, in Japanese patients with solid tumors. *Jpn. J. Clin. Oncol.* **2009**, *39*, 116–123. [CrossRef]
83. Sorafenib Summary of Product Characteristics. Available online: https://www.ema.europa.eu/en/documents/product-information/nexavar-epar-product-information_en.pdf (accessed on 15 June 2018).
84. Minami, H.; Kawada, K.; Ebi, H.; Kitagawa, K.; Kim, Y.I.; Araki, K.; Mukai, H.; Tahara, M.; Nakajima, H.; Nakajima, K. Phase I and pharmacokinetic study of sorafenib, an oral multikinase inhibitor, in Japanese patients with advanced refractory solid tumors. *Cancer Sci.* **2008**, *99*, 1492–1498. [CrossRef]
85. Blanchet, B.; Billemont, B.; Cramard, J.; Benichou, A.S.; Chhun, S.; Harcouet, L.; Ropert, S.; Dauphin, A.; Goldwasser, F.; Tod, M. Validation of an HPLC UV method for sorafenib determination in human plasma and application to cancer patients in routine clinical practice. *J. Pharm. Biomed. Anal.* **2009**, *49*, 1109–1114. [CrossRef]
86. Lathia, C.; Lettieri, J.; Cihon, F.; Gallentine, M.; Radtke, M.; Sundaresan, P. Lack of effect of ketoconazole-mediated CYP3A inhibition on sorafenib clinical pharmacokinetics. *Cancer Chemother. Pharmacol.* **2006**, *57*, 685–692. [CrossRef]
87. Pécuchet, N.; Lebbe, C.; Mir, O.; Billemont, B.; Blanchet, B.; Franck, N.; Viguier, M.; Coriat, R.; Tod, M.; Avril, M.F.; et al. Sorafenib in advanced melanoma: A critical role for pharmacokinetics? *Br. J. Cancer* **2012**, *107*, 455–461. [CrossRef]
88. Fukudo, M.; Ito, T.; Mizuno, T.; Shinsako, K.; Hatano, E.; Uemoto, S.; Kamba, T.; Yamasaki, T.; Ogawa, O.; Seno, H.; et al. Exposure-toxicity relationship of sorafenib in Japanese patients with renal cell carcinoma and hepatocellular carcinoma. *Clin. Pharmacokinet.* **2014**, *53*, 185–196. [CrossRef] [PubMed]
89. Boudou-Rouquette, P.; Ropert, S.; Mir, O.; Coriat, R.; Billemont, B.; Tod, M.; Cabanes, L.; Franck, N.; Blanchet, B.; Goldwasser, F. Variability of sorafenib toxicity and exposure over time: A pharmacokinetic/pharmacodynamic analysis. *Oncologist* **2012**, *17*, 1204–1212. [CrossRef] [PubMed]

Article
Population Pharmacokinetics of Valproic Acid in Pediatric and Adult Caucasian Patients

Paulo Teixeira-da-Silva [1,2,3,*], Jonás Samuel Pérez-Blanco [1,2,3,*], Dolores Santos-Buelga [1,2,3], María José Otero [2,3] and María José García [1,2,3]

1 Pharmaceutical Sciences Department, Universidad de Salamanca, 37007 Salamanca, Spain; sbuelga@usal.es (D.S.-B.); mjgarcia@usal.es (M.J.G.)
2 Institute of Biomedical Research of Salamanca (IBSAL), 37007 Salamanca, Spain; mjotero@saludcastillayleon.es
3 Pharmacy Service, University Hospital of Salamanca, 37007 Salamanca, Spain
* Correspondence: paulo@usal.es (P.T.-d.-S.); jsperez@usal.es (J.S.P.-B.)

Abstract: (1) Background: The aim of this study was to explore the valproic acid (VPA) pharmacokinetic characteristics in a large population of pediatric and adult Caucasian patients and to establish a robust population pharmacokinetic (PopPK) model. (2) Methods: A total of 2527 serum VPA samples collected from 1204 patients included in a therapeutic drug monitoring program were retrospectively analyzed. Patients were randomly assigned to either a model development group or an external evaluation group. PopPK analysis was performed on 1751 samples from 776 patients with NONMEM using a nonlinear mixed-effect modelling approach. The influence of demographic, anthropometric, treatment and comedication variables on the apparent clearance (CL/F) of VPA was studied. The bootstrap method was used to evaluate the final model internally. External evaluation was carried out using 776 VPA serum samples from 368 patients. (3) Results: A one-compartment model with first-order absorption and elimination successfully described the data. The final model included total body weight, age and comedication with phenytoin, phenobarbital and carbamazepine with a significant impact on VPA elimination. Internal and external evaluations demonstrated the good predictability of the model. (4) Conclusions: A PopPK model of VPA in Caucasian patients was successfully established, which will be helpful for model-informed precision dosing approaches in clinical patient care.

Keywords: drug interactions; therapeutic drug monitoring; epilepsy; NONMEM; population pharmacokinetics; valproic acid

1. Introduction

Valproic acid (VPA) is an antiepileptic drug (AED) that has been widely used in multiple seizure types and various neurological and psychiatric disorders since its serendipitous discovery in 1962 [1]. It is still considered a first-line option for treating generalized epilepsies [2].

There are several oral formulations on the market, differing in their rate of absorption. However, regardless of the formulation, VPA absorption is rapid and almost complete with a bioavailability greater than 90% [1]. The metabolism of VPA is mainly characterized by three routes: glucuronidation via uridine diphosphate glucuronosyltransferase (UGT) isoforms (50%), including UGT1A3/1A4/1A6/1A8/1A9/1A10/2B7; beta oxidation in mitochondria (40%); and cytochrome P450 (CYP)-mediated oxidation (10%), such as CYP2A6/2B6/2C9/2C19 [3–6]. Only a small amount of VPA is excreted unaltered in urine (1–3%). VPA serum apparent clearance (CL/F) varies from 6 to 10 mL/h/kg [6], with a half-life ranging from 12 to 16 h and from 8.6 to 12.3 h for adults and children, respectively [5].

Serum level monitoring was introduced as a result of the large interindividual variability (IIV) observed in the pharmacokinetic (PK) behavior of VPA, in order to individualize dosage regimens and to achieve a steady-state serum concentration between 50 and 100 mg/L [5]. It is essential to establish adequate and robust population PK (PopPK) models of VPA and to investigate the influence of potential covariates on its PK behavior, specially to quantify drug–drug interactions with other AEDs and the PK changes from childhood to adulthood. Traditional pharmacokinetic methods make it difficult to estimate pharmacokinetic parameters from clinically obtained sparse blood samples.

VPA exhibits saturable binding to serum proteins, which results in a higher unbound fraction at high serum concentrations [7]. Some studies included VPA dose with its influence on its CL/F, probably to capture this phenomenon [7–16]. However, this nonlinear PK behavior remains controversial [7], being highlighted as a potential confounding factor of the commonly known "Therapeutic Drug Monitoring (TDM) effect". In fact, in clinical setting, subjects with higher CL/F will have a lower concentration of the drug, and consequently higher doses will be administered and vice versa. That is why VPA dose is not recommended for consideration as a potential covariate in PopPK models based on sparse data from TDM [17].

Previous PopPK studies showed that total body weight (TBW), age, gender, genetic factors, VPA dose and comedication had a significant influence on VPA PK parameters [6–11,13–15,17–27]. However, few PopPK studies have been performed with a wide range of ages of Caucasian patients. This study was performed with the aim of exploring the PK characteristics of VPA in a large population of pediatric and adult Caucasian patients and developing a robust VPA PopPK model for improving current VPA therapeutic drug monitoring (TDM).

2. Materials and Methods

2.1. Study Design and Population Characteristics

Data from ambulatory patients (aged 0.11–92.9 years old) treated with VPA and followed by the TDM program of the University Hospital of Salamanca were retrospectively recruited for model development and external evaluation. Only mono- or dual therapies were considered, and the following exclusion criteria were applied: (1) missing laboratory data/treatment information/concentration data; (2) inaccurate medication or blood collection time records; (3) poor patient treatment adherence; (4) patients whose body mass index (BMI) was outside the range of 16.0–39.9 kg/m^2, in accordance with World Health Organization (WHO) indications (for patients under 18 years of age, the criterion used was three standard deviations from the means in the WHO tables for children) [28]; (5) nonsteady state achieved and (6) more than two AEDs administered concurrently.

Steady-state concentrations were assumed to have been reached a month after the initiation of treatment or a dose change. Treatment adherence was assessed by means of an interview with the attending health care provider. Demographic and anthropometric information (age, gender, height (HGT), TBW, body surface area (BSA), BMI,), disease information (seizure type and diagnosis), medication information (dosage forms, dosage regimens and administration time), comedication with another antiepileptic drug other than VPA (carbamazepine (CBZ), phenytoin (PHT), phenobarbital (PB), ethosuximide (ESM), lamotrigine (LTG), topiramate (TPM) and clobazam (CLB)) and the analytical technique used to determine serum concentrations were recorded for each patient.

All patients included in the study were randomly assigned to either a model development or a model external evaluation group in an approximate 2:1 proportion stratified by age groups (Table S1). The model development dataset consisted of 1751 serum concentration samples from 836 patients. In addition, 776 serum samples from 368 different patients were used as an external evaluation dataset. Table 1 shows a summary of the baseline characteristics of both the development and external evaluation datasets. No statistically significant differences ($p < 0.001$) were shown for any covariate considered across the two datasets considered.

Table 1. Baseline patients' characteristics.

Variable	Level	Development	External
Subjects (*n*)		836	368
Age (years)		33.22 ± 23.90; 32.42 (0.11–89.42)	33.48 ± 22.73; 31.58 (0.67–92.92)
Total body weight (kg)		55.82 ± 26.08; 60.00 (6.70–125.00)	58.07 ± 24.59; 62.00 (6.50–110.00)
Height (cm)		149.00 ± 28.58; 160.00 (62.00–194.00)	152.17 ± 26.50; 160.00 (69.00–194.00)
Body mass index * (kg/m^2)		23.04 ± 5.63; 23.31 (11.81–39.79)	23.36 ± 5.70; 23.36 (11.78–39.61)
Body surface area ** (m^2)		1.50 ± 0.50; 1.63 (0.36–2.52)	1.55 ± 0.47; 1.68 (0.35–2.39)
VPA daily dose (mg)		1107.13 ± 587.00; 1000.00 (150.00–4500.00)	1177.04 ± 625.21; 1000.00 (200.00–4500.00)
Gender, *n* (%)	Male	451 (53.9)	188 (51.1)
	Female	385 (46.1)	180 (48.9)

* body mass index [29]; ** body surface area [30]; VPA: valproic acid; SD: standard deviation. All continuous covariates are expressed as mean ± SD; median (minimum–maximum).

The final PopPK model was evaluated internally and externally using the development and external evaluation datasets, respectively, and for the last step, the two datasets (development and external evaluation) were merged for evaluating potential differences in the final PK parameter estimates. Thus, three types of datasets were used: the development, the external evaluation and the merged datasets. The effect of demographic, anthropometric and comedication variables on VPA CL/F was investigated.

2.2. Blood Sampling and Assay

VPA was administered orally in one of the following presentations: gastro-resistant tablets (200 mg and 500 mg), coated prolonged-release tablets (300 mg and 500 mg) or oral solution (200 mg/mL). The dose was adjusted in accordance with the observed VPA serum level, clinical efficacy and any adverse reactions. All of the blood samples were taken as a part of the routine TDM procedure. Fluorescent polarization immunoassay (FPIA) was used to determine serum VPA concentrations, using a fluorescence polarization analyzer (Abbott TDx analyzer) with an inter- and intra-assay variation coefficient of less than 10% and a limit of detection of 0.7 mg/L [31,32]. Normally, serum VPA concentrations were obtained at the end of the dosing interval and once the steady state had been reached.

2.3. Population Pharmacokinetic Modeling

NONMEM (v.7.5.1, ICON Development Solutions, Ellicott City, MD, USA), Perl-speaks-NONMEM (PsN) v.5.2.6. (Uppsala University, Sweden, http://psn.sourceforge.net), R v.4.1.2., RStudio v.2022.02.0+443 (RStudio, Boston, MA, USA) and Pirana v.3.0.0. (Certara, Princeton, NJ, USA, http://www.certara.com) were used to apply a nonlinear mixed-effect modeling methodology. The first-order conditional estimation method with interaction (FOCEI) was used. The log-transforming both sides (LTBS) approach was applied to the VPA concentrations [33]. Most concentrations (97.5%) in this study were steady-state trough concentrations (C_{min}^{ss}), which could not totally reflect the absorption and distribution process characteristics. Considering the type of sampling points (C_{min}^{ss} and sparse data) and information available in the literature, a one-compartment structural kinetic model with first-order absorption and elimination was chosen as the base structural PK model [8–10,14,15,17,24], and the absorption rate constant (Ka) was fixed at 2.64 h^{-1} for oral solution (syrup), 0.78 h^{-1} for gastro-resistant tablets and 0.38 h^{-1} for modified-release coated tablets based on previous information [7,8]. In the case formulation information in the clinical records was not available, oral solution and gastro-resistant tablets were considered for patients younger and older than 12 years old, respectively. PK parameters scaled to TBW were a priori included in the base model based on physiological reasons and previous knowledge [34]. A standard allometric scale based on TBW with a single exponential value of 0.75 was assumed for apparent clearance (CL/F), and a single exponential value of 1.0 was defined for apparent volume of distribution (V/F). Estimation of these exponents was also evaluated. Additional maturation functions for characterizing physiological changes in addition to those explained by body size were also investigated. Furthermore, the population value of V/F was fixed at 14 L for a typical patient of 70 kg in accordance with previous studies [5]. Although these assumptions could be considered a limitation, they enable the use of data generated during clinical practice (sparse data), and this constitutes the foundations of the utility of the PopPK approach developed by Beal and Sheiner in 1990 [35–37].

PK parameters were assumed log-normally distributed; thus, an exponential model was used to describe the interindividual variability (IIV) in CL/F. The residual unknown variability (RUV) was included as an additive error model after the natural logarithm transformation of measured drug concentrations and model predictions (which is equivalent as a proportional error in the natural scale) [33]. Additional error models, such as additive and combined, were also tested.

Plausible variables previously identified in the literature and with physiological significance were incorporated into the model for covariate screening and identification, by means of a stepwise strategy performed in PsN (p-forward = 0.05, p-backward = 0.01). In the forward step, the selected covariates were included in the base model one by one, and only those causing a decrease in the objective function value (OFV) > 3.84 (p = 0.05, χ^2 distribution with one degree of freedom) were incorporated into the full regression model. Covariates were removed one at a time in the backward elimination step performed on the final forward step model. A covariate resulting in an increased OFV of over 6.63 (p = 0.01, χ^2 distribution with one degree of freedom) was considered significant for CL/F prediction and was retained in the final PopPK model. All other covariates that did not meet this criterion were excluded. Linear and exponential functions were used to analyze continuous covariates, whereas the dichotomous categorical covariates were analyzed by estimating the change in the PK parameter with respect to the reference group (most common). Finally, a conditional function was used for categorical covariates with more than two groups [38].

2.4. Model Assessment and Evaluation

Model selection was guided by run convergence minimization with at least 2 significant digits in parameter estimates, a successful covariance step, changes in minimum objective function value (MOFV) for each nested model (p < 0.05, χ^2-test, and ΔOFV > 3.84), plausibility and precision of parameter estimates, evaluation of random effects (i.e., η and ε) shrinkage, reduction in IIV and/or RUV and visual inspection of standard diagnostic plots including goodness-of-fit plots (GOF). Performance of the final PopPK model was assessed by both internal and external evaluation. A bootstrap resampling technique from the development dataset was used to judge the reliability and stability of the final PopPK model developed in the study. A total of 1000 bootstrap-resampled datasets were generated from the original model development dataset, and each was individually fitted to the final PopPK model with PsN. All PK parameters were estimated in the 1000 bootstrap datasets, and the median and 95% confidence intervals (CI) of the parameters were compared with the estimates of the final PopPK model parameters.

The external evaluation (external evaluation dataset) of the model using different patients than those used for model development from a real (not simulated) population with similar characteristics to the population used for model development was carried out in three steps [39,40]:

(1) Evaluation of the predictive capacity of the final PopPK model developed in the external evaluation dataset, using the option MAXEVAL = 0 (Bayesian forecasting). The mean prediction error (MPE) and root mean squared prediction error (RMSE) were calculated to determine bias and precision, respectively [41]. These metrics were evaluated by age group to confirm the accurate and precise-model-based VPA predictions across the wide range of ages considered in this study.
(2) PK parameters' re-estimation with the merged dataset (model development together with external evaluation datasets) to confirm the stability of the final PK parameter estimates when different patients were considered.
(3) Visual inspection of the GOF generated when VPAs of external evaluation dataset are predicted through Bayesian forecasting (MAXEVAL = 0) based on a priori information relying on the final PopPK model developed.

3. Results

3.1. Population Pharmacokinetic Modeling

A one-compartment model was selected as the structural model to describe VPA PK profile. Age significantly influences CL/F, which was mainly captured by the inclusion of TBW in CL/F following allometric scaling principles (IIV of CL/F decreased by 41% when only considering TBW on CL/F).

Exponential and proportional error models for IIV and for RUV, respectively, successfully described the data (Table 2).

Table 2. PK parameters estimates (development, bootstrap and merged dataset re-estimation).

Parameter	Final Model (Development Dataset)			Re-Estimation Final Model (Merged Dataset)			Bootstrap ◊	
	Estimate	RSE (%)	Shkg (%)	Estimate	RSE (%)	Shkg (%)	Median	95% CI
Ka	Fixed *	-	-	-	-	-	-	-
CL/F	0.646	1.20	-	0.641	1.00	-	0.645	0.631–0.661
AGE	−0.0154	64.3	-	−0.0107	80.2	-	−0.0154	−0.034–0.004
CBZ	0.512	13.4	-	0.549	11.7	-	0.513	0.379–0.658
PB	0.386	23.2	-	0.349	21.1	-	0.398	0.232–0.623
PHT	0.640	24.2	-	0.642	17.8	-	0.638	0.361–0.966
V/F	Fixed **	-	-	-	-	-	-	-
IIV_CL/F (%)	26.8	5.50	19.0	26.4	4.50	19.0	26.6	23.8–29.8
RUV (%)	57.7	3.80	17.0	56.0	3.30	17.0	28.1	25.8–30.4

◊ Bootstrap n = 1000 with successful minimization and no problems for 994 models. * Absorption rate constant (Ka) was fixed at 2.64 h^{-1} for oral solution (syrup), to 0.78 h^{-1} for gastro-resistant tablets and to 0.38 h^{-1} for modified-release coated tablets based on previous information [7,8]. ** Apparent volume of distribution (V/F) was fixed at 14 L for a typical patient of 70 kg [5]. AGE: influence of age on CL/F; CBZ: influence of comedication with carbamazepine (CBZ) on apparent clearance (CL/F) (expressed as a proportion); CI, confidence interval; IIV_CL/F: interindividual variability (IIV) in CL/F (expressed as coefficient of variation in %); PB: influence of comedication with phenobarbital (PB) on CL/F (expressed as a proportion); PHT: influence of comedication with phenytoin (PHT) on CL/F (expressed as a proportion); RSE: relative standard error; RUV: residual unknown variability (expressed as coefficient of variation in %); Shkg: shrinkage. See Equations (1) and (2) for the final CL/F and V/F equations, respectively.

A visual inspection of the GOF plots allowed us to confirm an adequate description of the data except for subjects weighting less than 24 kg and/or younger than approximately 6 years old (data not shown). Therefore, additional evaluations of CL/F were carried out. Thus, the potential influence of age on VPA CL/F, were evaluated both as a standard maturation function collapsing at 2 years old (Hill equation) and as an exponential relationship centered on the age of 15, the cut-off point observed following a visual inspection of CL/F with respect to age. Finally, age was included on VPA CL/F following an exponential relationship as described in Equation (1), which, together with the comedications influence on CL/F identified in the covariate model evaluation procedure, considerably improved the GOF in the youngest pediatric subjects (Figure 1).

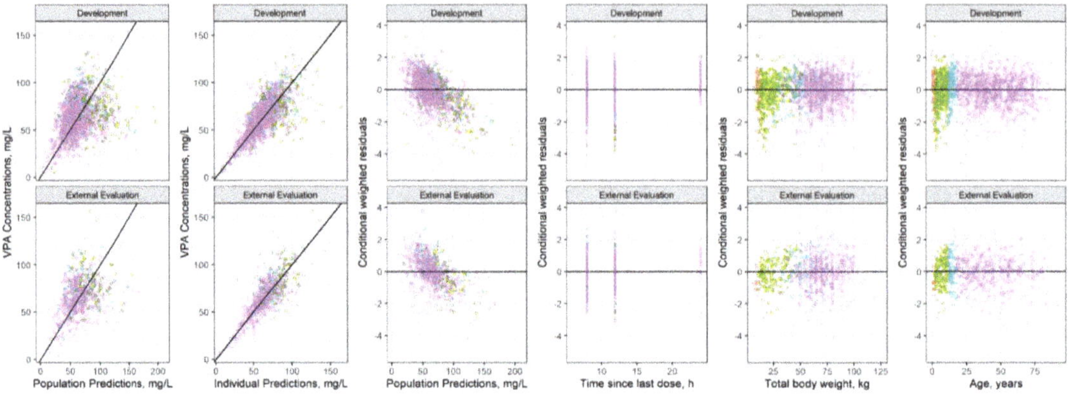

Figure 1. Goodness-of-fit plots for the development dataset (upper panels) and the external evaluation dataset (lower panels) colored by age classification (AGEC), • 28 d–2 y • 2–11 y • 12–18 y • >18 y.

The covariates fulfilling the statistical requirement for inclusion ($p < 0.001$) were, in addition to TBW as an allometric relationship: AGE centered on the age of 15 and introduced as a power function on CL/F and comedication with carbamazepine (CBZ), phenytoin (PHT) and phenobarbital (PB) (Equation (1)). Furthermore, the association with LTG and gender initially showed a statistically significant impact on CL/F ($p < 0.005$). However, these covariates were not retained in the final model due to the lack of clinical relevance, as the VPA CL/F was impacted by less than 10% in both cases. VPA V/F was finally described following an allometric scaling relationship with a value of 14 L for a typical adult patient (Equation (2)), as explained above.

$$\text{CL/F [L/h]} = 0.646 \, (\text{TBW}/70)^{0.75} \times 1.640^{\text{PHT}} \times 1.386^{\text{PB}} \times 1.521^{\text{CBZ}} \times (\text{AGE}/15)^{-0.0154} \quad (1)$$

$$\text{V/F [L]} = 14 \, (\text{TBW}/70)^1 \quad (2)$$

where TBW is the total body weight in kg, Age is the age in years and PHT, PB and CBZ represent comedications of phenytoin, phenobarbital and carbamazepine, respectively; these variables (comedication) take a value of 0 when absent and 1 when the drug is administered simultaneously with VPA.

These results highlight the requirement of VPA dose intensification in combination with other AEDs, especially in adults and very young children (1 year old), where VPA serum concentration can be reduced by approximately 50% compared to the VPA administered in monotherapy.

The estimated CL/F of VPA for a typical patient with a median TBW of 70 kg and absence of any comedication was 0.646 L/h. Compared to the corresponding base model, the IIV of CL/F decreased by about 48%, showing that the occurrence of these covariates effectively improves the fit of the data.

Given the sampling strategy routinely applied in TDM procedures (mainly C_{min}^{ss}), V/F was not able to be suitably estimated with sufficient physiological plausibility. Thus, V/F was fixed at 14 L for a standard adult patient of 70 kg [5].

3.2. Model Evaluation

The bootstrap results (Table 2) demonstrate the robustness of the PopPK model. The 95% confidence interval (CI) of parameter estimates showed satisfactory overlap. The final model proved to be highly stable, with a total of 99.6% bootstrap runs fitting successfully without problems to the new datasets generated by bootstrapping. The bootstrap estimates resembled those of the population with errors lower than 50% in all the parameters, except for the RUV value, potentially due to the sampling design.

All of the PK parameter estimates with the merged dataset (including both the development and the external datasets) were within the 95% CI of the PK parameters obtained in the bootstrap analysis (Table 2) (except the RUV, as previously mentioned), demonstrating the adequate predictive power of the proposed final model (Source code of the final model is available in Table S2).

The predictive performance of PopPK was assessed by means of a comparison between the concentrations observed in the external evaluation dataset and those predicted by the final model developed. Figure S1 shows an adequate distribution of the prediction errors calculated (mostly distributed within ±30%) in the external evaluation dataset through Bayesian estimation across all the different age classification groups supporting the correct model predictability along ages. In addition, Table 3 shows the calculated MPE and RMSE for population-predicted concentrations (PRED) and individual-predicted concentrations (IPRED). Estimation errors were acceptable in the PK parameters estimated for fixed (<20%) and random effects (<6%), as well as shrinkage values (<20%).

Table 3. Summary of precision and bias of the final model in the external evaluation dataset.

AGEC	28 d–2 y		2–11 y		12–18 y		>18 y	
	IPRED	PRED	IPRED	PRED	IPRED	PRED	IPRED	PRED
MPE, %	15.5	34.3	13.8	27.8	15.5	29.2	16.3	33.4
RMSE, %	18.2	37.5	19.6	37.8	19.7	36.4	23.7	56.8

AGEC: age classification group; MPE: median prediction error; RMSE: root mean squared prediction error. These metrics were calculated considering both the individual valproic-acid (VPA)-predicted concentrations (IPRED) and the population predicted concentrations (PRED).

In the case of the PK parameter quantifying the impact of the age on VPA CL/F, the standard error was high, which may limit its validity. However, bootstrap results confirm the value estimated in a largest dataset, supporting, together with the GOF, its inclusion in the final model. Internal evaluation by bootstrapping methodology demonstrated the good predictability of the final PopPK model developed (Table 3).

Figure 2 shows the evolution of steady-state plasma VPA concentrations in different scenarios: four age groups in mono- and dual therapy, with the antiepileptic drugs identified in the PopPK. The regimens shown were designed to achieve VPA concentrations within the acceptable therapeutic margins in monotherapy.

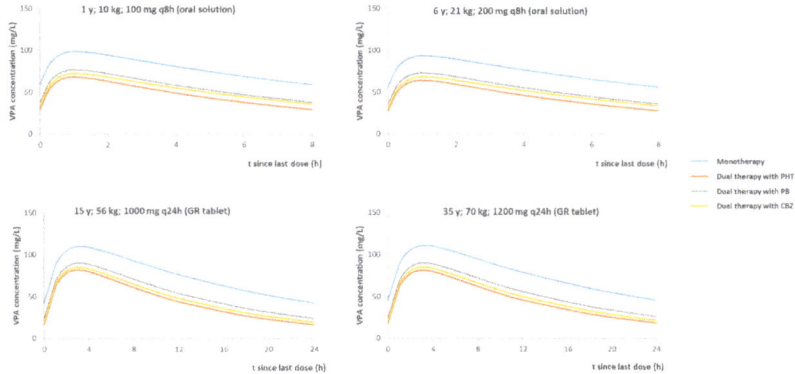

Figure 2. Valproic acid (VPA) concentration–time profiles simulated with the final model developed. The following acronyms represent the drug administered in each scenario: VPA monotherapy together with carbamazepine (CBZ), phenobarbital (PB) and phenytoin (PHT); GR: gastro-resistant.

4. Discussion

Individual differences in drug disposition could cause effective epilepsy management to fail. Traditionally, VPA TDM was routinely carried out in a large number of hospitals, which made it possible to individualize the dosage of this drug. To address the PK-guided TDM of VPA, robust and sufficiently evaluated and wide applicability (age and weight ranges), PopPK models are required to help optimize VPA dosage regimens. So reducing health care costs and improving treatment outcomes by using Bayesian algorithms and drug serum concentrations taken during routine clinical monitoring.

A number of studies have developed VPA PopPK models in epileptic patients [1,3,7–9,11,13–27,42–44]. Most of the previous PopPK models available were developed based on non-Caucasian populations, and some of them involved a small number of patients, which limits their usefulness in the clinical setting. Furthermore, one-third of the published PopPK models for VPA were not adequately evaluated at all, and several of the remaining PopPK models did not have an external evaluation performed [6], which is highly recommended by the European Medicines Agency (EMA) and the Food and Drug Administration (FDA) [45,46], especially with studies carried out with real-world patients.

The development of this PopPK model is justified by the need for a model that has been validated both internally and externally, making it possible to correctly estimate CL/F in both children and adults, and does not include DDV as a covariate, so that it may be used in dosage optimization.

Considering the large number of data available for model development and the wide range of ages included (0.1–92.9 years old), special caution was taken to characterize PK changes according to body size and years of life related to physiological maturation. In conclusion, the impact of total body weight on VPA CL/F following an allometric relationship together with age for correcting maturation processes, mainly in young infants, adequately described the large number of data considering the broad age spectrum (Figure 1). Gender showed a slight influence on CL/F. However, this difference was not considered clinically relevant (<10% change of VPA CL/F), and gender was not retained in the final model. This finding is in agreement with other studies that tested the gender covariate in the CL/F [1,3,7–9,11,13,14,18,21,23,26,42,44]. However, a few studies showed that gender had a significant effect on CL/F, reporting a reduction from 5.7% to 35.4% in women [10,16,19,24,27,43].

The most important factors affecting VPA PK are those related to their association with drugs that induce or inhibit its metabolism. Consequently, we studied the effect of the concomitant administration of classic AED (CBZ, PHT and PB) on VPA CL/F. To avoid the complexity of PK interactions caused by multiple-drug coadministration, the influence of a single AED when added to VPA treatment was analyzed. Therefore, the collected data correspond to either mono- or dual therapies.

CBZ, PHT and PB interact with VPA by inducing the metabolism of CYP3A4, CYP2C19, CYP2C9, UGT1A6, UGT1A9 and UGT2B7. This leads to a reduction in plasma VPA levels (CBZ: 39%; PHT and PB: 37%) [5]. Despite the low number of patients undergoing concomitant dual therapy (CBZ = 6.9%; PHT = 2.2% and PB = 2.3% in the development dataset), the effects of the association with CBZ, PHT and PB on the CL/F of VPA were highly determinant of the value of this parameter. In addition, association with LTG was initially included in the model following statistical criteria but was not retained in the final PopPK model due to the lack of clinical relevance, as CL/F of VPA was altered by less than 10%.

In dual therapy with CBZ, a typical VPA CL/F value was estimated at 0.0150 L/h, 0.0157 L/h, 0.818 L/h and 2.258 L/h for typical reference for patients aged 1 year old (mean weight 9.4 kg), 6 years old (mean weight 22.9 kg), 15 years old (mean weight 53.3 kg) and 35 years old (mean weight 73.5 kg), respectively, and 0.010 L/h, 0.103 L/h, 0.538 L/h and 1.484 L/h for the same patients when VPA was administered as monotherapy, resulting in an increase CL/F of about 52%, with the consequent reduction in VPA serum levels. These results are consistent with those calculated using models proposed by other authors, which estimate a 30–43% increase in the CL/F for patients between 5 and 15 years old [7,13,15,16,21,27] and a 40–42% increase for patients over 15 years of age [7,14,18].

In association with PHT, typical VPA CL/F values for the previously mentioned reference patients were estimated at 0.016 L/h, 0.169 L/h, 0.883 L/h and 2.434 L/h, respectively, resulting in an increase in CL/F of about 64%, similar to the 54% reported by Blanco-Serrano 1999 [14], but superior to the 11–43% reported by other authors [9,10,18,24].

In dual therapy with PB, typical VPA CL/F values for the previously mentioned reference patients were estimated at 0.014 L/h, 0.143 L/h, 0.746 L/h and 2.057 L/h, respectively, resulting in an increase in CL/F of about 39%. This is similar to the 24% and 36% reported by several authors [11,14]. However, this increase differs from values (10%, 11%, 12% and 57%) reported by other authors [9,10,16,21].

Considering the significant effect of dual therapy with CBZ, PHT and PB, it would be necessary to reduce the a priori dose of VPA by approximately 52%, 64% or 39% of the standard dose of VPA monotherapy, respectively, to obtain steady-state drug levels within the reference therapeutic range (C_{min}^{ss} = 50–100 mg/L). Despite the significance of these dual-therapeutic effects, no recommendations are given in the reference guidelines for VPA dosing adjustments in patients that take these AEDs in combination [47,48].

According to the literature [5], CLB inhibits the metabolism of VPA, while ESM increases it. However, this effect was not observed in the proposed models, probably due to the low representativeness of these covariates in our population sample, lower than 2% for all age group classifications.

Part of the CL/F IIV seen in the base model (60%) can be explained by the proposed final model. The remaining unexplained PK variability was still relatively large, justifying the need to perform TDM as a strategy to reduce individual PK uncertainty in order to assist in personalized VPA dosage regimens.

The tendency observed in the conditional weighted residuals with respect to population prediction (Figure 1) can be attributed to the fact that many data were taken from the post-monitoring stage, and this biases the residual profile due to the effect of TDM. However, this is not a model misspecification as all other goodness-of-fit measurements appear to indicate the suitability of the model [49].

Before they can be used to reliably optimize dosage, PopPK models must be validated. Both internal and external evaluation procedures were used to successfully assess the suitability of the developed PopPK model for application in dose individualization (Table 3), supporting its implementation in TDM procedures together with Bayesian forecasting according to the correct model performance, adequate precision, accuracy and prediction capability.

The typical population value of VPA CL/F in the monotherapy regimen in the final model was 0.010 L/h, 0.103 L/h, 0.5381 L/h and 1.484 L/h for typical patients of 1 year old (mean weight 9.4 kg), 6 years old (mean weight 22.9 kg), 15 years old (mean weight 53.3 kg) and 35 years old (mean weight 73.5 kg), respectively. These values were aligned with the previous value reported in the scientific literature, where the ranges of CL/F were 0.18–0.37 L/h and 0.22–0.53 L/h in patients younger than 5 years and patients between 6 and 14 years, respectively [1,3,7,10,11,13,15,16,19,21–23,27,42–44], and 0.38–0.93 L/h in patients ≥ 15 years [8–10,13,14,16–19,21–24,26,27,42,43]. VPA–protein binding decreases in patients aged over 65, and this increases the free fraction that may be distributed and eliminated, compensating the expected reduction in CL/F in elderly patients due to the inevitable deterioration of liver function with age. The differences found between VPA CL/F in adult and elderly patients were not as significant.

Our findings show the need to adjust the VPA dosage considering the dual therapies with CBZ, PHT or PB to reach therapeutic concentrations (C_{min}^{ss} ≥ 100 mg/L). This fact supports the need for CL/F's proper characterization in order to optimize VPA dosage regimens.

To the best of our knowledge, this PopPK model of VPA was developed in the largest Caucasian population used to date. The study presented in this manuscript includes a very wide range of ages and a sufficient representation of the most common antiepileptic dual therapies supporting its robustness and wide application in routine clinical practice to improve dosage optimization. Indeed, the VPA PopPK model proposed should be considered for model-informed precision dosing (MIPD) of this drug in Caucasian populations from pediatrics to adults.

Besides all the strengths of the research carried out, some limitations might be acknowledged, such as the retrospective and sparse sampling characteristics of the data, potentially limiting additional evaluations, such as unbound VPA concentrations, additional comedications not taken into account or proper estimation of Ka and V/F. However, the successful internal and external evaluations support the adequate descriptive and predictive capabilities of the final VPA PopPK model developed.

5. Conclusions

This study adequately characterized the CL/F of VPA in a large number of Caucasian patients across a very wide range of ages (from 0.1 to 89.4 years old) by using nonlinear mixed-effect modeling and assessing the influence of anthropomorphic, demographic and comedication factors on this parameter. The final PopPK model confirmed the influence of coadministration with carbamazepine, phenytoin and phenobarbital and it demonstrated good stability with an acceptable predictive ability in internal and external evaluations. Based on the final model, which includes development and external evaluation datasets, this PopPK model could be used in the design of a priori VPA dosage regimens and for model-informed precision dosing (MIPD) strategies to optimize VPA treatments in clinical patient management along with Bayesian algorithms during TDM procedures.

Supplementary Materials: The following supporting information can be downloaded at: https://www.mdpi.com/article/10.3390/pharmaceutics14040811/s1, Figure S1: Prediction error (PE) boxplot by age group calculated considering both the individual valproic-acid (VPA)-predicted concentrations (IPRED) and the population-predicted concentrations (PRED) using the final PopPK model developed and the external dataset, Table S1: Summary of number of subjects and valproic acid (VPA) concentrations by age group and dataset type, Table S2: Source code of the final model.

Author Contributions: Conceptualization, P.T.-d.-S. and D.S.-B.; Data curation, P.T.-d.-S. and J.S.P.-B.; Formal analysis, P.T.-d.-S., J.S.P.-B., D.S.-B. and M.J.G.; Investigation, M.J.O. and M.J.G.; Methodology, P.T.-d.-S., J.S.P.-B., D.S.-B., M.J.O. and M.J.G.; Project administration, D.S.-B. and M.J.O.; Resources, M.J.O.; Software, P.T.-d.-S. and J.S.P.-B.; Supervision, J.S.P.-B., D.S.-B., M.J.O. and M.J.G.; Validation, J.S.P.-B.; Visualization, J.S.P.-B.; Writing—original draft, P.T.-d.-S. and J.S.P.-B.; Writing—review and editing, D.S.-B., M.J.O. and M.J.G. All authors have read and agreed to the published version of the manuscript.

Funding: This research received no external funding.

Institutional Review Board Statement: The study was conducted in accordance with the Declaration of Helsinki and approved by the Institutional Review Board (or Ethics Committee) of University Assistance Complex of Salamanca (protocol code CEIm: PI 2022 03 977). This study was not registered in any clinical trial registry since this was not an interventional trial, and all enrolled participants received standard-of-care treatment.

Informed Consent Statement: Patient consent was waived, as this was a retrospective study design of coded samples obtained in routine clinical practice. In addition, obtaining informed consent was considered very difficult and would require unreasonable effort.

Data Availability Statement: Not applicable.

Acknowledgments: The authors would like to thank the patients, investigators and the medical, nursing and laboratory staff who participated in the clinical routine practice included in the present work.

Conflicts of Interest: The authors declare no conflict of interest.

References

1. Rodrigues, C.; Chhun, S.; Chiron, C.; Dulac, O.; Rey, E.; Pons, G.; Jullien, V. A Population Pharmacokinetic Model Taking into Account Protein Binding for the Sustained-Release Granule Formulation of Valproic Acid in Children with Epilepsy. *Eur. J. Clin. Pharmacol.* **2018**, *74*, 793–803. [CrossRef] [PubMed]
2. Tomson, T.; Battino, D.; Perucca, E. Valproic Acid after Five Decades of Use in Epilepsy: Time to Reconsider the Indications of a Time-Honoured Drug. *Lancet Neurol.* **2016**, *15*, 210–218. [CrossRef]
3. Xu, S.; Chen, Y.; Zhao, M.; Guo, Y.; Wang, Z.; Zhao, L. Population Pharmacokinetics of Valproic Acid in Epileptic Children: Effects of Clinical and Genetic Factors. *Eur. J. Pharm. Sci.* **2018**, *122*, 170–178. [CrossRef] [PubMed]
4. Ghodke-Puranik, Y.; Thorn, C.F.; Lamba, J.K.; Leeder, J.S.; Song, W.; Birnbaum, A.K.; Altman, R.B.; Klein, T.E. Valproic Acid Pathway: Pharmacokinetics and Pharmacodynamics. *Pharm. Genom.* **2013**, *23*, 236–241. [CrossRef] [PubMed]
5. Patsalos, P. *Antiepileptic Drug Interactions: A Clinical Guide*, 2nd ed.; Springer Science & Business Media: London, UK, 2012.
6. Methaneethorn, J. A Systematic Review of Population Pharmacokinetics of Valproic Acid. *Br. J. Clin. Pharmacol.* **2018**, *84*, 816–834. [CrossRef] [PubMed]
7. Ding, J.; Wang, Y.; Lin, W.; Wang, C.; Zhao, L.; Li, X.; Zhao, Z.; Miao, L.; Jiao, Z. A Population Pharmacokinetic Model of Valproic Acid in Pediatric Patients with Epilepsy: A Non-Linear Pharmacokinetic Model Based on Protein-Binding Saturation. *Clin. Pharm.* **2015**, *54*, 305–317. [CrossRef]
8. Methaneethorn, J. Population Pharmacokinetics of Valproic Acid in Patients with Mania: Implication for Individualized Dosing Regimens. *Clin. Ther.* **2017**, *39*, 1171–1181. [CrossRef] [PubMed]
9. Lin, W.W.; Jiao, Z.; Wang, C.L.; Wang, H.Y.; Ma, C.L.; Huang, P.F.; Guo, X.Z.; Liu, Y.W. Population Pharmacokinetics of Valproic Acid in Adult Chinese Epileptic Patients and Its Application in an Individualized Dosage Regimen. *Ther. Drug Monit.* **2015**, *37*, 76–83. [CrossRef] [PubMed]
10. Ogusu, N.; Saruwatari, J.; Nakashima, H.; Noai, M.; Nishimura, M.; Deguchi, M.; Oniki, K.; Yasui-Furukori, N.; Kaneko, S.; Ishitsu, T. Impact of the Superoxide Dismutase 2 Val16Ala Polymorphism on the Relationship between Valproic Acid Exposure and Elevation of γ-Glutamyltransferase in Patients with Epilepsy: A Population Pharmacokinetic-Pharmacodynamic Analysis. *PLoS ONE* **2014**, *9*, e111066. [CrossRef]
11. Correa, T.; Rodriguez, I.; Romano, S. Population Pharmacokinetics of Valproate in Mexican Children with Epilepsy. *Biopharm. Drug Dispos.* **2008**, *29*, 511–520. [CrossRef] [PubMed]
12. Fattore, C.; Messina, S.; Battino, D.; Croci, D., Mamoli, D.; Perucca, E. The Influence of Old Age and Enzyme Inducing Comedication on the Pharmacokinetics of Valproic Acid at Steady-State: A Case-Matched Evaluation Based on Therapeutic Drug Monitoring Data. *Epilepsy Res.* **2006**, *70*, 153–160. [CrossRef] [PubMed]
13. Desoky, E.S.E.L.; Fuseau, E.; Amry, S.E.L.D.; Cosson, V. Pharmacokinetic Modelling of Valproic Acid from Routine Clinical Data in Egyptian Epileptic Patients. *Eur. J. Clin. Pharmacol.* **2004**, *59*, 783–790. [CrossRef] [PubMed]
14. Blanco-Serrano, B.; Otero, M.J.; Santos-Buelga, D.; Garcia-Sanchez, M.J.; Serrano, J.; Dominguez-Gil, A. Population Estimation of Valproic Acid Clearance in Adult Patients Using Routine Clinical Pharmacokinetic Data. *Biopharm. Drug Dispos.* **1999**, *20*, 233–240. [CrossRef]
15. Serrano, B.B.; Sanchez, M.J.G.; Otero, M.J.; Buelga, D.S.; Serrano, J.; Dominguez-Gil, A. Valproate Population Pharmacokinetics in Children. *J. Clin. Pharm. Ther.* **1999**, *24*, 73–80. [CrossRef] [PubMed]
16. Yukawa, E.; To, H.; Ohdo, S.; Higuchi, S.; Aoyama, T. Population-Based Investigation of Valproic Acid Relative Clearance Using Nonlinear Mixed Effects Modeling: Influence of Drug-Drug Interaction and Patient Characteristics. *J. Clin. Pharmacol.* **1997**, *37*, 1160–1167. [CrossRef] [PubMed]
17. Vucicevic, K.; Miljkovic, B.; Pokrajac, M.; Prostran, M.; Martinovic, Z.; Grabnar, I. The Influence of Drug-Drug Interaction and Patients' Characteristics on Valproic Acid's Clearance in Adults with Epilepsy Using Nonlinear Mixed Effects Modeling. *Eur. J. Pharm. Sci.* **2009**, *38*, 512–518. [CrossRef]
18. Alqahtani, S.; Alandas, N.; Alsultan, A. Estimation of Apparent Clearance of Valproic Acid in Adult Saudi Patients. *Int. J. Clin. Pharm.* **2019**, *41*, 1056–1061. [CrossRef]
19. Ibarra, M.; Vazquez, M.; Fagiolino, P.; Derendorf, H. Sex Related Differences on Valproic Acid Pharmacokinetics after Oral Single Dose. *J. Pharm. Pharm.* **2013**, *40*, 479–486. [CrossRef]
20. Williams, J.H.; Jayaraman, B.; Swoboda, K.J.; Barrett, J.S. Population Pharmacokinetics of Valproic Acid in Pediatric Patients with Epilepsy: Considerations for Dosing Spinal Muscular Atrophy Patients. *J. Clin. Pharmacol.* **2012**, *52*, 1676–1688. [CrossRef]
21. Jankovic, S.M.; Milovanovic, J.R.; Jankovic, S. Factors Influencing Valproate Pharmacokinetics in Children and Adults. *Int. J. Clin. Pharmacol. Ther.* **2010**, *48*, 767–775. [CrossRef]
22. Jiang, D.; Bai, X.; Zhang, Q.; Lu, W.; Wang, Y.; Li, L.; Muller, M. Effects of CYP2C19 and CYP2C9 Genotypes on Pharmacokinetic Variability of Valproic Acid in Chinese Epileptic Patients: Nonlinear Mixed-Effect Modeling. *Eur. J. Clin. Pharmacol.* **2009**, *65*, 1187–1193. [CrossRef] [PubMed]
23. Jankovic, S.M.; Milovanovic, J.R. Pharmacokinetic Modeling of Valproate from Clinical Data in Serbian Epileptic Patients. *Methods Find Exp. Clin. Pharmacol.* **2007**, *29*, 673–679. [CrossRef] [PubMed]
24. Birnbaum, A.K.; Ahn, J.E.; Brundage, R.C.; Hardie, N.A.; Conway, J.M.; Leppik, I.E. Population Pharmacokinetics of Valproic Acid Concentrations in Elderly Nursing Home Residents. *Ther. Drug Monit.* **2007**, *29*, 571–575. [CrossRef] [PubMed]

25. Jiang, D.C.; Wang, L.; Wang, Y.Q.; Li, L.; Lu, W.; Bai, X.R. Population Pharmacokinetics of Valproate in Chinese Children with Epilepsy. *Acta Pharmacol. Sin.* **2007**, *28*, 1677–1684. [CrossRef] [PubMed]
26. Park, H.M.; Kang, S.S.; Lee, Y.B.; Shin, D.J.; Kim, O.N.; Lee, S.B.; Yim, D.S. Population Pharmacokinetics of Intravenous Valproic Acid in Korean Patients. *J. Clin. Pharm. Ther.* **2002**, *27*, 419–425. [CrossRef] [PubMed]
27. Yukawa, E.; Honda, T.; Ohdo, S.; Higuchi, S.; Aoyama, T. Detection of Carbamazepine-Induced Changes in Valproic Acid Relative Clearance in Man by Simple Pharmacokinetic Screening. *J. Pharm. Pharmacol.* **1997**, *49*, 751–756. [CrossRef] [PubMed]
28. World Health Organization Body Mass Index-for-Age (BMI-for-Age). Available online: https://www.who.int/toolkits/child-growth-standards/standards/body-mass-index-for-age-bmi-for-age (accessed on 8 February 2022).
29. Green, B.; Duffull, S.B. Development of a Dosing Strategy for Enoxaparin in Obese Patients. *Br. J. Clin. Pharmacol.* **2003**, *56*, 96–103. [CrossRef] [PubMed]
30. Mosteller, R.D. Simplified Calculation of Body-Surface Area. *N. Engl. J. Med.* **1987**, *317*, 1098. [CrossRef] [PubMed]
31. Lin, W.; Kelly, A.R. Determination of Valproic Acid in Plasma or Serum by Solid-Phase Column Extraction and Gas-Liquid Chromatography. *Ther. Drug Monit.* **1985**, *7*, 336–343. [CrossRef] [PubMed]
32. Sedman, A.J.; Molitoris, B.A.; Nakata, L.M.; Gal, J. Therapeutic Drug Monitoring in Patients with Chronic Renal Failure: Evaluation of the Abbott TDx Drug Assay System. *Am. J. Nephrol.* **1986**, *6*, 132–134. [CrossRef]
33. Mould, D.R.; Upton, R.N. Basic Concepts in Population Modeling, Simulation, and Model-Based Drug Development—Part 2: Introduction to Pharmacokinetic Modeling Methods. *CPT Pharmacomet. Syst. Pharmacol.* **2013**, *2*, 1–14. [CrossRef] [PubMed]
34. Back, H.M.; Lee, J.B.; Han, N.; Goo, S.; Jung, E.; Kim, J.; Song, B.; An, S.H.; Kim, J.T.; Rhie, S.J.; et al. Application of Size and Maturation Functions to Population Pharmacokinetic Modeling of Pediatric Patients. *Pharmaceutics* **2019**, *11*, 259. [CrossRef]
35. Aarons, L. Sparse Data Analysis. *Eur. J. Drug Metab. Pharmacokinet.* **1993**, *18*, 97–100. [CrossRef] [PubMed]
36. Aarons, L. Population Approaches/Sparse Data Analysis for Human Variability in Kinetics and Dynamics. *Environ. Toxicol. Pharmacol.* **1996**, *2*, 197–199. [CrossRef]
37. Aarons, L. Population Pharmacokinetics: Theory and Practice. *Br. J. Clin. Pharmacol.* **1991**, *32*, 669–670. [PubMed]
38. Simon, N. *Pharmacocinétique de Population: Introduction à Nonmem*; Groupe de Boeck: Marselle, France, 2006.
39. Bruno, R.; Vivier, N.; Vergniol, J.C.; De Phillips, S.L.; Montay, G.; Sheiner, L.B. A Population Pharmacokinetic Model for Docetaxel (Taxotere®): Model Building and Validation. *J. Pharmacokinet. Pharmacodyn.* **1996**, *24*, 153–172. [CrossRef] [PubMed]
40. Chen, C. Validation of a Population Pharmacokinetic Model for Adjunctive Lamotrigine Therapy in Children. *Br. J. Clin. Pharmacol.* **2000**, *50*, 135–145. [CrossRef] [PubMed]
41. Trocóniz, I.; Carreras, J.M.; Codina, H. 11. Farmacocinética poblacional. In *Tratado General de Biofarmacia y Farmacocinética. Vol. II, Vías de Administración de Fármacos: Aspectos Biofarmacéuticos, Farmacocinética no Lineal y Clínica*; Berrozpe, J., Lanao, J., Guitart, C., Eds.; Editorial Sintesis, S.A.: Madrid, Spain, 2013; pp. 319–363. ISBN 9788499589534.
42. Jakovljevic, M.B.; Jankovic, S.M.; Todorovic, N.; Milovanovic, J.R.; Jankovic, S. Pharmacokinetic Modelling of Valproate in Epileptic Patients. *Med. Pregl.* **2010**, *63*, 349–355. [CrossRef] [PubMed]
43. Yukawa, E. A Feasibility Study of the Multiple-Peak Approach for Pharmacokinetic Screening: Population-Based Investigation of Valproic Acid Relative Clearance Using Routine Clinical Pharmacokinetic Data. *J. Pharm. Pharmacol.* **1995**, *47*, 1048–1052. [CrossRef] [PubMed]
44. Botha, J.H.; Gray, A.L.; Miller, R. A Model for Estimating Individualized Valproate Clearance Values in Children. *J. Clin. Pharmacol.* **1995**, *35*, 1020–1024. [CrossRef]
45. European Medicines Agency. *Guideline on the Qualification and Reporting of Physiologically Based Pharmacokinetic (PBPK) Modelling and Simulation*; European Medicines Agency: London, UK, 2016. Available online: https://www.ema.europa.eu/en/documents/scientific-guideline/draft-guideline-qualification-reporting-physiologically-based-pharmacokinetic-pbpk-modelling_en.pdf (accessed on 12 January 2022).
46. Food and Drug Administration. *Guidance for Industry. Population Pharmacokinetics*; Food and Drug Administration: Silver Spring, MD, USA, 2019. Available online: https://www.fda.gov/media/128793/download (accessed on 12 January 2022).
47. Food and Drug Administration. *Medication Guide. DEPAKENE Safely and Effectively*; Food and Drug Administration: Silver Spring, MD, USA, 2019. Available online: https://www.accessdata.fda.gov/drugsatfda_docs/label/2016/018081s065_018082s048lbl.pdf (accessed on 12 January 2022).
48. European Medicines Agency. Assessment Report. Valproic Acid/Valproate Containing Medicinal Products. 2019. Available online: https://www.ema.europa.eu/en/documents/referral/valproate-article-31-referral-prac-assessment-report_en.pdf (accessed on 12 January 2022).
49. Ahn, J.E.; Birnbaum, A.K.; Brundage, R.C. Inherent Correlation between Dose and Clearance in Therapeutic Drug Monitoring Settings: Possible Misinterpretation in Population Pharmacokinetic Analyses. *J. Pharmacokinet. Pharmacodyn.* **2005**, *32*, 703–718. [CrossRef] [PubMed]

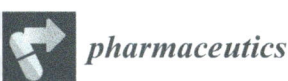

Article

Model-Informed Precision Dosing of Linezolid in Patients with Drug-Resistant Tuberculosis

Laurynas Mockeliunas [1,†], Lina Keutzer [1,†], Marieke G. G. Sturkenboom [2], Mathieu S. Bolhuis [2], Lotte M. G. Hulskotte [2], Onno W. Akkerman [3,4] and Ulrika S. H. Simonsson [1,*]

1. Department of Pharmaceutical Biosciences, Uppsala University, 75124 Uppsala, Sweden; laurynas.mockeliunas@farmbio.uu.se (L.M.); lina.keutzer@farmbio.uu.se (L.K.)
2. Department of Clinical Pharmacy and Pharmacology, University Medical Center Groningen, University of Groningen, 9713 GZ Groningen, The Netherlands; m.g.g.sturkenboom@umcg.nl (M.G.G.S.); m.s.bolhuis@umcg.nl (M.S.B.); l.m.g.hulskotte@student.rug.nl (L.M.G.H.)
3. Department of Pulmonary Diseases and Tuberculosis, University Medical Center Groningen, University of Groningen, 9713 GZ Groningen, The Netherlands; o.w.akkerman@umcg.nl
4. Tuberculosis Center Beatrixoord, University Medical Center Groningen, University of Groningen, 9751 ND Groningen, The Netherlands
* Correspondence: ulrika.simonsson@farmbio.uu.se
† These authors contributed equally to this work.

Citation: Mockeliunas, L.; Keutzer, L.; Sturkenboom, M.G.G.; Bolhuis, M.S.; Hulskotte, L.M.G.; Akkerman, O.W.; Simonsson, U.S.H. Model-Informed Precision Dosing of Linezolid in Patients with Drug-Resistant Tuberculosis. *Pharmaceutics* 2022, 14, 753. https://doi.org/10.3390/pharmaceutics14040753

Academic Editors: Jonás Samuel Pérez-Blanco and José Martínez Lanao

Received: 14 February 2022
Accepted: 28 March 2022
Published: 30 March 2022

Publisher's Note: MDPI stays neutral with regard to jurisdictional claims in published maps and institutional affiliations.

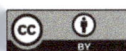

Copyright: © 2022 by the authors. Licensee MDPI, Basel, Switzerland. This article is an open access article distributed under the terms and conditions of the Creative Commons Attribution (CC BY) license (https://creativecommons.org/licenses/by/4.0/).

Abstract: Linezolid is an efficacious medication for the treatment of drug-resistant tuberculosis but has been associated with serious safety issues that can result in treatment interruption. The objectives of this study were thus to build a population pharmacokinetic model and to use the developed model to establish a model-informed precision dosing (MIPD) algorithm enabling safe and efficacious dosing in patients with multidrug- and extensively drug-resistant tuberculosis. Routine hospital therapeutic drug monitoring data, collected from 70 tuberculosis patients receiving linezolid, was used for model development. Efficacy and safety targets for MIPD were the ratio of unbound area under the concentration versus time curve between 0 and 24 h over minimal inhibitory concentration ($fAUC_{0-24h}$/MIC) above 119 and unbound plasma trough concentration (fC_{min}) below 1.38 mg/L, respectively. Model building was performed in NONMEM 7.4.3. The final population pharmacokinetic model consisted of a one-compartment model with transit absorption and concentration- and time-dependent auto-inhibition of elimination. A flat dose of 600 mg once daily was appropriate in 67.2% of the simulated patients from an efficacy and safety perspective. Using the here developed MIPD algorithm, the proportion of patients reaching the efficacy and safety target increased to 81.5% and 88.2% using information from two and three pharmacokinetic sampling occasions, respectively. This work proposes an MIPD approach for linezolid and suggests using three sampling occasions to derive an individualized dose that results in adequate efficacy and fewer safety concerns compared to flat dosing.

Keywords: tuberculosis; population pharmacokinetics; linezolid; auto-inhibition of linezolid elimination; model-informed precision dosing; simulation

1. Introduction

Rifampicin-resistant (including multidrug-resistant (MDR)) tuberculosis (TB) is still a global health threat, with close to half a million new cases annually [1]. MDR-TB is defined as resistant to both isoniazid and rifampicin and extensively drug-resistant (XDR) as resistant to isoniazid and rifampicin, plus any fluoroquinolone and at least one Group A drug (levofloxacin, moxifloxacin, bedaquiline, or linezolid). Treatment of these infections requires the use of second-line treatment, which is longer, associated with higher costs, increased toxicity, and has a success rate of merely 59% [2,3]. Currently, one of the core second-line anti-TB drugs used for the treatment of MDR- and XDR-TB is linezolid, a synthetic antibiotic from the oxazolidinone class, inhibiting the bacterial protein synthesis by binding to the 23S rRNA of 50S ribosomal subunit [4]. Its two main inactive metabolites are hydroxyethyl glycine and aminoethoxy acetic acid, excreted both renally (unchanged) and non-renally [4]. The efficacy of linezolid has been suggested to be related to the ratio of unbound area under the concentration versus time curve between 0 and 24 h over minimal inhibitory concentration ($fAUC_{0-24h}$/MIC) with a threshold above 119 [5,6]. As a potential safety target for linezolid in TB treatment, it has been suggested that the unbound plasma trough concentration (fC_{min}) should be below 1.38 mg/L [6,7] since the time above fC_{min} is assumed to be related to mitochondrial toxicity [8,9].

Treatment of MDR- and XDR-TB with linezolid (nowadays usually in combination with one of the later generation fluoroquinolones, bedaquiline, and another second-line anti-TB drug) [10] is much longer than the standard treatment of other indications with linezolid that have a maximum treatment length of 28 days, which has been shown to lead to more serious adverse events [6,10]. A common adverse event, especially during longer treatment, is myelosuppression (mainly thrombocytopenia, but also leukopenia and anemia). Peripheral and optic neuropathy, lactic acidosis, hepatotoxicity, and hypoglycemia occur more seldom but can be severe and irreversible (neuropathies) [6,11]. Linezolid's high toxicity during longer treatment contributes to a treatment discontinuation rate of 22.6% (141/624, based on 11 studies conducted between 2009 and 2018) [12]. One approach to reduce the risk of developing serious adverse events and minimize the risk of early treatment discontinuation is model-informed precision dosing (MIPD) [13]. MIPD is guided by patient characteristics, individual plasma drug concentrations, and a population pharmacokinetic (PK) or combined pharmacokinetic-pharmacodynamic (PKPD) model. The approach can be used in TB treatment to reduce the risk of treatment failure as well as toxicity [13–16]. The challenge in the treatment of MDR- and XDR-TB is to administer a linezolid dose that is highly efficacious with limited toxicity. MIPD can be used to support individual dose selection using a population PK model and targets for efficacy and safety.

The objectives of this work were to develop a population PK model, which, together with pre-set efficacy and safety targets, can be used to develop an MIPD algorithm enabling safe and efficacious dosing on an individual level.

2. Materials and Methods

2.1. Patients and Pharmacokinetic Data

Routine therapeutic drug monitoring (TDM) data from 70 MDR- or XDR-TB patients receiving linezolid was collected at the TB center Beatrixoord in Haren, University Medical Center Groningen (UMCG), The Netherlands, between 2007 and 2019. Due to the retrospective nature of this study and because TDM was already part of the routine treatment protocol in the TB center, the need for subjects to provide informed consent was waived by the Medical Ethical Review Board UMCG (METC 2013.492, ethical clearance date: 3 December 2013). Patient demographics, patient characteristics, linezolid total plasma concentrations, and linezolid dosing regimens were retrieved from the medical charts. A summary of patient demographics and characteristics is provided in Table 1. Linezolid was administered in combination with other anti-TB drugs for up to 542 days with oral daily doses (once daily (QD) or twice daily (BID)) ranging from 150 to 1200 mg. A summary of all regimens included in the analysis can be found in Table S1 (Supplementary Materials). Linezolid plasma concentrations were obtained at varying time points at up to seven independent sampling occasions in each patient. In most instances, a pre-dose sample was taken before drug administration. Plasma total linezolid concentrations were quantified using validated liquid chromatography coupled with the mass spectrometry (LC-MS/MS) (ThermoFisher, San Jose, CA, USA) method with a lower limit of quantification (LLOQ) of 0.05 mg/L [17].

Table 1. Demographics and covariates for patients included in the data set used for population pharmacokinetic model building.

Parameter	Unit	All Patients
N		70
Mean weight (range)	kg	61.2 (35.3–88.9)
Mean height (range)	m	1.70 (1.50–1.93)
Mean creatinine clearance (range)	mL/min	116.1 (40.7–150.0) [a]
Mean age (range)	years	32 (15–70)
Mean body mass index (range)	kg/m^2	21.2 (15.5–32.6)
No. of male sex	n (%)	38 (54.5)
No. with HIV	n (%)	5 (7.1)
No. with diabetes	n (%)	9 (12.9)
No. smoking	n (%)	26 (37.1)
No. alcohol abuse	n (%)	6 (8.6)
No. pregnancy	n (%)	3 (4.3)
No. from indicated WHO region	n (%)	
African region		10 (14.3)
Region of the Americas		2 (2.9)
Southeast Asia region		6 (8.6)
European region		27 (38.6)
Eastern Mediterranean region		15 (21.4)
Western Pacific region		10 (14.3)

[a] Calculated using the Cockcroft-Gault equation [18], using lean body weight instead of regular body weight for patients with BMI higher than 25 and with creatinine clearance truncated at 150 mL/min (13 patients had a calculated creatinine clearance above 150 mL/min). Age, bodyweight, body mass index, and creatinine plasma concentration were registered on the day of admission. WHO region–region based on World Health Organization (WHO) region classification describing origin of birth; ART–antiretroviral therapy; alcohol–alcohol abuse characterized by more than 1 or 2 glasses of alcohol/day and less than 2 days/week with no alcohol; n–number of patients.

2.2. Population Pharmacokinetic Model

A population pharmacokinetic model was developed based on data from 70 patients (811 observations). One individual's second sampling occasion was excluded from the analysis as the treatment with linezolid was stopped one day before sampling. There were two observations below LLOQ, which were set to LLOQ/2 since the usage of likelihood-based methods such as the M3 and M4 method [19] did not seem necessary in light of the sparseness of LLOQ data.

Model comparison during the modeling process was performed by comparing the objective function value (OFV) of two nested hierarchical models, where a decrease in OFV of 3.84 for one degree of freedom (addition or removal of one parameter) is considered to be statistically significant at a 5% significance level according to the chi-squared distribution (χ^2-distribution).

2.2.1. Structural Model Building

Different disposition models were evaluated, including one- and two-compartment models. In order to describe absorption, a first-order absorption with and without lag-time and a transit absorption model [20,21] were tested. Transit absorption was hard-coded with an increasing number of transit compartments (NN) until the most optimal number of compartments was reached [20,21], as described in Equations (1) and (2). Equation (1) represents the first absorption transit compartment, while Equation (2) represents all other transit compartments.

$$\frac{dA_1}{dt} = -k_{tr} \cdot A_1 \tag{1}$$

$$\frac{dA_n}{dt} = -k_{tr} \cdot A_{(n-1)} - k_{tr} \cdot A_n \tag{2}$$

k_{tr} is the transit rate constant calculated as k_{tr} = (NN + 1)/MTT, and MTT is the mean transit time (estimated). The amount of drug in a certain transit compartment is described by A_n, where n is the absorption compartment.

For drug elimination, linear elimination, Michaelis–Menten elimination kinetics, as well as different approaches to account for drug-induced auto-inhibition of elimination [22–24] were explored. The first evaluated approach describing auto-inhibition of elimination was developed for linezolid by Plock et al. [22], where an empirical inhibition compartment is introduced, i.e., the drug concentration in the inhibition compartment drives the auto-inhibition. Different previously published rate constant into the inhibition compartment (k_{IC}) and concentration in the inhibition compartment yielding half of clearance inhibition (IC_{50}) values [22,25,26] were evaluated, and the ones providing the best fit were fixed and retained in the model. The second approach, initially developed for itraconazole [23], describes clearance inhibition dependent on dose with an exponential function. Lastly, in a model originally developed for auto-induction of rifampicin elimination [24], the formation of an enzyme is described by a first-order enzyme degradation and zero-order formation rate in which enzyme formation is stimulated by the presence of the drug via a nonlinear (E_{max}) model. For description of linezolid elimination auto-inhibition, the approach was reversed by inhibiting the enzyme formation.

2.2.2. Stochastic Model Building

Different residual error models on a normal scale were explored, including additive, proportional and combined additive plus proportional models. All possible combinations of inter-individual variability (IIV) and inter-occasion variability (IOV) were tested on all structural parameters. IIVs and IOVs were modeled exponentially, assuming that individual parameter values are log-normally distributed. Correlations were tested between IIVs of absorption parameters.

2.2.3. Covariate Model Building

Allometric scaling of apparent clearance (*CL/F*) and apparent volume of distribution (*V/F*) was introduced using bodyweight as a descriptor for body size [27–29]. The exponents for the allometric relationships were fixed to 0.75 and 1 for *CL/F* and *V/F*, respectively [30], and the terms were scaled to 70 kg. The impact of additional covariates including age, sex, origin of birth (WHO region), HIV co-infection, diabetes, smoking, alcohol abuse, pre-emptive use of erythropoietin, creatinine clearance (calculated using the Cockcroft-Gault equation [18]) and the effects of concomitant P-glycoprotein (P-gp) inhibitors, P-gp inducers, CYP3A4 inhibitors, and CYP3A4 inducers were assessed using the automated stepwise covariate modeling (SCM) procedure in Perl-speaks-NONMEM (PsN) [31]. Values of calculated creatinine clearance above 150 mL/min were truncated to 150 mL/min. Only clinically plausible covariate relationships were explored (see Table S2, Supplementary Materials). Missing covariate information was handled by imputing the mean value of a covariate for continuous covariates and the mode for categorical covariates. Covariates were selected in a forward inclusion step at a statistical significance level of $p < 0.05$ and retained following a backward deletion step ($p < 0.01$). Statistically significant covariate relationships from the SCM were also assessed for clinical significance. Clinical significance was defined as a change in the typical parameter by more than 20% caused by the covariate effect for categorical covariates and 20% change from the median for the 10% and 90% percentiles of the continuous covariate. The covariates pregnancy, anti-retroviral therapy, and therapeutic use of erythropoietin were not evaluated since only 3, 4, and 0 patients, respectively, exhibited the particular covariate.

2.2.4. Model Evaluation

Prediction-corrected visual predictive checks (pcVPCs), goodness-of-fit (GOF) plots, scientific plausibility, and precision of model parameter estimates were evaluated. A 1000 sample sampling importance resampling (SIR) procedure was performed in PsN for the final model to obtain the 90% nonparametric confidence interval for all parameters in order to assess parameter uncertainty.

2.3. Model-Informed Precision Dosing Algorithm

An MIPD algorithm originally developed for dose individualization of rifampicin [15] was adapted for dose optimization of linezolid treatment in patients with MDR- and XDR-TB.

A simulated population of 1000 hypothetical patients was created by bootstrapping patient covariates, as well as individual MIC values from the original study population (patient characteristics, see Table 1).

For the MIPD algorithm, the $fAUC_{0-24h}/MIC > 119$ and $fC_{min} < 1.38$ mg/L were used as efficacy and safety targets [5,7], respectively, and the individualized dose should meet both the efficacy and the safety target.

In order to obtain observed linezolid plasma concentrations for the simulated patient population, the exposure following an initial dose of 600 mg QD was simulated for the first day of treatment. In the next step, these concentrations were used to compute individual PK parameters (empirical Bayes estimates (EBEs)), such as individual clearance or mean transit time. Based on the individual PK parameters, the individual $fAUC_{0-24h}/MIC$ and fC_{min} were derived following doses of 150 mg to 1200 mg QD and 150 mg to 600 mg BID (increments of 150 mg). The MIPD algorithm was then used to select the individual dose that meets the efficacy and safety target. In case both the efficacy and safety were reached, the lowest efficacious dose was selected. If two dosing regimens resulted in the same $fAUC_{0-24h}/MIC$, which is the case for the same daily dose administered once versus twice daily, the dosing regimen leading to the lower fC_{min} was chosen, ensuring safety. If efficacy but not safety was reached, the lowest efficacious dose was selected, and a warning was given regarding safety. If safety but not efficacy was attained, the highest dose was chosen, and an efficacy warning was given. If neither efficacy nor safety could be achieved, the highest dose was selected (1200 mg QD), and warnings regarding efficacy and safety were reported. The selected individual dose was then used for simulation of further sampling occasions using an adaptive dosing strategy. Using this workflow, in total, three PK sampling occasions on days 1, 8, and 15 of treatment were simulated using a sparse sampling (0, 2, and 5 h post dose) [32], updating the individual PK parameters at every occasion using the newly obtained linezolid plasma concentrations.

For transformation of simulated total AUC_{0-24h} and C_{min} to $fAUC_{0-24h}$ and fC_{min}, respectively, linearity in protein binding across the simulated plasma concentration range was assumed, and AUC_{0-24h} and C_{min} were multiplied by the fraction unbound (assumed to be 0.69) [33].

In order to evaluate the performance of the MIPD algorithm, the true individual doses were derived using information from all sampling occasions and a rich PK sampling for EBE estimation.

To compare the performance of the MIPD algorithm using different amounts of information for computation of the individual PK parameters, the relative bias (rBias) Equation (3) and relative root mean squared error (rRMSE) Equation (4) were calculated for $fAUC_{0-24h}/MIC$ and fC_{min} as follows:

$$rBias = \frac{1}{N} \sum_1^i \frac{\frac{predicted_i - observed_i}{predicted_i + observed_i}}{2} \times 100 \qquad (3)$$

$$rRMSE = \sqrt{\frac{1}{N}\sum_{1}^{i}\frac{(predicted_i - observed_i)^2}{\left(\frac{predicted_i + observed_i}{2}\right)^2}} \times 100 \qquad (4)$$

The relative dose prediction error (rDPE), evaluating the accuracy in dose prediction, was computed as follows Equation (5):

$$rDPE = \frac{predictedDD_i - trueDD_i}{trueDD_i} \times 100 \qquad (5)$$

where DD is the total daily dose.

2.4. Software

The data were analyzed with the non-linear mixed-effects modeling software NONMEM (v.7.4.3; Icon Development Solutions, Ellicott City, MD, USA) [34] using conditional estimation with interaction (FOCE-I). Data handling and visualization were performed in R (v.3.6.1; R Foundation for Statistical Computing, Vienna, Austria) [35]. Model diagnostics were generated using Xpose4 (v.4.6.1) [31] and prediction-corrected visual predictive checks (pcVPCs) were created with PsN (v.4.9.5) [31].

3. Results

3.1. Population Pharmacokinetic Model

The final population PK model consisted of a one-compartment disposition model since a two-compartment model did not describe the data statistically significantly better ($p > 0.05$). A transit absorption model including five transit compartments was statistically significantly superior to an absorption lag-time model. The addition of a sixth transit compartment did not improve the fit significantly. Incorporating Michaelis–Menten elimination kinetics did not improve the model fit (OFV: 1978.5) compared to a model with first-order elimination (OFV: 1974.9), and thus first-order kinetics were chosen for the description of linezolid elimination. Based on goodness-of-fit plots (GOF) plots and prediction-corrected visual predictive checks (pcVPCs), a slight underestimation at higher concentrations was observed, suggesting the need to explore concentration-dependent auto-inhibition of linezolid elimination. For that purpose, different models, including dose- and time-dependency [23] as well as concentration- and time-dependency [22,24], were tested to describe auto-inhibition of linezolid elimination. In the final model, the structure of a previously developed concentration- and time-dependent elimination model developed by Plock et al. [22] was implemented. The incorporated auto-inhibition model [22] consists of an empirical inhibition compartment. Depending on the concentration in the inhibition compartment (C_i), clearance (CL) from the central compartment (A_c) is inhibited, where CL is a fraction of the original uninhibited value at the first dose. Equations (6) and (7) describe the CL auto-inhibition:

$$\frac{dA_c}{dt} = k_a \cdot A_a - \frac{CL}{V_d} \cdot A_c \cdot \left(RCLF + (1 - RCLF) \cdot \left(1 - \frac{C_i}{IC_{50} + C_i}\right)\right) \qquad (6)$$

$$\frac{dC_i}{dt} = k_{IC} \cdot \left(\frac{A_c}{V_d} - C_i\right) \qquad (7)$$

where CL is the uninhibited clearance (L/h), A_a the linezolid amount in the absorption compartment (mg), A_c the linezolid amount in the central compartment (mg), C_i the linezolid concentration in the inhibition compartment (mg/L), k_a the absorption rate constant (h^{-1}), V_d the central volume of distribution (L), k_{IC} the rate constant into the inhibition compartment (1/h), RCLF the remaining CL fraction, and IC_{50} the concentration in the inhibition compartment leading to half of the maximum clearance inhibition (mg/L). The k_{IC} was fixed to the best fitting literature value of 0.0005 h^{-1} [25] and IC_{50} to 0.38 mg/L [25] due to the fact that most of the patient data in this study were captured in steady state, thus not enabling estimation of the inhibition parameters with sufficient precision.

The residual error model was a combined additive and proportional error on a normal scale. IIV in CL/F and mean transit time (MTT) were statistically significant, as well as IOV in CL/F, V/F, MTT, and k_a. Covariances were not found to be statistically significant between any of the parameters.

The parameters CL/F and V/F were allometrically scaled using bodyweight. Out of all explored covariates, HIV on CL/F, sex on k_a, administration of P-gp inhibitors on MTT were found to be both statistically and clinically significant.

The NONMEM code for the final model is given in Text S1 (Supplementary Materials). Goodness-of-fit plots are shown in Figure S1 (Supplementary Materials). The structure of the final model is schematically represented in Figure 1, and the final parameter estimates are provided in Table 2. The final model described the observed data well in all dose groups based on the precision in parameter estimates, GOFs, individual plots (not shown), and pcVPCs showing both the whole population (Figure 2) as well as strata for the different patient covariates (Figure S2, Supplementary Materials).

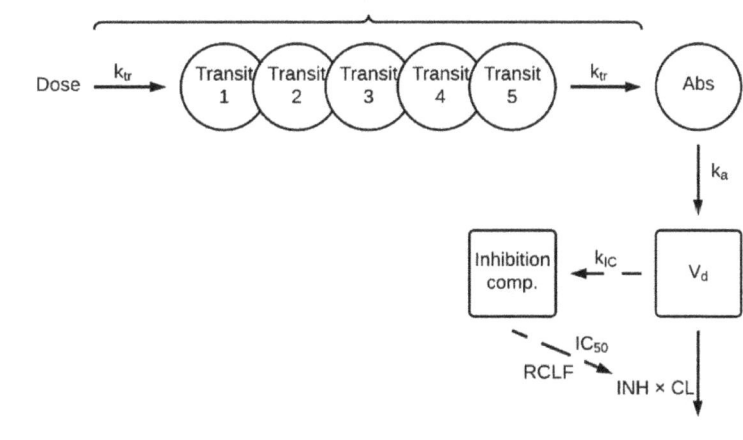

$$INH = RCLF + (1 - RCLF) \times (1 - C_{inhib.comp.}/(IC_{50} + C_{inhib.comp.}))$$

Figure 1. Schematic representation of the final linezolid population pharmacokinetic model. First, the dose is transferred into an absorption compartment (Abs) via five transit compartments (Transit 1–5), where k_{tr} is the transit rate constant describing the transfer between transit compartments, calculated as the number of transit compartments (NN) + 1 divided by the mean transit time (MTT). The drug is absorbed from Abs to the central compartment (indicated by V_d, the distribution volume of the central compartment), described by the absorption rate constant (k_a). Clearance (CL) from the central compartment is inhibited based on the linezolid plasma concentration ($C_{inhib.comp}$) in an empirical inhibition compartment (Inhibition comp.). The concentration- and time-dependency of the inhibition (INH) is described by the $C_{inhib.comp}$ leading to half of the maximum possible inhibition (IC_{50}) and a rate constant (k_{IC}) representing the transfer from the central into the inhibition compartment. The fraction of clearance remaining uninhibited is described by the parameter $RCLF$. The elimination of the drug is described by first-order kinetics, which is inhibited by INH.

Table 2. Parameter estimates from the final linezolid population pharmacokinetic model.

Parameter	Description	Estimate	90% CI [c]	RSE% [d]
CL/F (L/h/70 kg)	Apparent clearance (uninhibited)	6.3	5.6–7.0	6.4
V_d/F (L/70 kg)	Apparent volume of distribution	50.6	48.5–53.1	3.1
ka (h^{-1})	Absorption rate constant	1.8	1.5–2.1	13.8
MTT (h)	Mean transit time	0.53	0.44–0.61	10.6
k_{IC} (h^{-1})	Rate constant into the inhibition compartment	0.0005 FIX [e]	-	-
IC_{50} (mg/L)	Concentration in the inhibition compartment yielding half of clearance inhibition	0.38 FIX [e]	-	-
$RCLF$	Remaining clearance fraction uninhibited	0.798	0.69–0.92	11.3
Covariates				
HIV co-infection on CL/F	Effect of HIV co-infection on CL/F	0.43	0.07–0.90	122.0
Sex on k_a	Effect of sex on k_a	0.95	0.78–1.10	14.0
P-gp inhibitor on MTT	Effect of P-gp inhibitor on MTT	0.96	0.84–1.09	9.0
Inter-individual variability				
$IIV_{CL/F}$ (%CV) [a]	Inter-individual variability in apparent clearance (uninhibited)	0.26	0.21–0.31	13.0
IIV_{MTT} (%CV) [a]	Inter-individual variability in mean transit time	0.62	0.40–0.80	19.9
Inter-occasion variability				
$IOV_{CL/F}$ (%CV) [b]	Inter-occasion variability in apparent clearance (uninhibited)	0.27	0.23–0.30	9.0
$IOV_{V/F}$ (%CV) [b]	Inter-occasion variability in apparent volume of distribution	0.26	0.23–0.30	8.5
IOV_{ka} (%CV) [b]	Inter-occasion variability in absorption rate constant	0.93	0.71–1.16	15.2
IOV_{MTT} (%CV) [b]	Inter-occasion variability in mean transit time	0.69	0.53–0.85	13.4
Residual variability				
Proportional error (%)	Proportional residual error	0.054	0.045–0.065	12.5
Additive error (mg/L)	Additive residual error	0.53	0.483–0.570	7.0

[a] Inter-individual variability expressed as the standard deviation and in % of the parameter estimate. [b] Inter-occasion variability expressed as the standard deviation and in % of the parameter estimate. [c] 90% CI is the 90% percentile confidence interval obtained from a sampling importance resampling (SIR) procedure. [d] Standard errors expressed as relative standard errors (standard errors for omegas relative to their variance estimates). [e] Values obtained by a publication by Keel et al. [25]. IIV, inter-individual variability; IOV, inter-occasion variability; RSE, residual standard error.

3.2. MIPD Algorithm

An MIPD algorithm incorporating adaptive dosing was developed for individualized linezolid dosing in patients with MDR- and XDR-TB. The proposed MIPD workflow is illustrated in Figure 3.

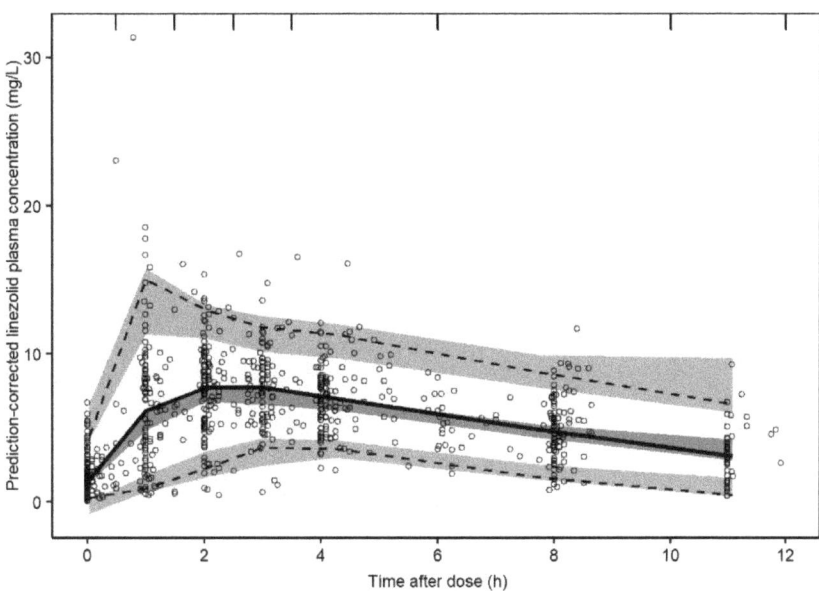

Figure 2. Prediction-corrected visual predictive check (pcVPC) of the final linezolid population pharmacokinetic model. The solid and dashed lines are the median, 2.5th and 97.5th percentiles of the observed data, respectively. The shaded areas (top to bottom) are the 95% confidence intervals of the 97.5th (light gray), median (gray), and 2.5th (light gray) percentiles of the simulated data based on 1000 simulations. Open circles are prediction-corrected observation points.

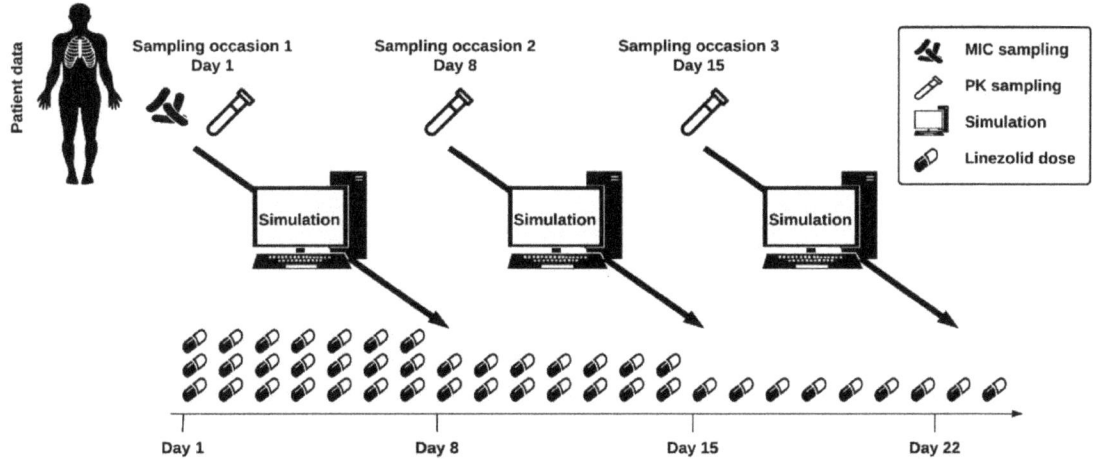

Figure 3. Model-informed precision dosing workflow. MIC determination is performed on day 1 of treatment and PK sampling on days 1, 8, and 15. A Bayesian forecast is then performed using the population PK model, patient characteristics, and individual linezolid plasma concentrations. Taking efficacy and safety into account, the dose is adjusted one week after PK sampling. MIC, minimal inhibitory concentration; PK, pharmacokinetics.

A flat dose of 600 mg QD led to efficacious and safe ($fAUC_{0-24h}$/MIC > 119 and fC_{min} < 1.38 mg/L) exposures in 67.2% of the simulated patients (17.6% of the patients did not meet the safety, 14.0%, not the efficacy, and 1.2% neither the efficacy nor the safety target) (Figure 4). Using the MIPD approach, both the efficacy and safety targets were met in 76.1%, 81.5%, and 88.2% of the simulated patients following dosing regimens derived based on information from one, two, or three PK sampling occasions, respectively. Using information from three occasions, 6.9% of the simulated patients did not meet the safety target, 4.6% did not meet the efficacy target, and 0.3% did not meet the safety nor the efficacy target (Figure 4). A Sankey plot (Figure S3, Supplementary Materials) was created showing individual dose adjustments for three consecutive PK sampling occasions, indicating that a significant part of the simulated patients received the appropriate dose when adjusted based on information from the first sampling occasion. All doses selected by the MIPD algorithm were QD doses since BID dosing would lead to a higher fC_{min}.

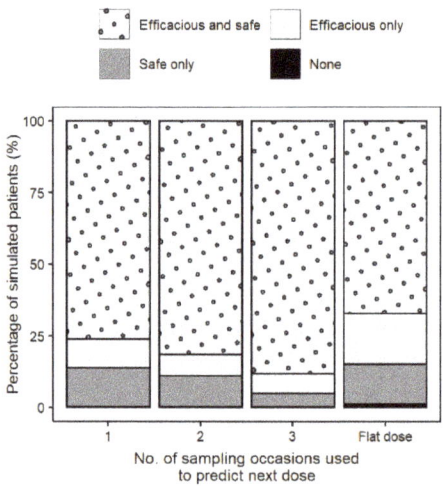

Figure 4. Percentage of patients reaching both efficacy and safety, only efficacy, only safety, and neither efficacy nor safety using information from one, two, and three sampling occasions to derive individual PK parameters. The true individual PK parameters were obtained from a rich sampling in order to derive the true optimal dose for comparison.

In order to determine how many sampling occasions are necessary to compute the individual PK parameters and subsequently predict the $fAUC_{0-24h}$/MIC and fC_{min} with sufficient accuracy and precision, the rRMSE and rBias were calculated for $fAUC_{0-24h}$/MIC and fC_{min} predictions based on information from one, two and three sampling occasions. Both the accuracy and precision in predictions of $fAUC_{0-24h}$/MIC (rBias: −5.0%, −2.1%, and −1.8%; rRMSE: 19.3%, 12.4%, and 8.1% for one, two, and three occasions) and fC_{min} (rBias: −8.9%, −2.7%, and −2.1%; rRMSE: 44.8%, 30.5%, and 20.2% for one, two and three occasions) improved when additional information was added.

The relative dose prediction error decreased with increasing information used to obtain individual parameters from sparse sampling (Figure 5), indicating that a higher percentage of simulated individuals received a dose closer to the true dose.

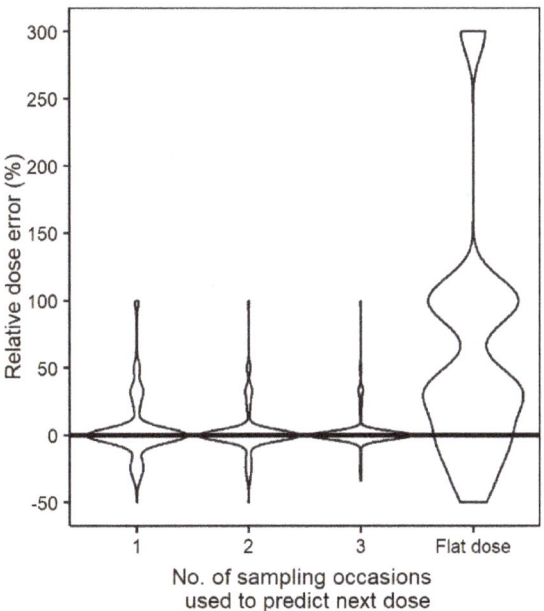

Figure 5. Violin plot showing the dose prediction error comparing the true dose to the individualized dose derived based on information from one, two, and three sampling occasions, as well as flat dosing of 600 mg QD for comparison.

4. Discussion

An MIPD workflow, using the here developed population PK model, was established, enabling safe and efficacious dosing on an individual level.

Several studies have shown that linezolid clearance decreases with increasing doses. This phenomenon has previously been described with either Michaelis–Menten elimination kinetics [36,37] or concentration- and time-dependent auto-inhibition of elimination [22,25,26]. In this work, Michaelis–Menten elimination kinetics was not supported by the data; however, the inclusion of a concentration- and time-dependent auto-inhibition of elimination described the data well, and its incorporation is crucial to be able to use the population PK model for MIPD before steady state is reached. The mechanism behind the auto-inhibition of linezolid elimination is not fully known yet. It is suggested that for the metabolite's hydroxyethyl glycine formation, reduced nicotinamide adenine dinucleotide phosphate (NADPH) is needed [22,38]. As linezolid inhibits cytochrome c-oxidase activity, it interrupts the synthesis of adenosine triphosphate (ATP), which is needed for nicotinamide adenine dinucleotide phosphate (NADP) reduction to NADPH [22]. Lack of NADPH results in decreased hydroxylinezolid formation, and thus, linezolid elimination is inhibited.

In this work, both statistical and clinical significance were considered when incorporating covariates in the model. Three covariates fulfilled both criteria, HIV co-infection on CL/F, sex on k_a, and coadministration of P-gp inhibitors on MTT (Table 2). Typical CL/F was 43% higher in patients with HIV co-infection, and the effect of the covariate on the apparent clearance could be explained by changes in kidney function or concomitant medication (Table 2). Typical k_a was 95% higher in females, possibly due to biological differences between men and women, such as differences in gastric pH, gastric fluid flow, intestinal motility, and gastric emptying [39]. Typical MTT was 96% higher in patients who received P-gp inhibitors. The imprecision in the estimated effect of HIV on CL/F was high, with a 90% confidence interval of 7–90% (Table 2), which is probably due to the low number of HIV patients in the study population (n = 5/70). The covariate was kept in the model since clearance is a parameter that can greatly influence plasma concentration. However, the effect of HIV on CL/F estimated here should be interpreted with caution and studied further. Allometric scaling, besides improving the model fit, was implemented in order to be able to apply the population PK model to a pediatric population.

Linezolid has high efficacy for the treatment of MDR- and XDR-TB and a low resistance development rate but is one of the most frequently reported anti-TB drugs to cause severe adverse events, which might require early termination of treatment [40]. A recent clinical trial investigating long-term linezolid treatment showed that toxicity was high, with 81% of the patients suffering from peripheral neuropathy and 48% from myelosuppression [8]. According to our simulations, a flat dosing regimen of 600 mg QD led to efficacious and safe exposures in 67.2% of the simulated patients, which is comparable to previous findings [5,6,41]. While some work suggests that 600 mg BID is needed to reach efficacy [42], other studies are in accordance with the here described findings. In the work by Millard et al. [6], the majority of simulated patients reached the safety target following doses of 300 mg QD, 300 mg BID, and 600 mg QD, but almost all subjects were above the safety threshold with a dose of 600 mg BID. Alghamdi et al. [41] also suggested that 600 mg QD is preferred in most patients with respect to safety. Furthermore, recent results from the ZeNix trial presented in Berlin 2021 [43] highlight that cure is achievable with 600 mg QD for 6 months, leading to less frequent adverse events compared to 1200 mg QD (38% vs. 24% for peripheral neuropathy and 22% vs. 2% for anemia) [43].

Besides studying the use of lower doses to increase safety, as in the ZeNix trial (NCT03086486), individualizing a patient's dose based on individual characteristics and drug exposure with MIPD can be used as a tool to increase efficacy and safety [13–16]. MIPD provides individual dose suggestions, which is different from classical TDM, where the achieved PK exposure after a dose is compared to a target without a precise dose suggestion apart from the information that a dose is too high or too low. The here proposed MIPD approach (Figure 3) ensures efficacy and safety on an individual level and can be applied at any time during treatment. Simulations of 1000 virtual patients showed that by using the MIPD approach, 88.2% reached efficacious and safe linezolid concentrations with an individualized dose obtained using information from three sampling occasions. After three sampling occasions, 6.9% of all simulated patients would get an efficacious but not safe dose (17.6% following a flat dose of 600 mg QD), 4.3% would get a safe but not efficacious dose (versus 14% for 600 mg QD flat dosing), and for 0.3% of the simulated patients, the dose would be considered neither safe nor efficacious (versus 1.2% for 600 mg QD flat dosing) (see Figure 4). Using information from three occasions resulted in 88.2% of simulated patients reaching both the efficacy and safety target (improvement of 6.7% compared to using information from two occasions), thus highlighting the importance of the third occasion (Figure 4). In all simulated patients, a QD dosing strategy was superior compared to BID due to the fact that the fC_{min} is lower following QD dosing. The superiority of a QD dosing strategy over BID has been shown previously [5,6,41] and could be advantageous to increase patient adherence.

There are some limitations to this work. Firstly, since retrospective TDM data from routine clinical care was analyzed and because patients were in their intensive phase of TB infection, selection bias might have been introduced. In addition, it was only possible to derive the dose prediction error for the total daily dose; thus, there was no distinction between QD and BID dosing. However, since a QD strategy was superior to BID in all simulated patients, it was not necessary here to compare the dose prediction error between QD versus BID strategies. Furthermore, the parameters describing the auto-inhibition of elimination were not identifiable in this work as the majority of samples were taken at steady state, and thus the parameters related to elimination auto-inhibition had to be fixed to values obtained from earlier studies [25]. In this work, efficacy and safety targets from earlier defined PKPD indices were used for dose selection. A simulation study by Kristoffersson et al. [44] showed that the use of longitudinal PKPD models can be more appropriate in certain situations than using PKPD indices. PKPD indices can further be influenced by uncertainty in the obtained MIC value, both due to intra- and inter-laboratory variability [45,46]. Since the MIC is determined in two-fold dilution steps, an error may lead to a substantial change in the PKPD index and, subsequently, dose selection. These findings indicate that MIPD based on a PKPD model might be more appropriate than based on PKPD indices, which should be investigated in further studies. Furthermore, the safety target has only been evaluated in one study with 38 participants [7], and the authors merely explored fC_{min} as a potential driver for toxicity. Other PK parameters such as AUC or C_{max} were not explored, and there is, therefore, a need to derive an updated individualized safety target based on PK data combined with clinical safety outcome data. Lastly, the developed MIPD approach should be validated in the clinic.

5. Conclusions

In conclusion, a linezolid population PK model for MDR- and XDR-TB patients was successfully developed. This work presents an MIPD workflow for linezolid, which can be used on any day of treatment, proposes to use three sparse sampling occasions to derive the individualized dose, and suggests that an individualized dose would be beneficial from an efficacy and safety perspective compared to a flat dose of 600 mg QD.

Supplementary Materials: The following supporting information can be downloaded at: https://www.mdpi.com/article/10.3390/pharmaceutics14040753/s1, Text S1 NONMEM model code for the final population pharmacokinetic model; Figure S1 Goodness-of-fit plots for the final population pharmacokinetic model; Figure S2 Prediction corrected visual predictive checks (pcVPC) for the final linezolid population pharmacokinetic model stratified on covariates; Figure S3 Sankey plot showing individual dose adjustments for three consecutive PK sampling occasions, each one week apart; Table S1 Summary of the different regimens included in the analysis dataset; Table S2 Covariate relationships evaluated in the population pharmacokinetic analysis.

Author Contributions: Conceptualization, L.K., L.M., L.M.G.H., M.G.G.S., M.S.B., O.W.A. and U.S.H.S.; methodology, L.K., L.M., L.M.G.H. M.G.G.S., M.S.B., O.W.A. and U.S.H.S.; software, L.K., L.M. and U.S.H.S.; validation, L.K., L.M., L.M.G.H., M.G.G.S., M.S.B., O.W.A. and U.S.H.S.; formal analysis, L.K., L.M. and U.S.H.S.; data curation, L.K., L.M. and U.S.H.S.; writing—original draft preparation, L.K. and L.M.; writing—review and editing, L.K., L.M., L.M.G.H., M.G.G.S., M.S.B., O.W.A. and U.S.H.S.; visualization, L.K. and L.M.; supervision, U.S.H.S. All authors have read and agreed to the published version of the manuscript.

Funding: This research received no external funding.

Institutional Review Board Statement: The study was conducted in accordance with the Declaration of Helsinki, and approved by the Medical Ethical Review Board UMCG (METC 2013.492, ethical clearance date: 3 December 2013).

Informed Consent Statement: Due to the retrospective nature of this study and because TDM was already part of the routine treatment protocol in the TB center, the need for subjects to provide informed consent was waived by the Medical Ethical Review Board UMCG (METC 2013.492, ethical clearance date: 3 December 2013).

Data Availability Statement: The data presented in this study are available on request from the corresponding author. The data are not publicly available due to privacy reasons, as this is sensitive personal patient data.

Acknowledgments: The computations were enabled by resources in project SNIC 2020-5-524 provided by the Swedish National Infrastructure for Computing (SNIC) at UPPMAX, partially funded by the Swedish Research Council through grant agreement no. 2018-05973.

Conflicts of Interest: The authors declare no conflict of interest.

References

1. *Global Tuberculosis Report 2019*; Licence: CC BY-NC-SA 3.0 IGO; World Health Organization: Geneva, Switzerland, 2019.
2. *Meeting Report of the WHO Expert Consultation on the Definition of Extensively Drug-Resistant Tuberculosis, 27–29 October 2020*; CC BY-NC-SA 3.0 IGO; World Health Organization: Geneva, Switzerland, 2021.
3. *Global Tuberculosis Report 2021*; Licence: CC BY-NC-SA 3.0 IGO; World Health Organization: Geneva, Switzerland, 2021.
4. Hashemian, S.M.; Farhadi, T.; Ganjparvar, M. Linezolid: A review of its properties, function, and use in critical care. *Drug Des. Dev. Ther.* **2018**, *12*, 1759–1767. [CrossRef]
5. Srivastava, S.; Magombedze, G.; Koeuth, T.; Sherman, C.; Pasipanodya, J.G.; Raj, P.; Wakeland, E.; Deshpande, D.; Gumbo, T. Linezolid Dose That Maximizes Sterilizing Effect While Minimizing Toxicity and Resistance Emergence for Tuberculosis. *Antimicrob. Agents Chemother.* **2017**, *61*, e00751-17. [CrossRef]
6. Millard, J.; Pertinez, H.; Bonnett, L.; Hodel, E.M.; Dartois, V.; Johnson, J.L.; Caws, M.; Tiberi, S.; Bolhuis, M.; Alffenaar, J.-W.C.; et al. Linezolid pharmacokinetics in MDR-TB: A systematic review, meta-analysis and Monte Carlo simulation. *J. Antimicrob. Chemother.* **2018**, *73*, 1755–1762. [CrossRef] [PubMed]
7. Song, T.; Lee, M.; Jeon, H.-S.; Park, Y.; Dodd, L.E.; Dartois, V.; Follman, D.; Wang, J.; Cai, Y.; Goldfeder, L.C.; et al. Linezolid Trough Concentrations Correlate with Mitochondrial Toxicity-Related Adverse Events in the Treatment of Chronic Extensively Drug-Resistant Tuberculosis. *EBioMedicine* **2015**, *2*, 1627–1633. [CrossRef]
8. Conradie, F.; Diacon, A.H.; Ngubane, N.; Howell, P.; Everitt, D.; Crook, A.M.; Mendel, C.M.; Egizi, E.; Moreira, J.; Timm, J.; et al. Treatment of Highly Drug-Resistant Pulmonary Tuberculosis. *N. Engl. J. Med.* **2020**, *382*, 893–902. [CrossRef] [PubMed]
9. Maartens, G.; Benson, C.A. Linezolid for Treating Tuberculosis: A Delicate Balancing Act. *EBioMedicine* **2015**, *2*, 1568–1569. [CrossRef]
10. *WHO Consolidated Guidelines on Drug-Resistant Tuberculosis Treatment*; Licence: CC BY-NC-SA 3.0 IGO; World Health Organization: Geneva, Switzerland, 2019.
11. Rao, G.G.; Konicki, R.; Cattaneo, D.; Alffenaar, J.-W.; Marriott, D.J.E.; Neely, M. Therapeutic Drug Monitoring Can Improve Linezolid Dosing Regimens in Current Clinical Practice: A Review of Linezolid Pharmacokinetics and Pharmacodynamics. *Ther. Drug Monit.* **2020**, *42*, 83–92. [CrossRef] [PubMed]
12. Singh, B.; Cocker, D.; Ryan, H.; Sloan, D.J. Linezolid for drug-resistant pulmonary tuberculosis. *Cochrane Database Syst. Rev.* **2019**, *3*, CD012836. [CrossRef]
13. Keizer, R.J.; ter Heine, R.; Frymoyer, A.; Lesko, L.J.; Mangat, R.; Goswami, S. Model-Informed Precision Dosing at the Bedside: Scientific Challenges and Opportunities. *CPT Pharmacomet. Syst. Pharmacol.* **2018**, *7*, 785–787. [CrossRef]
14. van Beek, S.W.; ter Heine, R.; Keizer, R.J.; Magis-Escurra, C.; Aarnoutse, R.E.; Svensson, E.M. Personalized Tuberculosis Treatment Through Model-Informed Dosing of Rifampicin. *Clin. Pharmacokinet.* **2019**, *58*, 815–826. [CrossRef]
15. Svensson, R.J.; Niward, K.; Davies Forsman, L.; Bruchfeld, J.; Paues, J.; Eliasson, E.; Schön, T.; Simonsson, U.S. Individualised dosing algorithm and personalised treatment of high-dose rifampicin for tuberculosis. *Br. J. Clin. Pharmacol.* **2019**, *85*, 2341–2350. [CrossRef]
16. Keutzer, L.; Simonsson, U.S.H. Individualized Dosing With High Inter-Occasion Variability Is Correctly Handled With Model-Informed Precision Dosing-Using Rifampicin as an Example. *Front. Pharmacol.* **2020**, *11*, 794. [CrossRef]
17. Harmelink, I.M.; Alffenaar, J.-W.; Wessels, A.M.A. A rapid and simple liquid chromatography-tandem mass spectrometry method for the determination of linezolid in human serum. *Eur. J. Hosp. Pharm.* **2008**, *14*, 3–7.
18. Cockcroft, D.W.; Gault, M.H. Prediction of creatinine clearance from serum creatinine. *Nephron* **1976**, *16*, 31–41. [CrossRef] [PubMed]
19. Beal, S.L. Ways to fit a PK model with some data below the quantification limit. *J. Pharmacokinet. Pharmacodyn.* **2001**, *8*, 481–504. [CrossRef] [PubMed]
20. Rousseau, A.; Léger, F.; Le Meur, Y.; Saint-Marcoux, F.; Paintaud, G.; Buchler, M.; Marquet, P. Population Pharmacokinetic Modeling of Oral Cyclosporin Using NONMEM: Comparison of Absorption Pharmacokinetic Models and Design of a Bayesian Estimator. *Ther. Drug Monit.* **2004**, *26*, 23–30. [CrossRef]
21. Savic, R.M.; Jonker, D.M.; Kerbusch, T. *Evaluation of a Transit Compartment Model Versus a Lag Time Model for Describing Drug Absorption Delay*; Abstr 513; Population Approach Group Europe: Uppsala, Sweden, 2004.
22. Plock, N.; Buerger, C.; Joukhadar, C.; Kljucar, S.; Kloft, C. Does linezolid inhibit its own metabolism? Population pharmacokinetics as a tool to explain the observed nonlinearity in both healthy volunteers and septic patients. *Drug Metab. Dispos.* **2007**, *35*, 1816–1823. [CrossRef] [PubMed]
23. Abuhelwa, A.Y.; Foster, D.J.R.; Mudge, S.; Hayes, D.; Upton, R.N. Population pharmacokinetic modeling of itraconazole and hydroxyitraconazole for oral SUBA-itraconazole and sporanox capsule formulations in healthy subjects in fed and fasted states. *Antimicrob. Agents Chemother.* **2015**, *59*, 5681–5696. [CrossRef] [PubMed]
24. Smythe, W.; Khandelwal, A.; Merle, C.; Rustomjee, R.; Gninafon, M.; Bocar Lo, M.; Sow, O.B.; Olliaro, P.L.; Lienhardt, C.; Horton, J.; et al. A semimechanistic pharmacokinetic-enzyme turnover model for rifampin autoinduction in adult tuberculosis patients. *Antimicrob. Agents Chemother.* **2012**, *56*, 2091–2098. [CrossRef] [PubMed]
25. Keel, R.A.; Schaeftlein, A.; Kloft, C.; Pope, J.S.; Knauft, R.F.; Muhlebach, M.; Nicolau, D.P.; Kuti, J.L. Pharmacokinetics of Intravenous and Oral Linezolid in Adults with Cystic Fibrosis. *Antimicrob. Agents Chemother.* **2011**, *55*, 3393–3398. [CrossRef] [PubMed]

26. Minichmayr, I.K.; Schaeftlein, A.; Kuti, J.L.; Zeitlinger, M.; Kloft, C. Clinical Determinants of Target Non-Attainment of Linezolid in Plasma and Interstitial Space Fluid: A Pooled Population Pharmacokinetic Analysis with Focus on Critically Ill Patients. *Clin. Pharmacokinet.* **2017**, *56*, 617–633. [CrossRef]
27. West, G.B.; Brown, J.H.; Enquist, B.J. A General Model for the Origin of Allometric Scaling Laws in Biology. *Science* **1997**, *276*, 122–126. [CrossRef]
28. West, G.; Brown, J.; Enquist, B. The Fourth Dimension of Life: Fractal Geometry and Allometric Scaling of Organisms. *Science* **1999**, *284*, 1677–1679. [CrossRef] [PubMed]
29. Holford, N.H. A size standard for pharmacokinetics. *Clin. Pharmacokinet.* **1996**, *30*, 329–332. [CrossRef] [PubMed]
30. Holford, N.H.G.; Anderson, B.J. Allometric size: The scientific theory and extension to normal fat mass. *Eur. J. Pharm. Sci.* **2017**, *109*, S59–S64. [CrossRef] [PubMed]
31. Keizer, R.J.; Karlsson, M.O.; Hooker, A. Modeling and Simulation Workbench for NONMEM: Tutorial on Pirana, PsN, and Xpose. *CPT Pharmacomet. Syst. Pharmacol.* **2013**, *2*, e50. [CrossRef] [PubMed]
32. Kamp, J.; Bolhuis, M.S.; Tiberi, S.; Akkerman, O.W.; Centis, R.; de Lange, W.C.; Kosterink, J.G.; van der Werf, T.; Migliori, G.B.; Alffenaar, J.-W.C. Simple strategy to assess linezolid exposure in patients with multi-drug-resistant and extensively-drug-resistant tuberculosis. *Int. J. Antimicrob. Agents* **2017**, *49*, 688–694. [CrossRef]
33. Pawsey, S.D.; Daley-Yates, P.T.R.; Wajszczuk, C.P. U-1007666 safety, toleration and pharmacokinetics after oral and intravenous administration. In *Abstracts of the First European Congress of Chemotherapy, Glasgow UK*; Abstract F151; Federation for the Societies for European Chemotherapy and Infection: London, UK, 1996.
34. Beal, S.; Sheiner, L.; Boeckmann, A.; Bauer, R. *NONMEM 7.4 Users Guides*; ICON plc.: Gaithersburg, MD, USA, 1989.
35. R Core Team. *R: A Language and Environment for Statistical Computing*; R Foundation for Statistical Computing: Vienna, Austria, 2015.
36. Cojutti, P.; Pai, M.P.; Pea, F. Population Pharmacokinetics and Dosing Considerations for the Use of Linezolid in Overweight and Obese Adult Patients. *Clin. Pharmacokinet.* **2018**, *57*, 989–1000. [CrossRef]
37. Beringer, P.; Nguyen, M.; Hoem, N.; Louie, S.; Gill, M.; Gurevitch, M.; Wong-Beringer, A. Absolute bioavailability and pharmacokinetics of linezolid in hospitalized patients given enteral feedings. *Antimicrob. Agents Chemother.* **2005**, *49*, 3676–3681. [CrossRef]
38. De Vriese, A.S.; Van Coster, R.; Smet, J.; Seneca, S.; Lovering, A.; Van Haute, L.L.; Vanopdenbosch, L.J.; Martin, J.-J.; Groote, C.C.-D.; Vandecasteele, S.; et al. Linezolid Induced Inhibition of Mitochondrial Protein Synthesis. *Clin. Infect. Dis.* **2006**, *42*, 1111–1117. [CrossRef]
39. Soldin, O.P.; Mattison, D.R. Sex differences in pharmacokinetics and pharmacodynamics. *Clin. Pharmacokinet.* **2009**, *48*, 143–157. [CrossRef]
40. *Guidelines for Treatment of Drug-Susceptible Tuberculosis and Patient Care*; Licence: CC BY-NC-SA 3.0 IGO; 2017 Update; World Health Organization: Geneva, Switzerland, 2017.
41. Alghamdi, W.A.; Al-Shaer, M.H.; An, G.; Alsultan, A.; Kipiani, M.; Barbakadze, K.; Mikiashvili, L.; Ashkin, D.; Griffith, D.E.; Cegielski, J.P.; et al. Population Pharmacokinetics of Linezolid in Tuberculosis Patients: Dosing Regimens Simulation and Target Attainment Analysis. *Antimicrob. Agents Chemother.* **2020**, *64*, e01174-20. [CrossRef]
42. Tietjen, A.K.; Kroemer, N.; Cattaneo, D.; Baldelli, S.; Wicha, S.G. Population pharmacokinetics and target attainment analysis of linezolid in multidrug-resistant tuberculosis patients. *Br. J. Clin. Pharmacol.* **2021**, *88*, 1835–1844. [CrossRef]
43. New Trial Results Show Effectiveness of BPaL Regimen for Highly Drug-Resistant TB Can Be Maintained with Reduced Dosing of Linezolid. TB Alliance n.d. Available online: https://www.tballiance.org.za/news/zenix-press-release-english (accessed on 19 November 2021).
44. Kristoffersson, A.N.; David-Pierson, P.; Parrott, N.J.; Kuhlmann, O.; Lave, T.; Friberg, L.E.; Nielsen, E.I. Simulation-Based Evaluation of PK/PD Indices for Meropenem Across Patient Groups and Experimental Designs. *Pharm. Res.* **2016**, *33*, 1115–1125. [CrossRef]
45. Mouton, J.W.; Meletiadis, J.; Voss, A.; Turnidge, J. Variation of MIC measurements: The contribution of strain and laboratory variability to measurement precision. *J. Antimicrob. Chemother.* **2018**, *73*, 2374–2379. [CrossRef]
46. Mouton, J.W.; Muller, A.E.; Canton, R.; Giske, C.G.; Kahlmeter, G.; Turnidge, J. MIC-based dose adjustment: Facts and fables. *J. Antimicrob. Chemother.* **2018**, *73*, 564–568. [CrossRef]

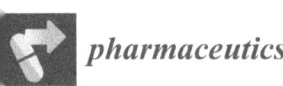

Article

Free and Open-Source Posologyr Software for Bayesian Dose Individualization: An Extensive Validation on Simulated Data

Cyril Leven [1,2,*], Anne Coste [3] and Camille Mané [1]

[1] Department of Biochemistry and Pharmaco-Toxicology, Brest University Hospital, 29200 Brest, France; camille.mane@chu-brest.fr
[2] Univ Brest, EA 3878, GETBO, 29200 Brest, France
[3] Infectious Diseases Department, Brest University Hospital, 29200 Brest, France; anne.coste@chu-brest.fr
* Correspondence: cyril.leven@chu-brest.fr

Abstract: Model-informed precision dosing is being increasingly used to improve therapeutic drug monitoring. To meet this need, several tools have been developed, but open-source software remains uncommon. Posologyr is a free and open-source R package developed to enable Bayesian individual parameter estimation and dose individualization. Before using it for clinical practice, performance validation is mandatory. The estimation functions implemented in posologyr were benchmarked against reference software products on a wide variety of models and pharmacokinetic profiles: 35 population pharmacokinetic models, with 4.000 simulated subjects by model. Maximum A Posteriori (MAP) estimates were compared to NONMEM post hoc estimates, and full posterior distributions were compared to Monolix conditional distribution estimates. The performance of MAP estimation was excellent in 98.7% of the cases. Considering the full posterior distributions of individual parameters, the bias on dosage adjustment proposals was acceptable in 97% of cases with a median bias of 0.65%. These results confirmed the ability of posologyr to serve as a basis for the development of future Bayesian dose individualization tools.

Keywords: clinical pharmacokinetics; dosage individualization; Bayesian dosing; therapeutic drug monitoring; Maximum A Posteriori

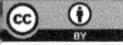

1. Introduction

Model-informed precision dosing (MIPD) is an emerging dosing paradigm in which mathematical models are used for dose optimization, using individual information such as a patient's age, organ function, and the results of therapeutic drug monitoring. Driven by the increasing importance of information technology in health care [1], MIPD is being promoted as a strategy to improve the efficiency of therapeutic drug monitoring and improve standards of care [2].

Because of the complexity of generic modeling software such as NONMEM, MIPD generally requires custom-made software tools tailored to the needs of clinical providers [1]. User-friendly software such as MWPharm [3], TDMx [4], and many others [5] have been developed to meet various needs. Some of this software is freely available, some allows specialist users to integrate their own models, and some has been validated for their predictive performance, but few tools combine all of these features. Software that utilizes publicly documented, accessible and reusable algorithms is even rarer.

Moreover, most of these software products rely only on Maximum A posteriori Bayesian Estimation (MAP-BE), assuming that the mode of the posteriori distribution leads to the prediction with the highest probability. However, Bayesian inference goes beyond point estimates: full posterior (conditional) distributions retain information about the uncertainty associated with individual parameter estimates. Taking this uncertainty into account helps to improve the quality of the predictions, and full Bayesian approaches have been shown superior to MAP-based approaches in dosing individualization [6].

The posologyr software has been developed to address these issues. Featuring Bayesian inference of individual parameters based on parametric nonlinear mixed-effects modeling, posologyr is a free R package [7], licensed under AGPLv3 [8] to guarantee external auditability and accessibility to the widest possible audience of R users.

The aim is for posologyr to be a reliable and open foundation for the development of future MIPD tools. To this end, the extensive validation of the predictive performance of the various implemented functions was an essential requirement.

2. Materials and Methods

2.1. Nonlinear Mixed Effects Models

Nonlinear mixed-effects models are frequently used for the analysis of pharmacokinetic data. They take into account different levels of variability, including inter-individual variability, by incorporating random effects [9]. The observations can be described using the following general nonlinear mixed-effects model implemented in the NONMEM software:

$$y_{ij} = f(x_{ij}, \psi_i) + g(x_{ij}, \psi_i, \varepsilon_{ij}) \quad (1)$$

for i from 1 to N, and for j from 1 to n_i. Where,

- y_{ij} is the jth observation of subject i;
- N is the number of subjects;
- n_i is the number of observations of subject i;
- f is the function defining the structural model;
- g is the function defining the residual error model;
- x_{ij} is the vector of regression variables;
- for subject i, the vector ψ_i is a vector of individual parameters:

$$\psi_i = H(\theta, c_i, \eta_i) \quad (2)$$

where,

  ○ θ is a vector of fixed effects;
  ○ c_i is a vector of covariates;
  ○ η_i is a vector of normally distributed random effects, of length k, with variance-covariance matrix Ω:

$$\eta_i \sim N(0, \Omega) \quad (3)$$

- The residual errors ε_{ij} are normally distributed random variables centered on 0, with variance Σ:

$$\varepsilon_{ij} \sim N(0, \Sigma) \quad (4)$$

In the Monolix software, the implementation of the residual error model differs, and the nonlinear mixed-effects model becomes:

$$y_{ij} = f(x_{ij}, \psi_i) + g(x_{ij}, \psi_i, \xi)\varepsilon_{ij} \quad (5)$$

where the residual error model is defined by the function g and some parameters ξ. The residual errors are then random variables with mean zero and variance one.

2.2. Estimation of Individual Parameters

2.2.1. General Strategy

In the context of MIPD, the aim is to determine the individual parameters ψ_i of a subject i, for which dosage personalization is needed. The estimation of individual parameters requires (i) a model for (y, ψ) with the prior estimates of θ, x_{ij}, the Ω variance covariance matrix, and, depending on the definition of the residual error model, either the Σ matrix, or the vector of parameters ξ; (ii) the input of the observed concentrations y, the measurement times t, the individual covariates, and the administration regimen; and (iii) algorithms capable of estimating and maximizing $p(\psi_i|y_i)$. The fixed effects of the population pharmacokinetic model are used as prior information, and the values of the individual random effects η_i are estimated a posteriori, taking advantage of the observed data.

2.2.2. Maximum A Posteriori

MAP estimation determines the vector of individual parameters with the highest probability, i.e., the mode of the posterior distribution. In NONMEM, it is performed during the POSTHOC step by minimizing the following objective function value (OFV), based on the log likelihood (LL) [10]:

$$\text{OFV}_i = -2\text{LL}(\eta_i) = \sum_j \left[\log \sigma^2_{ij} + \frac{(y_{ij} - f_{ij})^2}{\sigma^2_{ij}} \right] + \eta_i^T \Omega^{-1} \eta_i \qquad (6)$$

where σ^2_{ij} is the variance of the residual error for individual i at time j.

While most Bayesian forecasting tools rely on the MAP estimation, this approach does not necessarily predict the most probable outcome [6]. To provide a comprehensive uncertainty quantification, it may be desirable to compute the full posterior distributions, and not just point estimates such as the MAP.

2.2.3. Markov Chain Monte Carlo

While the probabilities of $p(\psi_i)$ or $p(\eta_i)$ cannot be directly calculated, Markov chain Monte Carlo (MCMC) methods allow this distribution to be sampled. The typical procedure is as follows: at each iteration of the algorithm, a new vector of individual parameters ψ_i is drawn from a proposal distribution. The new value is accepted with a probability that depends on $p(\psi_i)$ and on $p(y_i|\psi_i)$. After a transition period, the algorithm reaches a stationary state where the accepted samples come from the posterior probability distribution $p(\psi_i|y_i)$.

2.2.4. Sequential Importance Resampling

Particle filter algorithms, including Sequential Importance Resampling (SIR), are another class of algorithms that asymptotically draw samples from the posterior probability distribution, allowing for estimation of $p(\psi_i|y_i)$. The SIR algorithm, consists of 3 steps [11]:

1. Step 1 (sampling): a defined number M of parameters are sampled from a multivariate parametric proposal distribution;
2. Step 2 (importance weighting): weights are computed for each of the sampled vectors, using the likelihood of the data given the parameter vector, weighted by the likelihood of the parameter vector in the proposal distribution;
3. Step 3 (resampling): m parameter vectors are resampled from the M simulated vectors ($M > m$), with probabilities proportional to their weighting.

Each step of the algorithm can be parallelized: for the same number of samples, the time needed for estimation can be significantly reduced when compared to MCMC.

2.3. Implementation in Posologyr

The posologyr package (available at https://github.com/levenc/posologyr/, accessed on 15 January 2022) builds on the RxODE [12] simulation framework, using the Fortran package LSODA (Livermore Solver for Ordinary Differential Equations) for solving systems of differential equations. It does not depend on any non-free licensed software, such as NONMEM or Monolix, to run. Random effects of individual models (inter-individual, inter-occasion), and residual error models are implemented within posologyr; RxODE is employed as a deterministic simulation engine. For the MAP estimation, the OFV minimization is performed with the L-BFGS-B algorithm [13] included in the optim package, a limited-memory approximation of the Broyden–Fletcher–Goldfarb–Shanno algorithm (BFGS) allowing for box constraints. To avoid converging to a suboptimal local minimum of the OFV, initial values of the parameters are drawn from the multinormal distribution $\eta_i \sim N(0, \Omega)$. The MCMC algorithm of posologyr is an adaptation of the Metropolis–Hastings algorithm from the R package saemix [14], slightly modified to estimate the posterior distribution $p(\eta_i|y_i)$ and to use RxODE as a simulation engine. As in the Metropolis–Hastings algorithm featured in Monolix, three different distributions are used in turn with a (2,2,2) pattern for the proposal distribution: the population distribution, a unidimensional Gaussian random walk, or a multidimensional Gaussian random walk [15]. For the random walks, the variance of the Gaussian is automatically adapted to reach an optimal acceptance ratio. The number of iterations to be discarded following the burn-in period, the number of Markov chains, and the number of iterations per chain are user-defined. The SIR algorithm implemented in posologyr works by sampling from the multinormal distribution $N(0, \Omega)$ using the rmvnorm function of the mvtnorm package. The weightings are computed from the LL, i.e., $-0,5 \times OFV$, following the simultaneous simulation of the observations generated by the M individual parameter vectors from the sampling step. The initial number of samples M, and the number of draws m in the resampling step can be defined by the user.

2.4. Dosing Adjustment

In order to individualize treatments, posologyr features several dosage optimization functions based on individual parameter estimates. The posologyr::poso_dose_conc and posologyr::poso_dose_auc functions determine the optimal dose to reach, respectively, a target concentration at a given time, or a target area under the time-concentration curve (AUC) over a given duration. The optimization is based on the minimization of the square of the difference between the desired target (target concentration, target AUC) and the result of the successive simulations. The posologyr::poso_time_cmin function determines by simulation the time needed to reach a target concentration (typical application: the therapeutic drug monitoring of aminoglycoside treatment). Finally, the posology::poso_inter_cmin function estimates the optimal inter-dose interval to reliably achieve a target trough concentration between each administration. All these functions allow optimization from MAP estimates of individual parameters, but also from posterior distributions. In the latter case, the set of probable profiles is simulated using RxODE, and the proportion p of the distribution to be considered for optimization is set by the user. For example, for posologyr::poso_dose_auc with $p = 0.5$, posologyr will determine the optimal dose so that 50% of the probable profiles reach or exceed the target AUC.

2.5. Validation

2.5.1. Point Estimate: MAP

To allow for an extensive comparison of the performance of posologyr estimates and NONMEM POSTHOC estimates [16] (NONMEM version 7.4.4, Dublin, Ireland: ICON), the validation of the posologyr MAP algorithm was performed following the methodology proposed by Le Louedec et al. [17]. The 35 population pharmacokinetic models (Table 1) were transcribed for posologyr (an example is given in Appendix A): default monocompartmental with linear elimination, bicompartmental, with various absorption models (lag-time, zero order, first order, combination of zero and first order kinetics, bioavailability), with nonlinear Michaelis–Menten elimination associated or not with linear elimination, with time-varying covariates, different residual error models (additive, proportional, mixed, log-additive), with two types of observations (parent–metabolite model), and finally with increasing levels of inter-individual variability (with variances ranging from 0.2 to 2).

Table 1. Test models.

Model Characteristics		Model Number (Number of Estimated Parameters)	
		Oral Administration	IV Administration
Monocompartmental (default)		1 (3)	2 (2)
Absorption	Lag time	3 (4)	/
	Zero-order in Central compartment	4 (3)	/
	Zero-order in Depot compartment	5 (4)	/
	Dual 0- and 1st orders	6 (4)	/
	Dual 1st orders	7 (4)	/
	Bioavailability	8 (4)	/
Distribution	Bicompartmental	101 (4)	102 (3)
Elimination	Michaelis–Menten (K_M, V_{MAX})	201 (4)	202 (3)
	Cl + Michaelis–Menten (K_M)	203 (4)	204 (3)
	Cl + Michaelis–Menten (V_{MAX})	205 (4)	206 (3)
	Cl + Michaelis–Menten (K_M, V_{MAX})	207 (5)	208 (4)
Time-Varying Covariates	Time-varying Cl	301 (3)	302 (2)
Residual Error Model	Metabolite	401 (5)	402 (4)
	Additive	403 (3)	404 (2)
	Mixed	405 (3)	406 (2)
	Log-additive	407 (3)	408 (2)
Inter-individual Variability (variance)	0.4 on all parameters	501 (3)	/
	0.6 on all parameters	502 (3)	/
	0.8 on all parameters	503 (3)	/
	1 on all parameters	504 (3)	/
	2 on Cl, 0.2 on Ka, Vc	511 (3)	/
	2 on Cl, Ka, 0.2 on Vc	512 (3)	/
	2 on all parameters	513 (3)	/

Abbreviations: Cl, clearance; IV, intravenous 1 h infusion; Ka, absorption rate; KM, Michaelis–Menten constant; Vc, central volume of distribution; VMAX, maximum rate; /, not applicable.

For models with time-varying covariates, the interpolation of variables between observations was performed using the "next observation carried backward" (nocb) approach, similar to NONMEM. The data set simulated by mrgsolve [18] included 4000 subjects per model, or 140,000 subjects in total. They were equally divided into 4 administration and sampling schemes: single administration and rich sampling, single administration and sparse sampling, multiple administration and rich sampling, and multiple administration and sparse sampling. Doses of 10, 30, 60, 80, or 120 mg were administered to each group. To address the nondeterministic nature of the selection of initial η_i for OFV minimization, the pseudorandom generator seed was set to an identical value for all estimates using the set.seed function of R.

2.5.2. Conditional Distributions

The estimates of the posologyr MCMC and SIR algorithms were compared to the estimates of the MCMC algorithm from the conditional distributions task of Monolix (version 2021R1. Antony, France: Lixoft SAS, 2020). As the computational time per individual was significantly higher than for the validation of the MAP algorithm, the validation was performed on a subset of the test models and the simulated subjects. The conditional distributions were estimated based on 10,000 samples of each algorithm, for each parameter. The SIR algorithm was run with settings $M = 10^6$ samples, and with $m = 10^4$ resampling runs. The MCMC algorithm of posologyr was run with 2 Markov chains, each starting with 200 burn-in iterations, discarded before drawing 5000 samples from each chain. The models tested were as follows: the default single-compartment model with oral administration (model #1); the model with lag-time (#3); the model with dual zero and first order absorption (#6); the bicompartmental model with oral administration (#101); the model with nonlinear Michaelis–Menten elimination and oral administration (#201); the model with both linear and nonlinear Michaelis–Menten elimination with oral administration (#207); the model with time-dependent clearance and oral administration (#301); the model with mixed residual error (#405); the model with variance of the random effects set to 1 for all parameters (#504); and the model with variance of random effects equal to 2 (#513). For the model with time-varying covariates, the interpolation of variables between observations was performed using the "last observation carried forward" (locf) approach, similar to Monolix [19]. For model #405, the mixed residual error model was set to combined1 in Monolix. To test the different administration and sampling schemes, 20 subjects were estimated for each model (to test each administration/sampling cohort, and every dose level), i.e., 200,000 parameter samples estimated per algorithm. To ensure reproducibility of the experiments, the pseudorandom generator seed was set to an identical value for all estimates using the set.seed function of R for posologyr, and in the project settings for Monolix.

2.6. Performance Analysis

2.6.1. Point Estimate: MAP

To allow comparability of the results of the performance evaluation of the MAP algorithm of posologyr, the primary endpoints were identical to those proposed by Le Louedec et al. [17]. The maximum absolute difference was obtained between posologyr ($\eta_{ik,\,PGYR}$) and NONMEM ($\eta_{ik,NM}$) for each individual according to the following expressions:

$$\Delta \hat{\eta}_{ik} = \left| \hat{\eta}_{ik,PGYR} - \hat{\eta}_{ik,NM} \right| \qquad (7)$$

$$\Delta \hat{\eta}_i = \max(\Delta \hat{\eta}_{ik}) \qquad (8)$$

where k is the length of the vector $\hat{\eta}_i$. Based on this definition, several performance thresholds were defined. For $\Delta \hat{\eta}_i < 0.001$, the estimate was considered excellent because, assuming an individual exponential model, with a lognormal distribution of individual parameters around a population median value, the impact on the parameter estimate would be negligible: $\Delta \psi_i < 0.1\%$. For $\Delta \hat{\eta}_i > 0.095$, the estimate was considered discordant ($\Delta \psi_i > 10\%$). The other estimates were considered acceptable. Finally, for each estimate, the final result of the calculation of the OFV from the MAP estimates of posologyr was compared to the OFV computed from the NONMEM POSTHOC estimates.

2.6.2. Conditional Distributions

Because of the stochastic nature of the estimation algorithms, and because of the multivariate nature of the individual parameter vectors, the isolated posterior distributions were not directly compared using numerical criteria. The validation endpoints were the bias between the results of three different dosage adjustment functions built into posologyr, taking the optimizations based on the posterior distributions produced using Monolix as the reference. For each subject, and each function, the bias was calculated as follows:

$$bias = \left| \frac{Output_{algorithm} - Output_{Monolix}}{Output_{Monolix}} \right| \qquad (9)$$

where $Output_{Monolix}$ is the result of the dose adjustment function based on the distribution of individual parameters estimated using Monolix, and $Output_{algorithm}$ is the result of the same dose adjustment function based on the distribution of individual parameters estimated using either MCMC or SIR. One scenario per function was tested:

- Determination of the optimal dose to reach a concentration of 30 mg/L, 3 h after administration, with posologyr::poso_dose_conc;
- Determination of the optimal dose to achieve an AUC0-12h of 500 mg·h/L, with posologyr::poso_dose_auc;

- Determination of the time to reach a trough concentration below 0.5 mg/L after a 100 mg dose, with posologyr::poso_time_cmin.

The p proportion was set at 0.89 in all cases. For all outcomes, the bias was considered acceptable when ≤10%.

3. Results

3.1. Point Estimate: MAP

The performance of the posologyr MAP algorithm was satisfactory. The estimates were excellent in 98.7% of the cases. The median $\Delta \hat{\eta}_i$ was 7.70×10^{-6}, and only 0.58% of all estimates were discordant (Figure 1). Representative pharmacokinetic profiles of excellent and discordant estimates, compared with NONMEM profiles, are given in Appendix B (Figure A1).

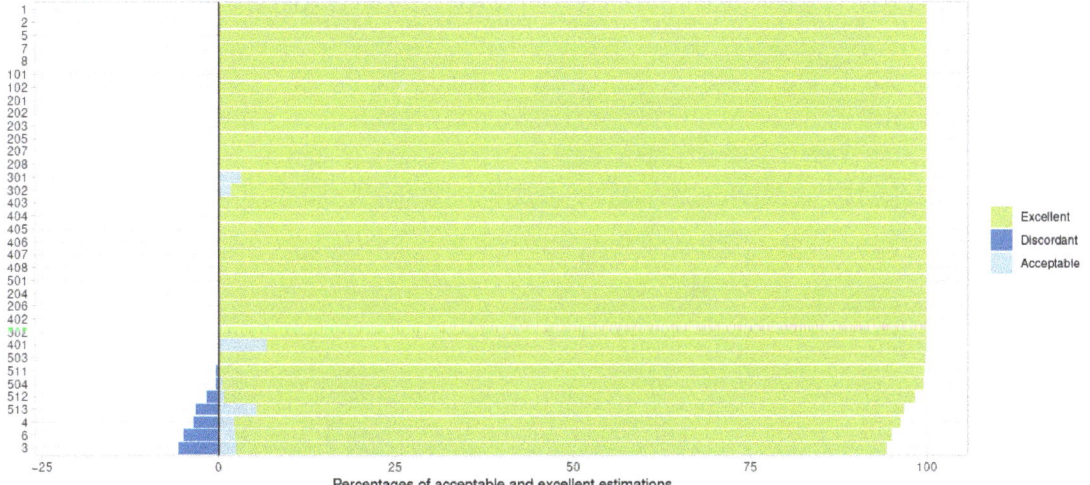

Figure 1. Performance of posologyr MAP estimation by test model. The negative percentages are the proportions of discordant estimates.

The greatest number of discordant estimates was observed for the models with lag-time (model #3), and those with zero order absorption in the central compartment (models #4 and #6). For these models, no discrepancies were found in the case of sparse sampling. In contrast, for the 6000 patients in models 3, 4, and 6 with rich sampling, 9.5% of the estimates were discordant. In the majority of these cases (402 of 570 subjects, or 70% of the estimates), the OFV associated with the posologyr estimate was lower than that calculated based on the NONMEM POSTHOC estimate, in support of a better performance of minimization when using posologyr, leading to the most likely value of $\hat{\eta}_i$. Discordant MAP estimates were also more frequently observed in models with increasing inter-individual variability (models #504, #511, #512 and #513), up to a maximum of 3.3% for model 513, irrespective of the administration or observation scheme. Again, for model #513, the posologyr OFVs were lower than the NONMEM POSTHOC estimate in most cases (24 subjects out of 4000, or 99.4%). Extending the above observation regarding OFV to all 140,000 simulated subjects, the estimates produced using posologyr were outperformed by the NONMEM POSTHOC estimate in only 0.14% of cases.

3.2. Posterior Distribution

The performance of the SIR algorithm was satisfactory. Using the posologyr::poso_dose_conc and posologyr::poso_dose_auc functions, the bias on dosage adjustment proposals based on SIR estimates was acceptable in 97% of cases (Figures 2 and 3). The median bias was 0.65% (minimum: 0.00%, maximum: 31.41%). Elimination time predictions using posologyr::poso_time_cmin were acceptable in 99.5% of cases (all but one subject) and the median bias was 0.14% (minimum: 0.00%, maximum: 23.16%).

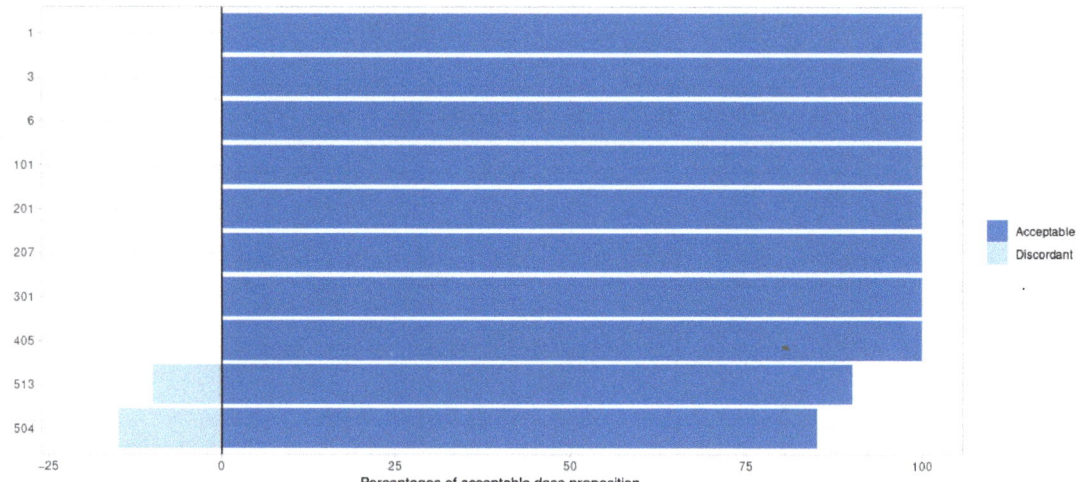

Figure 2. Adequacy of dose adaptation by tested model for a target AUC based on SIR posterior estimates. The negative percentages are the proportions of discordant propositions.

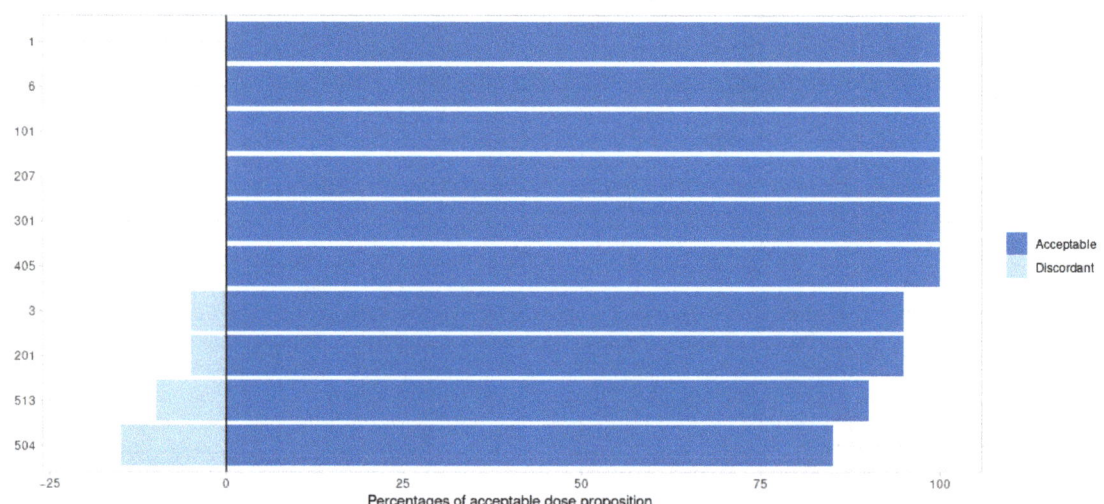

Figure 3. Adequacy of dose adaptation by tested model for a target concentration based on SIR posterior estimates. The negative percentages are the proportions of discordant propositions.

All outcomes considered, the greatest number of discordances between SIR and Monolix was observed for models with significant inter-individual variability (#504 and #513): 8.3%. For these subjects, proposals based on estimates from the MCMC algorithm implemented in posologyr were discordant with propositions based on Monolix estimates in 10.8% of cases. For the entire dataset, the estimates produced using MCMC exhibited 4.17% discrepancies with Monolix, with a median bias of 0.77%.

For illustration purposes, the density curves of the posterior distributions computed using the different algorithms for subject #1, model #003 are presented in Figure 4.

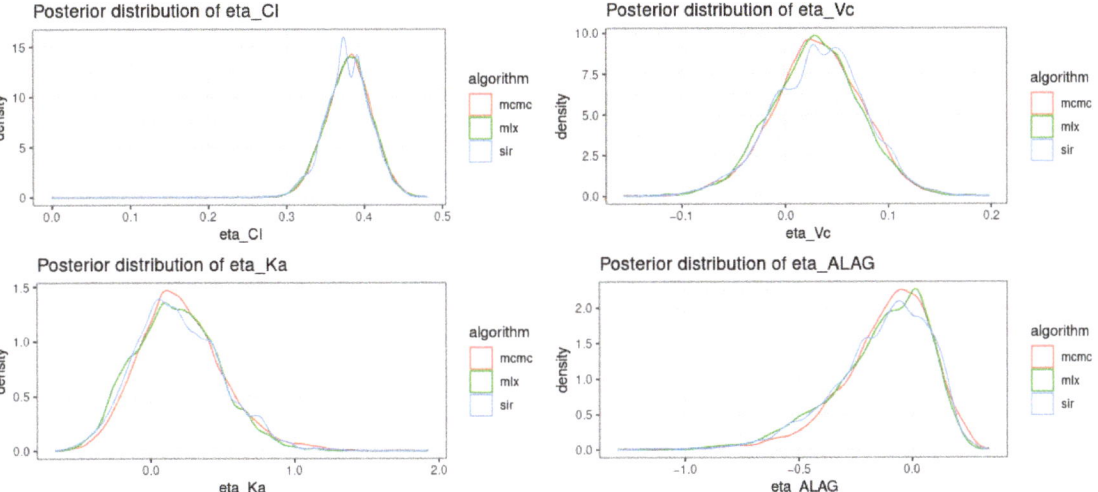

Figure 4. Density plots of the posterior distributions of η_i for subject #1 with model #003. mcmc, the MCMC algorithm implemented in posologyr; mlx, the MCMC algorithm of Monolix; sir, the SIR algorithm of posologyr; Cl, clearance; Ka, absorption rate; Vc, central volume of distribution; ALAG, lag-time.

4. Discussion

A free and open-source software has been developed to allow for the Bayesian individualization of treatments. The performance of posologyr for individual parameter estimation was benchmarked against NONMEM for MAP point estimates and against Monolix for the estimation of full posterior distributions of individual parameters.

The MAP optimization function of posologyr showed excellent performance compared to NONMEM for a wide variety of models and pharmacokinetic profiles. In particular, agreement with NONMEM's POSTHOC estimates was excellent for the single-compartment and two-compartment models, the models with nonlinear Michaelis–Menten elimination, the model with time-dependent clearance, and the various residual error models, for values of inter-individual variability lower than 1.

A greater number of discrepancies was observed for the different absorption models, especially following administration with lag-time. This type of model produces discontinuous time-concentration profiles, which to some degree may be responsible for difficulties in determining the optimal values of individual parameters [20]. An increasing, but small, number of discrepancies was also observed for increasing values of inter-individual variability. In these different cases, under the assumption that the OFV calculated from the estimated individual parameters [10] is a satisfactory reflection of the minimization performance, posologyr outperformed NONMEM's POSTHOC estimates for the majority of discordances.

The SIR algorithm implemented in posologyr demonstrated satisfactory performance on the evaluated scenarios. The estimates of the posterior distributions of individual parameters led to dose adjustment proposals comparable to those based on the Monolix estimates. The execution time of the different algorithms was not formally evaluated; however, the observations made during this study showed that the time required to obtain 10,000 samples was 15 times shorter with the SIR algorithm of posologyr than with the MCMC algorithm of posologyr. These results are reassuring with regard to the feasibility of developing a probabilistic MIPD tool in R, opening the door to personalized treatment options informed by knowledge of the uncertainty associated with individual parameter estimation [6]. Still, in this preliminary study, the simulated population tested was limited to 200 patients, with one scenario per function, and a single probability threshold; these exploratory results need to be confirmed before considering the application of this methodology to therapeutic drug monitoring. A thorough evaluation of the performance of SIR will be necessary in order to define the precise scope of its application according to model types, sampling schemes, and patient profiles. The evaluation of different sample sizes, and resampling numbers, would also allow for the optimization of runtime without foregoing estimation quality.

The posologyr software is, and will remain, free and open source under the AGPLv3 license [8]. Now available at https://github.com/levenc/posologyr (accessed on 15 January 2022), it is scheduled for release via the comprehensive R archive network (CRAN) soon. These decisions to make the software easy to distribute and to guarantee its external auditability serve the purpose for which posologyr was developed: to provide a foundation for future Bayesian dosage individualization tools.

Author Contributions: Conceptualization, C.L.; methodology, C.L., A.C. and C.M.; software, C.L.; validation, C.L., A.C. and C.M.; writing—original draft preparation, C.L, C.M.; writing—review and editing, C.L., A.C. and C.M.; All authors have read and agreed to the published version of the manuscript.

Funding: This research received no external funding.

Institutional Review Board Statement: Not applicable.

Informed Consent Statement: Not applicable.

Data Availability Statement: Data supporting the reported results can be found at https://github.com/levenc/posologyr-pharmaceutics (accessed on 15 January 2022).

Acknowledgments: We are thankful to Sasha Schutz for providing computing power useful for this work, and to Pauline Ménard for her insights throughout the development of posologyr.

Conflicts of Interest: The authors declare no conflict of interest.

Appendix A

Model #207 transcribed for posologyr, to match NONMEM estimates:

```
mod_run207 <- list(
  ppk_model   = RxODE::RxODE({
    centr(0) = 0;
    depot(0) = 0;

    TVVmax= THETA_Vmax;
    TVVc  = THETA_Vc;
    TVKa  = THETA_Ka;
    TVKm  = THETA_Km;
    TVCl  = THETA_Cl;

    Vmax  = TVVmax*exp(ETA_Vmax);
    Vc    = TVVc*exp(ETA_Vc);
    Ka    = TVKa*exp(ETA_Ka);
    Km    = TVKm*exp(ETA_Km);
    Cl    = TVCl*exp(ETA_Cl);

    Cc    = centr/Vc;
    Ke    = Cl/Vc;

    d/dt(depot)  = - Ka*depot;
```

```
            d/dt(centr)   =    Ka*depot - Vmax*(centr/Vc)/(Km+(centr/Vc)) - Ke*centr;
            d/dt(AUC)     =    Cc;
        }),
        error_model = function(f,sigma){
            dv <- cbind(f,1)
            g  <- diag(dv%*%sigma%*%t(dv))
            return(sqrt(g))
        },
        theta = c(THETA_Vmax=10000, THETA_Vc=70.0, THETA_Ka=1.0, THETA_Km=2500,
THETA_Cl=4.0),
        omega = lotri::lotri({ETA_Vmax + ETA_Vc + ETA_Ka + ETA_Km + ETA_Cl ~
            c(0.2    ,
              0      ,     0.2,
              0      ,     0,     0.2,
              0      ,     0,     0,     0.2,
              0      ,     0,     0,     0,     0.2)}),
        sigma       = lotri::lotri({prop + add ~ c(0.05,0.0,0.00)}))
```

Model #207 transcribed for posologyr, to match Monolix estimates:
```
mod_dist_run207 <- list(
    ppk_model   = RxODE::RxODE({
        centr(0) = 0;
        depot(0) = 0;

        TVVmax= THETA_Vmax;
        TVVc  = THETA_Vc;
        TVKa  = THETA_Ka;
        TVKm  = THETA_Km;
        TVCl  = THETA_Cl;

        Vmax  = TVVmax*exp(ETA_Vmax);
        Vc    = TVVc*exp(ETA_Vc);
        Ka    = TVKa*exp(ETA_Ka);
        Km    = TVKm*exp(ETA_Km);
        Cl    = TVCl*exp(ETA_Cl);

        Cc    = centr/Vc;
        Ke    = Cl/Vc;

        d/dt(depot)   = - Ka*depot;
        d/dt(centr)   =   Ka*depot - Vmax*(centr/Vc)/(Km+(centr/Vc)) - Ke*centr;
        d/dt(AUC)     =   Cc;
    }),
    error_model = function(f,sigma){
        g <- sigma[2] + sigma[1]*f
        return(g)
    },
    theta = c(THETA_Vmax=10000, THETA_Vc=70.0, THETA_Ka=1.0, THETA_Km=2500,
THETA_Cl=4.0),
        omega = lotri::lotri({ETA_Vmax + ETA_Vc + ETA_Ka + ETA_Km + ETA_Cl ~
            c(0.2    ,
              0      ,     0.2,
              0      ,     0,     0.2,
              0      ,     0,     0,     0.2,
```

$$\left.\begin{array}{cccccc} & 0 & , & 0, & 0, & 0, & 0.2)\}),\\ \text{sigma} & = c(\text{b\_prop}=0.05, \text{a\_add}=0.00) \end{array}\right)$$

Appendix B

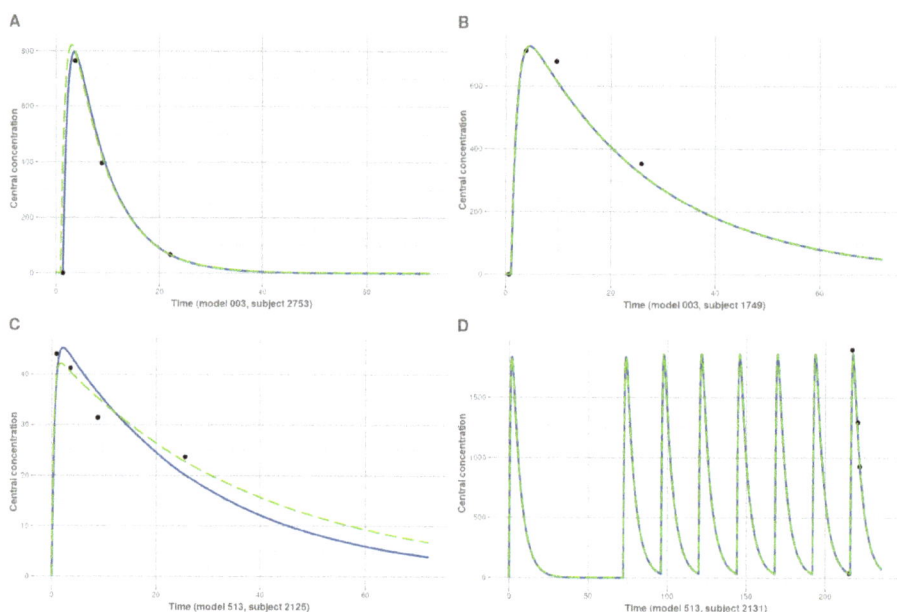

Figure A1. Simulated pharmacokinetic profiles from MAP estimates of posologyr (blue solid line) and NONMEM (green dashed line). (**A,C**): discordant profiles ($\Delta \hat{\eta}_i > 0.050$). (**B,D**): concordant profiles ($\Delta \hat{\eta}_i < 0.001$). Black dots: observed concentrations.

References

1. Keizer, R.J.; ter Heine, R.; Frymoyer, A.; Lesko, L.J.; Mangat, R.; Goswami, S. Model-Informed Precision Dosing at the Bedside: Scientific Challenges and Opportunities. *CPT Pharmacomet. Syst. Pharmacol.* **2018**, *7*, 785–787. [CrossRef] [PubMed]
2. Frymoyer, A.; Schwenk, H.T.; Zorn, Y.; Bio, L.; Moss, J.D.; Chasmawala, B.; Faulkenberry, J.; Goswami, S.; Keizer, R.J.; Ghaskari, S. Model-Informed Precision Dosing of Vancomycin in Hospitalized Children: Implementation and Adoption at an Academic Children's Hospital. *Front. Pharmacol.* **2020**, *11*, 551. [CrossRef]
3. Proost, J.H.; Meijer, D.K.F. MW/Pharm, an Integrated Software Package for Drug Dosage Regimen Calculation and Therapeutic Drug Monitoring. *Comput. Biol. Med.* **1992**, *22*, 155–163. [CrossRef]
4. Wicha, S.G.; Kees, M.G.; Solms, A.; Minichmayr, I.K.; Kratzer, A.; Kloft, C. TDMx: A Novel Web-Based Open-Access Support Tool for Optimising Antimicrobial Dosing Regimens in Clinical Routine. *Int. J. Antimicrob. Agents* **2015**, *45*, 442–444. [CrossRef] [PubMed]
5. Drennan, P.; Doogue, M.; van Hal, S.J.; Chin, P. Bayesian Therapeutic Drug Monitoring Software: Past, Present and Future. *Int. J. Pharmacokinet.* **2018**, *3*, 109–114. [CrossRef]
6. Maier, C.; Hartung, N.; de Wiljes, J.; Kloft, C.; Huisinga, W. Bayesian Data Assimilation to Support Informed Decision Making in Individualized Chemotherapy. *CPT Pharmacomet. Syst. Pharmacol.* **2020**, *9*, 153–164. [CrossRef] [PubMed]
7. R Core Team. *R: A Language and Environment for Statistical Computing*; R Foundation for Statistical Computing: Vienna, Austria, 2022.
8. GNU Affero General Public License—GNU Project—Free Software Foundation. Available online: https://www.gnu.org/licenses/agpl-3.0.en.html (accessed on 15 January 2022).
9. Bonate, P.L. Nonlinear Mixed Effects Models: Theory. In *Pharmacokinetic-Pharmacodynamic Modeling and Simulation*; Bonate, P.L., Ed.; Springer: Boston, MA, USA, 2011; pp. 233–301; ISBN 978-1-4419-9485-1.
10. Kang, D.; Bae, K.-S.; Houk, B.E.; Savic, R.M.; Karlsson, M.O. Standard Error of Empirical Bayes Estimate in NONMEM®VI. *Korean J. Physiol. Pharmacol. Off. J. Korean Physiol. Soc. Korean Soc. Pharmacol.* **2012**, *16*, 97–106. [CrossRef] [PubMed]

11. Dosne, A.-G.; Bergstrand, M.; Karlsson, M.O. An Automated Sampling Importance Resampling Procedure for Estimating Parameter Uncertainty. *J. Pharmacokinet. Pharmacodyn.* **2017**, *44*, 509–520. [CrossRef] [PubMed]
12. Wang, W.; Hallow, K.; James, D. A Tutorial on RxODE: Simulating Differential Equation Pharmacometric Models in R. *CPT Pharmacomet. Syst. Pharmacol.* **2016**, *5*, 3–10. [CrossRef] [PubMed]
13. Byrd, R.H.; Lu, P.; Nocedal, J.; Zhu, C. A Limited Memory Algorithm for Bound Constrained Optimization. *SIAM J. Sci. Comput.* **1995**, *16*, 1190–1208. [CrossRef]
14. Comets, E.; Lavenu, A.; Lavielle, M. Parameter Estimation in Nonlinear Mixed Effect Models Using Saemix, an R Implementation of the SAEM Algorithm. *J. Stat. Softw.* **2017**, *80*, 1–41. [CrossRef]
15. Conditional Distribution Calculation Using Monolix. Available online: https://monolix.lixoft.com/tasks/conditional-distribution/ (accessed on 15 January 2022).
16. Nonmem 7.4 Users Guides. Available online: https://nonmem.iconplc.com/#/nonmem744/guides (accessed on 15 January 2022).
17. Le Louedec, F.; Puisset, F.; Thomas, F.; Chatelut, É.; White-Koning, M. Easy and Reliable Maximum a Posteriori Bayesian Estimation of Pharmacokinetic Parameters with the Open-Source R Package Mapbayr. *CPT Pharmacomet. Syst. Pharmacol.* **2021**, *10*, 1208–1220. [CrossRef] [PubMed]
18. Elmokadem, A.; Riggs, M.M.; Baron, K.T. Quantitative Systems Pharmacology and Physiologically-Based Pharmacokinetic Modeling With Mrgsolve: A Hands-On Tutorial. *CPT Pharmacomet. Syst. Pharmacol.* **2019**, *8*, 883–893. [CrossRef] [PubMed]
19. Using Regression Variables in Monolix. Available online: https://monolix.lixoft.com/data-and-models/regressor/ (accessed on 15 January 2022).
20. Savic, R.M.; Jonker, D.M.; Kerbusch, T.; Karlsson, M.O. Implementation of a Transit Compartment Model for Describing Drug Absorption in Pharmacokinetic Studies. *J. Pharmacokinet. Pharmacodyn.* **2007**, *34*, 711–726. [CrossRef] [PubMed]

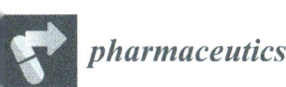

Article

Model-Based Equivalent Dose Optimization to Develop New Donepezil Patch Formulation

Woojin Jung [1,†], Heeyoon Jung [1,†], Ngoc-Anh Thi Vu [1,†], Gwan-Young Kim [2], Gyoung-Won Kim [2], Jung-woo Chae [1,*], Taeheon Kim [1,2,*] and Hwi-yeol Yun [1,*]

- [1] College of Pharmacy, Chungnam National University, Daejeon 34134, Korea; tnzo12@o.cnu.ac.kr (W.J.); hy93.jung@o.cnu.ac.kr (H.J.); ngocanhzunie@o.cnu.ac.kr (N.-A.T.V.)
- [2] Life Science Research Institute, Daewoong Pharmaceuticals, Yongin-si 17028, Korea; pharmrich@daewoong.co.kr (G.-Y.K.); kchemist@daewoong.co.kr (G.-W.K.)
- * Correspondence: jwchae@cnu.ac.kr (J.-w.C.); luluokj@gmail.com (T.K.); hyyun@cnu.ac.kr (H.-y.Y.)
- † These authors contributed equally to this work as first author.

Abstract: Donepezil patch was developed to replace the original oral formulation. To accurately describe the pharmacokinetics of donepezil and investigate compatible doses between two formulations, a population pharmacokinetic model for oral and transdermal patches was built based on a clinical study. Plasma donepezil levels were analyzed via liquid chromatography/tandem mass spectrometry. Non-compartmental analyses were performed to derive the initial parameters for compartmental analyses. Compartmental analysis (CA) was performed with NLME software NONMEM assisted by Perl-speaks-NONMEM, and R. Model evaluation was proceeded via visual predictive checks (VPC), goodness-of-fit (GOF) plotting, and bootstrap method. The bioequivalence test was based on a 2 × 2 crossover design, and parameters of AUC and C_{max} were considered. We found that a two-compartment model featuring two transit compartments accurately describes the pharmacokinetics of nine subjects administered in oral, as well as of the patch-dosed subjects. Through evaluation, the model was proven to be sufficiently accurate and suitable for further bioequivalence tests. Based on the bioequivalence test, 114 mg/101.3 cm^2–146 mg/129.8 cm^2 of donepezil patch per week was equivalent to 10 mg PO donepezil per day. In conclusion, the pharmacokinetic model was successfully developed, and acceptable parameters were estimated. However, the size calculated by an equivalent dose of donepezil patch could be rather large. Further optimization in formulation needs to be performed to find appropriate usability in clinical situations.

Keywords: donepezil; transdermal patch; equivalent dose optimization; model-based approaches

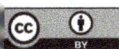

1. Introduction

Donepezil is frequently prescribed to treat Alzheimer's disease (AD). The drug enhances cognitive function by inhibiting acetylcholine esterase (which degrades acetylcholine), thus increasing acetylcholine concentrations in the central nervous system. This is thought to prevent further degeneration of brain function. Currently, donepezil is approved for the symptomatic treatment of AD, characterized by a long half-life in physiological conditions [1,2]. In several clinical trials, cholinesterase inhibitors (including donepezil) slowed long-term AD development and exhibited suitable tolerability and safety profiles [3–8]. Donepezil 5–10 mg daily is an approved treatment for mild to moderate AD, and a dose of 10–23 mg daily can be used to treat moderate to severe AD.

If a drug is to be taken orally, patient compliance is a major issue. AD patients suffer from cognitive dysfunction. Thus, efforts have been made to increase the efficacy of donepezil by modifying the formulations and using extended-release tablets and transdermal patches. In a previous study on medication-nonadherent AD patients, those with transdermal donepezil patches tended to be more compliant than patients on tablets or capsules [9]. A transdermal patch prolonged treatment duration and patient adherence and stabilized drug levels between dosing intervals. Moreover, the medication was readily controlled by attaching or removing patches. In addition, avoidance of gastrointestinal incompatibility and the first-pass effect of the liver offers huge benefits [10].

The most common method to prove bioequivalence between two different formulations is to perform two-one-sided tests (TOST) followed by non-compartmental analysis (NCA) [11]. Pharmacokinetic parameters such as AUC (area under plasma concentration curve) and C_{max} (peak concentration) are calculated for both sides. Their ratios are considered for determination. If the PK variability of a drug is high, the risk of a type I error increases. Models such as the non-linear mixed effect model (NLME) can quantify and distinguish between different kinds of variabilities represented as between-subject variability (BSV) and within-subject variability (WSV). The model-based bioequivalent approach is widely accepted in cases such as clinical trials with sparse sampling points, uneven samplings between individuals caused by missing values, drugs with a long half-life and high variabilities, and steady state-inducing studies [12].

When developing an extended-release donepezil formulation, it is essential to derive C_{max} and AUC values in bioequivalent doses. In general, transdermal patches exhibit PK profiles that differ from those of orally administered drugs. In transdermal dosing, the drug absorption process into the systemic circulation is slower than oral dosing in general, resulting in smaller gaps between concentration peaks and troughs in a similar administration condition. It is thus difficult to harmonize the C_{max} and AUC of a transdermal patch, which reduces the bioequivalence margin. PK profiling of transdermal drug delivery is compromised by high-level variability. Individual skin characteristics and metabolic differences affect drug diffusion.

As mentioned previously, NLME model-based, equivalent dose optimization not only yields optimal doses for bioequivalent trials but also facilitates dosing in clinical trials; this is model-informed drug discovery. Here we compared test transdermal formulation and reference oral formulation that differed in terms of the dosing schedule. Bioequivalence data were derived from the secondary PK parameters of an iterative, simulated clinical study. Then the optimal extended-release donepezil formulation was further investigated.

2. Materials and Methods

2.1. Clinical Study Design

A randomized, open-label, two-treatment, two-sequence, two-period (period I and II, washout period in between), two-way crossover comparative bioequivalence study was conducted in healthy male volunteers. The PK models of the donepezil patch and oral formulations were derived from the clinical data sets of the TL/WZ/19/001141 study, which adhered to the guidelines of the Declaration of Helsinki, good clinical practice, and the International Conference on Harmonization. Twelve healthy subjects aged 18–45 years with a body mass index 18.5–30.0 kg/m^2 were enrolled; all provided written informed consent. The clinical study protocol was approved by the institutional review board of Raptim Research Ltd. (Mumbai, India; IORG no. IORG0009526, DCGI reg. no. ECR/224/Indt/MH/2015/RR-18). Each subject was healthy on physical examination, medical history taken, and standard clinical laboratory tests. Exclusion criteria included any significant history or current evidence of malignancy; chronic infection; cardiovascular, renal, hepatic, ophthalmic, pulmonary, neurological, metabolic (endocrine), hematological, gastrointestinal, immunological, or psychiatric disease; and/or organ dysfunction. In addition, any history of allergy or hypersensitivity to or intolerance of donepezil or its excipients that, in the opinion of a clinical investigator, would compromise safety-triggered exclusion.

Donepezil dose for humans was decided from in vivo pre-clinical experiments with rats and minipigs in reference to in vitro skin permeability tests. The human equivalent dose for donepezil in the formulation was converted on the basis of body surface area.

We placed donepezil patches (108 mg/96 cm^2) on the torsos or backs of six test subjects for 1 week, followed by a washout period of at least 21 days (to exclude any carryover effect). The controls received donepezil tablets (Aricept; 10 mg) once a day for 1 week, a total of seven times of dose.

2.2. Preparation of Donepezil Patch

The donepezil-loaded patch was prepared using the solvent casting method reported in the previous experiment, with a slight modification (Jung et al., 2019). Oppanol® N100 (15%, w/w) was dissolved in toluene, while Oppanol® B15 and B12 were prepared at a concentration of 50% (w/w) in the mixture of toluene and n-heptane (1:1, w/w). Kristalex™ F85 hydrocarbon resin was dissolved in toluene to obtain a final concentration of 80% (w/w). These solutions were mixed with homomixer (HIVIS MIX model 2P-03, PROMIX, Japan) at 50 rpm for 2 h by varying the ratio of each component of the donepezil-containing patch. Then, the final solution was left for 1 h to remove air bubbles and set to a thickness of 100 or 200 μm applied to the release liner (Silicone-coated polyester film 7300A, Loparex, Cary, NC, USA), and dried at 90 °C for 10 min using labcoater (CH-8156, Mathis AG, Oberhasli, Switzerland). Backing membrane (Scotchpak™ 1012 PET film, 3M, St.Paul, MN, USA) was attached to the dried patch, and the patch was cut into 10 cm^2 (3.16 × 3.16 cm) or 20 cm^2 (4.47 × 4.47 cm) sizes and packed in an aluminum foil pouch (ALLS 819202, Amcor, Gent, Belgium). All patches were sealed with a bag sealer (Lovero, Wenzhou, Zhejiang, China) and stored at room temperature before use.

In summary, Oppanol® N100, B12, and B15 were used as an adhesive and Kristalex™ F85 hydrocarbon resin as a tackifier. BHT, LP300 or NMP, Kristalex™ F85, and mineral oil was used as stabilizer, permeation enhancer, tackifier, and plasticizer, respectively.

2.3. Quantitative Analysis of Donepezil in Plasma Using LC-MS/MS

Blood samples for donepezil assay were collected before dosing (within 2 h prior to administration) and 4, 8, 12, 24, 48, 70, 72, 74, 76, 80, 96, 120, 144, 168, 216, 264, and 312 h after administration. Samples were placed in prelabeled vacutainers with K3EDTA, centrifuged at 4000 rpm for 10 min at 5 °C, and the plasma stored at −80 °C. We determined plasma concentrations of donepezil using a high-performance liquid chromatography MS/MS system equipped with a pump (LC-30AD, Shimadzu, Kyoto, Japan) and an API3500 mass spectrometer. Donepezil and donepezil-d7 (internal standard) were separated on a reverse-phase C18 Gemini column (4.6 × 50 mm, 3 μm). The mobile phase was acetonitrile:5 mM ammonium acetate (90:10, v/v), and the flow rate was 0.6 mL/min. The oven temperature was 50 °C, and the injection volume was 5 μL. An electrospray ionization interface operating in the positive ion multiple reaction monitoring mode served as the ion source. The m/z values of the precursor/product ions of donepezil ranged from 380.2 to 91.0; the dwell time and collision energy were 200 ms and 48 V, respectively. The figures for donepezil-d7 were 387.2 to 98.1, 200 ms, and 45 V, respectively. The retention times of donepezil and IS were 1.32 and 1.28 min, respectively. The calibration curves were linear over the range 0.40–85.14 ng/mL. The curve precision and accuracy were 92.6–106.9 and 4.3%, respectively. The results of bioanalytical method validation were summarized in Supplementary Data (Tables S1 and S2 and Figure S1).

2.4. Model Development

Non-compartmental parameters were calculated with the R package ncappc [13]. We derived the C_{max}, T_{max}, AUC_{last}, AUC_{inf}, λ_z, half-life (based on Λ-z), V_z (volume of distribution, observed), and CL (clearance, observed). The parameter distributions were evaluated, and the results were used to set the initial parameters for CA.

When performing CA, an adequate model structure had chosen to describe the drug concentration profile for each formulation. Parameter estimation was performed with the first-order conditional estimation with interaction (FOCE-I) method. Interindividual variabilities were modeled exponentially, additively, and proportionally. In deciding the error model for residual variability, additive, proportional, and combined error models were tested [14]. We evaluated the adequacy of the parameters by calculating the decrease in the objective function value. Data analyses were performed with NLME software NONMEM (version 7.4; Icon Development Solutions, Ellicott City, MD, USA) assisted by Perl-speaks NONMEM (PsN; version 5.2.6), R (version 4.1.1), and Rstudio (version 1.4.1717).

Model evaluation was performed with PsN, and the R packages xpose and xpose4. We drew goodness-of-fit (GOF) plots (including conditional weighted residuals) and used a visual predictive check (VPC) to compare model predictions against observations. In terms of nonparametric diagnostics, bootstrap (1000 replicates) was performed to evaluate the precision of the final estimates.

2.5. Simulation to Optimize Equivalent Dose

The bioequivalence test of the oral and patch donepezil was based on a 2 × 2 crossover design. We simulated data for 200 patients (100 each in the oral and patch groups). The integrated donepezil PK model was used for simulation. The principal parameters used to evaluate bioequivalence are the AUC and C_{max} [15]. The plasma concentration-time values from simulation were analyzed with R version 1.4.1 to obtain the AUC and C_{max} for each patient 672 to 840 h after administration (when the level of donepezil would be in the steady state). We used an iterative process using various patch doses to determine the dose that was bioequivalent to 10 mg oral donepezil. AUC and C_{max} ratios within 0.8–1.25 of the 90% confidence intervals (CIs) served as the bioequivalence criteria [15].

3. Results

3.1. Subject Demographics and NCA

Twelve healthy volunteers were enrolled, but only nine completed the study. Three subjects (two in the test group and one in the control group) withdrew (for personal reasons) in periods I and II. Data from the nine who completed both periods were used to develop the PK model and for statistical analyses (Table 1). The test and reference products were safe and well tolerated by fasting subjects. Four adverse events were reported during the study, and one was reported during the post-study safety assessment. There was no serious adverse event or major concern.

Table 1. Demographic and baseline data (n = 09) of evaluable subjects.

Parameter	Age (yrs)	Weight (kg)	Height (cm)	BMI (kg/m^2)
Mean	29.56	66.11	165.94	24.00
SD	2.88	9.54	7.02	2.99
Median	30.00	63.10	168.40	24.67
Min	24.00	55.70	150.60	19.78
Max	33.00	80.90	173.60	27.33
%CV	9.73	14.43	4.23	12.46
Sex				
Male			09 (100%)	
Female			00	
Race				
Asian			09 (100%)	
Other			00	

Three subjects (two in the test group and another in the control group) withdrew from the study (for personal reasons) in periods I and II.

NCA was performed with data to 24 h after oral administration and with oral and patch data over the entire period. The C_{max}, T_{max}, and AUC values are listed in Table 2.

Table 2. NCA parameters by study group.

Parameters Mean (SD)	Oral (0–24 h)	Oral (0–312 h)	Patch (0–312 h)
C_{max}	20.26 (5.24)	53.86 (12.60)	28.62 (8.70)
T_{max}	3.11 (1.17)	146.33 (0.87)	106.67 (41.76)
AUC_{last}	286.62 (75.47)	6111.08 (2245.90)	5285.59 (1892.27)
AUC_{inf}	575.02 (242.57)	6873.40 (2772.54)	5909.34 (2291.77)
Λz	0.03 (0.01)	0.02 (0.01)	0.01 (0.0017)
HL	22.25 (4.95)	37.74 (11.60)	71.17 (11.95)
Vz	590 (130)	-	1080 (280)
Vss	-	560 (140)	-
Cl	20 (10)	10 (0.0030)	10 (0.0031)

SS: steady state, NS: non-steady state, C_{max}: peak concentration, T_{max}: peak time, AUC: area under curve, HL: half-life (based on Λ-z), Vz: volume of distribution (observed), Cl: clearance (observed), Vss: volume of distribution (steady state, observed).

3.2. Model Development

We developed a two-compartment PK model to describe the elimination of orally administered donepezil. The FOCE-I method best described the drug concentrations. The drug amount put in the gut is transferred to the central compartment at a first-order rate (Equation (1)).

$$\frac{dGUT}{dt} = -KA \cdot GUT, \quad (1)$$

where *GUT* stands for the drug amount disposed in the gut and *KA* for the rate of absorption in the gastrointestinal tract.

The drug disposed in skin by transdermal patch form passes through additional transit compartments; absorption by central compartments is thus delayed (Equation (2)). The drug amount that enters the skin (from the patch depot) was related to the patch dissolution percentage over time. We fit the relevant equation using in vitro data (Table S3). The amount of drug disposed on the skin is decided by coefficient driven from the difference between in vitro experiment and mean released amount measured by remains in the patch after clinical trial (Equation (3)).

$$\frac{dSKIN}{dt} = -KT \cdot SKIN,$$
$$\frac{dTR1}{dt} = KT \cdot SKIN - KT \cdot TR1, \quad (2)$$
$$\frac{dTR2}{dt} = KT \cdot TR1 - KT \cdot TR2,$$

$$Drug\ dissolution = \frac{78.257 \cdot Duration}{Duration + 8.481} \% \cdot Patch\ dose, \quad (3)$$

$$Disposed\ amount\ in\ skin = 0.74 \cdot Drug\ dissolution,$$

where *SKIN* stands for the drug amount disposed in the skin from the formulation, *KT* for the rate of drug transfer/absorption to the central compartment. *TR1* and *TR2* represent the amount of the drug in the middle of transition. In Equation (3), Duration means the time with patch attached in hours.

The central compartment receives drug amounts from both gut and skin, exchanges given amounts with the peripheral compartment, and eliminates at a rate of first-order kinetics (Equation (4))

$$\frac{dCENT}{dt} = KA \cdot SKIN + KT \cdot TR2 + KPC \cdot PERI - KCP \cdot CENT - KE \cdot CENT,$$

$$KE = CL/V_{cent},$$

$$KCP = Q/V_{cent}, \ KPC = Q/V_{peri},$$

(4)

where $CENT$ and $PERI$ stand for drug amount in central and peripheral compartment, KE for elimination constant, CL for clearance of oral and patch, V_{cent} and V_{peri} for central and peripheral compartments' volume of distribution. Q stands for intercompartmental clearance between central and peripheral compartments. The patch and oral doses are eliminated in the same compartment, but the clearances differ when the drug remains in the patch (Figure 1).

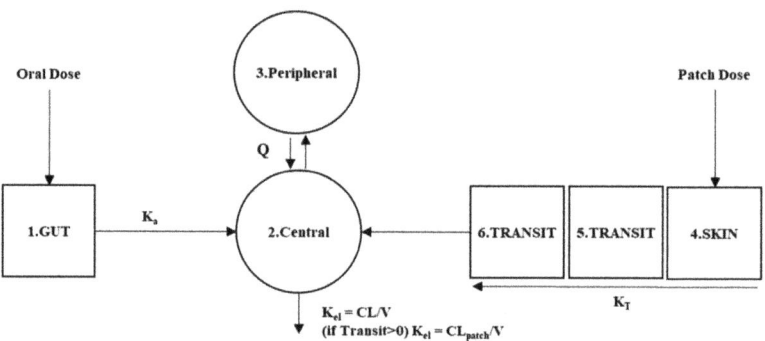

Figure 1. Compartmental scheme for oral and transdermal patch combined donepezil model used for bioequivalence test.

The GOF plots of observations versus predictions showed that the model predictions were reasonable. Most conditional weighted residual values were included within ±2, and the trends lay around zero (Figure S2). The VPC revealed that the model simultaneously handled both oral and patch administration of the drug (Figure 2). With 1000 newly generated data set with the bootstrap method, 992 successful runs were observed, indicating the model's robustness is sufficient. The model estimations are summarized in Table 3.

Table 3. The final parameter estimates of the donepezil integrated PK model.

	Parameter	Estimates (RSE%)	IIV (RSE%) [Shr%]	IIV in CV%
Oral	Ka (1/h)	0.0497 (25%)	0.00968 (28%) [51%]	9.9%
	CL (L/h)	10 (9%)	0.13 (12%) [0%]	37.3%
	Vc (L)	26.2 (35%)	0.198 (33%) [42%]	46.8%
	Q (L/h)	15.6 (33%)		
	Vp (L)	562 (11%)		
Patch	Kt (1/hr)	0.027 (9%)	0.02 (37%) [31%]	14.2%
		Residual variability (RSE%)		
Total	Additive error	2.89 (13%)		
	Proportional error	0.0795 (29%)		
	OFV	1443.703		

RSE: relative standard error, Shr: shrinkage, IIV: interindividual variability, CV: coefficient of variation, Ka: absorption rate constant, Vc: central volume of distribution, Vp: peripheral volume of distribution, Q: intercompartmental clearance, CL: clearance on central volume, Kt: rate constant for transit compartment.

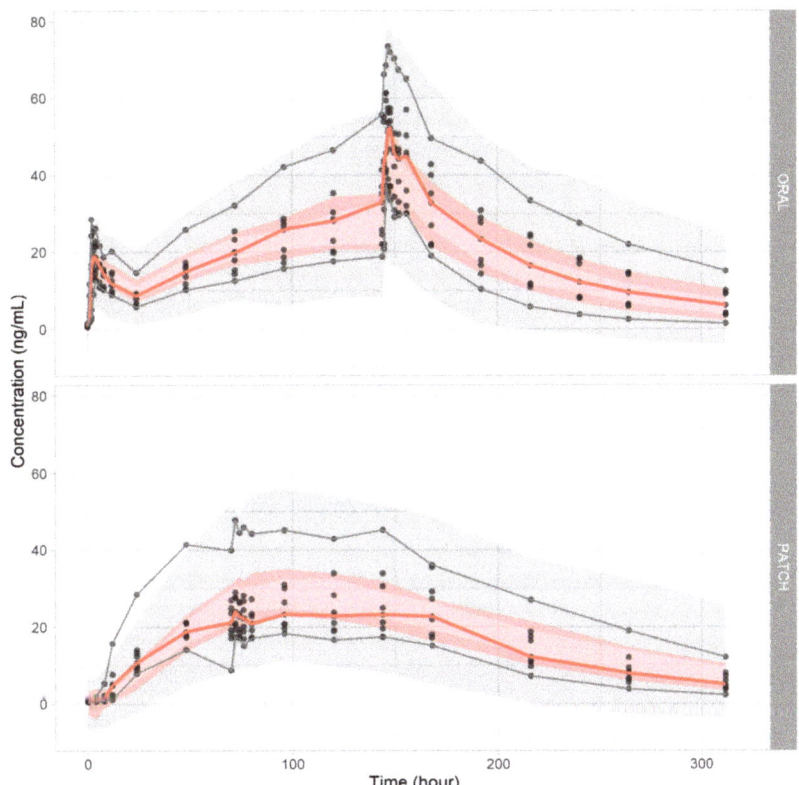

Figure 2. Visual predictive checks of donepezil in oral formulation (**upper panel**) and transdermal patch (**lower panel**).

3.3. Simulation to Optimize Equivalent Dose

The bioequivalence results summarized in Table 4 indicate that weekly patch doses from 114 mg/101.3 cm^2 to 146 mg/129.8 cm^2 were equivalent to the administration of 10 mg donepezil orally. Typical values used to assess bioequivalence (AUC and C$_{max}$ ratios) lay within 0.8- to 1.25-fold of the 90% CIs. The lower and upper 90% CI bounds for the AUC ratio were 85.61–97.06% for a 114 mg patch and 108.62–123.09% for a 146 mg patch. The C$_{max}$ ratios were 82.07–91.51% and 102.98–114.88% for 114 mg and 146 mg donepezil, respectively. The simulations for each bioequivalent dose are plotted in Figure 3.

Table 4. Results of the bioequivalence study on the simulation of the two donepezil formulations.

Range	Parameter	AUC	Cmax
Minimum (114 mg/101.3 cm^2)	CI 90% (Lower-Upper)	85.61–97.06	82.07–91.51
	RT Ratio (%Ref)	91.16	86.66
Maximum (146 mg/129.8 cm^2)	CI 90% (Lower-Upper)	108.62–123.09	102.98–114.88
	RT Ratio (%Ref)	115.63	108.77

CI: confidence interval, RT Ratio: equivalence ratio of test formulation to reference formulation, "Test" refers to patch donepezil dose, "Reference" refers to oral donepezil dose.

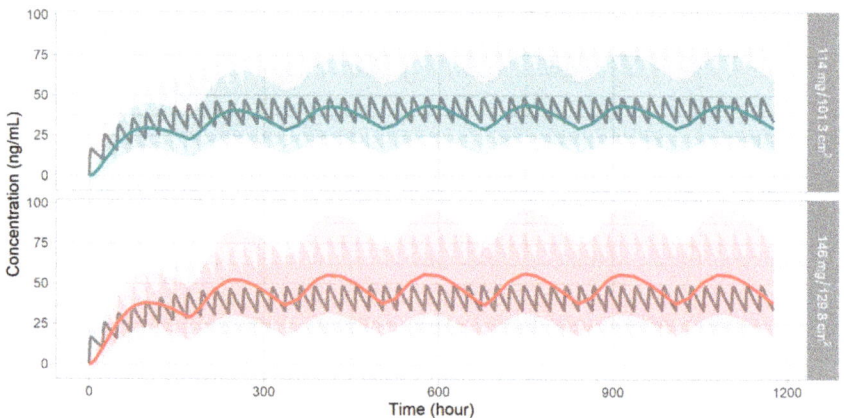

Figure 3. Simulated oral dose of donepezil 10 mg daily (gray line/area) and transdermal patch doses of 114 mg weekly (**upper**, green line/area) and 146 mg weekly (**lower**, red line/area). Lines: median predictions. Shaded areas: percentiles 5 to 95.

4. Discussion

The donepezil patch could replace the original oral formulation; the dosing frequency is thus reduced. The observed drug exposures (revealed by the C_{max} and AUC ratios) were slightly less than the predicted in vitro results, which indicates that adjustment of the patch dose may be required.

In this study, a population pharmacokinetic model of donepezil was developed as a two-compartment model for both oral and patch administration. Transit compartments were successfully applied for patch formulation to delay the arrival time to reach the central compartment. The same central compartment was used for both patch and oral dose, and its clearance was estimated as 10 L/h. A recent study using a population PK model of oral donepezil administration estimated an oral clearance of 12 L/h [16]. Another report stated that donepezil hydrochloride clearance was 9.65 L/h after administration of a 10 mg tablet [17]. The NCA PK parameters were 10 L/h (CLss) and 560 L (Vss) after oral administration of 10 mg drug. The Ka (absorption rate constant), Vc (central volume of distribution), Vp (peripheral volume of distribution), and Q (intercompartmental clearance) are listed in Table 2.

The VPC showed that the predictions were usually in agreement with the observations. However, the CIs for each percentile was rather wide, perhaps because of the intrinsic variability inherent in most of the transdermal formulation and estimation difficulties caused by flip-flop pharmacokinetics. It is thought that applying covariates of the study subject's skin condition would help minimize the variability of the model. However, bootstrapping (1000 replicates) showed that the model was reliable and robust. The GOF data suggested that the model was accurate in terms of both population and individual predictions. Plots of the GOF of the conditional and individual weighted residuals (CWRES and iWRES) by time showed that the residuals were evenly dispersed around the predictions. The model was appropriate for further simulation study.

In a previous study, Yoon et al. 2020, described oral and patch formulation in two different population models. The administered drugs in oral and transdermal route were cleared in different spaces with different clearances. The study focused on separately developing a descriptive model for both oral and patch formulation [18].

In this research, different PK profiles from formulations were described with one integrated model and showed better agreement with the reported drug parameters. The model can handle complicated dosing plans such as giving an oral titration period in patch study. In vitro dissolution data is applied in deciding patch delivered dose so that the model can deal with further experiments of modifications on formulation. Overall, a more simplified and generalized model for interpreting oral and patch formulation was made.

Finally, we performed bioequivalence testing of oral (10 mg) and patch donepezil using a 2 × 2 crossover design (100 patients/group, 200 in total). The test was performed on the simulated secondary NCA parameters. Iteration revealed that the patch-equivalent drug dose lays between 114 and 146 mg (patch sizes of 101.3 and 129.8 cm^2). Enhanced skin penetration or an increase in drug concentration would reduce the size of the patch, thus optimizing transdermal delivery of the drug by enhancing patient compliance.

For the first time, the inspection of appropriate patch doses satisfying the bioequivalence between two different formulations was performed. This model-informed bioequivalence assessment for different formulations was able to identify various kinds of variabilities and is expected to provide more accurate, interpretable data compared to the standard non-compartmental bioequivalence studies even in highly variable clinical situations.

5. Conclusions

To facilitate NCA-based bioequivalence testing, we built a population PK model for donepezil using data from nine healthy volunteers. We performed bioequivalence testing using secondary PK parameters derived from an iterative clinical simulation. A patch with 114–146 mg donepezil was equivalent to 10 mg oral donepezil.

Supplementary Materials: The following are available online at https://www.mdpi.com/article/10.3390/pharmaceutics14020244/s1, Table S1: Intra- and inter-day precision and accuracy values, Table S2: Stability of donepezil in human plasma, Table S3: Dissolution profile of oral and transdermal patch formulation, Figure S1: Representative chromatography of donepezil in human plasma ((A) double blank, (B) zero blank, (C) LLOQ, (D) sample obtained xx h after transdermal administration, and € sample obtained xx h after oral administration), Figure S2: Goodness-of-fit plot of model (A): Observation vs. population prediction, (B): Observation vs. individual prediction, (C): individual weighted residuals vs. individual predictions, (D): conditional weighted residuals vs. individual prediction, Figure S3: Pharmacokinetic profile of subjects with oral administration, Figure S4: Pharmacokinetic profile of subjects with transdermal patch administration.

Author Contributions: Conceptualization and methodology, W.J., H.J., N.-A.T.V., G.-Y.K., G.-W.K., J.-w.C., T.K. and H.-y.Y.; investigation, N.-A.T.V., G.-Y.K., G.-W.K., J.-w.C., T.K. and H.-y.Y.; data curation, G.-Y.K., G.-W.K., J.-w.C., T.K. and H.-y.Y.; modeling and simulation, W.J., H.J., N.-A.T.V., J.-w.C., T.K. and H.-y.Y.; statistical and graphical analysis, W.J., H.J., N.-A.T.V., J.-w.C., T.K. and H.-y.Y.; qualifying modeling, W.J., N.-A.T.V., J.-w.C., T.K. and H.-y.Y.; writing—original draft preparation, W.J., N.-A.T.V., J.-w.C., T.K. and H.-y.Y.; writing—review and editing, W.J., N.-A.T.V., J.-w.C., T.K. and H.-y.Y.; supervision, J.-w.C., T.K. and H.-y.Y.; project administration, J.-w.C., T.K. and H.-y.Y.; funding acquisition, H.-y.Y. and J.-w.C. All authors have read and agreed to the published version of the manuscript.

Funding: This research was funded by Chungnam National University and an Institute of Information and Communications Technology Planning and Evaluation grant funded by the government of the Republic of Korea (MSIT; no. 2020-0-01441, Artificial Intelligence Convergence Research Center, Chungnam National University).

Institutional Review Board Statement: The study protocol was reviewed and approved by the Institutional Review Board of the Raptim Research Ltd. (IORG no.: IORG0009526, DCGI reg. no.: ECR/224/Indt/MH/2015/RR-18, approved date: 5 June 2019) and performed in agreement with the Declaration of Helsinki and good clinical practice. A written informed consent form was signed by each volunteer before enrollment.

Informed Consent Statement: Informed consent was obtained from all subjects.

Data Availability Statement: Pharmacokinetic profiles of both oral and transdermal patch is available in Supplementary Materials (Figures S3 and S4).

Acknowledgments: This study was supported by Chungnam National University and an Institute of Information and Communications Technology Planning and Evaluation grant funded by the government of the Republic of Korea (MSIT; no. 2020-0-01441, Artificial Intelligence Convergence Research Center, Chungnam National University).

Conflicts of Interest: The authors declare no conflict of interest.

References

1. Jackson, S.; Ham, R.J.; Wilkinson, D. The safety and tolerability of donepezil in patients with Alzheimer's disease. *Br. J. Clin. Pharmacol. Suppl.* **2004**, *58*, 1–8. [CrossRef] [PubMed]
2. Small, G.W.; Rabins, P.V.; Barry, P.P.; Buckholtz, N.S.; DeKosky, S.T.; Ferris, S.H.; Finkel, S.I.; Gwyther, L.P.; Khachaturian, Z.S.; Lebowitz, B.D.; et al. Diagnosis and treatment of Alzheimer disease and related disorders: Consensus statement of the American Association for Geriatric Psychiatry, the Alzheimer's Association, and the American Geriatrics Society. *J. Am. Med. Assoc.* **1997**, *278*, 1363–1371. [CrossRef]
3. Winblad, B.; Wimo, A.; Engedal, K.; Soininen, H.; Verhey, F.; Waldemar, G.; Wetterholm, A.L.; Haglund, A.; Zhang, R.; Schindler, R. 3-Year study of donepezil therapy in Alzheimer's disease: Effects of early and continuous therapy. *Dement. Geriatr. Cogn. Disord.* **2006**, *21*, 353–363. [CrossRef] [PubMed]
4. Burns, A.; Rossor, M.; Hecker, J.; Gauthier, S.; Petit, H.; Möller, H.J.; Rogers, S.L.; Friedhoff, L.T. The effects of donepezil in Alzheimer's disease—Results from a multinational trial. *Dement. Geriatr. Cogn. Disord.* **1999**, *10*, 237–244. [CrossRef] [PubMed]
5. Whitehead, A.; Perdomo, C.; Pratt, R.D.; Birks, J.; Wilcock, G.K.; Evans, J.G. Donepezil for the symptomatic treatment of patients with mild to moderate Alzheimer's disease: A meta-analysis of individual patient data from randomised controlled trials. *Int. J. Geriatr. Psychiatry* **2004**, *19*, 624–633. [CrossRef] [PubMed]
6. Rogers, S.; Friedhoff, L. The efficacy and safety of donepezil in patients with AD: Results of a US Multicentre, Randomized, Double-Blind, Placebo-Controlled Trial. *Dement. Geriatr. Cogn. Disord.* **1996**, *7*, 293–303. [PubMed]
7. Rogers, S.L.; Doody, R.S.; Mohs, R.C.; Friedhoff, L.T.; The Donepezil Study Group. Donepezil Improves Cognition and Global Function in Alzheimer Disease: A 15-Week, Double-blind, Placebo-Controlled Study. *Arch. Intern. Med.* **1998**, *158*, 1021–1031.
8. Rogers, S.L.; Farlow, M.R.; Doody, R.S.; Mohs, R.; Friedhoff, L.T. A 24-week, double-blind, placebo-controlled trial of donepezil in patients with Alzheimer's disease. *Neurology* **1998**, *50*, 136–145. [CrossRef] [PubMed]
9. Molinuevo, J.L.; Arranz, F.J. Impact of transdermal drug delivery on treatment adherence in patients with Alzheimer's disease. *Expert Rev. Neurother.* **2012**, *12*, 31–37. [CrossRef] [PubMed]
10. Isaac, M.; Holvey, C. Transdermal patches: The emerging mode of drug delivery system in psychiatry. *Ther. Adv. Psychopharmacol.* **2012**, *2*, 255–263. [CrossRef] [PubMed]
11. Möllenhoff, K.; Loingeville, F.; Bertrand, J.; Nguyen, T.T.; Sharan, S.; Zhao, L.; Fang, L.; Sun, G.; Grosser, S.; Mentré, F.; et al. Efficient model-based bioequivalence testing. *Biostatistics* **2020**, *23*, 314–327. [CrossRef] [PubMed]
12. Hooker, A.C.; Chen, P.X.; Assawasuwannakit, P.; Karlsson, M.O. *Improved Bioequivalence Assessment through Model-Informed and Model-Based Strategies*; FDA: Silver Spring, MD, USA, 2020.
13. Acharya, C.; Hooker, A.C.; Türkyılmaz, G.Y.; Jönsson, S.; Karlsson, M.O. A diagnostic tool for population models using non-compartmental analysis: The ncappc package for R. *Comput. Methods Programs Biomed.* **2016**, *127*, 83–93. [CrossRef] [PubMed]
14. Proost, J.H. Combined proportional and additive residual error models in population pharmacokinetic modelling. *Eur. J. Pharm. Sci.* **2017**, *109*, S78–S82. [CrossRef] [PubMed]
15. FDA. *Guidance for Industry—Bioavailability and Bioequivalence Studies Submitted in NDAs or INDs—General Considerations*; Center for Drug Evaluation and Research: Silver Spring, MD, USA, 2014; Volume 24.
16. Choi, H.Y.; Kim, Y.H.; Hong, D.; Kim, S.S.; Bae, K.S.; Lim, H.S. Therapeutic dosage assessment based on population pharmacokinetics of a novel single-dose transdermal donepezil patch in healthy volunteers. *Eur. J. Clin. Pharmacol.* **2015**, *71*, 967–977. [CrossRef] [PubMed]
17. Choi, Y.; Rhee, S.; Jang, I.; Yu, K.; Yim, S.; Kim, B. Bioequivalence study of Donepezil hydrochloride in healthy Korean volunteers. *Transl. Clin. Pharmacol.* **2015**, *23*, 26–30. [CrossRef]
18. Yoon, S.K.; Bae, K.S.; Hong, D.H.; Kim, S.S.; Choi, Y.K.; Lim, H.S. Pharmacokinetic Evaluation by Modeling and Simulation Analysis of a Donepezil Patch Formulation in Healthy Male Volunteers. *Drug Des. Dev. Ther.* **2020**, *14*, 1729–1737. [CrossRef] [PubMed]

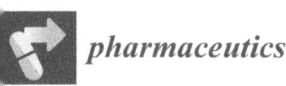

Article

Parametric and Nonparametric Population Pharmacokinetic Models to Assess Probability of Target Attainment of Imipenem Concentrations in Critically Ill Patients

Femke de Velde [1,*], Brenda C. M. de Winter [2], Michael N. Neely [3], Jan Strojil [4], Walter M. Yamada [3], Stephan Harbarth [5,6], Angela Huttner [5], Teun van Gelder [2], Birgit C. P. Koch [2], Anouk E. Muller [1,7] and on behalf of the COMBACTE-NET Consortium [†]

1. Department of Medical Microbiology and Infectious Diseases, Erasmus University Medical Center, 3000 CA Rotterdam, The Netherlands; anoukemuller@gmail.com
2. Department of Hospital Pharmacy, Erasmus University Medical Center, 3000 CA Rotterdam, The Netherlands; b.dewinter@erasmusmc.nl (B.C.M.d.W.); t.vangelder@erasmusmc.nl (T.v.G.); B.koch@erasmusmc.nl (B.C.P.K.)
3. Laboratory of Applied Pharmacokinetics, Keck School of Medicine, University of Southern California, Los Angeles, CA 90027, USA; mneely@chla.usc.edu (M.N.N.); wyamada@chla.usc.edu (W.M.Y.)
4. Department of Pharmacology, Palacky University, CZ-779 00 Olomouc, Czech Republic; jan.strojil@upol.cz
5. Division of Infectious Diseases, Faculty of Medicine, Geneva University Hospitals, 1205 Geneva, Switzerland; stephan.harbarth@hcuge.ch (S.H.); Angela.Huttner@hcuge.ch (A.H.)
6. Infection Control Program, Faculty of Medicine, Geneva University Hospitals, 1205 Geneva, Switzerland
7. Department of Medical Microbiology, Haaglanden Medical Centre, 2501 CK The Hague, The Netherlands
* Correspondence: femkedevelde@gmail.com
† Membership of the COMBACTE-NET Consortium is provided in the Acknowledgment.

Abstract: Population pharmacokinetic modeling and simulation (M&S) are used to improve antibiotic dosing. Little is known about the differences in parametric and nonparametric M&S. Our objectives were to compare (1) the external validation of parametric and nonparametric models of imipenem in critically ill patients and (2) the probability of target attainment (PTA) calculations using simulations of both models. The M&S software used was NONMEM 7.2 (parametric) and Pmetrics 1.5.2 (nonparametric). The external predictive performance of both models was adequate for eGFRs $\geq$ 78 mL/min but insufficient for lower eGFRs, indicating that the models (developed using a population with eGFR $\geq$ 60 mL/min) could not be extrapolated to lower eGFRs. Simulations were performed for three dosing regimens and three eGFRs (90, 120, 150 mL/min). Fifty percent of the PTA results were similar for both models, while for the other 50% the nonparametric model resulted in lower MICs. This was explained by a higher estimated between-subject variability of the nonparametric model. Simulations indicated that 1000 mg q6h is suitable to reach MICs of 2 mg/L for eGFRs of 90–120 mL/min. For MICs of 4 mg/L and for higher eGFRs, dosing recommendations are missing due to largely different PTA values per model. The consequences of the different modeling approaches in clinical practice should be further investigated.

Keywords: imipenem; population pharmacokinetic modeling; parametric; nonparametric; simulations

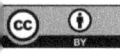

1. Introduction

Population pharmacokinetic (popPK) modeling and simulation is used to improve antibiotic dosing and clinical outcomes of infections. Antimicrobial efficacy is determined by the susceptibility of the drug in vitro (usually expressed as the minimal inhibitory concentration, MIC) and the exposure to the drug in vivo, which relies on the pharmacokinetics and the dose [1]. PopPK models describe the variability of exposure to a drug, and are therefore used to support dosing optimization. This optimization can take place in different ways: individualization of dosing via therapeutic drug monitoring (TDM) software, improving dosing regimens from the package insert (especially for specific subpopulations), and setting clinical breakpoints on a population level [2]. Clinical breakpoints are MICs that categorize microorganisms as susceptible or resistant to specific antibiotics [3].

Several popPK modeling methods are available. Statistically, they are classified as either parametric or nonparametric methods [2]. Parametric methods assume that the population parameter distribution is known, with unknown population parameter estimates [4]. Nonparametric methods make no assumption about the shapes of the underlying parameter distributions, by which, theoretically, subpopulations are more easily detected [5]. Many parametric and nonparametric popPK models are published in the literature, often accompanied by simulations of the model which lead to dosing recommendations [2]. Little is known about the differences in modeling and simulation results between parametric and nonparametric methods, which may influence dosing recommendations.

Previously, we described the development and results of parametric and nonparametric popPK models of imipenem in critically ill patients [6]. Both models described imipenem popPK well, and the population parameter estimates were similar. The same covariate was included: the CKD-EPI (Chronic Kidney Disease Epidemiology Collaboration) eGFR (estimated Glomerular Filtration Range) equation [7], which was unadjusted for body surface area, on elimination rate K_e. The estimated between-subject variability (BSV) was higher in the nonparametric model. External validation and simulations of both models were not yet performed.

Like other beta-lactams, the antibacterial effect of imipenem is determined by the percent of time of the dosing interval during which the free concentration remains above the MIC ($fT_{>MIC}$) [8]. Reported targets for beta-lactam antibiotics range from 20 to 100% $fT_{>MIC}$ to 100% $fT_{>5xMIC}$ [9–13]. Smaller preclinical and clinical studies suggest that the required targets seem to be the highest in cephalosporines, followed by penicillins, and then carbapenems [11,14]. Other M&S studies of imipenem in critically ill patients used targets of 20–100% $fT_{>MIC}$ [15–17]. The DALI study showed a significant association of positive clinical outcome (defined as no switch of addition of antibiotics needed) with 50% $fT_{>MIC}$ (OR 1.02) and 100% $fT_{>MIC}$ (OR 1.56) for eight beta-lactams in 361 critically ill patients [18]. However, this study did not distinguish between the three classes of beta-lactams. Due to the lack of consensus about the target, we chose to use two targets in this paper (50% $fT_{>MIC}$ and 100% $fT_{>MIC}$). A Swiss study in hospitalized patients treated with standard imipenem dosing regimens from the package insert found a trend towards increased clinical failure in case of trough levels < 2 mg/L (11% vs. 19%), indicating that the dosing could be optimized. Unfortunately, this study was underpowered to detect a significant difference [19].

The first objective of the current study was to determine which of the two previously described imipenem models [6] delivers the best Bayesian posterior estimates to predict the imipenem concentrations in an external independent database. The second objective was to determine the probability of target attainment (PTA) for several doses and estimated glomerular filtration rate (eGFR) values using simulations of both models.

2. Materials and Methods

2.1. Population PK Models

Two previously published parametric (using NONMEM 7.2) and nonparametric (using Pmetrics 1.5.2) population PK models of imipenem in critically ill patients were used for the analyses in this paper. The development and results of both models are described in detail elsewhere [6]. Both models included two distribution compartments and the absolute (unadjusted for body surface area) CKD-EPI eGFR [7] as a covariate on the elimination rate constant (K_e). The parameter estimates in both models were comparable, except from the estimated BSV, which was higher in the nonparametric model. The parameter estimates are displayed in Supplementary Table S1.

2.2. Population Used for Modeling

The models were built using imipenem PK data of 26 critically ill patients from a previously published prospective cohort study [20] in the intensive care unit (ICU) of the Geneva University Hospitals (Geneva, Switzerland). Inclusion criteria were suspected or documented severe bacterial infection and age between 18 and 60 years. Exclusion criteria were estimated glomerular filtration rate (eGFR) < 60 mL/min (measured by the Cockcroft–Gault equation [21]), Body Mass Index (BMI) < 18 or >30 kg/m^2, and pregnancy. None of the patients received continuous renal replacement therapy (CRRT). None of the patients used probenecid, which is the only drug that is known to influence imipenem concentrations [22]. The usual dosing regimen for imipenem/cilastatin was 500 mg/500 mg every 6 h, administered by intermittent intravenous infusion for 30 min.

Peak (approximately 15–30 min after end of infusion), intermediate (midway between two sequential administrations), and trough (approximately 15 min before the next dose) blood samples ($n = 138$) were collected on days 1, 2, 3, 4, and/or 6 of therapy; 47% was drawn on the second day. After centrifugation of the blood, MOPS [3-(N-morpholino)propanesulfonic acid], a stabilizing buffer that protects imipenem from degradation [23], was added to an equivalent volume of plasma. Imipenem plasma concentrations were analysed by high-performance liquid chromatography (HPLC), with ultraviolet (UV) detection at 298 nm. A median of three creatinine measures per patient were available.

Fewer than 10% [24] of all concentrations (13/138 = 9.4%) were below the limit of quantification (0.5 mg/L) and were excluded from the popPK analysis. All concentrations above the LOQ ($n = 125$) were included for popPK analysis.

2.3. Population Used for Validation

The external dataset consisted of imipenem PK data of 19 critically ill patients from a previously published prospective randomized study [25] in the ICU of the General University Hospital (Prague, Czech Republic). Inclusion criteria were hospital acquired pneumoniae (HAP) and age above 18 years. Exclusion criteria were carbapenem allergy, hepatic dysfunction (total serum bilirubin > 27 µmol/L), neutropenia (granulocytes < 500/mm^3), acute or chronic renal failure (serum creatinine > 280 µmol/L or CRRT), obesity (BMI > 35 kg/m^2 or weight > 110 kg), and pregnancy. None of the patients used probenecid.

Patients were randomized to receive either short infusion (bolus group) or extended infusion (extended group) of imipenem/cilastatin. Patients in the bolus group received 1 g/1 g imipenem/cilastatin every 8 h, administered by intermittent intravenous infusion for 30 min. Patients in the extended group received an initial loading dose of 1 g/1 g imipenem/cilastatin over 30 min, followed by an infusion of 500 mg/500 mg imipenem/cilastatin administered over 3 h every 6 h.

Blood samples ($n = 114$) were drawn on the second day of therapy: one sample prior to infusion and then at 0.33, 0.67, 4, 6, and 8 h (bolus group) or 2, 3.17, 4, 5, and 6 h (extended group). After centrifugation, MOPS buffer was added to an equivalent volume of plasma. Imipenem plasma concentrations were analysed by HPLC-UV at 313 nm. One creatinine measure per patient was available.

Fewer than 10% [24] of all concentrations (3/114 = 2.6%) were below the limit of quantification (0.26 mg/L) and were excluded from analysis. All concentrations above the LOQ ($n = 111$) were included for analysis.

2.4. External Validation

Imipenem concentrations of the external validation database were predicted using the parametric and nonparametric models. Subsequently, the prediction errors (individual predicted concentration minus observed concentration) and relative prediction errors (prediction error/observed concentration) were calculated. The prediction errors were also calculated using Monte Carlo simulations ($n = 1000$) of both models.

To visualize the external validation, plots with predicted versus observed concentrations and visual predictive checks (VPCs) were generated. For each VPC, a set of 1000 simulated datasets (using one of the popPK models developed with the modeling population) was created to compare the observed concentrations of the external validation database with the distribution of the simulated concentrations. Stratification on dose (500 mg and 1000 mg) and eGFR (measured by the CKD-EPI equation unadjusted for BSA) was applied. For eGFR, stratification in three groups (19–46, 50–89, and 90–178 mL/min) and two groups (19–59 and 79–178 mL/min) was performed. These ranges were chosen to create equal groups.

2.5. Simulations

Monte Carlo simulations were performed using the final models. The three imipenem dosing regimens from the package insert [22,26] were evaluated: 500 mg every 6 h (q6h), 1000 mg every 8 h (q8h), and 1000 mg q6h, each for a predefined eGFR (measured by the CKD-EPI equation unadjusted for BSA) of 150, 120, and 90 mL/min. The infusion rate was 1000 mg/h for each dosing regimen. Five thousand subjects were simulated for each combination of dosing regimen and eGFR. For each simulated concentration–time profile, the $fT_{>MIC}$ was calculated for MICs of 0.015–64 mg/L. The unbound imipenem concentrations were calculated from the total concentration using a fixed value for protein binding of 20% [22]. Subsequently, the probability of target attainment (PTA) for 50% and 100% $fT_{>MIC}$ was calculated. A PTA threshold of 97.5% [3] was chosen.

2.6. Software

Parametric population PK modeling and simulation was performed using NONMEM (version 7.2, ICON Development Solutions, Ellicott City, MD, USA), Intel Visual Fortran Compiler XE 14.0 (Santa Clara, CA, USA), RStudio (version 1.1.456; RStudio, Boston, MA, USA, 2018), R (version 3.5.1; R foundation, Vienna, Austria, 2018), XPose (version 4.6.1; Uppsala University, Department of Pharmaceutical Biosciences, Uppsala, Sweden, 2018), PsN (version 4.6.0; Uppsala University, Department of Pharmaceutical Biosciences, Uppsala, Sweden, 2016), and Pirana [27] (version 2.9.4; Certara, Princeton, NJ, USA, 2018). The $fT_{>MIC}$ and PTA were calculated using Excel 2013.

Nonparametric population PK modeling, simulation, and calculation of $fT_{>MIC}$ and PTA was performed using Pmetrics version 1.5.2 (Laboratory of Applied Pharmacokinetics and Bioinformatics, Los Angeles, CA, USA) [28], Intel Visual Fortran Compiler XE 14.0 (Santa Clara, CA, USA), RStudio (version 1.1.456), and R (version 3.5.1). The raw VPC data were imported from Pmetrics into PsN (version 4.6.0) using the Pirana interface [27] to generate VPCs with the same layout as NONMEM. VPC plots were subsequently created using XPose (version 4.6.1) within RStudio (version 1.1.456).

3. Results

3.1. Population

Demographic and clinical characteristics of the population (*n* = 26) used to build the popPK models and of the validation population (*n* = 19) are summarized in Table 1. None of the patients received continuous renal replacement therapy (CRRT). The medians of the APACHE II score and age were higher in the validation group compared to the modeling population. The median eGFR was lower in the validation group. Six validation subjects had an absolute CKD-EPI eGFR lower than the minimum of 51 mL/min in the modeling group, while one validation subject had an eGFR above the maximum of 172 mL/min in the modeling population. The other characteristics were comparable between the two groups.

Table 1. Demographic and clinical characteristics of the population (*n* = 26) used to build the popPK models and of the validation population (*n* = 19). APACHE, Acute Physiology and Chronic Health Evaluation; eGFR, estimated Glomerular Filtration Range; CKD-EPI, Chronic Kidney Disease Epidemiology Collaboration; BMI, Body Mass Index; BSA, Body Surface Area.

Parameter	Modeling Population	Validation Population
Male, *n* (%)	18 (69)	14 (74)
APACHE II score, median (range)	22 (7–35)	26 (13–42)
Age (years), median (range)	51 (25–59)	64 (26–90)
Creatinine at inclusion (µmol/L), median (range)	59 (28–108)	98 (44–235)
eGFR CKD-EPI at inclusion (ml/min/1.73 m^2), median (range)	116 (50–143)	73 (20–145)
eGFR absolute CKD-EPI at inclusion, unadjusted for BSA (ml/min), median (range)	119 (51–172)	79 (19–178)
Height (cm), median (range)	175 (155–190)	170 (150–190)
Total bodyweight (kg), median (range)	75 (50–107)	78 (45–110)
BMI (kg/m^2), median (range)	25 (18–35)	28 (18–34)
BSA (m^2), median (range)	1.89 (1.51–2.23)	1.92 (1.40–2.29)
Presumed infection, *n* (%)		
Respiratory tract infection	16 (62)	19 (100)
Intra-abdominal infection	4 (15)	-
Bloodstream infection	3 (12)	-
Surgical site infection	1 (4)	-
Meningitis	1 (4)	-
Gynecological infection	1 (4)	-

3.2. External Validation

The graphs of individual and population predicted concentrations plotted against the observed concentrations of the external dataset (Figure 1) were comparable for the two models. Both models showed good predictive performance for 500 mg as well as 1000 mg, except for concentrations higher than approximately 20 mg/L for the 1000 mg dose (see also the visual predictive checks (VPCs) in Figure 2). The same deviation of the peak concentration was still shown in VPCs without samples during infusion (data not shown).

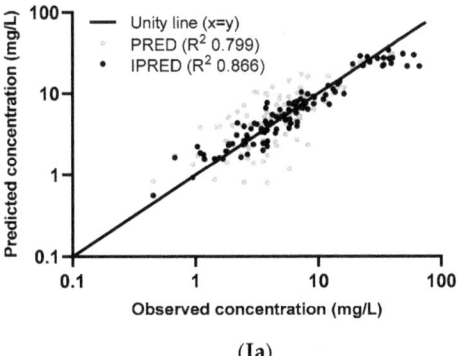

(**Ia**)

Figure 1. *Cont.*

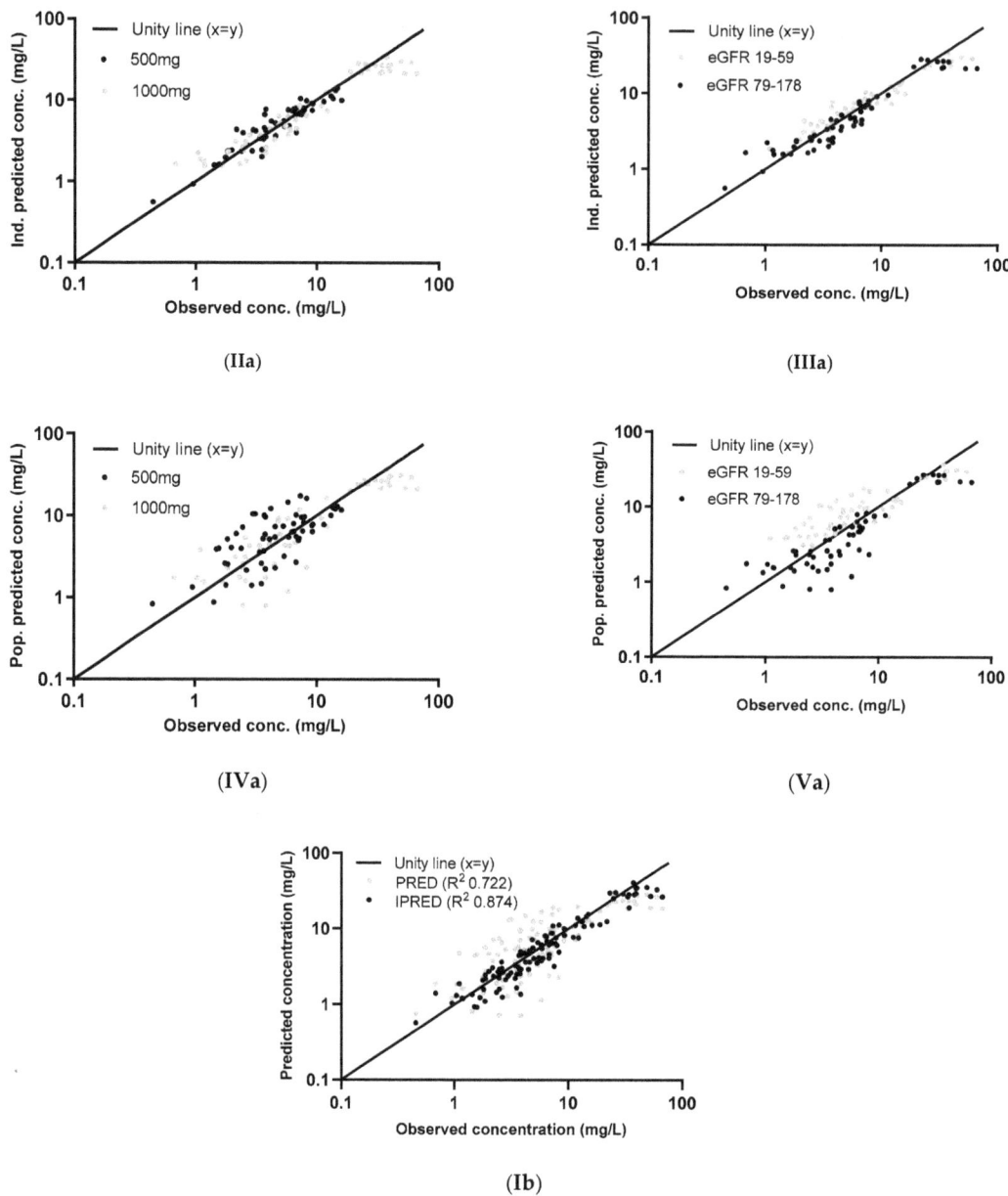

Figure 1. Cont.

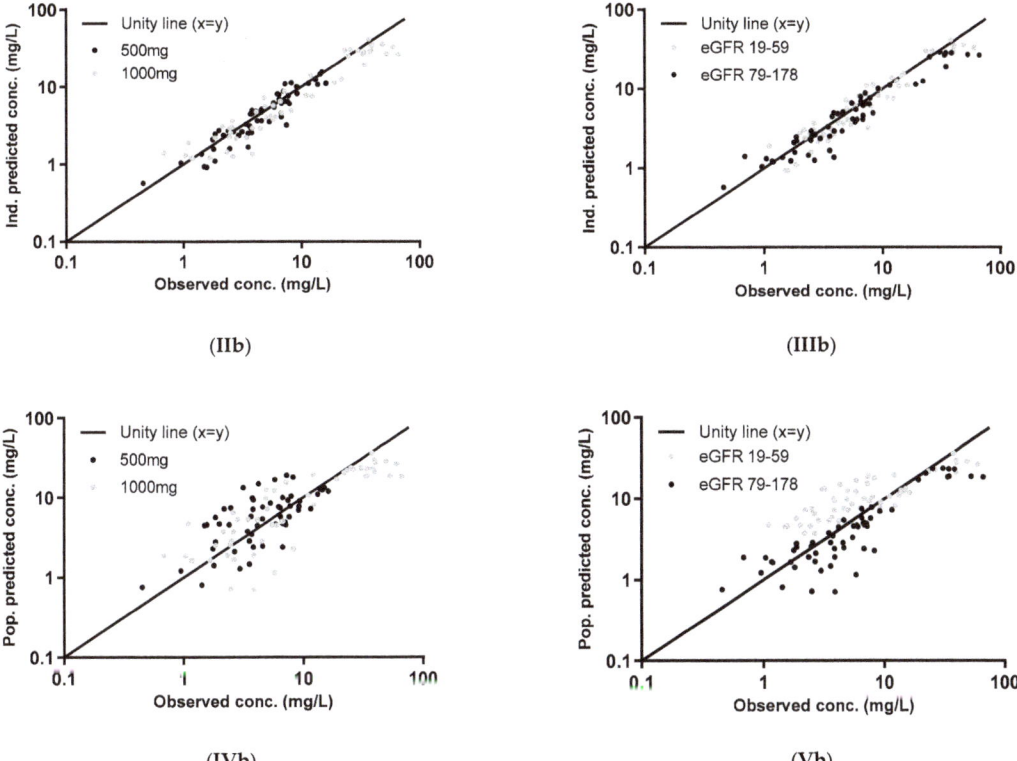

Figure 1. Individual (I [IPRED], II, and III) and population (I (PRED), IV, and V) concentrations, predicted using the parametric model (**a**) and the nonparametric model (**b**), plotted against the observed concentrations of the external dataset. The two dose groups, 500 mg and 1000 mg, are differentiated in graphs II and IV and two eGFR groups (measured by the CKD-EPI unadjusted for BSA) in graphs III and V. The log-transformed concentrations of the parametric model (**a**) are back transformed for an easier comparison with the untransformed concentrations in the figures of the nonparametric model (**b**).

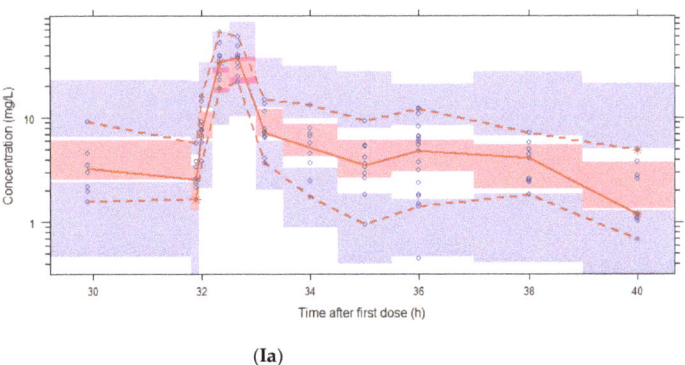

(**Ia**)

Figure 2. *Cont.*

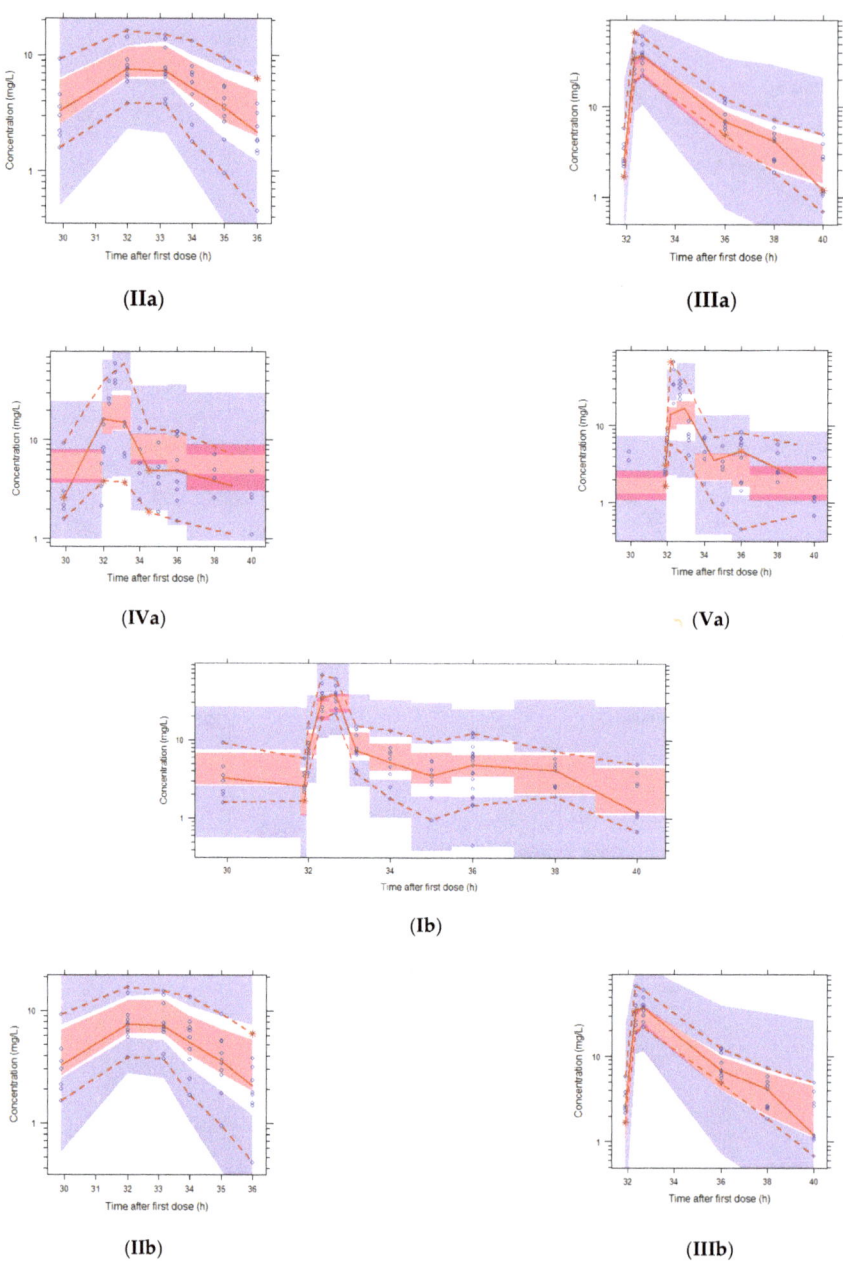

Figure 2. *Cont.*

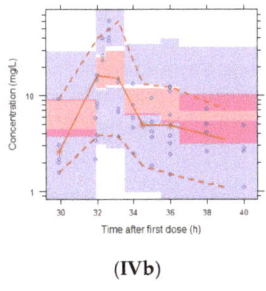
(IVb)

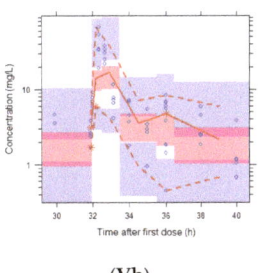
(Vb)

Figure 2. Visual Predictive Checks (VPCs) of both models using the external validation database. Circles: observed concentrations. Upper, middle, and lower lines: 95th, 50th, and 5th percentile of observations. Shaded areas: 95%CI of the corresponding percentiles of predictions. I: both dose regimens, II: 500 mg, III: 1000 mg, IV: eGFR 20–59 mL/min, V: eGFR 79–178 mL/min. The log-transformed concentrations of the parametric model (**a**) are back transformed for an easier comparison with the untransformed concentrations in the figures of the nonparametric model (**b**).

The VPCs with eGFR stratification on three groups were unclear due to the small group size (data not shown). Stratification on the two eGFR groups was better, but the VPC plots are still not optimal due to the different sampling times of both dosing groups, which were equally distributed among the eGFR groups (see Figure 2). The individual plots in Figures 1 and 2, with stratification on the two eGFR groups, show that the predictive performance for eGFRs of 19–59 mL/min ($n = 9$) was worse than for eGFRs of 79–178 mL/min ($n = 10$). The VPCs show that both models predict too high concentrations for the trough levels of the low eGFR group. The median relative prediction error (Table 2) was higher for trough levels in the low eGFR group (parametric: 83% and nonparametric: 88%) than in the high eGFR group (−24% and −19%). These prediction errors were comparable for the 500 mg and 1000 mg in each eGFR group (data not shown).

Table 2. Prediction errors of the parametric and nonparametric popPK models using the external validation database (111 concentrations). The prediction errors were also calculated after 1000 simulations (111.000 concentrations) of both models. In the last 4 columns, a selection of the simulations (trough levels only) per eGFR group are shown. PE = prediction error (mg/L) = individual predicted concentration—observed concentration. RPE = relative prediction error (%) = prediction error/observed concentration.

KERRYPNX	External Database 111 Concentrations		Simulations 1000 × 111 Concentrations		Simulations (Selection) 1000 × 17 trough eGFR19-59		Simulations (Selection) 1000 × 18 trough eGFR79-178	
Parametric	PE (mg/L)	RPE (%)	PE (mg/L)	RPE (%)	PE (mg/L)	RPE (%)	PE (mg/L)	RPE (%)
97.5%	3.83	105	8.97	252	9.74	360	2.03	225
75%	0.61	19	1.97	56	3.92	167	0.38	31
50%	−0.02	−1	−0.04	−1	2.13	83	−0.50	−24
25%	−1.52	−20	−2.20	−31	0.72	23	−1.64	−53
2.5%	−30.55	−52	−28.63	−74	−3.16	−41	−3.15	−82
Nonparametric	PE (mg/L)	RPE (%)	PE (mg/L)	RPE (%)	PE (mg/L)	RPE (%)	PE (mg/L)	RPE (%)
97.5%	3.89	54	30.68	594	28.96	996	7.08	564
75%	0.51	15	3.22	83	5.66	221	0.80	58
50%	−0.43	−9	0.02	0.5	2.24	88	−0.33	−19
25%	−1.74	−29	−2.47	−39	0.32	11	−1.56	−56
2.5%	−25.99	−58	−24.77	−79	−4.15	−63	−3.36	−91

The median prediction error and median relative prediction error after 1000 simulations were similar to the single external validation for both models (Table 2), although the 97.5–2.5% range is larger after the simulations using the nonparametric model. The wider distribution of the nonparametric model is also shown in the VPCs in Figure 2.

The proportion of observations between the 5th and 95th simulated percentiles in the VPCs in Figure 2 are: 96% (Ia), 95% (IIa), 94% (IIIa), 81% (IVa), 88% (Va), 96% (Ib), 97% (IIb), 96% (IIIb), 81% (IVb), and 95% (Vb).

3.3. Simulations

The highest MICs with a probability of target attainment (PTA) >97.5% for a target of 50% and 100% $fT_{>MIC}$ attained by several imipenem dosing regimens and eGFR values of 150, 120, 90 mL/min are shown in Table 3 for both models. Fifty percent of the MICs calculated using the parametric model were equal to those calculated by the nonparametric model and the other half of the MICs were lower for the nonparametric model. The PTAs for the full MIC profile from 0.015 to 64 mg/L are shown in Supplementary Table S2.

Table 3. The highest MIC for which a probability of target attainment (PTA) of 97.5% is reached at targets of 50% and 100% $fT > MIC$ by several imipenem dosing regimens and eGFR values (measured by the CKD-EPI equation unadjusted for BSA) of 150, 120, and 90 mL/min. The PTAs were calculated by Monte Carlo simulations (n = 5000) using parametric and nonparametric popPK models.

eGFR (ml/min)	Dose Regimen	Target $fT_{>MIC}$	Highest MIC (mg/L) with PTA > 97.5%	
			Parametric	Nonparametric
150	500 mg q6h	100%	0.125	0.06
	1000 mg q8h	100%	0.125	0.03
	1000 mg q6h	100%	0.25	0.125
	500 mg q6h	50%	0.5	0.25
	1000 mg q8h	50%	0.5	0.5
	1000 mg q6h	50%	1	1
120	500 mg q6h	100%	0.125	0.125
	1000 mg q8h	100%	0.25	0.06
	1000 mg q6h	100%	0.25	0.25
	500 mg q6h	50%	0.5	0.5
	1000 mg q8h	50%	1	0.5
	1000 mg q6h	50%	2	1
90	500 mg q6h	100%	0.25	0.25
	1000 mg q8h	100%	0.25	0.25
	1000 mg q6h	100%	0.5	0.5
	500 mg q6h	50%	1	0.5
	1000 mg q8h	50%	1	1
	1000 mg q6h	50%	2	1

4. Discussion

The external validation of parametric and nonparametric popPK models of imipenem in critically ill patients showed that the predictive performance of both models was sufficient in patients with high eGFRs (79–178 mL/min). However, the models could not be extrapolated to patients with lower eGFRs, as they were hardly included in the population used to build the model. The PTA simulations using both models were therefore performed for eGFR ≥ 90 mL/min only. Fifty percent of the PTA calculations resulted in similar MICs for both models, while the other half of the simulations resulted in lower MICs for the nonparametric model.

Our external validation simulations showed that the median PE and RPE were comparable for both models, although the ranges of the PE and RPE were wider for the nonparametric model. This was also shown in the VPCs and can be explained by the higher BSV in the nonparametric model. In contrast to the external validation simulations, the original external validation (without simulations) showed higher medians of the PE and RPE for the nonparametric model. However, the mean PEs (−1.9 mg/L parametric and −1.8 mg/L nonparametric) were similar. Given the similar external validation simulation results, this deviation of median PEs and RPEs might be caused by the small study size.

The poor predictive performance for low eGFRs can be explained by the paucity of subjects with renal impairment in the modeling population. Only 1 of 26 patients in the modeling population (n = 26) had an eGFR lower than 90 mL/min, while this applied to 12 of 19 patients in the validation population. After the external validation showed that both popPK models could not be extrapolated to low eGFRs, we decided to perform the PTA simulations for eGFR ≥ 90 mL/min only, deviating from the original plan to also simulate for lower eGFRs. The cut-off of 90 mL/min was chosen from a practical point of view, in line with the package inserts [22,26] instead of the eGFR ranges from the VPCs (19–59 and 79–178 mL/min), which were chosen to create two equal groups. The popPK models are still applicable to a high proportion of critically ill patients. Augmented renal clearance (defined as increased renal elimination of circulating solutes and drugs as compared with normal baseline [29]) has been reported in approximately 30–65% of critically ill patients [30].

The VPCs stratified on dose showed for both models a good predictive performance for the 500 and 1000 mg regimens, except for peak concentrations (C_{max}) for the 1000 mg dose. This dose could not be tested during popPK modeling because the modeling population only used 500 mg. The higher than predicted C_{max} is not likely to be explained by nonlinear PK [22,31]. The most probable reasons for the C_{max} deviation are the critical timing of the peak samples and the variable PK in critically ill patients [32], which is also shown by others [31,33–35]. However, it is important to realize that, instead of C_{max}, the trough level is relevant for the targets of 50–100% $fT_{> MIC}$. Importantly, the simulations did not show different prediction errors for trough levels after 500 mg and 1000 mg. Therefore, we decided to include 1000 mg dose regimens in the PTA simulations.

Our external validation findings emphasise the importance of such a validation when popPK models are used to optimize dosing strategies based on PTA simulations, or to individualize dosing by therapeutic drug monitoring software. PopPK model publications often not include external validation. A survey of the literature revealed that only for 7% of popPK models published between 2002 and 2004 (n = 324) was an external evaluation performed [36]. To our knowledge, a more recent survey does not exist.

Our simulations showed that 50% of the PTA results were comparable for both models, while the other half resulted in lower MICs for the nonparametric model, although the majority (7/9 = 78%) differed by only one dilution. The lower MICs could be caused by a higher estimated BSV of the popPK parameter values in the nonparametric model, leading to a wider range of concentrations. It is impossible to judge which of the models represents the "truth". The parametric model could have included too little variability or the nonparametric model could be too flexible. Probably, the truth is somewhere in between. We compared our simulation results with other published M&S studies of imipenem in critically ill patients, of which one was based on a parametric model [15] and two on nonparametric models [16,17]. Despite differences in parameter estimates, our finding of higher MICs with the parametric model was confirmed by these papers [15–17]. Similar to two studies [15,17], we showed that it is difficult to reach high MICs from 1 mg/L with an increased target of 100% $fT_{> MIC}$, which confirms again that more prospective studies about the required target of beta-lactams in critically ill patients are needed. The regression analysis of the original study [20], with four beta-lactams from which we analysed a subgroup, did not find a significant association between clinical failure and trough levels below 2 mg/L, indicating that an elevated target of 100% $fT_{>MIC}$ might not be necessary in this population. Even a larger study was underpowered to find a significant association between clinical failure and troughs below 2 mg/L [19]. Importantly, the latter study [19] proved that fear about toxicity at high doses of 3–4 g/day is unnecessary, as patients receiving these doses did not have increased toxicity compared to the standard dose of 2 g/day.

Based on the 50% $fT_{>MIC}$ target simulations, we conclude that a high dose of 1000 mg q6h is required to maximize the probability to reach MICs of 2 mg/L (e.g., for *Enterobacterales* [37]) in critically ill patients with eGFRs of 90–120 mL/min, although the PTAs using the nonparametric model were below the 97.5% cut-off but still above 90% (see Supplementary Table S2). This is in line with the American prescribing information [26]. However, they recommend this dosing regimen also for MICs of 4 mg/L (e.g., for *Pseudomonas aeruginosa*), similar to the European product characteristics [22], although these brochures are of course not specifically dedicated to critically ill patients. Considering our simulation results, it is difficult to give dosing recommendations for MICs of 4 mg/L, and also for higher MICs of 2 mg/L and eGFRs of 150 mL/min, because the PTA values differ largely per modeling approach. For example, for 1000 mg q6h, eGFR 90, 50% $fT_{>MIC}$, and MIC 4 mg/L, the PTA was 90% for the parametric model and 63% for the nonparametric model (see also Supplementary Table S2). Dosing regimens may look acceptable following the parametric model, while the nonparametric model might plead for increased dosing. As previously stated, the truth may be somewhere in between. One of the objectives of our study was to determine which of the two previously described imipenem models delivers the best Bayesian posterior estimates to predict the imipenem concentrations in an external independent database. It was not possible to assign a winner, because the external predictive performance of both models was adequate. However, as the dosing simulations based on the models show different results, more research on this topic is clearly needed. Until now, we recommend all readers of M&S papers to be aware of the consequences of the chosen modeling approach before implementing the dosing recommendations of these papers in clinical practice.

Few studies comparing parametric and nonparametric M&S are available in the literature. Precluding the studies with currently outdated software [38–41], we found eight comparison studies [42–49]. For three of these studies, the parameters of both models could not be compared due to a different model structure [42,43] or unreported values [46]. The majority of the remaining five comparison studies showed comparable parameter estimates of both models [45,47–49], although the BSV of the parametric estimates was often higher for the nonparametric model [44,45,47], similar to our findings. The three comparison studies that performed an external validation of both models concluded that the nonparametric models provided the lowest relative prediction error (RPE) for concentrations [46] and area under the curve [43,44], although for one of the latter studies [44], the RPE of the concentrations was similar. Our external validation showed a comparable RPE for both models after simulations, reflecting a good predictive performance of both models. PTA calculations using both modeling approaches were only performed by one previous study [48], which concluded that the PTA versus MIC profiles (based on 10,000 simulations) were similar. This seems to be caused by the similar parameter estimates and BSV of these models. Contrary to the latter study, our PTA simulations show different results for both modeling approaches, which could be explained by the higher BSV of our nonparametric model.

This paper has a few limitations. The main limitation is that the modeling population did not include 1000 mg dose regimens as well as patients with impaired renal function. A drawback of the validation population was that only 12 patients matched the eGFR range of the modeling population (51–172 mL/min). Another limitation is that the simulations were performed with a fixed value of protein binding because only total drug concentrations were available. However, the consequences seem to be low given the small protein binding of 20% [22].

5. Conclusions

The external predictive performance of parametric and nonparametric popPK models of imipenem in critically ill patients was adequate for subjects with high eGFRs, but insufficient for low eGFRs. This was explained by a paucity of subjects with renal impairment in the modeling population. External validation of popPK models is important to test the possibility of extrapolation to other populations. The PTA simulations of both models indicated that 1000 mg q6h is suitable to reach MICs of 2 mg/L in critically ill patients with eGFRs of 90–120 mL/min. However, for MICs of 2 mg/L and an eGFR of 150 mL/min, and for MICs of 4 mg/L, dosing recommendations could not be given because the PTA values differed largely per modeling approach. The consequences of the different modeling approaches in clinical practice should be further investigated.

Supplementary Materials: The following are available online at https://www.mdpi.com/article/10.3390/pharmaceutics13122170/s1, Table S1: Population parameter estimates; Table S2: Probabilities of target attainment (PTA) simulations.

Author Contributions: Conceptualization, F.d.V., B.C.M.d.W., M.N.N., J.S., W.M.Y., S.H., A.H., T.v.G., B.C.P.K. and A.E.M.; acquisition of data, J.S., S.H. and A.H.; formal analysis, F.d.V., B.C.M.d.W., T.v.G., B.C.P.K. and A.E.M.; writing—original draft preparation, F.d.V.; writing—review and editing, B.C.M.d.W., M.N.N., J.S., W.M.Y., S.H., A.H., T.v.G., B.C.P.K. and A.E.M. All authors have read and agreed to the published version of the manuscript.

Funding: This research was funded by the Innovative Medicines Initiative Joint Undertaking under grant agreement no. [115523], resources of which are composed of financial contribution from the European Union's Seventh Framework Programme (FP7/2007–2013) and EFPIA companies' in-kind contribution. The research leading to these results was conducted as part of the COMBACTE-NET consortium. For further information please refer to http://www.combacte.com/, accessed on 8 November 2021. The popPK models were developed using data of a cohort study funded by a Research and Development Grant awarded by the Geneva University Hospitals in 2009 [PRD 09-II-025]. AH was partially supported by the EU-funded project AIDA [grant Health-F3-2011-278348]. The external validation was performed using data of a study supported by the Internal Grant Agency of Palacky University (Olomouc, Czech Republic) [IGA UPOL2014 LF 008].

Institutional Review Board Statement: The study performed in the Geneva University Hospitals was conducted according to the guidelines of the Declaration of Helsinki and approved by the Geneva University Hospitals Ethics Committee (NAC 09-117). The study performed in the General University Hospital of Prague was conducted according to the guidelines of the Declaration of Helsinki, and approved by the local institutional Research Ethics Committee of General University Hospital (Prague, Czech Republic) [no. 1547/09 S-IV].

Informed Consent Statement: For the study performed in the Geneva University Hospitals, the Ethics Committee waived the requirement for informed consent from patients who were unconscious or otherwise unable to understand the study protocol, given its observational nature. For the study performed in the General University Hospital of Prague, written informed consent was not required from the subjects prior to inclusion because both regimens are considered standard clinical practice, but a subsequent written consent for analysis of the data was obtained from the subjects after recovery from unconsciousness.

Data Availability Statement: The data presented in this study are available on request from the corresponding author. The data are not publicly available due to controlled access requirements for clinical trial data.

Acknowledgments: The authors thank Johan W. Mouton for his contribution to the study design and all inspiring discussions about the data interpretation. Unfortunately, he was not able to read the first version of the manuscript. We are very sad that Mouton passed away on 9 July 2019. We thank Elodie von Dach (Geneva University Hospitals) for her extensive work recruiting patients and entering the data. Full membership of the COMBACTE-NET Consortium is available on the website: https://www.combacte.com/about/about-combacte-net-detail/ (accessed on 8 November 2021).

Conflicts of Interest: F.d.V., B.C.M.d.W., M.N.N., J.S., A.H. and A.E.M. declare that they have no conflict of interest. B.K. has received research funding from ZonMw (Dutch governmental support) and Teva. S.H. has received honoraria from Sandoz for participation in a Scientific Advisory Board. T.v.G. has received honoraria as consultant/speaker from Aurinia Pharma, Vitaeris, Roche Diagnostics, Novartis, Astellas, and Chiesi, and grant support for transplant related studies from Chiesi and Astellas. None of the EFPIA partners involved in the COMBACTE-NET consortium have a conflict of interest; none of them contributed to this article.

References

1. Mouton, J.W.; Ambrose, P.G.; Canton, R.; Drusano, G.L.; Harbarth, S.; MacGowan, A.; Theuretzbacher, U.; Turnidge, J. Conserving antibiotics for the future: New ways to use old and new drugs from a pharmacokinetic and pharmacodynamic perspective. *Drug Resist. Updates* **2011**, *14*, 107–117. [CrossRef]
2. De Velde, F.; Mouton, J.W.; de Winter, B.C.M.; van Gelder, T.; Koch, B.C.P. Clinical applications of population pharmacokinetic models of antibiotics: Challenges and perspectives. *Pharmacol. Res.* **2018**, *134*, 280–288. [CrossRef]
3. Mouton, J.W.; Brown, D.F.; Apfalter, P.; Canton, R.; Giske, C.G.; Ivanova, M.; MacGowan, A.P.; Rodloff, A.; Soussy, C.J.; Steinbakk, M.; et al. The role of pharmacokinetics/pharmacodynamics in setting clinical MIC breakpoints: The EUCAST approach. *Clin. Microbiol. Infect.* **2012**, *18*, E37–E45. [CrossRef] [PubMed]
4. Racine-Poon, A.; Wakefield, J. Statistical methods for population pharmacokinetic modelling. *Stat. Methods Med. Res.* **1998**, *7*, 63–84. [CrossRef]
5. Tatarinova, T.; Neely, M.; Bartroff, J.; van Guilder, M.; Yamada, W.; Bayard, D.; Jelliffe, R.; Leary, R.; Chubatiuk, A.; Schumitzky, A. Two general methods for population pharmacokinetic modeling: Non-parametric adaptive grid and non-parametric Bayesian. *J. Pharmacokinet. Pharmacodyn.* **2013**, *40*, 189–199. [CrossRef]
6. De Velde, F.; de Winter, B.C.M.; Neely, M.N.; Yamada, W.M.; Koch, B.C.P.; Harbarth, S.; von Dach, E.; van Gelder, T.; Huttner, A.; Mouton, J.W.; et al. Population Pharmacokinetics of Imipenem in Critically Ill Patients: A Parametric and Nonparametric Model Converge on CKD-EPI Estimated Glomerular Filtration Rate as an Impactful Covariate. *Clin. Pharmacokinet.* **2020**, *59*, 885–898. [CrossRef] [PubMed]
7. Levey, A.S.; Stevens, L.A.; Schmid, C.H.; Zhang, Y.L.; Castro, A.F., 3rd; Feldman, H.I.; Kusek, J.W.; Eggers, P.; Van Lente, F.; Greene, T.; et al. A new equation to estimate glomerular filtration rate. *Ann. Intern. Med.* **2009**, *150*, 604–612. [CrossRef]
8. Ambrose, P.G.; Bhavnani, S.M.; Rubino, C.M.; Louie, A.; Gumbo, T.; Forrest, A.; Drusano, G.L. Pharmacokinetics-pharmacodynamics of antimicrobial therapy: It's not just for mice anymore. *Clin. Infect. Dis.* **2007**, *44*, 79–86. [CrossRef]
9. Crandon, J.L.; Luyt, C.E.; Aubry, A.; Chastre, J.; Nicolau, D.P. Pharmacodynamics of carbapenems for the treatment of Pseudomonas aeruginosa ventilator-associated pneumonia: Associations with clinical outcome and recurrence. *J. Antimicrob. Chemother.* **2016**, *71*, 2534–2537. [CrossRef] [PubMed]
10. Ariano, R.E.; Nyhlen, A.; Donnelly, J.P.; Sitar, D.S.; Harding, G.K.; Zelenitsky, S.A. Pharmacokinetics and pharmacodynamics of meropenem in febrile neutropenic patients with bacteremia. *Ann. Pharmacother.* **2005**, *39*, 32–38. [CrossRef] [PubMed]
11. Roberts, J.A.; Abdul-Aziz, M.H.; Lipman, J.; Mouton, J.W.; Vinks, A.A.; Felton, T.W.; Hope, W.W.; Farkas, A.; Neely, M.N.; Schentag, J.J.; et al. Individualised antibiotic dosing for patients who are critically ill: Challenges and potential solutions. *Lancet Infect. Dis.* **2014**, *14*, 498–509. [CrossRef]
12. Li, C.; Du, X.; Kuti, J.L.; Nicolau, D.P. Clinical pharmacodynamics of meropenem in patients with lower respiratory tract infections. *Antimicrob. Agents Chemother.* **2007**, *51*, 1725–1730. [CrossRef] [PubMed]
13. Muller, A.E.; Punt, N.; Mouton, J.W. Optimal exposures of ceftazidime predict the probability of microbiological and clinical outcome in the treatment of nosocomial pneumonia. *J. Antimicrob. Chemother.* **2013**, *68*, 900–906. [CrossRef]
14. Craig, W.A. Pharmacokinetic/pharmacodynamic parameters: Rationale for antibacterial dosing of mice and men. *Clin. Infect. Dis.* **1998**, *26*, 1–10. [CrossRef]
15. Couffignal, C.; Pajot, O.; Laouenan, C.; Burdet, C.; Foucrier, A.; Wolff, M.; Armand-Lefevre, L.; Mentre, F.; Massias, L. Population pharmacokinetics of imipenem in critically ill patients with suspected ventilator-associated pneumonia and evaluation of dosage regimens. *Br. J. Clin. Pharmacol.* **2014**, *78*, 1022–1034. [CrossRef] [PubMed]
16. Sakka, S.G.; Glauner, A.K.; Bulitta, J.B.; Kinzig-Schippers, M.; Pfister, W.; Drusano, G.L.; Sorgel, F. Population pharmacokinetics and pharmacodynamics of continuous versus short-term infusion of imipenem-cilastatin in critically ill patients in a randomized, controlled trial. *Antimicrob. Agents Chemother.* **2007**, *51*, 3304–3310. [CrossRef]
17. Suchankova, H.; Lips, M.; Urbanek, K.; Neely, M.N.; Strojil, J. Is continuous infusion of imipenem always the best choice? *Int. J. Antimicrob. Agents* **2017**, *49*, 348–354. [CrossRef] [PubMed]
18. Roberts, J.A.; Paul, S.K.; Akova, M.; Bassetti, M.; De Waele, J.J.; Dimopoulos, G.; Kaukonen, K.M.; Koulenti, D.; Martin, C.; Montravers, P.; et al. DALI: Defining antibiotic levels in intensive care unit patients: Are current beta-lactam antibiotic doses sufficient for critically ill patients? *Clin. Infect. Dis.* **2014**, *58*, 1072–1083. [CrossRef]

19. Bricheux, A.; Lenggenhager, L.; Hughes, S.; Karmime, A.; Lescuyer, P.; Huttner, A. Therapeutic drug monitoring of imipenem and the incidence of toxicity and failure in hospitalized patients: A retrospective cohort study. *Clin. Microbiol. Infect.* **2019**, *25*, 383.e1–383.e4. [CrossRef]
20. Huttner, A.; Von Dach, E.; Renzoni, A.; Huttner, B.D.; Affaticati, M.; Pagani, L.; Daali, Y.; Pugin, J.; Karmime, A.; Fathi, M.; et al. Augmented renal clearance, low beta-lactam concentrations and clinical outcomes in the critically ill: An observational prospective cohort study. *Int. J. Antimicrob. Agents* **2015**, *45*, 385–392. [CrossRef]
21. Cockcroft, D.W.; Gault, M.H. Prediction of creatinine clearance from serum creatinine. *Nephron* **1976**, *16*, 31–41. [CrossRef]
22. Merck Sharp & Dohme BV. Summary of Product Characteristics Tienam 500/500mg Powder for Solution for Infusion. Haarlem, The Netherlands, 2020. Available online: https://www.geneesmiddeleninformatiebank.nl/smpc/h11089_smpc.pdf (accessed on 8 November 2021).
23. Legrand, T.; Chhun, S.; Rey, E.; Blanchet, B.; Zahar, J.R.; Lanternier, F.; Pons, G.; Jullien, V. Simultaneous determination of three carbapenem antibiotics in plasma by HPLC with ultraviolet detection. *J. Chromatogr. B Analyt. Technol. Biomed. Life Sci.* **2008**, *875*, 551–556. [CrossRef] [PubMed]
24. Byon, W.; Smith, M.K.; Chan, P.; Tortorici, M.A.; Riley, S.; Dai, H.; Dong, J.; Ruiz-Garcia, A.; Sweeney, K.; Cronenberger, C. Establishing best practices and guidance in population modeling: An experience with an internal population pharmacokinetic analysis guidance. *CPT Pharmacomet. Syst. Pharmacol.* **2013**, *2*, e51. [CrossRef]
25. Lips, M.; Siller, M.; Strojil, J.; Urbanek, K.; Balik, M.; Suchankova, H. Pharmacokinetics of imipenem in critically ill patients during empirical treatment of nosocomial pneumonia: A comparison of 0.5-h and 3-h infusions. *Int. J. Antimicrob. Agents* **2014**, *44*, 358–362. [CrossRef]
26. Merck Sharp & Dohme Corp. Prescribing Information Primaxin (Imipenem and Cilastatin) for Injection, for Intravenous Use. USA, NJ, Whitehouse Station. 2018. Available online: https://www.merck.com/product/usa/pi_circulars/p/primaxin/primaxin_iv_pi.pdf (accessed on 8 November 2021).
27. Keizer, R.J.; Karlsson, M.O.; Hooker, A. Modeling and Simulation Workbench for NONMEM: Tutorial on Pirana, PsN, and Xpose. *CPT Pharmacomet. Syst. Pharmacol.* **2013**, *2*, e50. [CrossRef] [PubMed]
28. Neely, M.N.; van Guilder, M.G.; Yamada, W.M.; Schumitzky, A.; Jelliffe, R.W. Accurate detection of outliers and subpopulations with Pmetrics, a nonparametric and parametric pharmacometric modeling and simulation package for R. *Ther. Drug Monit.* **2012**, *34*, 467–476. [CrossRef] [PubMed]
29. Baptista, J.P.; Neves, M.; Rodrigues, L.; Teixeira, L.; Pinho, J.; Pimentel, J. Accuracy of the estimation of glomerular filtration rate within a population of critically ill patients. *J. Nephrol.* **2014**, *27*, 403–410. [CrossRef]
30. Hobbs, A.L.; Shea, K.M.; Roberts, K.M.; Daley, M.J. Implications of Augmented Renal Clearance on Drug Dosing in Critically Ill Patients: A Focus on Antibiotics. *Pharmacotherapy* **2015**, *35*, 1063–1075. [CrossRef] [PubMed]
31. Belzberg, H.; Zhu, J.; Cornwell, E.E., 3rd; Murray, J.A.; Sava, J.; Salim, A.; Velmahos, G.C.; Gill, M.A. Imipenem levels are not predictable in the critically ill patient. *J. Trauma* **2004**, *56*, 111–117. [CrossRef]
32. Roberts, J.A.; Lipman, J. Pharmacokinetic issues for antibiotics in the critically ill patient. *Crit. Care Med.* **2009**, *37*, 840–851, quiz 859. [CrossRef]
33. Jaruratanasirikul, S.; Sudsai, T. Comparison of the pharmacodynamics of imipenem in patients with ventilator-associated pneumonia following administration by 2 or 0.5 h infusion. *J. Antimicrob. Chemother.* **2009**, *63*, 560–563. [CrossRef]
34. Novelli, A.; Adembri, C.; Livi, P.; Fallani, S.; Mazzei, T.; De Gaudio, A.R. Pharmacokinetic evaluation of meropenem and imipenem in critically ill patients with sepsis. *Clin. Pharmacokinet.* **2005**, *44*, 539–549. [CrossRef]
35. Abhilash, B.; Tripathi, C.D.; Gogia, A.R.; Meshram, G.G.; Kumar, M.; Suraj, B. Pharmacokinetic/pharmacodynamic profiling of imipenem in patients admitted to an intensive care unit in India: A nonrandomized, cross-sectional, analytical, open-labeled study. *Indian J. Crit. Care Med.* **2015**, *19*, 587–592. [CrossRef]
36. Brendel, K.; Dartois, C.; Comets, E.; Lemenuel-Diot, A.; Laveille, C.; Tranchand, B.; Girard, P.; Laffont, C.M.; Mentre, F. Are population pharmacokinetic and/or pharmacodynamic models adequately evaluated? A survey of the literature from 2002 to 2004. *Clin. Pharmacokinet.* **2007**, *46*, 221–234. [CrossRef]
37. European Committee on Antimicrobial Susceptibility Testing Breakpoint Tables for Interpretation of MICs and Zone Diameters, Version 11.0. 2021. Available online: www.eucast.org (accessed on 8 November 2021).
38. Launay-Iliadis, M.C.; Bruno, R.; Cosson, V.; Vergniol, J.C.; Oulid-Aissa, D.; Marty, M.; Clavel, M.; Aapro, M.; Le Bail, N.; Iliadis, A. Population pharmacokinetics of docetaxel during phase I studies using nonlinear mixed-effect modeling and nonparametric maximum-likelihood estimation. *Cancer Chemother. Pharmacol.* **1995**, *37*, 47–54. [CrossRef]
39. Vermes, A.; Mathot, R.A.; van der Sijs, I.H.; Dankert, J.; Guchelaar, H.J. Population pharmacokinetics of flucytosine: Comparison and validation of three models using STS, NPEM, and NONMEM. *Ther. Drug Monit.* **2000**, *22*, 676–687. [CrossRef]
40. Patoux, A.; Bleyzac, N.; Boddy, A.V.; Doz, F.; Rubie, H.; Bastian, G.; Maire, P.; Canal, P.; Chatelut, E. Comparison of nonlinear mixed-effect and non-parametric expectation maximisation modelling for Bayesian estimation of carboplatin clearance in children. *Eur. J. Clin. Pharmacol.* **2001**, *57*, 297–303. [CrossRef]
41. de Hoog, M.; Schoemaker, R.C.; van den Anker, J.N.; Vinks, A.A. NONMEM and NPEM2 population modeling: A comparison using tobramycin data in neonates. *Ther. Drug Monit.* **2002**, *24*, 359–365. [CrossRef]

42. Woillard, J.B.; Debord, J.; Benz-de-Bretagne, I.; Saint-Marcoux, F.; Turlure, P.; Girault, S.; Abraham, J.; Choquet, S.; Marquet, P.; Barin-Le Guellec, C. A Time-Dependent Model Describes Methotrexate Elimination and Supports Dynamic Modification of MRP2/ABCC2 Activity. *Ther. Drug Monit.* **2017**, *39*, 145–156. [CrossRef]
43. Woillard, J.B.; Lebreton, V.; Neely, M.; Turlure, P.; Girault, S.; Debord, J.; Marquet, P.; Saint-Marcoux, F. Pharmacokinetic tools for the dose adjustment of ciclosporin in haematopoietic stem cell transplant patients. *Br. J. Clin. Pharmacol.* **2014**, *78*, 836–846. [CrossRef] [PubMed]
44. Premaud, A.; Weber, L.T.; Tonshoff, B.; Armstrong, V.W.; Oellerich, M.; Urien, S.; Marquet, P.; Rousseau, A. Population pharmacokinetics of mycophenolic acid in pediatric renal transplant patients using parametric and nonparametric approaches. *Pharmacol. Res.* **2011**, *63*, 216–224. [CrossRef]
45. Bustad, A.; Terziivanov, D.; Leary, R.; Port, R.; Schumitzky, A.; Jelliffe, R. Parametric and nonparametric population methods: Their comparative performance in analysing a clinical dataset and two Monte Carlo simulation studies. *Clin. Pharmacokinet.* **2006**, *45*, 365–383. [CrossRef]
46. Baverel, P.G.; Savic, R.M.; Wilkins, J.J.; Karlsson, M.O. Evaluation of the nonparametric estimation method in NONMEM VI: Application to real data. *J. Pharmacokinet. Pharmacodyn.* **2009**, *36*, 297–315. [CrossRef] [PubMed]
47. Carlsson, K.C.; van de Schootbrugge, M.; Eriksen, H.O.; Moberg, E.R.; Karlsson, M.O.; Hoem, N.O. A population pharmacokinetic model of gabapentin developed in nonparametric adaptive grid and nonlinear mixed effects modeling. *Ther. Drug Monit.* **2009**, *31*, 86–94. [CrossRef]
48. Bulitta, J.B.; Landersdorfer, C.B.; Kinzig, M.; Holzgrabe, U.; Sorgel, F. New semiphysiological absorption model to assess the pharmacodynamic profile of cefuroxime axetil using nonparametric and parametric population pharmacokinetics. *Antimicrob. Agents Chemother.* **2009**, *53*, 3462–3471. [CrossRef] [PubMed]
49. Bulitta, J.B.; Landersdorfer, C.B.; Huttner, S.J.; Drusano, G.L.; Kinzig, M.; Holzgrabe, U.; Stephan, U.; Sorgel, F. Population pharmacokinetic comparison and pharmacodynamic breakpoints of ceftazidime in cystic fibrosis patients and healthy volunteers. *Antimicrob. Agents Chemother.* **2010**, *54*, 1275–1282. [CrossRef] [PubMed]

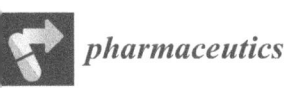

Article

Development of a Model-Informed Dosing Tool to Optimise Initial Antibiotic Dosing—A Translational Example for Intensive Care Units

Ferdinand Anton Weinelt [1,2], Miriam Songa Stegemann [3,4], Anja Theloe [5], Frieder Pfäfflin [3,4], Stephan Achterberg [3], Lisa Schmitt [1,2], Wilhelm Huisinga [6], Robin Michelet [1], Stefanie Hennig [1,7,8] and Charlotte Kloft [1,*]

1. Department of Clinical Pharmacy and Biochemistry, Institute of Pharmacy, Freie Universitaet Berlin, 12169 Berlin, Germany; ferdinand.weinelt@fu-berlin.de (F.A.W.); lisa.ehmann@fu-berlin.de (L.S.); robin.michelet@fu-berlin.de (R.M.); stefanie.hennig@certara.com (S.H.)
2. Graduate Research Training Program PharMetrX, 12169 Berlin, Germany
3. Department of Infectious Diseases and Respiratory Medicine, Charité-Universitaetsmedizin Berlin, Corporate Member of Freie Universitaet Berlin, Humboldt-Universitaet zu Berlin, Berlin Institute of Health, 10117 Berlin, Germany; miriam.stegemann@charite.de (M.S.S.); frieder.pfaefflin@charite.de (F.P.); stephan.achterberg@charite.de (S.A.)
4. Antimicrobial Stewardship, Charité-Universitaetsmedizin Berlin, Corporate Member of Freie Universitaet Berlin, Humboldt-Universitaet zu Berlin, Berlin Institute of Health, 10117 Berlin, Germany
5. Pharmacy Department, Charité-Universitaetsmedizin Berlin, Corporate Member of Freie Universitaet Berlin, Humboldt-Universitaet zu Berlin, Berlin Institute of Health, 10117 Berlin, Germany; anja.theloe@charite.de
6. Institute of Mathematics, University of Potsdam, 14476 Potsdam, Germany; huisinga@uni-potsdam.de
7. School of Clinical Sciences, Faculty of Health, Queensland University of Technology, Brisbane 4000, Australia
8. Certara, Inc., Princeton, NJ 08540, USA
* Correspondence: charlotte.kloft@fu-berlin.de; Tel.: +49-30-838-50656

Abstract: The prevalence and mortality rates of severe infections are high in intensive care units (ICUs). At the same time, the high pharmacokinetic variability observed in ICU patients increases the risk of inadequate antibiotic drug exposure. Therefore, dosing tailored to specific patient characteristics has a high potential to improve outcomes in this vulnerable patient population. This study aimed to develop a tabular dosing decision tool for initial therapy of meropenem integrating hospital-specific, thus far unexploited pathogen susceptibility information. An appropriate meropenem pharmacokinetic model was selected from the literature and evaluated using clinical data. Probability of target attainment (PTA) analysis was conducted for clinically interesting dosing regimens. To inform dosing prior to pathogen identification, the local pathogen-independent mean fraction of response (LPIFR) was calculated based on the observed minimum inhibitory concentrations distribution in the hospital. A simple, tabular, model-informed dosing decision tool was developed for initial meropenem therapy. Dosing recommendations achieving PTA > 90% or LPIFR > 90% for patients with different creatinine clearances were integrated. Based on the experiences during the development process, a generalised workflow for the development of tabular dosing decision tools was derived. The proposed workflow can support the development of model-informed dosing tools for initial therapy of various drugs and hospital-specific conditions.

Keywords: model-informed dosing tool; intensive care unit; antibiotic therapy; antimicrobial stewardship; meropenem; pathogen susceptibility

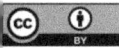

1. Introduction

Rational antibacterial therapy requires more than the appropriate choice of the antibiotic drug. Equally important are dosing regimens leading to an effective drug exposure linked to improved clinical success [1,2]. In intensive care unit (ICU) patients, the selection of an appropriate dosing regimen for an individual patient is challenging. The broad range of pathophysiological changes leads to high pharmacokinetic (PK) variability, which results in substantial differences in drug exposures between patients receiving the same dosing regimen [3–7]. To address these challenges, drug concentration measurements in combination with model-informed Bayesian dosing software have been suggested to monitor and, if needed, adjust dosing in this patient [8,9]. Unfortunately, in many hospitals, reliable, timely, and frequent concentration measurements of antibiotic drugs other than aminoglycosides are not implemented, and the use of Bayesian dosing software to inform subsequent dose adaptation is not common [10,11]. The lack of specialist expertise and structured processes, the costs for software and bioanalysis, and inconsistent global, national, and local regulations (e.g., concerning liability) impede the widespread implementation of model-informed Bayesian dosing software [12]. If software-based tools and frequent concentration measurements are not feasible, one promising alternative to individualise antibiotic therapy is tabular model-informed dosing tools or algorithms. These dosing tools can provide adequate initial dosing regimens for a wide range of patients, based on their patient characteristics and PK models of the drugs. In this context, existing PK models could be leveraged for a local patient population to circumvent the need for further PK studies.

Commonly, at the start of antibiotic therapy, neither the pathogen nor its susceptibility to the antibiotic are known. In many cases, both remain unknown during the course of antibiotic therapy [13]. Thus, patients without determined pathogen and its susceptibility are empirically treated based on the reported PK/pharmacodynamics (PD) breakpoints of the suspected pathogens [14]. The timely initiation of adequate empiric therapy is associated with decreased mortality rates, decreased length of hospitalisation, and decreased health care costs in patients with severe infections [15]. However, this strategy does usually not utilise available knowledge of a hospital regarding the susceptibility of local pathogens, and thus, it accepts the risk of unnecessary high or low and possibly toxic or ineffective antibiotic concentrations.

Meropenem is a broad-spectrum antibiotic frequently used to treat severe infections in ICU patients. It is considered to be a safe and well-tolerated antibiotic drug [16]. However, changes in meropenem PK in chronic disease patients, such as chronic kidney disease, can increase the risk for ineffective or toxic meropenem exposure [17]. The antimicrobial activity of meropenem is linked to the time period of the unbound concentration exceeding the minimum inhibitory concentration (MIC) of a pathogen. Therefore, the PK/PD index is $fT_{>MIC}$ [18]. Recently, a concentration measurement program for beta-lactam antibiotics at selected ICUs of Charité-Universitaetsmedizin Berlin, a tertiary care centre with a total of >3000 in-patient beds, was initiated. Observational unpublished data from that program showed >60% of measured minimum meropenem concentrations outside the locally defined target range of one to five times MIC. Consequently, the main goal of the present study was to improve the initial meropenem therapy in ICU patients and to optimise antibiotic dosing prior to pathogen detection. Hence, this study (i) aims to develop a tabular model-informed dosing tool to optimise initial therapy of the antibiotic meropenem at Charité-Universitaetsmedizin Berlin and for this (ii) investigated how to integrate previously observed, yet unexploited local pathogen susceptibility information into dosing decisions. Ultimately, a generalised workflow for the development of tabular model-informed dosing decision tools for initial antibiotic therapy to foster their implementation at the point-of-care was developed.

2. Materials and Methods

2.1. Patient Population and Meropenem Concentration Measurements

For the development of the model-informed dosing tool, 306 routine blood samples, dosing information immediately prior to sampling, and patient-specific data of 81 ICU patients receiving meropenem therapy at two ICUs (Department of Infectious Diseases and Respiratory Medicine; Department of Surgery) at Charité-Universitaetsmedizin Berlin were collected (approval: Charité Ethics Committee, EA4/053/19). For a subset of 34 patients with 66 samples, the full dosing history was recorded.

Meropenem concentrations were determined by Labor Berlin (Labor Berlin—Charité Vivantes GmbH, Berlin). Samples were sent to the laboratory within 1 h, centrifuged, and stored at −20 °C until plasma meropenem concentrations were measured After protein precipitation with methanol, meropenem concentration was quantified using high-performance liquid chromatography (C8 reverse phase column and a 4 min step-elution gradient (0.2% HCOOH/MeOH)) coupled with tandem mass spectrometry (electrospray ionisation (ESI+) in multiple reaction monitoring). The used bioanalytical method was validated according to the protocol of the Society of Toxicological and Forensic Chemistry (GTFCh) showing good analytical performance (inaccuracy: $\leq\pm5.9\%$ relative error, imprecision: $\leq 6.3\%$ coefficient of variation, calibration range: 2–30 µg/mL).

2.2. Pharmacokinetic Model Selection, Reduction, and Evaluation

Exclusively minimum meropenem concentrations and only 66 samples including the full dosing history were available. As a consequence, the PK data were unsuitable for PK model development. Instead, a published PK model was selected, evaluated for its appropriateness, and applied for the development of the dosing decision tool. The selection of the PK model was based on a high similarity of patient characteristics between the local study population and the model-underlying population.

To ensure the adequacy of the selected PK model for the new patient population, it was evaluated using median prediction errors and normalised prediction distribution errors (NPDEs) [19,20]. Model-predicted concentrations were obtained by 500 stochastic simulations based on the design and patient characteristics in the subset with full dosing history. To include parameter uncertainty, stochastic simulations were repeated for 1000 PK parameter sets obtained by bootstrapping of the dataset and re-estimation of the PK model. To assess possible deviations of the NPDEs from the standard normal distribution, the Wilcoxon signed rank test (mean $\neq 0$), Fisher ratio test (variance $\neq 1$), and Shapiro–Wilks test (normality assumption) were used. Simulations and bootstrap analyses were performed using NONMEM 7.4.3 (ICON Development Solutions, Ellicott City, MD, USA) and PsN version 4.7.0) [21]. NPDEs were analysed using the npde package (v. 2.0) in R/Rstudio (v. 3.5.0/v. 1.1.447) [22].

2.3. Pharmacokinetic/Pharmacodynamic Targets

Based on current literature evidence, the PK/PD target for ICU patients receiving short-time or prolonged meropenem infusions was defined as $100\%fT_{>MIC}$, while for patients receiving continuous meropenem infusions, it was defined as $100\%fT_{>4*MIC}$ to prevent steady-state meropenem concentrations within the mutant selection window [23,24]. The mutant selection window refers to a range of antibiotic drug concentrations in which only the growth of the most susceptible strains of a pathogen is suppressed. As a consequence, a growth advantage is provided to already available less susceptible strains in the pathogen population. Over a longer period of time, drug concentrations within the mutant selection window increase the proportion of less susceptible pathogens and thus the risk for resistant mutations to prevail [25]. Given that $100\%fT_{>MIC}$ cannot be achieved for an intravenous drug infusion on the first day of therapy, the attainment of a target of $98\%fT_{>MIC}$ was assessed. Total concentrations were evaluated due to the low ($\approx 2\%$) protein binding of meropenem [26]. Furthermore, to assess target attainment based on a single observed minimum meropenem concentration and to limit toxicities arising from high minimum meropenem concentrations, an additional target was introduced: the target range for minimum plasma concentrations was defined to be 1–5xMIC [27].

2.4. Development of the Dosing Decision Tool

2.4.1. Selection and Evaluation of Dosing Regimens

Dosing regimens were preselected based on their feasibility to integrate into local clinical routine. To reduce the number of eligible dosing regimens emerging from the possible combinations of the four variables (loading dose, infusion dose, infusion duration, dosing interval), deterministic simulations were performed. Comparing the dosing regimens, those achieving higher predicted minimum meropenem concentrations were further considered. The remaining dosing regimens (Table 1) were evaluated for probability of target attainment (PTA); for each dosing regimen and patient, the meropenem concentration time profile was predicted 1000 times (Monte Carlo simulations), and the probability to attain the PK/PD target was calculated for each individual MIC value). PTA was computed for treatment days 1 and 2 across target concentrations values ranging from 1 to 32 mg/L and creatinine clearance values were estimated according to Cockcroft and Gault (CLCRCG) [28] ranging from 10 to 300 mL/min (10–150 mL/min in steps of 10 mL/min, above in steps of 50 mL/min). PK model parameter uncertainty was incorporated by repeating each Monte Carlo simulation and the respective PTA analysis 1000 times using the PK parameter sets obtained from a non-parametric bootstrap. A dosing regimen leading to a PTA $\geq$ 90% for the median of the 1000 computed PTA values was considered adequate [29]. All dosing regimens reaching a PTA $\geq$ 90% were further ranked according to higher probability of minimum concentrations being in the defined target range (1–5xMIC) and subsequently according to lower total daily dose. Thus, for each CRCLCG group and MIC value, a single dosing recommendation was derived.

Table 1. Meropenem dosing regimens investigated in probability of target attainment analysis for potential inclusion in the dosing decision tool.

Dosing Regimen	Dose Per Infusion [mg]	Infusion Duration [h]	Dosing Interval [h]	Total Daily Dose [mg]
1	1000	4	6	4000
2	1000	4	8	3000
3	1000	4	12	2000
4	2000	4	6	8000
5	2000	4	8	6000
6	2000	4	12	4000
7	3000	4	6	12,000
8	3000	4	8	9000
9	3000	4	12	6000
10	4000	4	6	16,000
11	4000	4	8	12,000
12	4000	4	12	8000
13	4000	24	24	4000
14	6000	24	24	6000
15	8000	24	24	8000

All dosing regimens were administered in combination with a 1000 mg meropenem loading dose; *Grey*: Dosing regimen selected for the developed dosing tool.

2.4.2. Integration of Locally Available Pathogen Information

As a high number of antibiotic therapies are initiated prior to pathogen detection, dosing recommendations accounting for this situation were developed. Based on the PTA results and the pathogen-independent MIC distribution observed at Charité-Universitaetsmedizin Berlin in the previous year, the local pathogen-independent mean fraction of response (LPIFR) was introduced as metric for each dosing regimen: To determine the LPIFR for a dosing regimen ($LPIFR_{DR}$), first, the PTA for each investigated MIC level ($PTA_{MIC,DR}$) was multiplied by the relative MIC frequency ($\frac{n_{MIC}}{N_{MIC,total}}$; n_{MIC} = number of MIC values observed at a MIC level, $N_{MIC,total}$ = total number of observed MIC values) at this level in the distribution of MIC values in patients treated at Charité-Universitaetsmedizin Berlin.

Next, the resulting MIC-frequency weighted PTA values were summarised per dosing regimen (Equation (1)):

$$LPIFR_{DR} = \sum_{MIC}\left(PTA_{MIC,DR} \times \frac{n_{MIC}}{N_{MIC,total}}\right). \quad (1)$$

An LPIFR of ≥90% was considered adequate. Within each CRCLCG group, dosing regimens with a LPIFR ≥ 90% were selected and ranked by lower total daily dose.

2.5. Retrospective Evaluation of the Dosing Decision Tools Using Real Patient Data

Prior to implementation into clinical practice, the developed dosing decision tool was evaluated using the observed local patient population. The total daily dose of the dosing regimens recommended by the dosing decision tool for the local study population was compared to the total daily dose of the actual administered dosing regimens. For this purpose, the dataset of the local study population was stratified based on target attainment (above, below, and in the defined target range of 1–5xMIC) and the administered and recommended daily dose were compared.

3. Results

3.1. Pharmacokinetic Model Selection, Reduction, and Evaluation

A PK model developed by Ehmann et al. was selected for evaluation based on the high similarity in patient characteristics between the population used for model development and the local study population (Table 2 and Supplementary Material S1, Figure S1) [30]. The two-compartment model included a piecewise linear relation between CLCRCG and clearance (CL), a power relation between body weight and the central volume of distribution (V1), and a linear relation between serum albumin concentration and the peripheral volume of distribution (V2). Of these three covariates, Ehmann et al. demonstrated that only CLCRCG had a clinically relevant impact on PTA [30]. Therefore, for the development of the dosing tool, CLCRCG was kept as the only covariate in the model.

Table 2. Overview of patient characteristics.

Patient Characteristic	Charité Universitätsmedizin-Berlin	Ehmann et al.
Categorical	n (%)	n (%)
No. of patients	81	42
No. of meropenem samples	306	1376
Male	55 (67.9)	27 (56.3)
No. of extracorporeal membrane oxygenation	8 (9.88)	6 (12.5)
Continuous (unit)	Median (5th–95th percentile)	Median (5th–95th percentile)
Age (years)	64.0 (40.0–81.0)	55.5 (32.0–69.9)
Weight (kg)	75.0 (48.0–116)	70.5 (47.4–121)
Creatinine clearance [#] (mL/min)	74.4 (24.7–253)	80.8 (24.8–191)
Serum albumin concentration (g/dL)	2.68 (2.00–3.60)	2.80 (2.20–3.56)

[#] Calculated using Cockcroft–Gault formula [28]. Creatinine clearance and serum albumin concentration determined on sample level, all other characteristics determined on patient level.

This new reduced PK model was a two-compartment model with first-order elimination, interindividual variability on CL, V1 and V2, inter-occasion variability on CL, and a combined proportional and additive residual variability model (Supplementary Material S1, Figure S2). For this new reduced model, the PK parameters were re-estimated using the original dataset of the full model [30]. CL was shown to linearly increase with increasing CLCRCG up to an inflection point of 154 mL/min. An extensive internal model evaluation of the reduced model demonstrated high parameter accuracy and precision, robustness and predictive performance and, thus, applicability of the PK model to the new population (Supplementary Material S1, Text and Figure S3).

In Figure 1, prediction errors are plotted against observed meropenem concentrations in the 34 ICU patients with full dosing history. The median prediction error across all observations was −1.2 mg/L, indicating a slight bias towards underprediction. The 50% prediction error interval ranging from −3.5 to +2.5 mg/L indicated acceptable precision for the ICU patient population the model was applied to with a single outlier (Figure 1). Other samples of the same patient showed acceptable prediction errors, and therefore, this sample was excluded from the subsequent NPDE analysis. While the overall NPDE distribution did not significantly differ from the standard normal distribution (global adjusted p-value: 0.0976), the Wilcoxon signed-rank test revealed a significant (p-value 0.0325) deviation from a mean of 0 and therefore confirmed a small bias (NPDE mean: 0.296; detailed results: Supplementary Material S1, Tables S2 and S3; Figure S4).

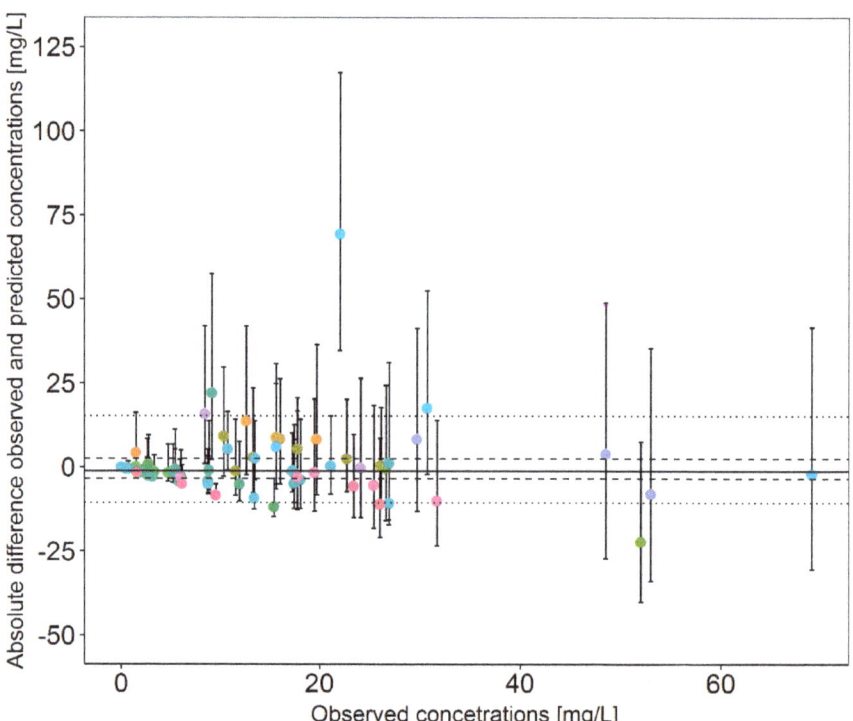

Figure 1. Absolute prediction error (mg/L) plotted against observed meropenem concentrations (n = 66) when predicting concentration based on the reduced pharmacokinetic model for the data in the subset. Points: median prediction error per sample. Colours: individual patients (i = 34). Error bar: 90% prediction interval of prediction error per sample. Solid horizontal line: median prediction error. Dashed line: 50% prediction interval of median prediction error. Dotted line: 90% prediction interval of median prediction error.

3.2. Development of the Dosing Decision Tool

3.2.1. Selection and Evaluation of Dosing Regimens

Deterministic simulations demonstrated that 2000 mg loading doses provided little further benefit over 1000 mg loading doses, the latter being sufficient to reach minimum meropenem concentrations above minimum meropenem concentrations in steady state (Figure 2A). Furthermore, short-term (0.5 h) infusions were inferior to prolonged infusions (4 h) with short-term infusions generally having higher maximum and lower minimum concentrations for the same daily dose (Figure 2B). Consequently, dosing regimens with a 2000 mg loading dose and short-term infusions were not further considered for PTA analysis. PTA analysis of the 15 remaining dosing regimens (Table 1) showed that for prolonged (4 h) infusions, four-times-daily dosing (i.e., a 6 h dosing interval) reached higher PTA values with lower total daily doses than three-times-daily dosing (Table 3). Furthermore, four-times-daily dosing of prolonged infusions (4 h) reached higher PTA values than continuous infusions with the same total daily dose, which was due to the higher targets for continuous infusions (Table 3). For pathogens with MIC ≥ 8 mg/L in patients with augmented renal clearance (≥150 mL/min), none of the investigated dosing regimens reached a PTA ≥ 90%.

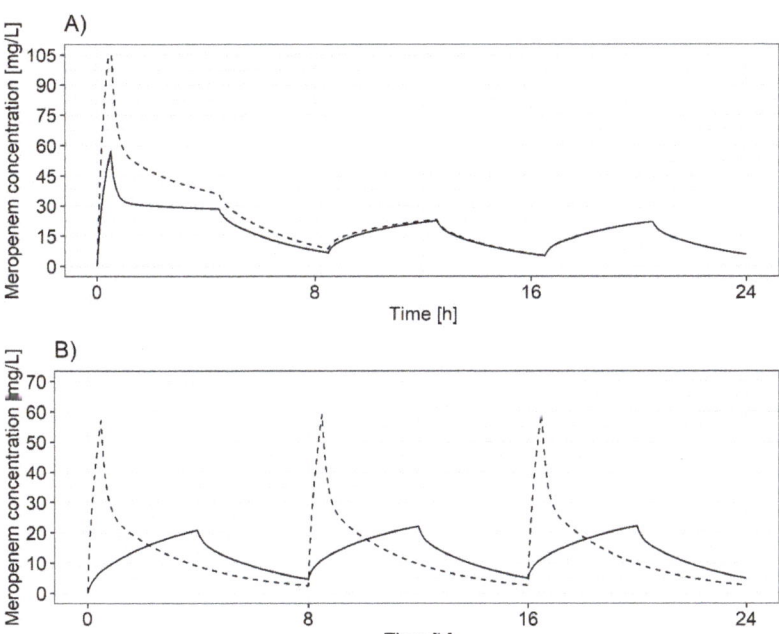

Figure 2. Predicted meropenem concentration–time profiles based on deterministic simulations using the reduced population pharmacokinetic model for a patient with creatinine clearance of 80.8 mL/min. (**A**) After either a 1000 (solid line) or a 2000 mg (dashed line) loading dose followed by prolonged (4 h) 1000 mg meropenem infusions with a dosing interval of 8 h. (**B**) After either a short-term (0.5 h; dashed line) or a prolonged (4 h; solid line) 1000 mg meropenem infusion administered every 8 h.

Table 3. Probability of target attainment for different dosing regimens administered to a patient with a creatinine clearance according to Cockroft–Gault of 120 mL/min and infected by a pathogen with a minimum inhibitory concentration of 4 mg/L for meropenem.

Total Daily Dose [mg]	Probability of Target Attainment, %		
	PI, 6 h Interval	PI, 8 h Interval	CI, 24 h Interval
4000	75.0	-	16.2
6000	-	58.0	67.7
8000	97.0	-	67.6
9000	-	76.8	-
12,000	99.4	-	-

Abbreviations: PI: Prolonged (4 h) infusion, CI: Continuous infusion.

Finally, dosing recommendations stratified by patient's CLCRCG and determined MIC were summarised in a single concise table (Figure 3).

Creatinine clearance [mL/min] (Cockcroft-Gault)	Dosing regimens* targeting minimum meropenem plasma concentrations [mg/L] of:							Creatinine clearance [mL/min] (Cockcroft-Gault)
	No MIC determined#	1†	2†	4†	8†	12†	16†	32†	
10	1 g MERO, q12h	1 g MERO, q12h	1 g MERO, q12h	1 g MERO, q12h	1 g MERO, q12h	1 g MERO, q8h	1 g MERO, q8h	1 g MERO, q6h	10
20					1 g MERO, q8h	1 g MERO, q6h	2 g MERO, q6h	20
30					1 g MERO, q8h	1 g MERO, q6h			30
40				1 g MERO, q8h	1 g MERO, q6h		2 g MERO, q6h	3 g MERO, q6h	40
50	1 g MERO, q8h		1 g MERO, q8h			2 g MERO, q6h		4 g MERO, q6h	50
60							3 g MERO, q6h		60
70		1 g MERO, q8h		1 g MERO, q6h	2 g MERO, q6h				70
80						3 g MERO, q6h	4 g MERO, q6h		80
90									90
100					3 g MERO, q6h	4 g MERO, q6h			100
110			1 g MERO, q6h					NO regimen reaching 90% PTA	110
120				2 g MERO, q6h					120
130									130
140	1 g MERO, q6h				4 g MERO, q6h		NO regimen reaching 90% PTA		140
150		1 g MERO, q6h				NO regimen reaching 90% PTA			150
175									175
200			2 g MERO, q6h	3 g MERO, q6h	4 g MERO, q6h Only PTA of 87% is reached!				200
250									250
300									300
Lower daily dose ←		1 g MERO q12h	1 g MERO q8h	1 g MERO q6h	2 g MERO q6h	3 g MERO q6h	4 g MERO q6h		→ Higher daily dose

daily dose ≤ 6 g
daily dose > 6 g and ≤12 g
daily dose > 12 g

*All prolonged infusions (4 h) with 1 g loading dose.
†90% of patients reach the targeted minimum meropenem concentration using the suggested dosing regimens.
#Based on the local pathogen-independent mean fraction of response (see page 2).
CAUTION: use only if no resistent bacteria (MIC > 8 mg/L) are expected.

Figure 3. Front page of the developed dosing decision tool for initial meropenem dosing in intensive care patients. Dosing recommendations are stratified for creatinine clearance according to Cockroft and Gault and target (minimal meropenem concentration or local pathogen-independent mean fraction of response (LPIFR), see text) MERO: meropenem; q6h: every 6 h dosing; q8h; every 8 h dosing; q12h: every 12 h dosing; PTA: probability of target attainment; MIC: minimal inhibitory concentration.

3.2.2. Integration of Locally Available Pathogen Information

If the pathogen and its MIC value are not known at the time of dosing selection, two options are implemented in the dosing tool: an empirical dosing regimen based on non-species related EUCAST breakpoints for meropenem or a dosing regimen based on the LPIFR metric and pathogen-independent MIC distribution data from ICUs at Charité-Universitaetsmedizin Berlin. A short summary of both options was added on the backside of the dosing decision table (Supplementary Material S2). Compared to targeting the pathogen independent 'susceptible/susceptible at increased exposure' (2 mg/L) or the 'susceptible at increased exposure/resistant' (8 mg/L) EUCAST breakpoints, the LPIFR substantially reduced the drug exposure in patients while still assuring a desired percentage of 90% of patients being above the PK/PD target of $98\%T_{>MIC}$. Based on the LPIFR, the daily dose for a patient with a creatinine clearance of 120 mL/min was 4000 mg, whereas there was a three-fold higher dose of 12,000 mg when targeting the EUCAST susceptible at increased exposure/resistant breakpoint (8 mg/L).

3.3. *Retrospective Evaluation of the Dosing Decision Tools Using Real Patient Data*

Of the 306 meropenem samples of the local study population, 46 (15.0%) were found to be below and 160 (52.3%) were found to be above the defined target range. The retrospective application of the developed tool recommended a change in dosing for the majority (77%) of patients with concentrations observed outside the target range (Figure 4). For 72% of the patients with minimum meropenem concentration below the target range, the developed dosing tool recommended an increased daily dose, while for 78% of the patients with samples above the target range, a lower daily dose was recommended.

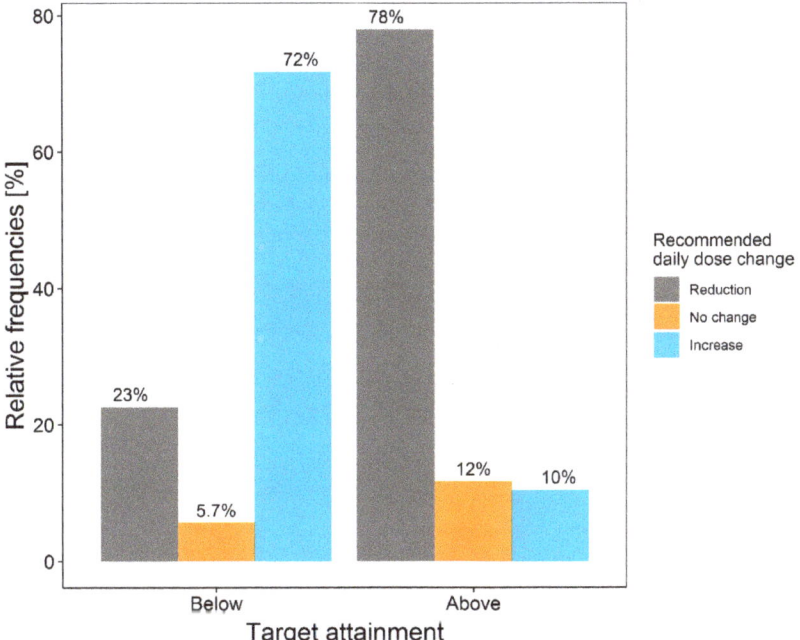

Figure 4. Frequency of daily meropenem dose adjustments by comparing the recommended daily dose to the actual administered daily dose at Charité-Universitaetsmedizin Berlin, stratified by non-attainment of the target range of the administered dosing regimen. Of 306 samples, 46 were below and 160 were above the target range.

4. Discussion

A concise dosing decision tool for initial meropenem dosing incorporating local susceptibility data was developed for the specific local needs. Additionally, a generalised workflow that can be used as blueprint for the development of such a dosing decision tool at the point-of-care was derived based on our experiences (Figure 5). After the identification of the elevated risk of inadequate antibiotic drug exposure in ICU patients, a local collaboration was established to assess and, if needed, improve antibiotic dosing. The close interprofessional collaboration between the antimicrobial stewardship (AMS) team, infectious disease specialists, critical care specialists, pharmacists, the clinical laboratory and pharmacometricians proved to be a vital part of the development process and should enable best adaptation to the local clinical routine. Bi-weekly meetings of the study team enabled continuous discussions, feedback, and adjustments throughout each step of the course of action.

As a mandatory prerequisite, the external PK model evaluation assured good predictive performance between the developed tool and the local patient population. The slight bias of the PK model to underpredict observed meropenem concentrations led to slightly lower PTA values for each dosing regimen and can be considered as an additional safety margin. The first evaluation of the dosing decision tool using retrospectively collected data suggests a substantial potential to improve target attainment. For 72% of the patients with concentrations below the target, a dose increase was recommended, and for 78% of the patients with concentrations above the target, a dose reduction was recommended. The suggested reduction of daily dose for 23% of samples below the target is due to the recommendation of four-times-daily dosing instead of the three-times-daily dosing being administered: This more frequent administration of meropenem achieved higher PTA values despite reduced daily doses (Table 3). At the same time, the suggested increase in daily dose for 10% of the sample above the target range is mostly likely due to the selected PK model: The safety margin included in the PK model leads to more conservative, higher dosing recommendations to guarantee effective drug exposure. Additionally, in both cases, the high PK variability observed in critically ill patients renders a perfect recommendation for all patients untenable. To conclude, the retrospective evaluation highlighted the potential of the tool to improve meropenem therapy in critically ill patients. As next step, a prospective clinical trial should investigate the impact of the dosing decision tool on target attainment. The approach and workflow presented can improve acceptance and therefore the implementation of model-informed dosing decision tools at the point-of-care.

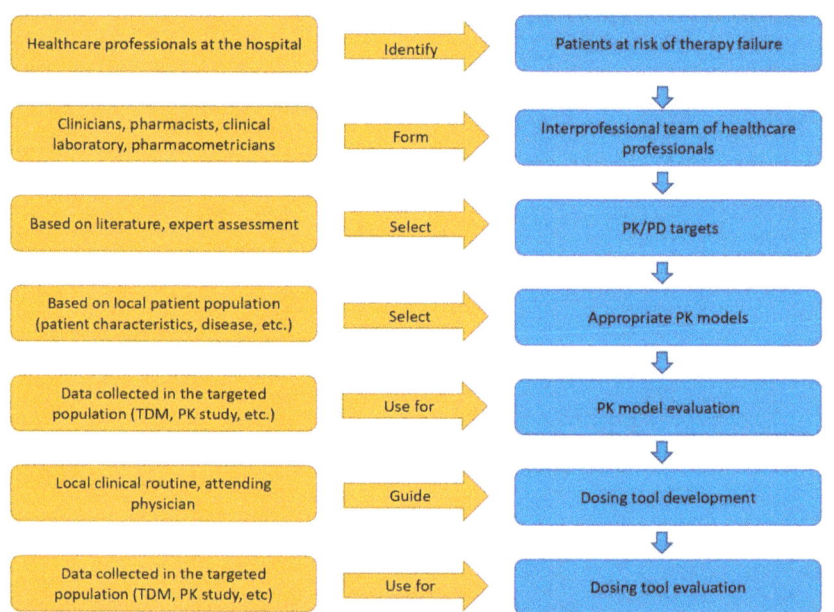

Figure 5. Steps (blue) considered in the generalised workflow development of a tabular precision dosing tool for initial therapy together with recommendations (yellow) to support each step.

All recommended dosing regimens included a 1000 mg loading dose to ensure an immediate achievement of sufficiently high meropenem concentrations at the start of antibiotic therapy. Regardless of the loading dose used (1000 mg vs. 2000 mg), the minimum meropenem concentration after the first maintenance dose was higher than or equal to minimum concentrations in steady state. Therefore, a 2000 mg loading dose showed no additional benefit compared to a 1000 mg loading dose and was considered to be an unnecessary higher drug exposure for patients and thus not retained in the dosing tool. Due to the different PK/PD targets for prolonged and continuous infusions, prolonged infusions provided higher target attainment for the same daily dose and as a consequence represent all integrated dosing regimen. In order to keep an explicit and clear structure in the dosing decision tool, only one dosing regimen was incorporated for each individual CLCRCG and MIC value. Overall, only six different initial dosing regimens (Table 2) were included in the dosing decision tool. This simplicity aims to achieve an initial dose individualisation to optimise dosing in ICU patients while maintaining a level of standardisation and avoiding complication of the ICU ward process. One further important note on the integrated dosing regimen: The dosing regimens selected and integrated into the tool were selected based on their ability to reach a predefined PK target. As a consequence, high daily doses (up to 16 g) are included in the tool for high target concentrations. However, for such high targets, a change in antibiotic should be considered.

A further feature in the dosing decision tool is the use of local, hospital-specific and pathogen-independent MIC values. The LPIFR metric facilitates dosing based on not only patient characteristics but additionally on local bacterial susceptibility conditions in the hospital. While we foresee that this approach is a valuable opportunity to reduce unnecessary high meropenem dosing, we also strongly advise to apply it with caution: As local MIC distributions can vary over time, these need to be monitored and dosing suggestions based on LPIFR need to be updated regularly. Furthermore, in the rare event of a pathogen with high MIC values (>8–32 mg/L), the risk of target non-attainment could be underestimated until the MIC is determined. Therefore, it is vital to communicate those limitations to the decision-making team and encourage a dosing increase or change of antibiotic if higher MIC values are expected. In general, the dosing regimen recommendations based on the LPIFR metric should only be used as long as there is no further information about the pathogen (e.g., MIC) available. Furthermore, patients receiving renal replacement therapy (RRT), obese patients, and paediatric patients were not included in the PK model development and evaluation. Consequently, the derived dosing recommendations do not apply to those patient populations but only to adult critically ill patients.

For critically ill patients receiving antibiotics, drug measurements linked with Bayesian dosing software have been recommended for dose individualisation [3]. To date, this very promising approach could not always be implemented into clinical practice. Individualised meropenem therapy guided by concentration measurements is still only available in very few hospitals [10]. As an alternative, tabular dosing decision tools based on PTA analysis of an evaluated PK model can be used for initial dosing. Furthermore, these tabular dosing decision tools can provide dosing recommendations prior to the first drug measurement to improve dosing in this especially crucial time window of antibiotic drug therapy [31].

To optimise meropenem dosing, several complementary model-based tools or algorithms exist: the MeroRisk calculator supports the identification of critically ill patients at risk of suboptimal exposure and different model-based algorithms or nomograms provide dosing suggestions [30,32,33]. Unfortunately, none of the tools matched our local conditions and objectives: The dosing regimens frequently used at Charité-Universitaetsmedizin Berlin were either not included in the available tools or were part of a multitude of dosing regimen recommendations complicating the daily use of the tool. Furthermore, the risk of reaching toxic minimum concentrations was not considered in those other tools, and an evaluation of the underlying PK models would have been necessary. Most likely, this situation is similar for a wide range of drugs, model-based tools, and hospitals. Even when model-based tools or PK models are available for a specific drug in a specific patient population, the selected target or the clinical setting might hinder implementation and use. In those situations, local initiatives are needed to develop a dosing decision tool fit for the situation on site. As presented in our example, routine drug measurements can be used to evaluate published PK models instead of conducting expensive clinical trials to develop new PK models as the basis for new tools. Furthermore, by employing the LPIFR, antibiotic dosing prior to pathogen detection can be adapted to local susceptibility patterns. Even though tools developed to fit local conditions might be more difficult to transfer to other institutions, we believe the advantages of local initiatives clearly outweigh this drawback. The approach with the generalised workflow (Figure 5) may serve as a blueprint to a wide range of hospitals, patient populations, and drugs to develop a sophisticated dosing decision tool providing optimised initial dosing adapted for local conditions and objectives.

Supplementary Materials: The following are available online at https://www.mdpi.com/article/10.3390/pharmaceutics13122128/s1, Supplementary Material S1: Pharmacokinetic model selection, reduction and evaluation, Supplementary Material S2: Dosing decision tool.

Author Contributions: Conceptualisation: F.A.W., S.H., C.K., methodology: F.A.W., L.S., S.H., C.K.; software: F.A.W.; validation: F.A.W., formal analysis: F.A.W.; investigation F.A.W., M.S.S., A.T., F.P., S.H.; data curation: F.A.W., S.A.; writing—original draft preparation: F.A.W.; writing—review and editing: M.S.S., A.T., F.P., S.A., L.S., W.H., R.M., S.H., C.K.; visualisation: F.A.W.; supervision: C.K.; project administration: M.S.S. All authors have read and agreed to the published version of the manuscript.

Funding: S.H. was partly supported by the Alexander von Humboldt Foundation, Germany, during this project.

Institutional Review Board Statement: The study was conducted according to the guidelines of the Declaration of Helsinki, and approved by the Institutional Review Board (or Ethics Committee) of Charité-Universitaetsmedizin Berlin (protocol code EA4/053/19, date of approval: 17 April 2019).

Informed Consent Statement: Patient consent was waived due to the retrospective evaluation of data from routine samples in the context of research without intervention.

Data Availability Statement: The data presented in the study are available at reasonable request from the corresponding author.

Acknowledgments: Lukas Duebel is acknowledged for support in data acquisition, Peggy Kiessling for laboratory support, Alexander Uhrig, and Ralf Lorenz for clinical support and Agata Mikolajewska for support of the study design. The authors thank the High-Performance Computing Service of ZEDAT at Freie Universitaet Berlin (https://www.fu-berlin.de/sites/high-performance-computing/index.html, last accessed date: 1 December 2021) for high-performance computing capacities.

Conflicts of Interest: C.K. and W.H. report grants from an industry consortium (AbbVie Deutschland GmbH & Co. KG, AstraZeneca, Boehringer Ingelheim Pharma GmbH & Co. KG, Grünenthal GmbH, F. Hoffmann-La Roche Ltd., Merck KGaA and SANOFI) for the PharMetrX program. C.K. reports grants for the Innovative Medicines Initiative-Joint Undertaking ("DDMoRe"), Diurnal Ltd., the Federal Ministry of Education and Research within the Joint Programming Initiative on Antimicrobial Resistance Initiative (JPIAMR) and from the European Commission within in the Horizon 2020 framework programme ("FAIR"), all outside the submitted work.

References

1. Levy Hara, G.; Kanj, S.S.; Pagani, L.; Abbo, L.; Endimiani, A.; Wertheim, H.F.L.; Amábile-Cuevas, C.; Tattevin, P.; Mehtar, S.; Lopes Cardoso, F.; et al. Ten Key Points for the Appropriate use of Antibiotics in Hospitalised Patients: A Consensus from the Antimicrobial Stewardship and Resistance Working Groups of the International Society of Chemotherapy. *Int. J. Antimicrob. Agents* **2016**, *48*, 239–246. [CrossRef] [PubMed]
2. Roberts, J.A.; Paul, S.K.; Akova, M.; Bassetti, M.; De Waele, J.J.; Dimopoulos, G.; Kaukonen, K.M.; Koulenti, D.; Martin, C.; Montravers, P.; et al. DALI: Defining Antibiotic Levels in Intensive Care Unit Patients: Are Current ß-lactam Antibiotic Doses Sufficient for Critically Ill Patients? *Clin. Infect. Dis.* **2014**, *58*, 1072–1083. [CrossRef] [PubMed]
3. Roberts, J.A.; Abdul-Aziz, M.H.; Lipman, J.; Mouton, J.W.; Vinks, A.A.; Felton, T.W.; Hope, W.W.; Farkas, A.; Neely, M.N.; Schentag, J.J.; et al. Individualised Antibiotic Dosing for Patients Who are Critically Ill: Challenges and Potential Solutions. *Lancet Infect. Dis.* **2014**, *14*, 498–509. [CrossRef]
4. McKenzie, C. Antibiotic dosing in critical illness. *J. Antimicrob. Chemother.* **2011**, *66*, 25–31. [CrossRef]
5. Vossen, M.G.; Ehmann, L.; Pferschy, S.; Maier-Salamon, A.; Haidinger, M.; Weiser, C.; Wenisch, J.M.; Saria, K.; Kajahn, C.; Jilch, S.; et al. Elimination of Doripenem during Dialysis and Pharmacokinetic Evaluation of Posthemodialysis Dosing for Patients Undergoing Intermittent Renal Replacement Therapy. *Antimicrob. Agents Chemother.* **2018**, *62*, e02430-17. [CrossRef]
6. Kees, M.G.; Minichmayr, I.K.; Moritz, S.; Beck, S.; Wicha, S.G.; Kees, F.; Kloft, C.; Steinke, T. Population Pharmacokinetics of Meropenem during Continuous Infusion in Surgical ICU patients. *J. Clin. Pharmacol.* **2016**, *56*, 307–315. [CrossRef]
7. Minichmayr, I.K.; Schaeftlein, A.; Kuti, J.L.; Zeitlinger, M.; Kloft, C. Clinical Determinants of Target Non-Attainment of Linezolid in Plasma and Interstitial Space Fluid: A Pooled Population Pharmacokinetic Analysis with Focus on Critically Ill Patients. *Clin. Pharmacokinet.* **2017**, *56*, 617–633. [CrossRef]
8. Felton, T.W.; Hope, W.W.; Roberts, J.A. How Severe Is Antibiotic Pharmacokinetic Variability in Critically Ill Patients and What Can Be Done about it? *Diagn. Microbiol. Infect. Dis.* **2014**, *79*, 441–447. [CrossRef] [PubMed]
9. Roberts, J.A.; Ulldemolins, M.; Roberts, M.S.; McWhinney, B.; Ungerer, J.; Paterson, D.L.; Lipman, J. Therapeutic Drug Monitoring of β-Lactams in Critically Ill Patients: Proof of Concept. *Int. J. Antimicrob. Agents* **2010**, *36*, 332–339. [CrossRef]
10. Tabah, A.; de Waele, J.; Lipman, J.; Zahar, J.R.; Cotta, M.O.; Barton, G.; Timsit, J.F.; Roberts, J.A. The ADMIN-ICU Survey: A Survey on Antimicrobial Dosing and Monitoring in ICUs. *J. Antimicrob. Chemother.* **2015**, *70*, 2671–2677. [CrossRef] [PubMed]
11. Paviour, S.; Hennig, S.; Staatz, C.E. Usage and Monitoring of Intravenous Tobramycin in Cystic Fibrosis in Australia and the UK. *J. Pharm. Pract. Res.* **2016**, *46*, 15–21. [CrossRef]

12. Darwich, A.S.; Ogungbenro, K.; Vinks, A.A.; Powell, J.R.; Reny, J.; Marsousi, N.; Daali, Y.; Fairman, D. Why Has Model-Informed Precision Dosing Not Yet Become Common Clinical Reality? Lessons from the Past and a Roadmap for the Future. *Clin. Pharmacol. Ther.* **2017**, *101*, 646–656. [CrossRef] [PubMed]
13. Liebchen, U.; Paal, M.; Scharf, C.; Schroeder, I.; Grabein, B.; Zander, J.; Siebers, C.; Zoller, M. The ONTAI Study—A Survey on Antimicrobial Dosing and the Practice of Therapeutic Drug Monitoring in German Intensive Care Units. *J. Crit. Care* **2020**, *60*, 260–266. [CrossRef]
14. EuCAST. EuCAST Breakpoints. The European Committee on Antimicrobial Susceptibility Testing. 2018. Available online: https://eucast.org/fileadmin/src/media/PDFs/EUCAST_files/Breakpoint_tables/v_8.0_Breakpoint_Tables.pdf (accessed on 3 December 2021).
15. Ewig, S.; Höffken, G.; Kern, W.; Rohde, G.; Flick, H.; Krause, R.; Ott, S.; Bauer, T.; Dalhoff, K.; Gatermann, S.; et al. Behandlung von erwachsenen Patienten mit ambulant erworbener Pneumonie und Prävention—Update 2016. *Pneumologie* **2016**, *70*, 151–200. [CrossRef]
16. Linden, P. Safety Profile of Meropenem: An Updated Review of Over 6000 Patients Treated with Meropenem. *Drug Saf.* **2007**, *30*, 657–668. [CrossRef]
17. Chimata, M.; Nagase, M.; Suzuki, Y.; Shimomura, M.; Kakuta, S. Pharmacokinetics of Meropenem in Patients with Various Degrees of Renal Function, Including Patients with End-Stage Renal Disease. *Antimicrob. Agents Chemother.* **1993**, *37*, 229–233. [CrossRef] [PubMed]
18. Nicolau, D.P. Pharmacokinetic and Pharmacodynamic Properties of Meropenem. *Clin. Infect. Dis.* **2008**, *47*, S32–S40. [CrossRef]
19. Brendel, K.; Comets, E.; Laffont, C.; Laveille, C.; Mentré, F. Metrics for External Model Evaluation with an Application to the Population Pharmacokinetics of Gliclazide. *Pharm. Res.* **2006**, *23*, 2036–2049. [CrossRef]
20. Mentré, F.; Escolano, S. Prediction Discrepancies for the Evaluation of Nonlinear Mixed-Effects Models. *J. Pharmacokinet. Pharmacodyn.* **2006**, *33*, 345–367. [CrossRef]
21. Lindbom, L.; Pihlgren, P.; Jonsson, N. PsN-Toolkit—A Collection of Computer Intensive Statistical Methods for Non-Linear Mixed Effect Modeling Using NONMEM. *Comput. Methods Progr. Biomed.* **2005**, *79*, 241–257. [CrossRef]
22. Comets, E.; Brendel, K.; Mentré, F. Computing Normalised Prediction Distribution Errors to Evaluate Nonlinear Mixed-Effect Models: The NPDE Add-On Package for R. *Comput. Methods Progr. Biomed.* **2007**, *90*, 154–166. [CrossRef] [PubMed]
23. Li, C.; Du, X.; Kuti, J.L.; Nicolau, D.P. Clinical Pharmacodynamics of Meropenem in Patients with Lower Respiratory Tract Infections. *Antimicrob. Agents Chemother.* **2007**, *51*, 1725–1730. [CrossRef]
24. Ariano, R.E.; Zelenitsky, S.A.; Nyhlén, A.; Sitar, D.S. An Evaluation of an Optimal Sampling Strategy for Meropenem in Febrile Neutropenics. *J. Clin. Pharmacol.* **2005**, *45*, 832–835. [CrossRef]
25. Drlica, K. The Mutant Selection Window and Antimicrobial Resistance. *J. Antimicrob. Chemother.* **2003**, *52*, 11–17. [CrossRef] [PubMed]
26. Craig, W.A. The Pharmacology of Meropenem, a New Carbapenem Antibiotic. *Clin. Infect. Dis.* **1997**, *24*, S266–S275. [CrossRef]
27. Guilhaumou, R.; Benaboud, S.; Bennis, Y.; Dahyot-Fizelier, C.; Dailly, E.; Gandia, P.; Goutelle, S.; Lefeuvre, S.; Mongardon, N.; Roger, C.; et al. Optimization of the Treatment with Beta-Lactam Antibiotics in Critically Ill Patients—Guidelines from the French Society of Pharmacology and Therapeutics (Société Française de Pharmacologie et Thérapeutique—SFPT) and the French Society of Anaesthesia. *Crit. Care* **2019**, *23*, 1–20. [CrossRef]
28. Cockcroft, D.W.; Gault, M.H. Prediction of Creatinine Clearance from Serum Creatinine. *Nephron* **1976**, *16*, 31–41. [CrossRef] [PubMed]
29. European Medicines Agency Committee for Medicinal Products for Human Use (CHMP). Guideline on the Use of Pharmacokinetics and Pharmacodynamics in the Development of Antimicrobial Medicinal Products. 2016, pp. 1–17. Available online: https://www.ema.europa.eu/en/documents/scientific-guideline/guideline-use-pharmacokinetics-pharmacodynamics-development-antimicrobial-medicinal-products_en.pdf (accessed on 10 May 2021).
30. Ehmann, L.; Zoller, M.; Minichmayr, I.K.; Scharf, C.; Huisinga, W.; Zander, J.; Kloft, C. Development of a Dosing Algorithm for Meropenem in Critically Ill Patients Based on a Population Pharmacokinetic/Pharmacodynamic Analysis. *Int. J. Antimicrob. Agents* **2019**, *54*, 309–317. [CrossRef]
31. Harbarth, S.; Garbino, J.; Pugin, J.; Romand, J.A.; Lew, D.; Pittet, D. Inappropriate Initial Antimicrobial Therapy and Its Effect on Survival in a Clinical Trial of Immunomodulating Therapy for Severe Sepsis. *Am. J. Med.* **2003**, *115*, 529–535. [CrossRef] [PubMed]
32. Ehmann, L.; Zoller, M.; Minichmayr, I.K.; Scharf, C.; Maier, B.; Schmitt, M.V.; Hartung, N.; Huisinga, W.; Vogeser, M.; Frey, L.; et al. Role of Renal Function in Risk Assessment of Target Non-Attainment after Standard Dosing of Meropenem in Critically Ill Patients: A Prospective Observational Study. *Crit. Care* **2017**, *21*, 1–14. [CrossRef] [PubMed]
33. Minichmayr, I.K.; Roberts, J.A.; Frey, O.R.; Roehr, A.C.; Kloft, C.; Brinkmann, A. Development of a Dosing Nomogram for Continuous-Infusion Meropenem in Critically Ill Patients Based on a Validated Population Pharmacokinetic Model. *J. Antimicrob. Chemother.* **2018**, *73*, 1330–1339. [CrossRef] [PubMed]

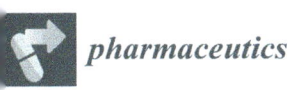

Article

Pseudomonas aeruginosa Susceptibility in Spain: Antimicrobial Activity and Resistance Suppression Evaluation by PK/PD Analysis

Ana Valero [1,2], Alicia Rodríguez-Gascón [1,3], Arantxa Isla [1,3], Helena Barrasa [4,5], Ester del Barrio-Tofiño [6], Antonio Oliver [6], Andrés Canut [3,7,*] and María Ángeles Solinís [1,3,*]

[1] Pharmacokinetic, Nanotechnology and Gene Therapy Group (PharmaNanoGene), Faculty of Pharmacy, Centro de Investigación Lascaray Ikergunea, University of the Basque Country UPV/EHU, Paseo de la Universidad 7, 01006 Vitoria-Gasteiz, Spain; avalero@fhp.cat (A.V.); alicia.rodriguez@ehu.eus (A.R.-G.); arantxa.isla@ehu.eus (A.I.)
[2] Pharmacy Service, Fundació Sant Hospital, Passeig Joan Brudieu 8, 25700 La Seu d'Urgell, Spain
[3] Bioaraba, Microbiology, Infectious Disease, Antimicrobial Agents, and Gene Therapy, 01006 Vitoria-Gasteiz, Spain
[4] Instituto de Investigación Sanitaria Bioaraba, 01006 Vitoria-Gasteiz, Spain; helena.barrasagonzalez@osakidetza.eus
[5] Intensive Care Unit, Araba University Hospital, Osakidetza Basque Health Service, 01006 Vitoria-Gasteiz, Spain
[6] Microbiology Service, Hospital Son Espases, Instituto de Investigación Sanitaria Illes Balears (IdISBa), 07120 Palma de Mallorca, Spain; ester.delbarrio@ssib.es (E.d.B.-T.); antonio.oliver@ssib.es (A.O.)
[7] Microbiology Service, University Hospital of Araba, Osakidetza Basque Health Service, 01006 Vitoria-Gasteiz, Spain
* Correspondence: andres.canutblasco@osakidetza.eus (A.C.); marian.solinis@ehu.eus (M.Á.S.); Tel.: +34-945-0075-60 (A.C.); +34-945-013-469 (M.Á.S.)

Abstract: *Pseudomonas aeruginosa* remains one of the major causes of healthcare-associated infection in Europe; in 2019, 12.5% of invasive isolates of *P. aeruginosa* in Spain presented combined resistance to ≥3 antimicrobial groups. The Spanish nationwide survey on *P. aeruginosa* antimicrobial resistance mechanisms and molecular epidemiology was published in 2019. Based on the information from this survey, the objective of this work was to analyze the overall antimicrobial activity of the antipseudomonal antibiotics considering pharmacokinetic/pharmacodynamic (PK/PD) analysis. The role of PK/PD to prevent or minimize resistance emergence was also evaluated. A 10,000-subject Monte Carlo simulation was executed to calculate the probability of target attainment (PTA) and the cumulative fraction of response (CFR) considering the minimum inhibitory concentration (MIC) distribution of bacteria isolated in ICU or medical wards, and distinguishing between sample types (respiratory and non-respiratory). Ceftazidime/avibactam followed by ceftolozane/tazobactam and colistin, categorized as the Reserve by the Access, Watch, Reserve (AWaRe) classification of the World Health Organization, were the most active antimicrobials, with differences depending on the admission service, sample type, and dose regimen. Discrepancies between EUCAST-susceptibility breakpoints for *P. aeruginosa* and those estimated by PK/PD analysis were detected. Only standard doses of ceftazidime/avibactam and ceftolozane/tazobactam provided drug concentrations associated with resistance suppression.

Keywords: *Pseudomonas aeruginosa*; pharmacokinetic/pharmacodynamic (PK/PD) analysis; Monte Carlo simulation; antimicrobial resistance; probability of target attainment (PTA); cumulative fraction of response (CFR)

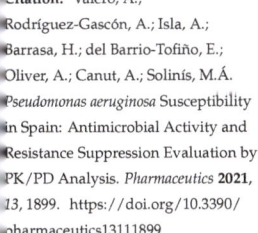

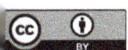

1. Introduction

The World Health Organization (WHO) has declared antimicrobial resistance as one of the top 10 global public health threats facing humanity [1]. The emergence of resistance to multiple antimicrobial agents in pathogenic bacteria has become a significant public health concern, as there are few, or even sometimes a complete lack of, effective antimicrobial agents available for infections caused by these bacteria. This fact is especially relevant considering that, in the last 10 years, no new group of antibiotics has been marketed in Europe [2].

P. aeruginosa is an opportunistic pathogen that is difficult to treat and eradicate, because it has evolved multiple mechanisms of resistance categorized as intrinsic, acquired, or adaptive [3]. In fact, it has an extraordinary ability to develop resistance to nearly all antimicrobials available either by chromosomal mutations or by acquisition of localized genes in transferable elements [4].

P. aeruginosa remains one of the major causes of healthcare-associated infection in Europe, and according to the EARS-Net report 2019, in Spain, 12.5% of invasive isolates of *P. aeruginosa* presented combined resistance to ≥ 3 antimicrobial groups [5]. In the ENVIN-HELICS national registry 2019 (Spanish National ICU-Acquired Infection Surveillance Study), *P. aeruginosa* was the second most frequently isolated microorganism, just behind *Escherichia coli*, as a cause of nosocomial infections in intensive care units (ICUs), and the third most frequent (after *E. coli* and *Staphylococcus aureus*) in community-acquired infections requiring ICU admission [6]. Del Barrio-Tofiño et al. [7] published in 2019 the Spanish nationwide survey on *P. aeruginosa* antimicrobial resistance mechanisms and molecular epidemiology. This study showed that up to 26.2% of the isolates were classified as multidrug-resistant (MDR: non-susceptibility to at least one agent in at least three antibiotic classes), 17.3% as extensively drug-resistant (XDR: non-susceptibility to at least one agent in all, but one or two antibiotic classes), and 0.1% as pandrug resistant (PDR: non-susceptibility to all agents in all antimicrobial categories). ICU isolates were more frequently MDR/XDR than those from other wards. DTR (difficult-to-treat resistance) is a novel classifier of antimicrobial co-resistance that integrates the impact of resistance into antibiotic choices [8]. Recently, the Infectious Diseases Society of America published a guidance for the treatment of DTR-*P. aeruginosa* [9].

The optimization of the use of antimicrobial agents is one of the five strategic objectives included in the global action plan endorsed in 2015 by the World Health Assembly to face antimicrobial resistance [10]. The major indicator of the effect of the antibiotics (pharmacodynamics, PD) is the minimum inhibitory concentration (MIC), but antimicrobial optimization also requires information about the time evolution of the antibiotic concentration in the patients (pharmacokinetics, PK). Pharmacokinetic/pharmacodynamic (PK/PD) analysis has been applied in recent years to optimize therapy, with the aim of maximizing the efficacy and reducing side effects of new and old antibiotics, as well as minimizing the emergence of resistance [11,12]. Currently, it is clearly established that inadequate exposure to antimicrobials can lead to the amplification of resistant subpopulations. The generation of resistant mutants within a bacterial population is an inevitable event, but it is possible to intervene to avoid or reduce the amplification of such subpopulation, and thus to preserve the activity of antimicrobials [13]. Different strategies have been implemented in hospital care to optimize the antimicrobial dosage regimens [14] and, in this context, PK/PD analysis has become an essential tool to be included in antimicrobial stewardship programs [15].

Therefore, based on the information of the large-scale Spanish nationwide survey on *P. aeruginosa* molecular epidemiology and antimicrobial resistance, the objective of this work was to analyze the overall antimicrobial activity of the antipseudomonal antibiotics considering PK/PD criteria. The antimicrobial therapy optimization by PK/PD analysis was applied separately for ICU and medical ward isolates, as well as distinguishing between respiratory and non-respiratory isolates, to support the selection of the appropriate antimicrobial and predicting the dosage regimen with a higher probability of success. A secondary objective was to evaluate the role of PK/PD analysis to prevent or minimize the emergence of resistance to these antimicrobials.

2. Materials and Methods

2.1. Antimicrobials and Pharmacokinetic Data

Tables 1 and 2 show the evaluated antimicrobials, their dosage regimens according to the European Committee on Antimicrobial Susceptibility Testing (EUCAST) [16], and the PK parameters in ICU and medical ward patients, respectively. Population PK parameters were obtained from the literature. Prospective studies performed in critically ill and in medical ward patients with infections were selected.

Table 1. Pharmacokinetic parameters for each antimicrobial agent from published studies among critically ill patients (mean ± standard deviation).

Antimicrobial Agent	Dosing Regimen	Infusion Time (h)	Vd (L)	Cl (L/h)	Ke (h^{-1})	Fu	References
Amikacin	25–30 mg/kg q 24 h	0.5	36.27 ± 8.34	5.58 ± 1.56			[17]
Aztreonam	2 g q 6 h	2–3	27.20 ± 20.80	9.60 ± 5.00		0.72	[18]
Cefepime	2 g q 8 h	0.5–3	21.80 ± 5.10	7.62 ± 1.98		0.85	[19,20]
Ceftazidime	2 g q 8 h / 1 g q 4 h	0.5–3	18.90 ± 9.00		0.27 ± 0.21	0.80	[21]
Ceftazidime/ avibactam	2/0.5 g q 8 h	2	34.78 ± 10.49 / 50.81 ± 14.32	6.14 ± 3.80 / 11.09 ± 6.78		0.90 / 0.92	[22–24]
Ceftolozane/ tazobactam	1/0.5 g q 8 h / 2/1 g q 8 h	1	20.40 ± 3.70 / 32.40 ± 10.00	7.20 ± 3.20 / 25.40 ± 9.40		0.79 / 0.70	[25,26]
Ciprofloxacin	400 mg q 8 h	1		13.60 ± 5.80			[27]
Colistin	150 mg q 12 h	0.5		2.92 ± 2.72			[28]
Imipenem	1 g q 6 h	1–2	28.70 ± 9.70	11.40 ± 3.53		0.80	[29]
Meropenem	2 g q 8 h	0.5–3	22.70 ± 3.70	13.60 ± 2.08		0.98	[30]
Piperacillin/ tazobactam	4/0.5 g q 6 h	0.5–4	19.40 ± 7.76	13.80 ± 4.77		0.75	[31]
Tobramycin	6–7 mg/kg q 24 h	0.5	17.50 ± 5.25		0.25 ± 0.01		[32]

Vd: volume of distribution; Cl: total clearance; Ke: elimination rate constant; Fu: unbound fraction.

Table 2. Dosing regimen and pharmacokinetic parameters for each antimicrobial agent from published studies in non-critically ill patients (mean ± standard deviation).

Antimicrobial Agent	Dosing Regimen	Infusion Time (h)	Vd (L)	Cl (L/h)	AUC (mg/L · h)	Fu	References
Amikacin	25–30 mg/kg q 24 h	0.5	15.80 ± 3.50	5.87 ± 0.98			[33]
Aztreonam	2 g q 6 h	2–3	0.14 ± 0.04 (L/kg)	4.41 ± 0.63		0.40	[34]
Cefepime	1 g q 8 h / 2 g q 12 h	0.5–3	0.28 ± 0.25 (L/kg)	7.00 ± 4.30		0.80	[35]
Ceftazidime	1 g q 8 h	0.5–3	15.75 ± 1.50	6.96 ± 1.08		0.90	[36]
Ceftazidime/ avibactam	2/0.5 g q 8 h	2	18.70 ± 1.65 / 25.30 ± 4.43	7.53 ± 1.28 / 12.30 ± 1.96		0.90 / 0.92	[24,37]
Ceftolozane/ tazobactam	1/0.5 g q 8 h / 2/1 g q 8 h	1	13.50 ± 2.83 / 18.20 ± 4.55	4.76 ± 1.13 / 20.51 ± 4.40		0.79 / 0.70	[38–40]
Ciprofloxacin	400 mg q 12 h	1			20.80 ± 5.70		[41]
Colistin	150 mg q 12 h	0.5		2.92 ± 0.10			[42]
Imipenem	500 mg q 6 h	1–2	16.50 ± 3.75	10.50 ± 1.38		0.90	[43]
Meropenem	1 g q 8 h	0.5–3	20.25 ± 3.00	14.40 ± 1.80		0.92	[43]
Piperacillin/ tazobactam	4/0.5 g q 8 h	0.5–4	11.25 ± 1.50	10.22 ± 2.12		0.70	[43]
Tobramycin	6–7 mg/kg q 24 h	0.5	20.50 ± 11.40	5.19 ± 0.91			[44,45]

Vd: volume of distribution; Cl: total clearance; AUC: area under the curve; Fu: unbound fraction.

2.2. Microbiological Data

Microbiological data (MIC distributions) were extracted from the Spanish nationwide survey study about *P. aeruginosa* isolates collected from 51 participating hospitals, covering all 17 Spanish regions during October 2017 [7], carried out by the GEMARA-SEIMC/REIPI group [46]. The collection included up to 30 consecutive health care-associated non-duplicated (one per patient) *P. aeruginosa* clinical isolates from respiratory, urinary, blood-stream, skin and soft tissue, and osteo-articular, as well as other sample types, and ICU, medical ward, surgical ward, emergency room, and other sources were recorded for each isolate.

Isolates were classified according to the admission service (ICU or medical wards) and according to the sample type (respiratory and non-respiratory). Respiratory samples were collected from tracheal aspirate, bronchial aspiration, sputum, bronchoalveolar lavage, pleural fluid, and bronchial brushing in ICU. In medical wards, the origin of these samples was the same as that from patients from the ICU and nasopharyngeal aspirate and sputum (from cystic fibrosis patients). Based on the location, 91.5% of isolates were collected outside the ICU (only 8.5% of isolates were from ICU). Most samples from ICU patients were from respiratory sources (58.3%); by contrast, most samples collected from medical ward patients were from non-respiratory sources (69.4%).

Susceptibility was recalculated according to the EUCAST breakpoints 2021 [16]. It is important to consider that, in 2019, EUCAST changed definitions of susceptibility testing categories, and intermediate (I-category) was defined as susceptible at increased exposure. Concerning antipseudomonal antimicrobials included in this study, aztreonam, cefepime, ceftazidime, ciprofloxacin, imipenem, and piperacillin/tazobactam are included in this new I-category. The EUCAST breakpoint for imipenem changed from 8 mg/L in 2018 to 4 mg/L in 2021. Table 3 shows the susceptibility rate of *P. aeruginosa* strains classified by admission service and sample location.

Table 3. Percentage of *P. aeruginosa* susceptible strains in 2017, classified by admission service and sample location, according to the Spanish nationwide survey [7] and applying EUCAST clinical breakpoints [16].

	Susceptibility (%)					
	ICU			Medical Ward Patients		
Antimicrobial Agent and Dosing Regimen	Total	Respiratory	Non-Respiratory	Total	Respiratory	Non-Respiratory
Amikacin	91 **	93 **	90 **	92 **	96 **	97 **
Aztreonam	70	64	77	*87*	*87*	*87*
Cefepime	67	69	65	*80*	72	*82*
Ceftazidime	64	67	60	*81*	79	*83*
Ceftazidime/avibactam	*85*	*87*	*83*	95 **	96 **	95 **
Ceftolozane/tazobactam	*81*	*87*	73	96 **	95 **	96 **
Ciprofloxacin	52	46	60	62	55	65
Colistin	95 **	96 **	94 **	95 **	96 **	94 **
Imipenem	55	57	52	75	72	75
Meropenem	71	73	69	*80*	*87*	*87*
Piperacillin/tazobactam	57	57	58	75	73	76
Tobramycin	74	75	73	*84*	*84*	*85*

** susceptibility ≥90%; *underlined and in italics*, susceptibility ≥80% and <90%.

2.3. PK/PD Analysis and Monte Carlo Simulation

Depending on the activity pattern of the antimicrobial, three different PK/PD indices have been defined as the best descriptors of clinical efficacy [12]: (i) for concentration-dependent activity antimicrobials, the ratio of the total or free-drug maximum concentration (C_{max}) to the MIC (C_{max}/MIC) or the area under the total or free-drug concentration–time curve, typically over a 24 h period, to the MIC (AUC_{24h}/MIC); (ii) for time-dependent patterns, the percentage of time the free drug concentration remains above the MIC throughout the dosage interval (%$fT_{>MIC}$); and (iii) AUC_{24h}/MIC concentration-dependent with time-dependence antibiotics [11,47].

Table 4 shows the PK/PD indexes and the magnitude of the targets associated with the success of therapy for each antimicrobial. For time-dependent pattern antimicrobials, steady-state concentration (C_{ss}) > 4 × MIC was selected as the primary endpoint to evaluate the suitability of the continuous infusion dosage regimens in ICU patients [48].

Table 4. Pharmacokinetic/pharmacodynamics (PK/PD) index and target magnitude for each antimicrobial agent.

Antimicrobial Agent	PK/PD Target	References
Amikacin	C_{max}/MIC > 10	[49]
Aztreonam	%$fT_{>MIC}$ > 60	[18]
Cefepime	%$fT_{>MIC}$ > 70	[50]
Ceftazidime	%$fT_{>MIC}$ > 70	[12]
Ceftazidime/avibactam	%$fT_{>MIC}$ > 50% %fT > 1 mg/L > 50%	[23]
Ceftolozane/tazobactam	%$fT_{>MIC}$ > 60% %fT > 1 mg/L > 20%	[25,26]
Ciprofloxacin	$fAUC_{24h}$/MIC > 125	[51]
Colistin	$fAUC_{24h}$/MIC > 25–35	[52]
Imipenem	%$fT_{>MIC}$ > 40	[12]
Meropenem	%$fT_{>MIC}$ > 40	[51]
Piperacillin/tazobactam	%$fT_{>MIC}$ > 50	[41]
Tobramycin	C_{max}/MIC > 10	[36]
Time-dependent antimicrobials Continuous infusion	C_{ss} > 4 × MIC	[48]

%$fT_{>MIC}$: Percentage of time that the antimicrobial free serum concentration remained above the MIC; %fT > 1 mg/L: cumulative percentage over a 24 h period that the free drug concentration exceeded a 1 mg/L threshold concentration; $fAUC_{24h}$: area under the free drug concentration–time curve over a 24 h period; C_{max}: maximum drug plasma concentration; MIC: minimum inhibitory concentration; C_{ss}: steady-state concentration.

PK/PD indices and the defined targets for suppression of the emergence of resistance are presented in Table 5.

With the defined PK/PD targets, the probability of target attainment (PTA) and the cumulative fraction of response (CFR) were calculated by Monte Carlo simulation with Oracle® Crystal Ball Fusion Edition v.11.1.2.3.500 software (Oracle Inc., Redwood City, CA, USA) and using 10,000 random iterations of the data. Logarithmic transformation was applied to the mean and the standard deviation of all pharmacokinetic parameters to normalize their distributions, whereas protein binding was included as a fixed value.

Table 5. The pharmacokinetic/pharmacodynamic (PK/PD) indices reported to suppress the emergence of antibiotic resistance for *P. aeruginosa*.

Antimicrobial	PK/PD Index	PK/PD Index Magnitude		References
		Total Drug	Free Drug	
Cefepime	C_{min}/MIC		≥ 3.8	[53]
Ceftazidime	$\%fT_{>MIC}$		≥ 100	[54]
Ceftazidime/avibactam	$\%fT_{>MIC}$		≥ 87	[55]
Ceftolozane/tazobactam	$\%fT_{>MIC}$	≥ 80		[56]
Piperacillin/tazobactam	C_{min}/MIC		≥ 5	[57]
Meropenem	C_{min}/MIC		≥ 3.8	[53]
Imipenem	AUC_{24}/MIC	$= 140$		[58]
Ciprofloxacin	$fAUC_{24}/MIC$	≥ 385		[59]

C_{min}: minimum concentration; MIC: minimum inhibitory concentration; $\%fT_{>MIC}$: percentage of time that the antimicrobial-free serum concentration remains above the MIC; AUC_{24h}: area under the concentration–time curve from 0 h to 24 h.

2.3.1. Probability of Target Attainment (PTA) Estimation

PTA is the probability that a specific value of the PK/PD index associated with the efficacy of the antibiotic is achieved at a certain MIC [12]. PTA was calculated using the following equations:

- Time-dependent activity antimicrobials;
- IV infusion.

$$\%fT_{>MIC} = [(t_2 + t_i) - t_1] \cdot \frac{100}{\tau} \quad (1)$$

where $\%fT_{>MIC}$ is the proportion of time that the free serum concentration remains above the MIC at steady state (%) over a dosage interval, t_1 (h) corresponds to the time at which the free serum concentration reached the MIC during the infusion phase; t_2 (h) corresponds to the post-infusion time at which the free serum concentration equaled the MIC in the elimination phase; and τ is the dosage interval. The times t_1 and t_2 were calculated as follows:

$$t_1 = \frac{(MIC - fC_{min,ss})}{(fC_{max,ss} - fC_{min,ss})} t_{inf} \quad (2)$$

$$t_2 = \ln\left(\frac{fC_{max,ss}}{MIC}\right) \cdot \frac{Vd}{Cl} \quad (3)$$

where Ke is the elimination rate constant.

The minimum and maximum serum concentrations of unbound drug (mg/L) at steady state, $fC_{min,ss}$ and $fC_{max,ss}$, respectively, were estimated according to the following equations using the total clearance (Cl), volume of distribution (Vd), infusion time (t_i), dosage interval (τ), total dose administered (D), and unbound fraction (f_u):

$$fC_{min,ss} = fC_{max,ss} \cdot e^{-\frac{Cl}{Vd} \cdot (\tau - t_i)} \quad (4)$$

$$fC_{max,ss} = f_u \cdot \frac{D}{Cl \cdot t_i} \cdot (1 - e^{-\frac{Cl}{Vd} \cdot t_i}) \cdot \frac{1}{1 - e^{-\frac{Cl}{Vd} \cdot \tau}} \quad (5)$$

- Continuous infusion

$$C_{ss} = \frac{k_0}{Cl} \quad (6)$$

where C_{ss} is the steady-state concentration, k_0 is the infusion rate, and Cl is the total clearance.

- Concentration–time-dependent antimicrobials;
- C_{max}/MIC: ratio of the maximum drug plasma concentration divided by the MIC.

$$C_{max} = \frac{k_o \cdot \left(1 - e^{\left(-\frac{Cl}{Vd} \cdot t_i\right)}\right)}{Cl \cdot \left(1 - e^{\left(-\frac{Cl}{Vd} \cdot \tau\right)}\right)} \quad (7)$$

where ko is the infusion rate, Ke is the elimination rate constant, t_i is the infusion time, Cl is the total clearance, and τ is the dosage interval.

- AUC_{24h}/MIC: ratio of the area under the antimicrobial concentration–time curve for 24 h divided by the MIC.

$$AUC_{24h} = \frac{D}{Cl} \quad (8)$$

where AUC_{24h} is the area under the serum concentration–time curve over 24 h.

PTA values (%) were calculated for each dosage regimen for both ICU and medical ward dose regimens for an MIC range from 0.0125 to 512 mg/L. Considering that the actual PTA in an individual patient may be significantly different from what would be concluded from a conventional simulation [60], 95% confidence intervals were calculated as the range from the 2.5th to the 97.5th percentile of the set of estimated values.

The dosage regimens were considered successful if PTA was ≥90%, whereas a PTA ≥80%, but <90% was associated with moderate probabilities of success [61].

2.3.2. Calculation of the Cumulative Fraction of Response (CFR)

CFR is the expected probability of success of a dosage regimen against bacteria in the absence of the specific value of MIC, thus the population distribution of MICs is used [12]. It was calculated using Equation (9):

$$CFR = \sum_{i=1}^{n} PTAi \times Fi \quad (9)$$

where CFR (%) results from the total sum of the products of the PTA at a certain MIC times the frequency (Fi) of isolates of microorganism exhibiting that MIC over the range of susceptible pathogens. The range of MIC concentrations tested for each antimicrobial includes dilutions below the susceptibility breakpoint; therefore, it is adequate to estimate CFR.

The CMI ranges evaluated for each antimicrobial were as follows: amikacin (2–128 mg/L), aztreonam (2–56 mg/L), cefepime and ceftazidime (1–128 mg/L), ceftazidime/avibactam and ceftolozane/tazobactam (0.5–64 mg/L), ciprofloxacin (0.125–32 mg/L), colistin (0.5–16 mg/L), imipenem (0.5–64 mg/L), meropenem (0.5–128 mg/L), piperacillin/tazobactam (4–512 mg/L), and tobramycin (0.25–64 mg/L).

The 95% confidence intervals were calculated as the range from the 2.5th to the 97.5th percentile of the set of estimated values.

A CFR ≥80%, but <90% was associated with moderate probabilities of success, whereas a CFR ≥90% was considered as optimal against that bacterial population [12].

2.3.3. Calculation of the Joint Probability of PK/PD Target Attainment

Joint PTA, calculated for beta-lactam and beta-lactamase inhibitor combinations, are defined as the simultaneous attainment of each individual PTA [23]. It was calculated by determining first if, in each simulated population, the PTA for the beta-lactamase inhibitor is achieved. If this threshold was met, the joint PTA is considered to be the calculated beta-lactam.

3. Results

Figures 1 and 2 feature the PTA values calculated by Monte Carlo simulation, considering the EUCAST breakpoints (including susceptible and intermediate categories), at MIC values ranging from 0.125 mg/L to 512 mg/L for each antimicrobial dosage regimen recommended in both ICU and medical wards. PTA values collected in the Supporting Information (Tables S1 and S2) include the 95% confidence interval.

For ICU dosage regimens, PTAs higher than 90% were obtained with ceftazidime/avibactam, cefepime, ceftazidime, ceftolozane/tazobactam imipenem, meropenem, and piperacillin/tazobactam depending on the dose regimen, although, in the case of cefepime, ceftazidime, and piperacillin/tazobactam, only when they are administered as extended infusion. PTA values were under 80% for amikacin and aztreonam, covering MICs up to 4 mg/L and 2 mg/L, respectively, far from the clinical breakpoint (16 mg/L). For medical ward regimen dosages, PTAs higher than 90% were observed for aztreonam, the two new combinations of cephalosporins with beta-lactamase inhibitor, colistin, imipenem, meropenem, and piperacillin/tazobactam, if extended infusion (4 h) is considered. All other antimicrobials showed PTA values under 80% for all dosage regimens evaluated. Tobramycin administered at 7 mg/kg q 24 h showed a PTA value of 72%, although the 95% confidence interval ranged from 69% to 84%, that is, including values corresponding to moderate probabilities of target attainment (>80–90%).

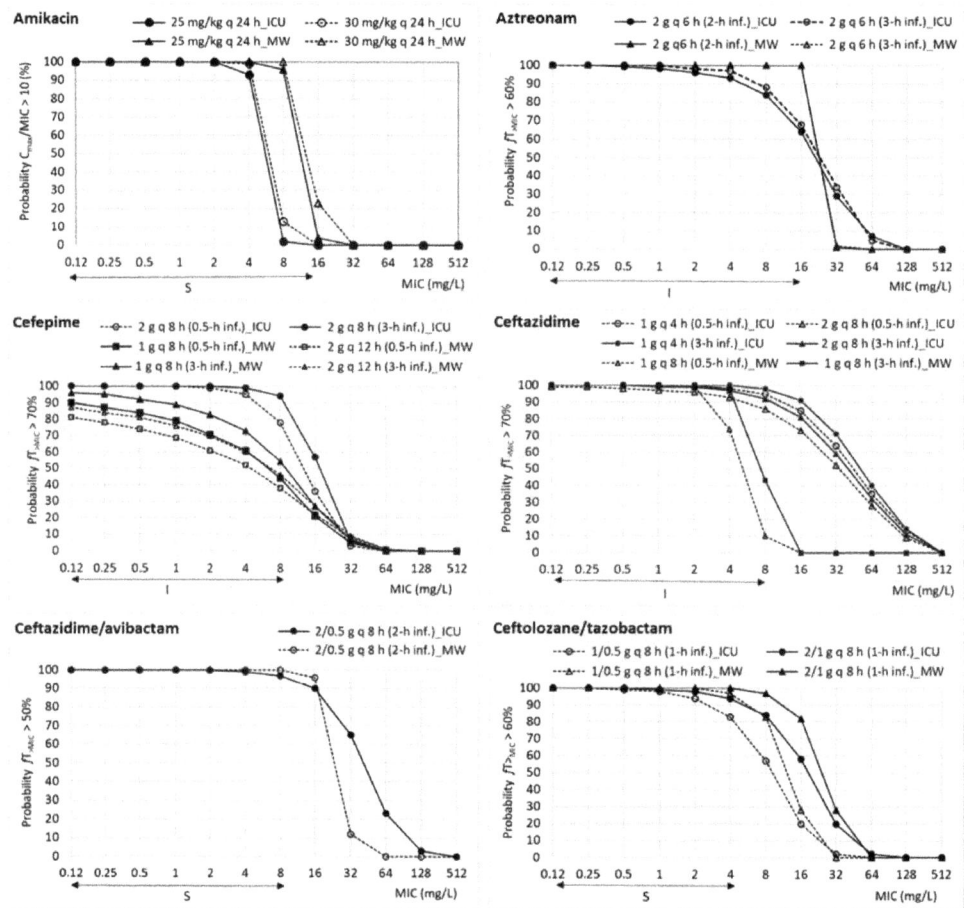

Figure 1. Estimated probability of target attainment (PTA) values for different dosing regimens in both ICU and medical ward patients for amikacin, aztreonam, cefepime, ceftazidime, ceftazidime/avibactam, and ceftolozane/tazobactam. The solid horizontal lines indicate MIC covered by the clinical EUCAST breakpoints (including susceptible and intermediate categories) of *P. aeruginosa* for each antimicrobial. ICU: intensive care unit; MW: medical ward; S: susceptible; I: intermediate category (susceptible at increased exposure).

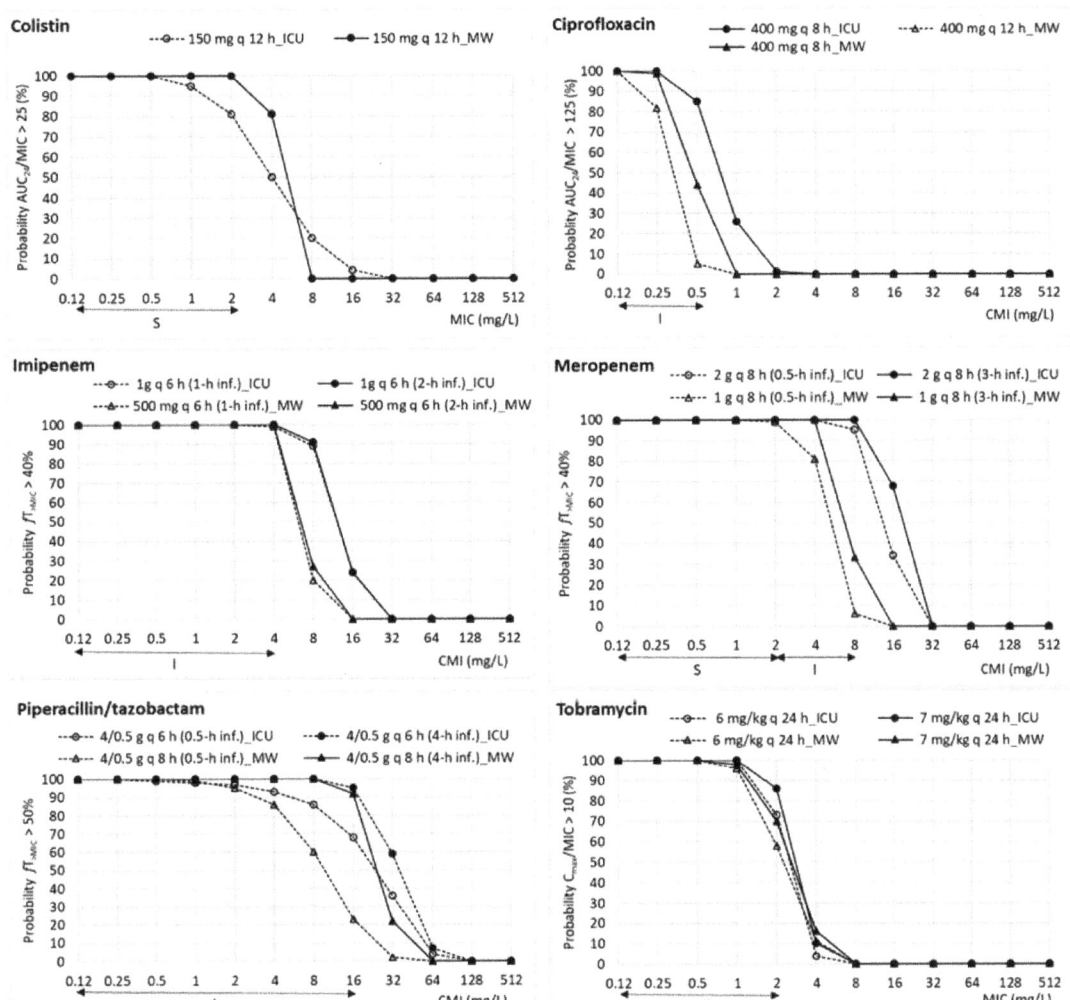

Figure 2. Estimated probability of target attainment (PTA) values for different dosing regimens in both ICU and medical ward patients for colistin, ciprofloxacin, imipenem, meropenem, piperacillin/tazobactam, and tobramycin. The solid horizontal lines indicate MIC covered by the clinical EUCAST breakpoints (including susceptible and intermediate categories) of *P. aeruginosa* for each antimicrobial. ICU: intensive care unit; MW: medical ward; S: susceptible; I: intermediate category (susceptible at increased exposure).

Table 6 features the CFR values obtained, including the 2.5th and 97.5th percentiles, considering the MIC distribution of the isolates classified by admission service and sample location. CFR values estimated from the MIC profile of ICU isolates were below 75% for most antimicrobial regimens, and only ceftazidime/avibactam showed a CFR > 90% (95%), although, with colistin, it was 89%. Only moderate probabilities of success were obtained with ceftolozane/tazobactam (both dosage regimens), ceftazidime (dose 1 g q 4 h, both standard and extended infusion), and meropenem. CFR for amikacin was 71%, despite its high susceptibility values (>90%).

Table 6. Cumulative fraction of response (CFR) calculated for all dosing regimens classified by admission service and sample location. Numbers in parentheses indicate the 2.5th and 97.5th percentiles.

Antimicrobial Agent and Dosing Regimen	CFR (%)					
	ICU			Medical Ward Patients		
Amikacin	Total	Respiratory	Non-Respiratory	Total	Respiratory	Non-Respiratory
25 mg/kg q 24 h	71 (68–74)	77 (75–79)	63 (60–66)	92 (91–94) **	88 (86–90) *	94 (93–96) **
30 mg/kg q 24 h	72 (69–75)	81 (78–84)	67 (64–70)	92 (91–94) **	90 (88–92) **	95 (94–97) **
Aztreonam						
2 g q 6 h (2 h inf.)	65 (62–69)	62 (59–65)	70 (67–73)	86 (83–87) *	85 (83–87) *	87 (84–89) *
2 g q 6 h (3 h inf.)	69 (66–71)	66 (64–70)	71 (68–74)	86 (84–88) *	85 (83–87) *	87 (85–89) *
Cefepime						
1 g q 8 h (0.5 h inf.)				57 (54–60)	51 (48–54)	53 (50–57)
2 g q 12 h (0.5 h inf.)				48 (45–51)	45 (42–48)	46 (43–49)
2 g q 8 h (0.5 h inf.)	68 (71–61)	67 (64–69)	65 (62–68)			
1 g q 8 h (3 h inf.)				63 (59–66)	59 (56–62)	65 (62–68)
2 g q 12 h (3 h inf.)				53 (49–55)	53 (51–55)	55 (53–59)
2 g q 8 h (3 h inf.)	77 (75–80)	76 (73–78)	73 (70–75)			
Ceftazidime						
1 g q 4 h (0.5 h inf.)	80 (78–83) *	83 (81–86) *	78 (75–81)			
1 g q 8 h (0.5 h inf.)				68 (65–70)	63 (60–66)	64 (60–66)
2 g q 8 h (0.5 h inf.)	76 (74–79)	76 (73–79)	72 (69–75)			
1 g q 4 h (3 h inf.)	85 (82–87) *	85 (83–87)	81 (78–83) *			
1 g q 8 h (3 h inf.)				73 (71–76)	75 (72–77)	74 (72–77)
2 g q 8 h (3 h inf.)	79 (76–82)	81 (79–83) *	77 (74–80)			
Ceftazidime/avibactam						
2/0.5 g q 8 h (2 h inf.)	95 (94–97) **	98 (97–99) **	93 (92–95) **	97 (96–98) **	98 (97–98) **	97 (96–99) **
Ceftolozane/tazobactam						
1/0.5 g q 8 h (1 h inf.)	84 (81–86) *	85 (82–87) *	81 (78–83) *	95 (94–96) **	92 (91–94) **	96 (95–98) **
2/1 g q 8 h (1 h inf.)	86 (84–88) *	92 (91–94) **	83 (81–86) *	96 (95–97) **	95 (94–96) **	97 (95–98) **
Ciprofloxacin						
400 mg q 12 h				53 (50–57)	43 (40–47)	58 (55–61)
400 mg q 8 h	54 (51–57)	48 (45–50)	59 (56–63)			
Colistin						
150 mg q 12 h	89 (86–90) *	88 (86–90) *	88 (87–90) *	95 (94–96) **	95 (94–97) **	94 (93–95) **
Imipenem						
500 mg q 6 h (1 h inf.)				75 (72–78)	75 (73–77)	78 (76–80)
1 g q 6 h (1 h inf.)	77 (74–79)	83 (81–85) *	77 (75–80)			
500 mg q 6 h (2 h inf.)				77 (75–80)	75 (73–78)	78 (75–80)
1 g q 6 h (2 h inf.)	81 (79–84) *	83 (81–85) *	76 (73–79)			
Meropenem						
1 g q 8 h (0.5 h inf.)				79 (77–82)	80 (77–82) *	80 (78–84) *
2 g q 8 h (0.5 h inf.)	77 (74–80)	79 (77–82)	73 (71–76)			
1 g q 8 h (3 h inf.)				84 (81–86) *	82 (80–84) *	83 (81–86) *
2 g q 8 h (3 h inf.)	82 (79–84) *	86 (84–88) *	77 (75–80)			

Table 6. Cont.

Antimicrobial Agent and Dosing Regimen	CFR (%)					
	ICU			Medical Ward Patients		
Amikacin	Total	Respiratory	Non-Respiratory	Total	Respiratory	Non-Respiratory
Piperacillin/tazobactam						
4/0.5 g q 8 h (0.5 h inf.)				51 (48–54)	50 (46–54)	50 (47–53)
4/0.5 g q 6 h (0.5 h inf.)	53 (49–56)	52 (49–56)	55 (52–59)			
4/0.5 g q 8 h (4 h inf.)				79 (76–82)	75 (73–78)	76 (74–79)
4/0.5 g q 6 h (4 h inf.)	64 (61–67)	67 (64–70)	68 (64–70)			
Tobramycin						
6 mg/kg q 24 h	72 (69–75)	72 (69–75)	71 (68–75)	81 (79–84) *	80 (78–83) *	81 (79–83) *
7 mg/kg q 24 h	70 (67–73)	71 (69–74)	72 (69–75)	82 (79–84) *	82 (79–84) *	83 (81–85) *

** susceptibility ≥90%; * susceptibility ≥80% and <90%; inf: infusion time.

Table 7 shows the probability to reach the suppression of the emergence of antimicrobial resistance, taking into account the MIC distribution of the isolates against the studied antimicrobials. For ICU patients, with the dosage regimens used in clinical practice, no treatment allows to obtain probabilities higher than 90%. Ceftazidime/avibactam reaches a probability of 89% (87–91%) and the highest dose of ceftolozane/tazobactam reaches 86% (84–88%). For medical ward patients, values > 90% were reached only with ceftolozane/tazobactam and ceftazidime/avibactam.

Table 7. Cumulative fraction of response (CFR) calculated for all dosing regimens considering PK/PD indices to suppress the emergence of resistance. Numbers in parentheses indicate the 2.5th and 97.5th percentiles.

Antimicrobial Agent and Dosing Regimen	CFR (%)	
	ICU	Medical Ward Patients
Cefepime		
1 g q 8 h (0.5 h inf.)		20 (18–23)
2 g q 12 h (0.5 h inf.)		14 (12–16)
2 g q 8 h (0.5 h inf.)	10 (9–12)	
1 g q 8 h (3 h inf.)		19 (17–22)
2 g q 12 h (3 h inf.)		16 (14–19)
2 g q 8 h (3 h inf.)	19 (17–21)	
Ceftazidime		
1 g q 4 h (0.5 h inf.)	78 (76–81)	
1 g q 8 h (0.5 h inf.)		26 (23–29)
2 g q 8 h (0.5 h inf.)	65 (62–68)	
1 g q 4 h (3 h inf.)	81 (79–84) *	
1 g q 8 h (3 h inf.)		51 (48–54)
2 g q 8 h (3 h inf.)	69 (66–72)	
Ceftazidime/avibactam		
2/0.5 g q 8 h (2 h inf.)	89 (87–91) *	91 (90–93) **
Ceftolozane/tazobactam		
1/0.5 g q 8 h (1 h inf.)	77 (75–80)	96 (95–97) **
2/1 g q 8 h (1 h inf.)	86 (84–88) *	97 (97–98) **

Table 7. *Cont.*

Antimicrobial Agent and Dosing Regimen	CFR (%)	
	ICU	Medical Ward Patients
Ciprofloxacin		
400 mg q 12 h		0 (0–0)
400 mg q 8 h	36 (33–39)	
Imipenem		
500 mg q 6 h		0 (0–0)
1 g q 6 h	42 (39–45)	
Meropenem		
1 g q 8 h (0.5 h inf.)		0 (0–0)
2 g q 8 h (0.5 h inf.)	5 (4–7)	
1 g q 8 h (3 h inf.)		1 (0–2)
2 g q 8 h (3 h inf.)	15 (13–18)	
Piperacillin/tazobactam		
4/0.5 g q 8 h (0.5 h inf.)		0 (0–0)
4/0.5 g q 6 h (0.5 h inf.)	2 (1–3)	
4/0.5 g q 8 h (4 h inf.)		0 (0–0)
4/0.5 g q 6 h (4 h inf.)	8 (7–10)	

** CFR $\geq$ 90%; * CFR $\geq$ 80% and < 90%; inf: infusion time.

4. Discussion

P. aeruginosa is among the antimicrobial-resistant gram-negative bacteria challenging current health care. The establishment of programs of antimicrobial activity surveillance integrating local epidemiologic is essential to guide clinicians towards appropriate empiric treatments. The incorporation of PK/PD analysis into these programs affords a valuable complementary tool for a rational antimicrobial and dosage regimen selection. The Spanish nationwide survey on *P. aeruginosa* antimicrobial resistance mechanisms and molecular epidemiology [7] showed that the highest susceptibility rates in both ICU and medical ward isolates were detected for amikacin, ceftazidime/avibactam, ceftolozane/tazobactam, and colistin and, except for these last three antimicrobials, a high prevalence of XDR phenotypes and resistance was documented. In this work, the overall antimicrobial activity of the antipseudomonal antibiotics was assessed by PK/PD analysis to estimate the probability of success of the treatments, incorporating the variability of the pharmacokinetic parameters and the bacterial population. Ceftazidime/avibactam, followed by ceftolozane/tazobactam and colistin, were the most active antimicrobials, with differences depending on the admission service, sample type, and dose regimen. Furthermore, the new combinations of cephalosporins with beta-lactamase inhibitors provided drug exposures associated with resistance suppression at recommended doses.

Standard surveillance indices based on MIC values are insufficient to detect changes in antimicrobial agents´ overall activity, as some less obvious variations in MIC distribution may result in treatment efficacy loss. In this regard, different studies on *P. aeruginosa* [40,62,63] highlight that the susceptibility rates and the probability of treatment success estimated by the PK/PD analysis are complementary tools that should be considered together to guide antimicrobial therapy. Our results (Figures 1 and 2) show relevant discrepancies between EUCAST-susceptibility breakpoints and those estimated by PK/PD analysis, defined as the highest MIC value at which a high probability of target attainment is obtained (PTA $\geq$ 90%). In this sense, the EMA also defends the use of PTA to predict whether a treatment may be useful against a specific microorganism, and underlines its relevance for the treatment of infections caused by multi-resistant bacteria [61]. Besides, in 2019, EUCAST implemented changes to the definitions of susceptibility testing categories to emphasize the relationship between breakpoints and exposure of the organism for the agent at the site of infection, even recommending extended infusions for some time-dependent antimicrobials. As can be observed in Figures 1 and 2 and Supplementary Tables S1 and S2, prolonged infusions of time-dependent antimicrobials enhance PTA against non-susceptible *P. aeruginosa* isolates, thus being a potential therapeutic option for infections due to multidrug-resistant microorganisms. However, in our study, this fact was relevant only for piperacillin/tazobactam. A recent systematic review [64] concluded that, prior to the implementation of prolonged infusion of antipseudomonal beta-lactam regimens, institutions should consider its advantage according to multiple variables including local incidence of *P. aeruginosa* infections, MIC distributions, pharmacokinetic variables, and PTA, as well as implementation challenges.

The Spanish nationwide survey [7] also indicated a complex scenario with major differences in local epidemiology, including carbapenemase production, that need to be acknowledged in order to guide antimicrobial therapy. The estimation of CFRs allows estimating the probability of success for a treatment without knowledge of the susceptibility of the specific isolate responsible for the infection, but taking into account the MIC distribution of a particular institution or hospital wards or regions/countries [11]. Overall, a lack of concordance between susceptibility and CFR values was detected, especially relevant in ICU. With the exception of amikacin, discordances in ICU show higher values of CFR than susceptibility rates. Therefore, taking into account the MIC distribution of UCI isolates in Spain, PK/PD analysis predicts, for the recommended dose regimens, a probability of treatment success higher than that expected if only the susceptibility data are considered. On the contrary, considering the isolates from medical wards, when discrepancies are detected, susceptibility percentages are higher than the CFRs calculated, which may justify treatment failures when dosing selection is based on the susceptibility rate without considering the antibiotic exposure. These results emphasize the importance of taking into account the susceptibility MIC distribution of the isolates of the geographical area or hospital setting and the PK/PD analysis to support empiric therapy.

Monte Carlo simulations were also performed to calculate CFR in ICU for time-dependent antimicrobials administered as continuous infusion at the highest doses, except for ceftazidime/avibactam, with a CFR value of 95% at the recommended dose, and imipenem due to stability concerns. All antimicrobials evaluated, except for ceftolozane/tazobactam (CFR 85%), provided low CFR values (< 60%) at the PK/PD endpoint of $C_{ss} > 4 \times$ MIC. The low values could be due to the restrictive target selected; however, this endpoint would allow for maximal bacterial killing and protection against bacterial regrowth considering that critically ill patients are vulnerable to suboptimal dosage and represent a source of selection of resistance to antibiotics [52]. These results agree with those obtained in other studies [65] reporting the target attainment of beta-lactam antibiotics in critically ill patients.

Regarding sample location, recently, Abuhussain et al. [66] conducted a study on the in vitro potency of antipseudomonal beta-lactams against blood and respiratory isolates of *P. aeruginosa* from ICU and non-ICU patients; these authors concluded that the blood sample isolates were more susceptible. In our study, no relevant differences were observed in susceptibility and CFR values between respiratory and non-respiratory isolates, although, for ceftolozane/tazobactam, the susceptibility of respiratory ICU strains was higher than that of non-respiratory ones. In this regard, for ICU isolates, respiratory and non-respiratory, ceftazidime/avibactam was able to attain CFR > 90%, and a high dose of ceftolozane/tazobactam, indicated for hospital-acquired pneumonia including ventilator-associated pneumonia [24], provided CFR > 90% only for respiratory infections.

As a final point, PK/PD analysis based on the MIC distributions of the Spanish national survey was applied to estimate the probability of the suppression of the emergence of resistance to the different antimicrobial dosage regimens. Different works have reported the required antimicrobial PK/PD indices to suppress the emergence of *P. aeruginosa* antibiotic resistance [53–59], although no standardized methods are currently established to determine the antibiotic exposure for the attainment of resistance suppression. In our study, none of the dosage regimens commonly used in ICU patients were able to attain high probabilities of resistance suppression, although ceftazidime/avibactam and ceftolozane/tazobactam 2/1 g q 8 h provide moderate probabilities (>80–90%). These new antimicrobial combinations were the only ones able to provide concentrations associated with the suppression of resistance at dosage regimens recommended for medical ward (CFR > 90%). Different studies have also concluded that the exposure required for resistance suppression is usually much higher than that to assess the treatment efficacy [11,54]. Consequently, to avoid resistance, the use of alternative dosage strategies should be considered, such as extended or continuous infusions, or the use of some antibiotic combinations for which in vitro studies have demonstrated a clear advantage [47].

With the aim of emphasizing the importance of antimicrobial appropriate use, supporting the development of tools for antibiotic management, and to reduce bacterial resistance, in 2019, the WHO released the Access, Watch, Reserve (AWaRe) classification [67], which categorizes the antibiotics into different stewardship groups. All antipseudomonals evaluated in this study are included in the Watch or Reserve category, except amikacin (Access). Apart from aztreonam, three other antimicrobials are held in reserve, ceftazidime/avibactam, ceftolozane/tazobactam, and colistin, which, in this work, were found to be the three most active against *P. aeruginosa* in terms of susceptibility and CFR, and only the two combinations are able to suppress the emergence of resistance at standard doses.

Finally, this study presents some limitations: (i) PK/PD analysis was carried out using the mean PK parameter and their variability, without considering the possible influence of covariates on the PK behavior of the drugs; (ii) PK information was extracted from studies carried out in critically ill patients and in hospital ward patients and available in the literature; and (iii) many of existing studies determining the exposure required to suppress the emergence of resistance were conducted in vitro, and we have not found the PK/PD indices required to suppress specifically the emergence of resistance of *P. aeruginosa* for all antimicrobials.

5. Conclusions

Considering the susceptibility rate and PK/PD criteria, the most active antimicrobial against *P. aeruginosa* was ceftazidime/avibactam, followed by ceftolozane/tazobactam and colistin, all of them categorized as Reserve by the AWaRe WHO classification. Noteworthy discrepancies between EUCAST-susceptibility breakpoints for *P. aeruginosa* and those estimated by PK/PD analysis were observed, as well as a lack of concordance between *P. aeruginosa* isolates susceptibility and CFR values. Our results also highlight the importance of considering the local susceptibility profile, such as the admission service of the patient or the sample location, as well as the PK/PD analysis to support empiric therapy. In this sense, prolonged infusions of time-dependent antimicrobials enhance PTA against non-susceptible *P. aeruginosa* isolate. Furthermore, antimicrobial stewardship programs need to consider not only the efficacy, but also the capacity to suppress resistance emergence to select the proper treatment, in terms of optimal choice of drug and dosage regimen. In this work, based on PK/PD analysis, only standard doses of ceftazidime/avibactam and ceftolozane/tazobactam provided drug concentrations associated with resistance suppression, confirming the need to use different dosage regimens or alternative therapeutic strategies to prevent or minimize resistance emergence.

Supplementary Materials: The following are available online at https://www.mdpi.com/article/10.3390/pharmaceutics13111899/s1, Table S1: Probability target attainment (PTA) (%) at each value of minimum inhibitory concentration (MIC) in ICU patients. Numbers in parenthesis indicate the 2.5th and 97.5th percentiles. The solid vertical lines indicate the intercept with the EUCAST clinical breakpoints of *P aeruginosa*. Grey shading indicates PTA > 90%. Table S2: Probability target attainment (PTA) (%) at each value of minimum inhibitory concentration (MIC) in medical ward patients. Numbers in parenthesis indicate the 2.5th and 97.5th percentiles. The solid vertical lines indicate the intercept with the EUCAST clinical breakpoints of *P aeruginosa*. Grey shading indicates PTA > 90%.

Author Contributions: Conceptualization, A.C., A.R.-G. and M.Á.S.; methodology, A.V. and A.I.; software A.V. and A.I. validation, H.B., E.d.B.-T. and A.O.; formal analysis, A.V., A.C. and M.Á.S.; investigation, A.V. and A.R.-G.; resources, E.d.B.-T., A.O. and M.Á.S.; data curation, A.I. writing—original draft preparation, A.V., A.C. and M.Á.S.; writing—review and editing, A.R.-G., A.I. and H.B.; visualization, A.I.; supervision, A.C. and M.Á.S.; project administration, A.R.-G.; funding acquisition, A.R.-G. and M.Á.S. All authors have read and agreed to the published version of the manuscript.

Funding: This research was funded by the UPV/EHU (GIU 20/048).

Institutional Review Board Statement: Not applicable.

Informed Consent Statement: Not applicable.

Data Availability Statement: All data are available in the main text.

Acknowledgments: Thanks to the GEMARA-SEIMC/REIPI *Pseudomonas* study group and the Comité Español del Antibiograma (COESANT) for kindly providing us with the *Pseudomonas aeruginosa* susceptibility database. A. Valero thanks Universia Foundation for her doctoral grant.

Conflicts of Interest: The authors declare no conflict of interest.

References

1. World Health Organization. Antimicrobial Resistance. Available online: https://www.who.int/health-topics/antimicrobial-resistance (accessed on 12 May 2021).
2. Jorda, A.; Zeitlinger, M. Preclinical Pharmacokinetic/Pharmacodynamic Studies and Clinical Trials in the Drug Development Process of EMA-Approved Antibacterial Agents: A Review. *Clin. Pharmacokinet.* **2020**, *59*, 1071–1084. [CrossRef]
3. Azam, M.W.; Khan, A.U. Updates on the pathogenicity status of *Pseudomonas aeruginosa*. *Drug Discov. Today* **2018**, *24*, 350–359. [CrossRef]
4. Oliver, A.; Mulet, X.; López-Causapé, C.; Juan, C. The increasing threat of *Pseudomonas aeruginosa* high-risk clones. *Drug Resist. Updates* **2015**, *21–22*, 41–59. [CrossRef]
5. European Centre for Disease Prevention and Control. Surveillance of Antimicrobial Resistance in Europe. Surveillance Report 2019. Available online: https://www.ecdc.europa.eu/sites/default/files/documents/Country%20summaries-AER-EARS-Net%20202019.pdf (accessed on 12 May 2021).
6. Estudio Nacional de Vigilancia de Infección Nosocomial en Servicios de Medicina Intensiva. Informe 2019. Available online: https://hws.vhebron.net/envin-helics/Help/Informe%20ENVIN-UCI%202019.pdf (accessed on 12 May 2021).
7. Del Barrio-Tofiño, E.; Zamorano, L.; Cortes-Lara, S.; López-Causapé, C.; Sánchez-Diener, I.; Cabot, G.; Bou, G.; Martínez-Martínez, L.; Oliver, A.; Galán, F.; et al. Spanish nationwide survey on *Pseudomonas aeruginosa* antimicrobial resistance mechanisms and epidemiology. *J. Antimicrob. Chemother.* **2019**, *74*, 1825–1835. [CrossRef]
8. Kadri, S.S.; Adjemian, J.; Lai, Y.L.; Spaulding, A.B.; Ricotta, E.; Prevots, D.R.; Palmore, T.N.; Rhee, C.; Klompas, M.; Dekker, J.P.; et al. Difficult-to-Treat Resistance in Gram-negative Bacteremia at 173 US Hospitals: Retrospective Cohort Analysis of Prevalence, Predictors, and Outcome of Resistance to All First-line Agents. *Clin. Infect. Dis.* **2018**, *67*, 1803–1814. [CrossRef] [PubMed]
9. Tamma, P.D.; Aitken, S.L.; Bonomo, R.A.; Mathers, A.J.; van Duin, D.; Clancy, C.J. Infectious Diseases Society of America Guidance on the Treatment of Extended-Spectrum β-lactamase Producing Enterobacterales (ESBL-E), Carbapenem-Resistant Enterobacterales (CRE), and *Pseudomonas aeruginosa* with Difficult-to-Treat Resistance (DTR-*P. aeruginosa*). *Clin. Infect. Dis.* **2020**, *72*, e169–e183.
10. World Health Organization. Global Action Plan. Available online: https://www.who.int/antimicrobial-resistance/global-action-plan/en/ (accessed on 12 May 2021).
11. Rodríguez-Gascón, A.; Solinís, M.; Isla, A. The Role of PK/PD Analysis in the Development and Evaluation of Antimicrobials. *Pharmaceutics* **2021**, *13*, 833. [CrossRef]
12. Asín-Prieto, E.; Rodríguez-Gascón, A.; Isla, A. Applications of the pharmacokinetic/pharmacodynamic (PK/PD) analysis of antimicrobial agents. *J. Infect. Chemother.* **2015**, *21*, 319–329. [CrossRef]
13. Blondeau, J.; Hansen, G.; Metzler, K.; Hedlin, P. The Role of PK/PD Parameters to Avoid Selection and Increase of Resistance: Mutant Prevention Concentration. *J. Chemother.* **2004**, *16*, 1–19. [CrossRef]
14. Owens, R.C.; Bulik, C.C.; Andes, D. Pharmacokinetics–pharmacodynamics, computer decision support technologies, and antimicrobial stewardship: The compass and rudder. *Diagn. Microbiol. Infect. Dis.* **2018**, *91*, 371–382. [CrossRef]
15. de Velde, F.; Mouton, J.W.; de Winter, B.C.; van Gelder, T.; Koch, B. Clinical applications of population pharmacokinetic models of antibiotics: Challenges and perspectives. *Pharmacol. Res.* **2018**, *134*, 280–288. [CrossRef] [PubMed]
16. The European Committee on Antimicrobial Susceptibility Testing. Breakpoint Tables for Interpretation of MICs and Zone Diameters, Version 10.0. 2021. Available online: www.eucast.org/clinical_breakpoints/ (accessed on 12 May 2021).

17. Zazo, H.; Martín-Suárez, A.; Lanao, J.M. Evaluating amikacin dosage regimens in intensive care unit patients: A pharmacokinetic/pharmacodynamic analysis using Monte Carlo simulation. *Int. J. Antimicrob. Agents* **2013**, *42*, 155–160. [CrossRef] [PubMed]
18. Ramsey, C.; MacGowan, A.P. A review of the pharmacokinetics and pharmacodynamics of aztreonam. *J. Antimicrob. Chemother.* **2016**, *71*, 2704–2712. [CrossRef]
19. Lipman, J.; Wallis, S.; Rickard, C. Low Plasma Cefepime Levels in Critically Ill Septic Patients: Pharmacokinetic Modeling Indicates Improved Troughs with Revised Dosing. *Antimicrob. Agents Chemother.* **1999**, *43*, 2559–2561. [CrossRef]
20. Gonçalves-Pereira, J.; Póvoa, P. Antibiotics in critically ill patients: A systematic review of the pharmacokinetics of β-lactams. *Crit. Care* **2011**, *15*, R206. [CrossRef] [PubMed]
21. Benko, A.S.; Cappelletty, D.M.; Kruse, J.A.; Rybak, M.J. Continuous infusion versus intermittent administration of ceftazidime in critically ill patients with suspected gram-negative infections. *Antimicrob. Agents Chemother.* **1996**, *40*, 691–695. [CrossRef] [PubMed]
22. Sherwin, K.B.; Zhuang, L.; Sy, S.K.B.; Zhuang, L.; Sy, S.; Derendorf, H. Clinical Pharmacokinetics and Pharmacodynamics of Ceftazidime–Avibactam Combination: A Model-Informed Strategy for its Clinical Development. *Clin. Pharmacokinet.* **2018**, *58*, 545–564.
23. Stein, G.E.; Smith, C.L.; Scharmen, A.; Kidd, J.M.; Cooper, C.; Kuti, J.; Mitra, S.; Nicolau, D.P.; Havlichek, D.H. Pharmacokinetic and Pharmacodynamic Analysis of Ceftazidime/Avibactam in Critically Ill Patients. *Surg. Infect.* **2019**, *20*, 55–61. [CrossRef]
24. European Medicines Agency. Zavicefta 2 g/0.5 g Powder for Concentrate for Solution for Infusion. Summary of Product Characteristics (SPC). Available online: https://www.ema.europa.eu/en/documents/product-information/zavicefta-epar-product-information_en.pdf (accessed on 2 June 2021).
25. Sime, F.B.; Lassig-Smith, M.; Starr, T.; Stuart, J.; Pandey, S.; Parker, S.L.; Wallis, S.C.; Lipman, J.; Roberts, J.A. Population Pharmacokinetics of Unbound Ceftolozane and Tazobactam in Critically Ill Patients without Renal Dysfunction. *Antimicrob. Agents Chemother.* **2019**, *63*, e01265-19. [CrossRef]
26. Kakara, M.; Larson, K.; Feng, H.-P.; Shiomi, M.; Yoshitsugu, H.; Rizk, M.L. Population pharmacokinetics of tazobactam/ceftolozane in Japanese patients with complicated urinary tract infection and complicated intra-abdominal infection. *J. Infect. Chemother.* **2019**, *25*, 182–191. [CrossRef]
27. Conil, J.-M.; Georges, B.; de Lussy, A.; Khachman, D.; Seguin, T.; Ruiz, S.; Cougot, P.; Fourcade, O.; Houin, G.; Saivin, S. Ciprofloxacin use in critically ill patients: Pharmacokinetic and pharmacodynamic approaches. *Int. J. Antimicrob. Agents* **2008**, *32*, 505–510. [CrossRef] [PubMed]
28. Garonzik, S.M.; Li, J.; Thamlikitkul, V.; Paterson, D.; Shoham, S.; Jacob, J.; Silveira, F.P.; Forrest, A.; Nation, R.L. Population Pharmacokinetics of Colistin Methanesulfonate and Formed Colistin in Critically Ill Patients from a Multicenter Study Provide Dosing Suggestions for Various Categories of Patients. *Antimicrob. Agents Chemother.* **2011**, *55*, 3284–3294. [CrossRef] [PubMed]
29. Lipš, M.; Šiller, M.; Strojil, J.; Urbánek, K.; Balík, M.; Suchánková, H. Pharmacokinetics of imipenem in critically ill patients during empirical treatment of nosocomial pneumonia: A comparison of 0.5-h and 3-h infusions. *Int. J. Antimicrob. Agents* **2014**, *44*, 358–362. [CrossRef]
30. Isla, A.; Canut, A.; Arribas, J.; Asín-Prieto, E.; Rodríguez-Gascón, A. Meropenem dosing requirements against *Enterobacteriaceae* in critically ill patients: Influence of renal function, geographical area and presence of extended-spectrum β-lactamases. *Eur. J. Clin. Microbiol. Infect. Dis.* **2016**, *35*, 511–519. [CrossRef]
31. Li, C.; Kuti, J.L.; Nightingale, C.H.; Mansfield, D.L.; Dana, A.; Nicolau, D.P. Population pharmacokinetics and pharmacodynamics of piperacillin/tazobactam in patients with complicated intra-abdominal infection. *J. Antimicrob. Chemother.* **2005**, *56*, 388–395. [CrossRef]
32. Peris-Marti, J.F.; Borras-Blasco, J.; Rosique-Robles, J.D.; Gonzalez-Delgado, M. Evaluation of once daily tobramycin dosing in critically ill patients through Bayesian simulation. *J. Clin. Pharm. Ther.* **2004**, *29*, 65–70. [CrossRef] [PubMed]
33. Barbhaiya, R.H.; Knupp, C.A.; Pfeffer, M.; Pittman, K.A. Lack of pharmacokinetic interaction between cefepime and amikacin in humans. *Antimicrob. Agents Chemother.* **1992**, *36*, 1382–1386. [CrossRef]
34. Scully, B.E.; Swabb, E.A.; Neu, H.C. Pharmacology of aztreonam after intravenous infusion. *Antimicrob. Agents Chemother.* **1983**, *24*, 18–22. [CrossRef]
35. Tam, V.H.; McKinnon, P.S.; Akins, R.L.; Drusano, G.L.; Rybak, M.J. Pharmacokinetics and Pharmacodynamics of Cefepime in Patients with Various Degrees of Renal Function. *Antimicrob. Agents Chemother.* **2003**, *47*, 1853–1861. [CrossRef]
36. Frei, C.R.; Wiederhold, N.P.; Burgess, D.S. Antimicrobial breakpoints for Gram-negative aerobic bacteria based on pharmacokinetic–pharmacodynamic models with Monte Carlo simulation. *J. Antimicrob. Chemother.* **2008**, *61*, 621–628. [CrossRef] [PubMed]
37. Bensman, T.J.; Wang, J.; Jayne, J.; Fukushima, L.; Rao, A.P.; D'Argenio, D.Z.; Beringer, P.M. Pharmacokinetic-Pharmacodynamic Target Attainment Analyses To Determine Optimal Dosing of Ceftazidime-Avibactam for the Treatment of Acute Pulmonary Exacerbations in Patients with Cystic Fibrosis. *Antimicrob. Agents Chemother.* **2017**, *61*, e00988-17. [CrossRef] [PubMed]
38. Monogue, M.L.; Pettit, R.S.; Muhlebach, M.; Cies, J.J.; Nicolau, D.P.; Kuti, J.L. Population Pharmacokinetics and Safety of Ceftolozane-Tazobactam in Adult Cystic Fibrosis Patients Admitted with Acute Pulmonary Exacerbation. *Antimicrob. Agents Chemother.* **2016**, *60*, 6578–6584. [CrossRef] [PubMed]

39. Rodríguez-Núñez, O.; Periañez-Parraga, L.; Oliver, A.; Munita, J.M.; Boté, A.; Gasch, O.; Nuvials, X.; Dinh, A.; Shaw, R.; Lomas, J.M.; et al. Higher MICs (>2 mg/L) Predict 30-Day Mortality in Patients With Lower Respiratory Tract Infections Caused by Multidrug- and Extensively Drug-Resistant *Pseudomonas aeruginosa* Treated With Ceftolozane/Tazobactam. *Open Forum Infect. Dis.* **2019**, *6*, ofz416. [CrossRef]
40. European Medicines Agency. Zerbaxa (Ceftolozane/Tazobactam) 1 g/0.5 g Powder for Concentrate for Solution for Infusion. Summary of Product Characteristics (SPC). Available online: https://www.ema.europa.eu/en/documents/product-information/zerbaxa-epar-product-information_en.pdf (accessed on 5 June 2021).
41. Zelenitsky, S.A.; Rubinstein, E.; Ariano, R.E.; Zhanel, G.G.; Hoban, D.J.; Adam, H.J.; Karlowsky, J.A.; Baxter, M.R.; Nichol, K.A.; Lagacé-Wiens, P.R.S.; et al. Integrating pharmacokinetics, pharmacodynamics and MIC distributions to assess changing antimicrobial activity against clinical isolates of *Pseudomonas aeruginosa* causing infections in Canadian hospitals (CANWARD). *J. Antimicrob. Chemother.* **2013**, *68*, i67–i72. [CrossRef]
42. Couet, W.; Grégoire, N.; Gobin, P.; Saulnier, P.J.; Frasca, D.; Marchand, S.; Mimoz, O. Pharmacokinetics of Colistin and Colistimethate Sodium After a Single 80-mg Intravenous Dose of CMS in Young Healthy Volunteers. *Clin. Pharmacol. Ther.* **2011**, *89*, 875–879. [CrossRef] [PubMed]
43. Asín-Prieto, E.; Isla, A.; Canut, A.; Gascón, A.R. Comparison of antimicrobial pharmacokinetic/pharmacodynamic breakpoints with EUCAST and CLSI clinical breakpoints for Gram-positive bacteria. *Int. J. Antimicrob. Agents* **2012**, *40*, 313–322. [CrossRef]
44. Zelenitsky, S.A.; Harding, G.K.M.; Sun, S.; Ubhi, K.; Ariano, R.E. Treatment and outcome of *Pseudomonas aeruginosa* bacteraemia: An antibiotic pharmacodynamic analysis. *J. Antimicrob. Chemother.* **2003**, *52*, 668–674. [CrossRef]
45. Guglielmo, B.J.; Flaherty, J.F.; Woods, T.M.; LaFollette, G.; Gambertoglio, J.G. Pharmacokinetics of cefoperazone and tobramycin alone and in combination. *Antimicrob. Agents Chemother.* **1987**, *31*, 264–266. [CrossRef]
46. Grupo de Estudio de los Mecanismos de Acción y de las Resistencias a los antimicrobianos. GEMARA-SEIMC. Available online: https://www.seimc.org/ (accessed on 12 May 2021).
47. Heffernan, A.J.; Sime, F.; Lipman, J.; Roberts, J.A. Individualising Therapy to Minimize Bacterial Multidrug Resistance. *Drugs* **2018**, *78*, 621–641. [CrossRef]
48. Abdul-Aziz, M.H.; Dulhunty, J.M.; Bellomo, R.; Lipman, J.; Roberts, J.A. Continuous beta-lactam infusion in critically ill patients: The clinical evidence. *Ann. Intensiv. Care* **2012**, *2*, 37. [CrossRef]
49. Kashuba, A.D.; Nafziger, A.N.; Drusano, G.L.; Bertino, J.S. Optimizing aminoglycoside therapy for nosocomial pneumonia caused by gram-negative bacteria. *Antimicrob. Agents Chemother.* **1999**, *43*, 623–629. [CrossRef]
50. Drusano, G.L. Antimicrobial pharmacodynamics: Critical interactions of 'bug and drug'. *Nat. Rev. Genet.* **2004**, *2*, 289–300. [CrossRef] [PubMed]
51. DeRyke, C.A.; Kuti, J.L.; Nicolau, D.P. Reevaluation of current susceptibility breakpoints for Gram-negative rods based on pharmacodynamic assessment. *Diagn. Microbiol. Infect. Dis.* **2007**, *58*, 337–344. [CrossRef]
52. Tängdén, T.; Martín, V.R.; Felton, T.W.; Nielsen, E.I.; Marchand, S.; Brüggemann, R.J.; Bulitta, J.; Bassetti, M.; Theuretzbacher, U.; Tsuji, B.T.; et al. The role of infection models and PK/PD modelling for optimising care of critically ill patients with severe infections. *Intensiv. Care Med.* **2017**, *43*, 1021–1032. [CrossRef]
53. Tam, V.H.; Chang, K.-T.; Zhou, J.; Ledesma, K.R.; Phe, K.; Gao, S.; Van Bambeke, F.; Sánchez-Díaz, A.M.; Zamorano, L.; Oliver, A.; et al. Determining β-lactam exposure threshold to suppress resistance development in Gram-negative bacteria. *J. Antimicrob. Chemother.* **2017**, *72*, 1421–1428. [CrossRef]
54. Sumi, C.D.; Heffernan, A.J.; Lipman, J.; Roberts, J.A.; Sime, F.B. What Antibiotic Exposures Are Required to Suppress the Emergence of Resistance for Gram-Negative Bacteria? A Systematic Review. *Clin. Pharmacokinet.* **2019**, *58*, 1407–1443. [CrossRef]
55. Crandon, J.L.; Schuck, V.J.; Banevicius, M.A.; Beaudoin, M.-E.; Nichols, W.W.; Tanudra, M.A.; Nicolau, D.P. Comparative In Vitro and In Vivo Efficacies of Human Simulated Doses of Ceftazidime and Ceftazidime-Avibactam against *Pseudomonas aeruginosa*. *Antimicrob. Agents Chemother.* **2012**, *56*, 6137–6146. [CrossRef] [PubMed]
56. VanScoy, B.D.; Mendes, R.E.; Castanheira, M.; McCauley, J.; Bhavnani, S.M.; Jones, R.N.; Friedrich, L.V.; Steenbergen, J.N.; Ambrose, P.G. Relationship between Ceftolozane-Tazobactam Exposure and Selection for *Pseudomonas aeruginosa* Resistance in a Hollow-Fiber Infection Model. *Antimicrob. Agents Chemother.* **2014**, *58*, 6024–6031. [CrossRef] [PubMed]
57. Bergen, P.J.; Bulitta, J.B.; Kirkpatrick, C.; Rogers, K.E.; McGregor, M.J.; Wallis, S.C.; Paterson, D.; Lipman, J.; Roberts, J.; Landersdorfer, C.B. Effect of different renal function on antibacterial effects of piperacillin against *Pseudomonas aeruginosa* evaluated via the hollow-fibre infection model and mechanism-based modelling. *J. Antimicrob. Chemother.* **2016**, *71*, 2509–2520. [CrossRef]
58. Firsov, A.A.; Gilbert, D.; Greer, K.; Portnoy, Y.A.; Zinner, S.H. Comparative Pharmacodynamics and Antimutant Potentials of Doripenem and Imipenem with Ciprofloxacin-Resistant *Pseudomonas aeruginosa* in an In Vitro Model. *Antimicrob. Agents Chemother.* **2011**, *56*, 1223–1228. [CrossRef]
59. Maciá, M.D.; Borrell, N.; Segura, M.; Gómez, C.; Pérez, J.L.; Oliver, A. Efficacy and Potential for Resistance Selection of Antipseudomonal Treatments in a Mouse Model of Lung Infection by Hypermutable *Pseudomonas aeruginosa*. *Antimicrob. Agents Chemother.* **2006**, *50*, 975–983. [CrossRef] [PubMed]
60. Colin, P.; Eleveld, D.J.; Jonckheere, S.; Van Bocxlaer, J.; De Waele, J.; Vermeulen, A. What about confidence intervals? A word of caution when interpreting PTA simulations. *J. Antimicrob. Chemother.* **2016**, *71*, 2502–2508. [CrossRef] [PubMed]

61. European Medicines Agency (EMA-CHMP). Guideline on the Use of Pharmacokinetics and Pharmacodynamics in the Development of Antimicrobial Medicinal Products (EMA/CHMP/594085/2015). London, UK, 2016. Available online: https://www.ema.europa.eu/en/documents/scientific-guideline/guideline-use-pharmacokinetics-pharmacodynamics-development-antimicrobial-medicinal-products_en.pdf (accessed on 5 June 2021).
62. Valero, A.; Isla, A.; Rodríguez-Gascón, A.; Calvo, B.; Canut, A.; Solinís, M. Pharmacokinetic/pharmacodynamic analysis as a tool for surveillance of the activity of antimicrobials against *Pseudomonas aeruginosa* strains isolated in critically ill patients. *Enfermedades Infecciosas y Microbiología Clínica* **2018**, *37*, 380–386. [PubMed]
63. Valero, A.; Isla, A.; Rodríguez-Gascón, A.; Canut, A.; Solinís, M. Susceptibility of *Pseudomonas aeruginosa* and antimicrobial activity using PK/PD analysis: An 18-year surveillance study. *Enfermedades Infecciosas y Microbiología Clínica* **2019**, *37*, 626–633. [CrossRef]
64. Thabit, A.K.; Hobbs, A.L.; Guzman, O.E.; Shea, K.M. The Pharmacodynamics of Prolonged Infusion β-Lactams for the Treatment of *Pseudomonas aeruginosa* Infections: A Systematic Review. *Clin. Ther.* **2019**, *41*, 2397–2415. [CrossRef]
65. Abdulla, A.; Dijkstra, A.; Hunfeld, N.G.M.; Endeman, H.; Bahmany, S.; Ewoldt, T.M.J.; Muller, A.E.; Van Gelder, T.; Gommers, D.; Koch, B.C.P. Failure of target attainment of beta-lactam antibiotics in critically ill patients and associated risk factors: A two-center prospective study (EXPAT). *Crit. Care* **2020**, *24*, 1–12. [CrossRef]
66. Abuhussain, S.S.A.; Sutherland, C.A.; Nicolau, D.P. In vitro potency of antipseudomonal β-lactams against blood and respiratory isolates of *P. aeruginosa* collected from US hospitals. *J. Thorac. Dis.* **2019**, *11*, 1896–1902. [CrossRef]
67. World Health Organization. The 2019 Who Aware Classification of Antibiotics for Evaluation and Monitoring of Use. Geneva, Switzerland, 2019. (WHO/EMP/IAU/2019.11). Licence: CC BY-NC-SA 3.0 IGO. Available online: https://apps.who.int/iris/handle/10665/327957 (accessed on 12 May 2021).

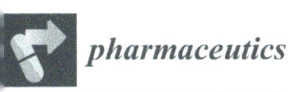

Article

Population Pharmacokinetics of Meropenem in Critically Ill Korean Patients and Effects of Extracorporeal Membrane Oxygenation

Dong-Hwan Lee [1,†], Hyoung-Soo Kim [2,†], Sunghoon Park [3], Hwan-il Kim [3], Sun-Hee Lee [2] and Yong-Kyun Kim [4,*]

1. Department of Clinical Pharmacology, Hallym University Sacred Heart Hospital, Hallym University College of Medicine, Anyang 14066, Korea; dhlee97@hallym.or.kr
2. Department of Thoracic and Cardiovascular Surgery, Hallym University Sacred Heart Hospital, Hallym University College of Medicine, Anyang 14066, Korea; cskhs99@hallym.or.kr (H.-S.K.); shlee1425@hallym.or.kr (S.-H.L.)
3. Division of Pulmonary, Allergy and Critical Care Medicine, Department of Internal Medicine, Hallym University Sacred Heart Hospital, Hallym University College of Medicine, Anyang 14066, Korea; f2000tj@hallym.or.kr (S.P.); hwanil@hallym.or.kr (H.-i.K.)
4. Division of Infectious Diseases, Department of Internal Medicine, Hallym University Sacred Heart Hospital, Hallym University College of Medicine, Anyang 14066, Korea
* Correspondence: amoureuxyk@hallym.or.kr; Tel.: +82-31-380-3724; Fax: +82-31-380-1555
† D.-H.L. and H.-S.K. contributed equally to this work as co-first authors.

Abstract: Limited studies have investigated population pharmacokinetic (PK) models and optimal dosage regimens of meropenem for critically ill adult patients using the probability of target attainment, including patients receiving extracorporeal membrane oxygenation (ECMO). A population PK analysis was conducted using non-linear mixed-effect modeling. Monte Carlo simulation was used to determine for how long the free drug concentration was above the minimum inhibitory concentration (MIC) at steady state conditions in patients with various degrees of renal function. Meropenem PK in critically ill patients was described using a two-compartment model, in which glomerular filtration rate was identified as a covariate for clearance. ECMO did not affect meropenem PK. The simulation results showed that the current meropenem dosing regimen would be sufficient for attaining $40\%fT_{>MIC}$ for *Pseudomonas aeruginosa* at MIC $\leq$ 4 mg/L. Prolonged infusion over 3 h or a high-dosage regimen of 2 g/8 h was needed for MIC > 2 mg/L or in patients with augmented renal clearance, for a target of $100\%fT_{>MIC}$ or $100\%fT_{>4\times MIC}$. Our study suggests that clinicians should consider prolonged infusion or a high-dosage regimen of meropenem, particularly when treating critically ill patients with augmented renal clearance or those infected with pathogens with decreased in vitro susceptibility, regardless of ECMO support.

Keywords: meropenem; population pharmacokinetics; critically ill patient; adult; extracorporeal membrane oxygenation; Monte Carlo simulation

Citation: Lee, D.-H.; Kim, H.-S.; Park, S.; Kim, H.-i.; Lee, S.-H.; Kim, Y.-K. Population Pharmacokinetics of Meropenem in Critically Ill Korean Patients and Effects of Extracorporeal Membrane Oxygenation. *Pharmaceutics* **2021**, *13*, 1861. https://doi.org/10.3390/pharmaceutics13111861

Academic Editors: Jonás Samuel Pérez-Blanco and José Martínez Lanao

Received: 30 September 2021
Accepted: 1 November 2021
Published: 4 November 2021

Publisher's Note: MDPI stays neutral with regard to jurisdictional claims in published maps and institutional affiliations.

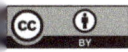

Copyright: © 2021 by the authors. Licensee MDPI, Basel, Switzerland. This article is an open access article distributed under the terms and conditions of the Creative Commons Attribution (CC BY) license (https://creativecommons.org/licenses/by/4.0/).

1. Introduction

Antibiotic treatment is a major factor in determining the survival of critically ill patients diagnosed with sepsis. Altered pharmacokinetics (PK) in these patients is a major obstacle for clinicians when determining an adequate antibiotic dosage regimen [1]. The "third spacing" phenomenon caused by vasodilation and capillary leakage in sepsis patients increases the volume of distribution and lowers the drugs' serum concentration, especially for hydrophilic antimicrobials [1,2], such as β-lactams and aminoglycoside, that are more affected by pathophysiological changes than lipophilic drugs [3].

Meropenem, a carbapenem β-lactam agent with a wide spectrum of activity against Gram-positive and Gram-negative pathogens, is used for the treatment of severe infections caused by multidrug-resistant organisms in intensive care unit (ICU) patients, including those on extracorporeal membrane oxygenation (ECMO) support [4–7]. A large heterogeneity was observed in the volume of distribution (over two-fold) in sepsis patients admitted to the ICU and receiving meropenem [3]. ECMO may further complicate PK changes in volume of distribution and clearance [8,9], which highlights the need for optimizing meropenem dosage in adult patients on ECMO. However, the effects of ECMO on the optimal dosage for meropenem have not been elucidated. Limited studies have performed population PK modelling and evaluated the pharmacodynamic (PD) alterations associated with ECMO [10–12]. Moreover, knowledge regarding the PK/PD profile of meropenem during ECMO and its clinical relevance for different ethnicities is also limited.

This study aimed to construct a population PK model for meropenem in critically ill Korean adult patients, including those receiving ECMO, to explore the effects of ECMO on meropenem PK. Moreover, we investigated optimal dosage regimens of meropenem by assessing the probability of PK/PD target attainment for various regimens using Monte Carlo simulations.

2. Methods

2.1. Patients

This prospective study was conducted in Hallym University Sacred Heart Hospital (840-bed university-affiliated tertiary referral hospital), Anyang, South Korea, from September 2020 to April 2021. Clinical indications for meropenem included: empirical management of sepsis from unknown source, nosocomial infections, and prophylactic administration for patients undergoing ECMO. Patients with a history of β-lactam allergy or a positive skin test result for meropenem were excluded. The demographic factors between the ECMO and the non-ECMO groups were compared. If meeting normality, the t-test was performed; otherwise, the Wilcoxon rank-sum test was used.

2.2. ECMO Apparatus

The ECMO system used was the Permanent Life Support (PLS) System (MAQUET, Rastatt, Germany), which consists of a broad range of HLS Cannulae and the Rotaflow Console. The PLS Set includes the PLS-i Oxygenator. A total of 1 L of plasma solution or normal saline was infused into the circuit, and the total circuit volume was 500–600 mL.

2.3. Study Design

Patients were able to participate at any time after the initiation of meropenem administration. Patients received 500 or 1000 mg of meropenem for 30 min every 8 or 12 h via intravenous (IV) infusion. Five blood samples were collected after the first dose following patients' enrollment, and two samples were collected at steady state after four or five consecutive doses. The planned sampling times for model development were as follows: (1) immediately before dosing, (2) 0.5, 1, 4, and 8 h after the start of the infusion for the 8 h interval, and (3) 0, 0.5, 1, 6, and 12 h after the start of the infusion for the 12 h interval. Samples were collected before (trough level) and 30 min after (peak level) the fourth or fifth dosage, for model validation.

2.4. Meropenem Assay

Meropenem plasma concentrations were analyzed using high-performance liquid chromatography (HPLC)–tandem mass spectrometry (MS). The HPLC system consisted of a prominence LC-20A System (Shimadzu, Japan) and a Gemini C_{18} column (Kinetex; Phenomenex, Torrance, CA, USA). The MS detection was conducted using a hybrid triple quadrupole/Linear Ion trap mass spectrometer (API4000 QTRAP; SCIEX, Framingham, MA, USA). Briefly, a 100 μL aliquot of plasma sample was pipetted into a centrifuge tube. Next, 100 μL of acetonitrile containing an internal standard (20 μg/mL, ceftazidime) was added to the tube and then vortexed for 1 min. After centrifugation at 12,000 rpm for 2 min, the supernatant was transferred to another centrifuge tube, and 100 μL of 0.1%

formic acid was added to the tube. An aliquot of 10 µL was injected into the LC–MS/MS system. The lower limit of quantitation was 0.2 mg/L. The assay results were linear over a range from 0.2 to 200 mg/L ($R^2 = 0.99$). Intraday precision and accuracy of the validation concentration range (0.5, 5, and 50 mg/L) analyzed using standard samples were 2.98–3.92% and 96.53–110.07%, respectively. Interday precision and accuracy of the validation concentration range (0.5, 5, and 50 mg/L) analyzed using standard samples for 3 days were 0.5–2.7% and 89.9–100.0%, respectively.

2.5. Population PK Analysis

Population PK modeling was implemented using the Nonlinear-mixed effects modelling software (NONMEM® 7.5, ICON Development Solutions, Elliot City, MD, USA). The first-order conditional estimation with interaction (FOCEI) method was used to estimate measured (fixed) and unexplained (random) effect parameters. FOCEI allows the interaction between the inter-individual variability (IIV, η) of PK parameters and the residual variability (RV) of measured concentrations. RV was caused by inter-individual variability, measurement error, assay error, and model misspecification. One-, two-, and three-compartment structural models were investigated using the PK model library in NONMEM. All PK processes were assumed to follow first-order kinetics rather than zero-order infusion. The PK parameter was defined as $θ_i = θ \times \exp(η_i)$, where $θ$ is the typical value of the PK parameter, $θ_i$ is an individual PK parameter, and $η_i$ is a random effect associated with IIV, which is assumed to have a normal distribution with a mean of 0 and a variance of $ω^2$. Proportional, additive, or combined proportional and additive error models were tested for RV, which was assumed to have a normal distribution with a mean of 0 and a variance of $σ^2$. A power parameter was tested to allow for nonlinear heteroscedastic variances [13].

Models were evaluated and selected based on NONMEM objective function values (OFVs), precision of parameter estimates (relative standard errors), shrinkage of IIV, and diagnostic goodness-of-fit plots. In a log-likelihood ratio test, a decrease in the OFV (ΔOFV) between two nested models, having 1 degree of freedom greater than 3.84 or 2 degrees of freedom greater than 5.99, was considered statistically significant at $p < 0.05$ for model improvement. Diagnostic plots included the following four plots: conditional weighted residuals (CWRES) vs. time, CWRES vs. model-predicted population concentration (PRED), observation vs. PRED, and observation vs. model-predicted individual concentration.

Perl-speaks-NONMEM software (PSN, version 5.2.6, available online: https://uupharmacometrics.github.io/PsN, accessed on 17 June 2021)) was used for searching covariates, evaluating a model with visual predictive check and conducting nonparametric bootstrap to obtain 95% confidence intervals (CIs). To search significant covariates for the PK parameters, stepwise forward inclusion and backward exclusion processes were conducted. Statistical significance was set at $p < 0.01$ (ΔOFV < -6.635 for 1 degree of freedom) for inclusion and $p < 0.001$ (ΔOFV > 10.83 for 1 degree of freedom) for exclusion. A significant covariate should have both statistical significance and clinical relevance. The tested covariates for structural PK parameters were age, sex, height, weight, body surface area (BSA), serum albumin level, serum protein level, serum creatinine level, serum cystatin C level, primary diagnosis, comorbidity, renal function, ECMO type (veno–arterial (VA) or veno–venous (VV)), and ECMO flow rate. The renal function was calculated by applying Chronic Kidney Disease Epidemiology Collaboration (CKD-EPI), modified CKD-EPI, Modification of Diet in Renal Disease (MDRD), modified MDRD, and Cockcroft-Gault (CG) formulations to determine the total clearance (CL). The modified CKD-EPI and MDRD estimates were adjusted using individual BSA values, where BSA was calculated by applying the Du Bois formula. Visual predictive check with prediction and variability correction (VPC$_{PVC}$) was performed using PSN by comparing the final PK model with the measured plasma concentrations with 80% prediction intervals from 1000 virtual datasets. Nonparametric bootstrapping was performed to investigate the stability of the final PK model. The median and 95% confidence interval for the estimates of bootstrap samples (n = 2000) were generated to evaluate the parameter estimates of the final PK model. R software (version 4.0.4, available online: www.rproject.org, accessed on 11 March 2021) was used for the postprocessing of model output and visualization.

The individual PK parameters between ECMO and non-ECMO groups were compared. If meeting normality, an independent t-test was used; otherwise, Wilcoxon rank-sum test was used.

2.6. Assessment of Prediction Performance

The predictive performance of the final PK model was assessed visually using the relative prediction error (rPE) vs. the observed concentration plot and numerically using the relative bias (rBias) for accuracy and the relative root-mean-square error (rRMSE) for precision.

$$\text{rPE} = \frac{C_P - C_O}{C_O}$$

$$\text{rBias} = 100\% \frac{1}{N} \sum_i \frac{C_P - C_O}{C_O}$$

$$\text{rRMSE} = 100\% \sqrt{\frac{1}{N} \sum_i \frac{(C_P - C_O)^2}{C_O^2}}$$

where C_O indicates the observed concentrations, and C_P v the predicted concentrations.

2.7. PD Target Attainment

Four Monte Carlo simulations were implemented. The first simulation was conducted to explore the adequacy of the recommended dosage regimen (for a creatinine clearance [CL_{CR}] > 50 mL/min, 1 g every 8 h by i.v. infusion; for a CL_{CR} of 26–50 mL/min, 1 g every 12 h by i.v. infusion; for a CL_{CR} of 10–25 mL/min, 500 mg every 12 h by i.v. infusion; for a CL_{CR} < 10 mL/min, 500 mg every 24 h i.v. infusion) when treating adult patients infected with *Pseudomonas aeruginosa* (*P. aeruginosa*). A total of 10,000 individual PK parameters were generated for virtual patients assuming a log-normal distribution for each parameter with the typical parameter values and the IIV of the final PK model. The selected covariate, glomerular filtration rate (eGFR) estimated using the CKD-EPI equation, was generated assuming a log-normal distribution within the range of 0 to 130 mL/min. Patients were treated empirically without knowing the pathogen, while minimum inhibitory concentration (MIC) values were generated using the clinical breakpoint distribution of MICs set by the European Committee on Antimicrobial Susceptibility Testing. They were randomly assigned to the 10,000 virtual patients. The steady-state concentration–time profiles of the virtual patients were generated using the simulated individual PK parameters and the recommended dosage regimen.

The antimicrobial activity of meropenem is related to the cumulative percentage of a 24 h period during which the free drug (unbound to protein, f) concentration exceeds the MIC for a pathogen, in steady-state condition ($fT_{>MIC}$). The parameter f was fixed at 98%. The tested treatment targets were 40%$fT_{>MIC}$, 100%$fT_{>MIC}$, and 100%$fT_{>4xMIC}$. A dosage strategy was considered adequate if the probability of target attainment (PTA) was greater than or equal to 90%. The PTAs for treatment target were compared for various combinations of renal function, MICs, and dosage regimen of the patients.

The second, third, and fourth simulations were conducted to determine the optimal dosage regimen for 40%$fT_{>MIC}$, 100%$fT_{>MIC}$, and 100%$fT_{>4xMIC}$ as treatment targets, respectively. A total of 1000 individual PK parameters were generated for virtual patients assuming a log-normal distribution for each parameter, whereas the covariate was generated by applying a uniform distribution within the range 0 to 170 mL/min. The patients were divided into the six renal function groups (0 < CL_{CR} ≤ 10, 10 < CL_{CR} ≤ 25, 25 < CL_{CR} ≤ 50, 50 < CL_{CR} ≤ 90, 90 < CL_{CR} ≤ 130, and 130 < CL_{CR} ≤ 170 mL/min). Steady-state concentration–time profiles of the 1000 virtual patients were generated for various combinations of the three doses (0.5, 1, and 2 g), two dosing intervals (8 and 12 h), four infusion times (0.5, 1, 2, and 3 h), and MICs (0.060, 0.125, 0.25, 0.5, 1, 2, 4, 8, and 16 mg/L).

3. Results

3.1. Patient Characteristics

The demographic and clinical characteristics of the 26 patients are described in Table 1. Eight adult patients received ECMO (veno–arterial (VA) ECMO, n = 7; veno–venous (VV) ECMO, n = 1). One of the 18 patients in the non-ECMO group and one of the eight patients in the ECMO group received continuous renal replacement therapy. Patients on ECMO support were younger (median age, interquartile range [IQR]; 64.0 [56.3–66.5] vs. 72.0 [66.0–80.3] days; $p = 0.0167$). The severity scores, including the APACHE II (median [IQR]; 12 [10–14] vs. 10 [7–14]; $p = 0.0321$) and SOFA scores (median [IQR]; 9.50 [8.00–12.5] vs. 5.00 [3.00–7.75]; $p = 0.0051$), were significantly higher in patients in the ECMO group compared to those in the non-ECMO group.

Table 1. Patients' characteristics (median (IQR)).

Parameter	ECMO (n = 8)	Non-ECMO (n = 18)	p-Value
ECMO type	VA 7/VV 1		
CRRT	Yes 3/No 5	Yes 1/No 17	
Sex	male 4/female 4	male 14/female 4	
Age (year)	64.0 (56.3–66.5)	72.0 (66.0–80.3)	0.0167 [c]
Height (cm)	162 (153–169)	165 (156–170)	0.6544 [d]
Weight (kg)	63.5 (61.9–66.3)	54.4 (50.5–64.5)	0.1731 [d]
Body surface area (m^2)	1.67 (1.61–1.75)	1.63 (1.51–1.72)	0.5074 [c]
ICU duration (days)	25.0 (6.00–43.5)	6.50 (4.00–17.8)	0.1249 [d]
APACHE II	21.0 (19.5–22.5)	16.0 (12.0–18.0)	0.0321 [c]
SOFA	9.50 (8.00–12.5)	5.00 (3.00–7.75)	0.0051 [c]
BUN (mg/dL)	26.9 (22.0–33.0)	22.6 (10.8–46.6)	0.8675 [d]
Scr (mg/dL)	0.820 (0.518–1.15)	0.615 (0.458–1.43)	0.9557 [d]
Cystatin C (mg/dL)	1.48 (1.43–1.90)	1.34 (0.985–1.86)	0.5411 [c]
Albumin (g/dL)	3.00 (2.83–3.20)	2.55 (2.30–2.98)	0.0364 [c]
Protein (g/dL)	5.15 (4.88–5.75)	5.05 (4.70–5.75)	0.5448 [d]
CL$_{CR}$, Cockcroft-Gault (mL/min)	76.9 (59.5–105)	73.4 (32.7–92.6)	0.4367 [d]
GFR, MDRD (mL/min/1.73 m^2)	86.9 (67.1–132)	111 (47.5–160)	0.9119 [c]
GFR, modified MDRD (mL/min) [b]	88.7 (67.0–115)	95.1 (45.0–153)	0.8676 [d]
GFR, CKD-EPI (mL/min/1.73 m^2)	87.7 (70.0–105)	91.6 (45.6–103)	0.7145 [c]
GFR, modified CKD-EPI (mL/min) [b]	82.4 (70.0–94.9)	77.7 (43.6–97.0)	0.5883 [c]

IQR, interquartile range; ECMO, extracorporeal membrane oxygenation; VA, veno–arterial; VV, veno–venous; CRRT, continuous renal replacement therapy; APACHE II, Acute Physiology and Chronic Health Evaluation; SOFA, sequential organ failure assessment; BUN, serum blood urea nitrogen level; Scr; serum creatinine level; CL$_{CR}$, creatinine clearance; GFR, glomerular filtration rate; MDRD, Modification of Diet in Renal Disease; CKD-EPI, Chronic Kidney Disease Epidemiology Collaboration. [b] The modified MDRD and CKD-EPI equations adjusted to individual BSA are GFR (mL/min) = GFR (MDRD or CKD-EPI) × (BSA/1.73 m^2). [c] Independent t-test. [d] Wilcoxon rank-sum test.

3.2. Population PK Analysis

A total of 125 samples were used to develop a population PK model, and 44 samples to validate the final model. The concentration–time profile of meropenem was best described by a two-compartment model. The NONMEM OFVs for one-, two-, and three-compartment models were 689.840, 6540.693, and 640.694, respectively.

The structural parameters for the two-compartment model were total clearance (CL), central volume of distribution (V$_C$), peripheral volume of distribution (V$_P$), and intercompartmental clearance (Q) between V$_C$ and V$_P$. The inter-individual variability (IIV) was estimated for CL, V1, and V2 (Table 2). In the final PK model (OFV 611.402), GFR was estimated using the CKD-EPI equation and identified as a statistically significant covariate of CL. The IIV for CL was reduced from 55.2% to 31.4% after the covariate were included. ECMO therapy did not affect the meropenem PK in this study.

Table 2. Population PK parameter estimates for meropenem.

Parameter	Estimates	RSE (%) [Shrinkage (%)]	Bootstrap Median (95% CI)
Structural model			
CL = $\theta_1 \times (1 + \theta_2 \times (CE - 91.57))$			
θ_1 (L/h)	6.37	7.41	6.32 (5.42–7.23)
θ_2	0.00925	10.3	0.00932 (0.00680–0.0110)
V_C (L)	9.07	12.2	8.97 (3.92–12.0)
Q (L/h)	10.7	21.5	10.6 (4.73–31.0)
V_P (L)	7.91	13.6	8.17 (5.35–11.1)
Inter-individual variability			
CL (%)	31.4	15.8 [3.70]	29.9 (18.0–38.7)
V_C (%)	43.6	22.5 [14.7]	41.0 (0.000–95.4)
V_P (%)	36.6	21.0 [41.3]	34.5 (0.000–55.7)
Residual variability			
Proportional error (%)	24.6	29.3 [24.2]	24.1 (10.3–41.5)
Power parameter	0.865	10.0	0.897 (0.533–1.38)

ECMO, extracorporeal membrane oxygenation; RSE, relative standard error; CL, total clearance; θ_1, typical population value for CL; θ_2, covariate coefficient for CE; V_C, central volume of distribution; V_P, peripheral volume of distribution; Q, inter-compartmental clearance between V_C and V_P; CE, glomerular filtration rate estimated by CKD-EPI equation.

The PK parameter estimates were not significantly different between the ECMO and the non-ECMO groups (Table 3). Residual error was well described using a proportional error model. The power parameter for RV reduced the relative standard error (RSE) of the IIV for CL from 27.3% to 22.5%. When IIV was expressed as a standard deviation, if the RSE of IIV exceeded 25%, it was not significant.

Table 3. Comparison of population PK parameter estimates between the ECMO and the non ECMO groups.

Parameter	ECMO	non ECMO	p-Value
CL	6.34 (4.84–7.92)	5.05 (3.43–7.37)	0.5782 [b]
V_C (L)	8.37 (7.35–8.89)	8.53 (7.21–11.7)	0.6567 [c]
V_P (L)	8.11 (7.75–8.86)	8.28 (6.55–8.64)	0.4258 [b]
V_{SS} (L)	16.2 (15.6–17.9)	17.2 (14.7–21.0)	0.6140 [b]

ECMO, extracorporeal membrane oxygenation; CL, total clearance; V_C, central volume of distribution; V_P, peripheral volume of distribution; V_{SS}, steady-state volume of distribution. [b] Independent t-test. [c] Wilcoxon rank-sum test.

The diagnostic goodness-of-fit plots for the final PK model are depicted in Figure 1. Conditional weighted residuals (CWRES) were randomly distributed around the x-axis, indicating no systemic deviation in the structural model (Figure 1a) or in the residual error model (Figure 1b); most of them remained within ±2 times the normalized standard deviation. The observation values were randomly distributed around the line of identity, indicating no evidence of misspecification of the structural, IIV, or RV model (Figure 1c,d).

VPC_{PVC} is shown in Figure 2, where most of the observations fall within the 80% prediction interval of the simulated concentrations, and the observed 10th, 50th, and 90th percentiles are overlaid with 95% CIs of the simulated 10th, 50th, and 90th percentiles. This plot suggests that the final PK model correctly explained the data and had appropriate predictive performance. The time course for individual observed, individual predicted, and population predicted concentrations is shown in Figure S1.

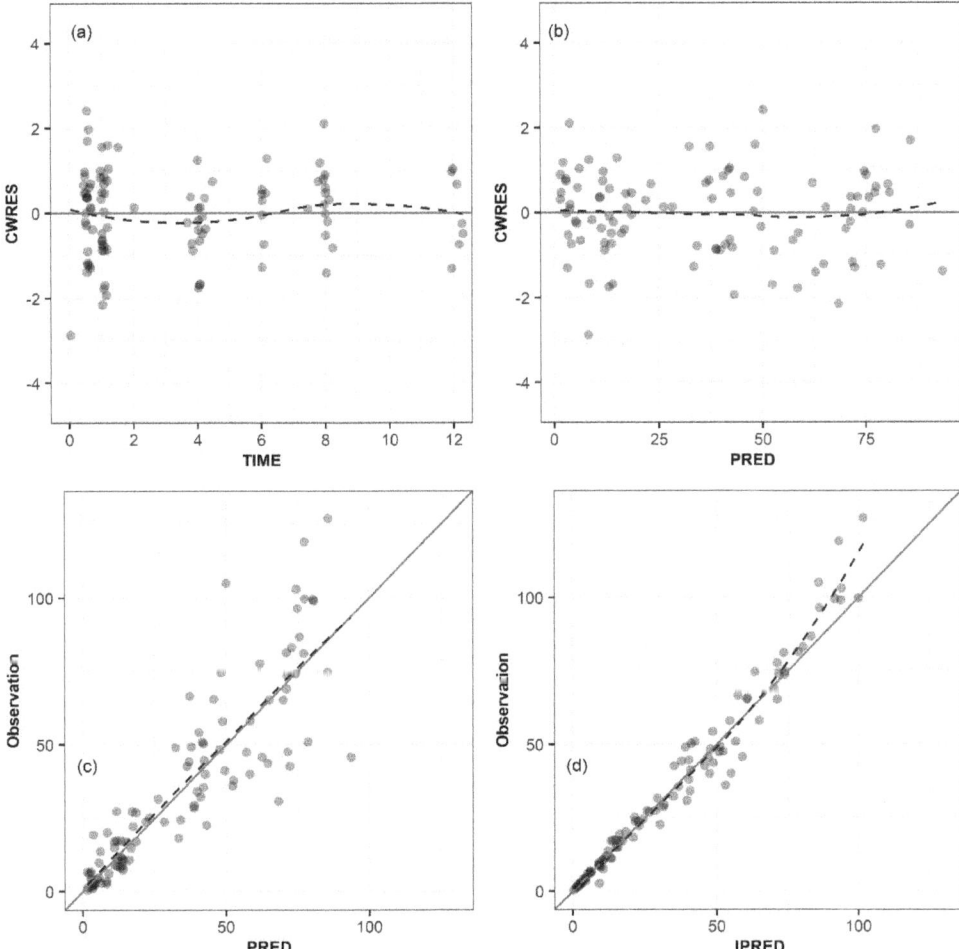

Figure 1. Goodness–of–fit plots. (**a**) Conditional weighted residuals (CWRES) versus time, (**b**) CWRES versus population predicted concentration (PRED), (**c**) observed concentration versus PRED, and (**d**) observed concentration versus individual predicted concentration. The dashed lines indicate smooth curves.

3.3. Assessment of Prediction Performance

Figure S2 displays the relative prediction error (rPE) vs. the observed concentration. As shown, most values are distributed around the x-axis. When the concentration exceeded 50 mg/L, underprediction was observed. When all subjects were included, the relative bias (rBias) and relative root-mean-square error (rRMSE) were 17.5% and 91.5%, respectively. However, when two subjects with extreme outliers were excluded, the rBias and rRMSE were 1.59% and 29.4%, respectively.

3.4. PD Target Attainment

Figure 3 shows the PTA of empirical therapy using the current dosage regimen in the first simulation. The recommended dosage regimen achieved 90% PTA at 40%$fT_{>MIC}$ when the MIC was less than 8 mg/L; however, it did not achieve 90% PTA at 100%$fT_{>MIC}$ when the MIC was greater than 0.25 mg/L. If the target was 100%$fT_{>4 \times MIC}$, the current regimen could not reach the 90% PTA regardless of the MIC.

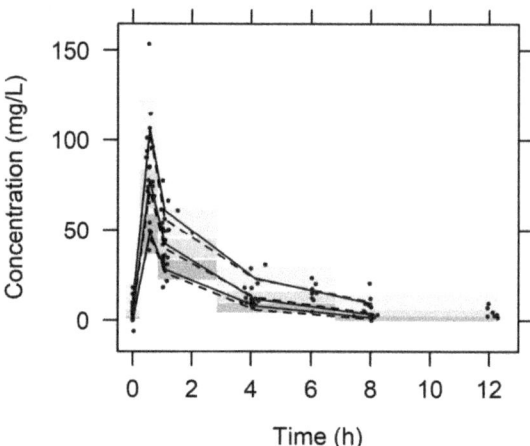

Figure 2. Visual predictive check plot. Plots from virtual concentrations of 1000 simulated datasets. Closed circles, observed serum meropenem concentrations; solid lines, the 10th, 50th, and 90th percentiles of observations; dashed lines, the 10th, 50th, and 90th percentiles of simulated serum meropenem concentrations; shaded areas, 95% confidence intervals for each percentiles of simulated concentrations.

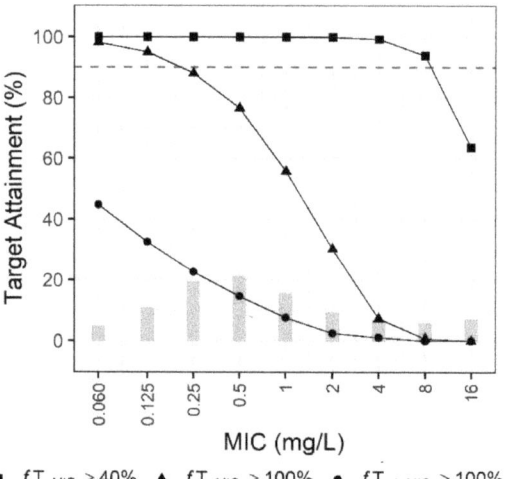

■ $fT_{>MIC} \geq 40\%$ ▲ $fT_{>MIC} \geq 100\%$ ● $fT_{>4 \times MIC} \geq 100\%$

Figure 3. Probabilities of target attainment (PTA) of empirical therapy using the current dosage regimen for patients with an eGFR of 0–130 mL/min/1.73 m². Bars indicate the MIC distribution for *P. aeruginosa*.

In the second simulation, optimal dosage regimens were explored to achieve PTA > 90% at 40%$fT_{>MIC}$ (Figure 4). In the case of patients with an eGFR of 26–50 mL/min/1.73 m², a regimen of 1 g every 12 h using i.v. infusion over 30 min could attain a 90% PTA when the MIC was 4 mg/L. However, a dosage regimen of 0.5 g every 12 h was also appropriate for patients in this study. As expected, a prolonged infusion enhanced the PTA. For patients with eGFR values of 90–130 mL/min/1.73 m², a dosage regimen of 1 g every 12 h using i.v. infusion over 2 h was optimum when the MIC was 4 mg/L, whereas 30 min or 1 h of infusion was not.

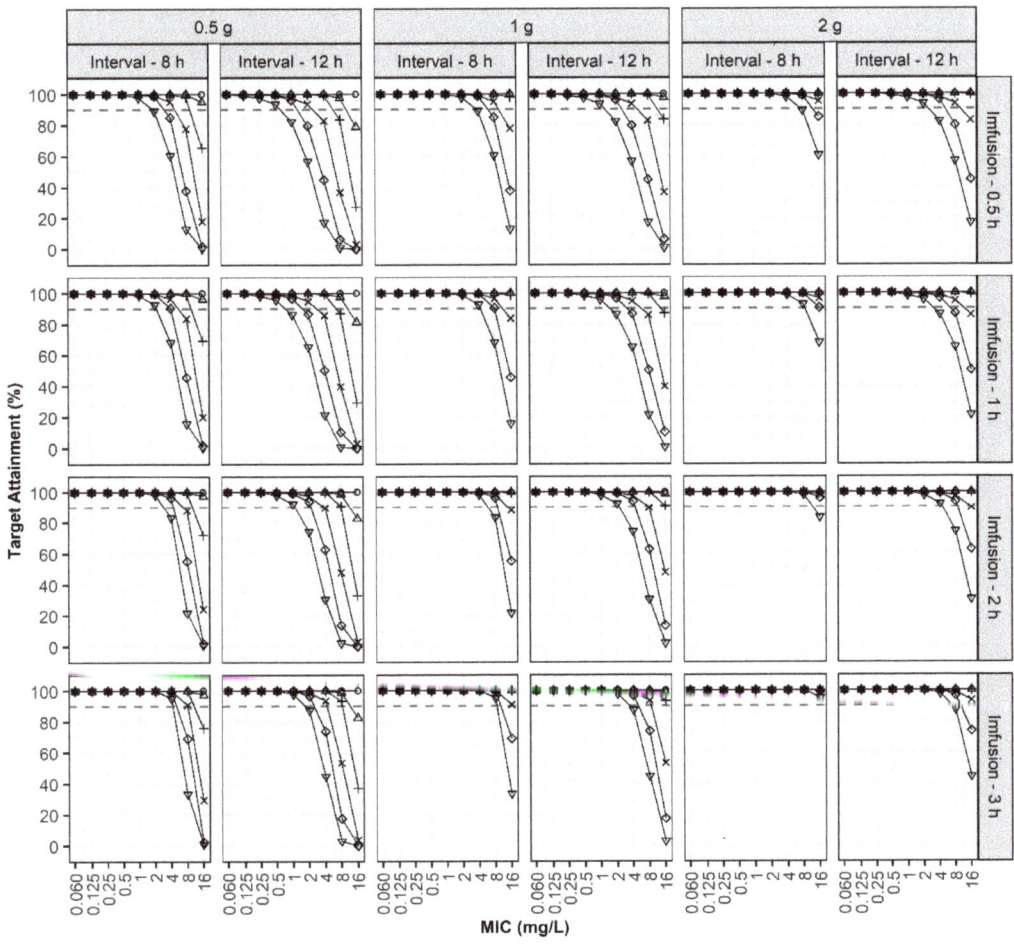

Figure 4. PTAs (40%$fT_{>MIC}$). Simulation results with three doses (0.5, 1, and 2 g), two dosing intervals (8 and 12 h), four infusion times (0.5, 1, 2, and 3 h), various degrees of renal function, and various MICs.

In the third simulation, optimal dosage regimens were explored to achieve PTA > 90% at 100%$fT_{>MIC}$ (Figure 5). In the case of patients with an eGFR of 50–90 mL/min/1.73 m², a regimen of 1 g every 8 h using i.v. infusion over 30 min or prolonged infusion over 3 h could attain a 90% PTA when the MIC was 1 mg/L and 2 mg/L, respectively. For patients with augmented renal clearance (eGFR values of 130–170 mL/min/1.73 m²), a regimen of 1 g every 8 h using prolonged i.v. infusion over 3 h was optimum only when the MIC was equal to or less than 0.25 mg/L, and a high-dosage regimen of 2 g every 8 h using prolonged i.v. infusion over 3 h was optimum when the MIC was less than 1 mg/L.

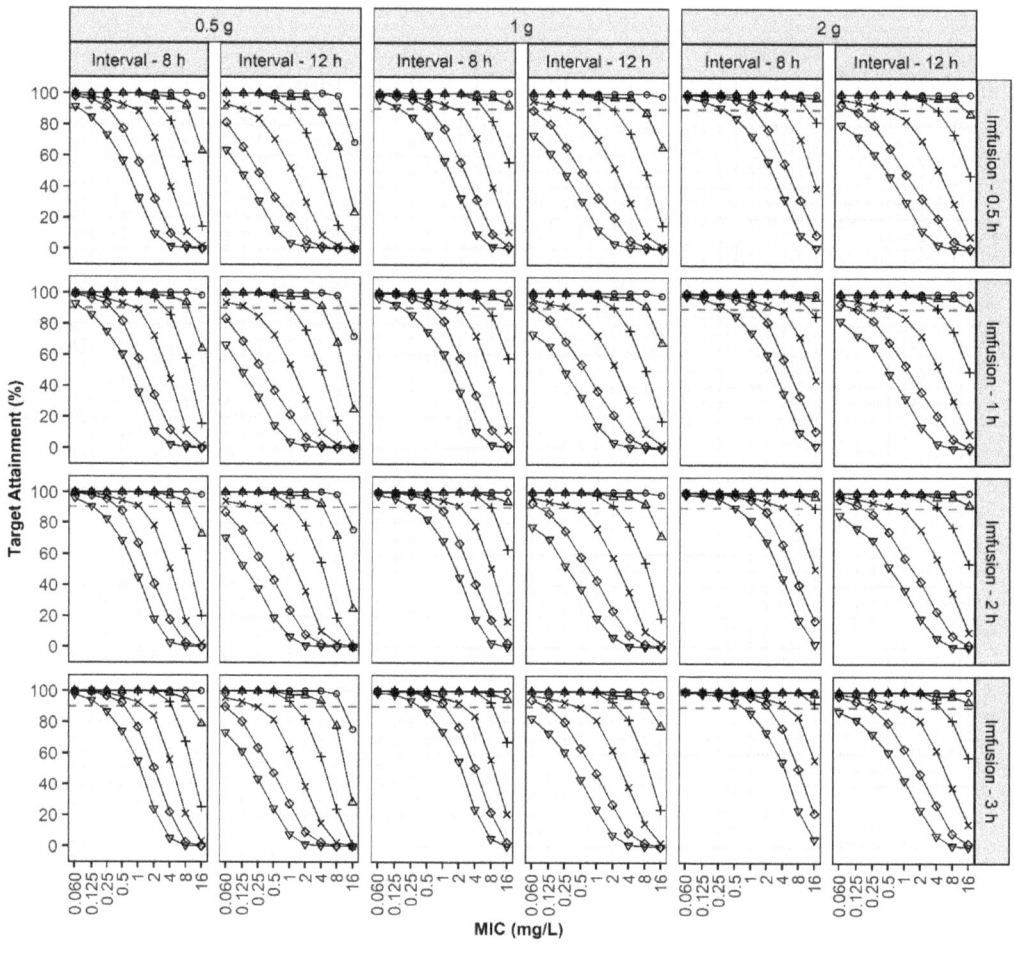

Figure 5. PTAs (100%$fT_{>MIC}$). Simulation results with three doses (0.5, 1, and 2 g), two dosing intervals (8 and 12 h), four infusion times (0.5, 1, 2, and 3 h), various degrees of renal function, and various MICs.

In the fourth simulation, optimal dosage regimens were explored to achieve PTA > 90% at 100%$fT_{>4XMIC}$ (Figure 6). In the case of patients with an eGFR of 50–90 mL/min/1.73 m², a regimen of 1 g every 8 h using i.v. infusion over 30 min could attain a 90% PTA when the MIC was ≤0.25 mg/L, and the high-dosage regimen of 2 g every 8 h using prolonged i.v. infusion over 3 h could attain a 90% PTA when the MIC was ≤1 mg/L. For patients with augmented renal clearance (eGFR values of 130–170 mL/min/1.73 m²), the high-dosage regimen of 2 g every 8 h using prolonged i.v. infusion over 3 h was optimum only when the MIC was less than 0.25 mg/L.

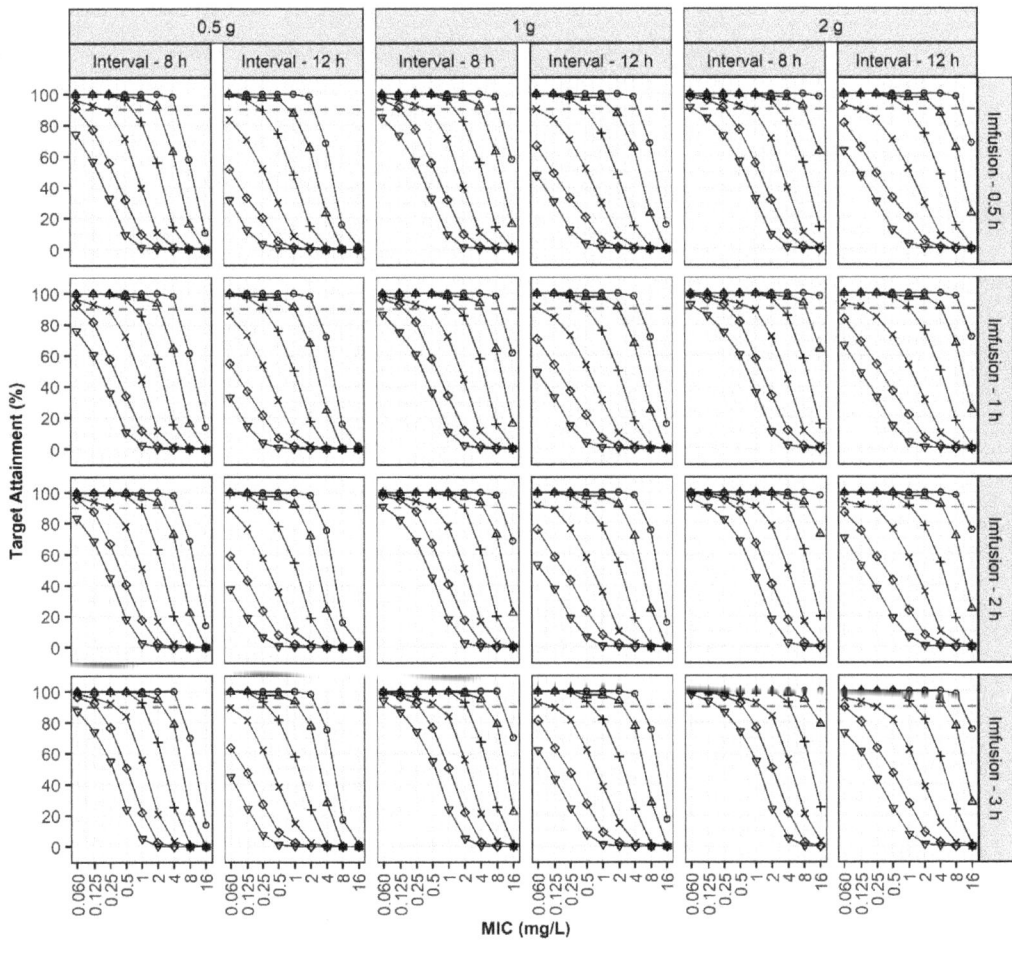

Figure 6. PTAs (100%$fT_{>4\times MIC}$). Simulation results with three doses (0.5, 1, and 2 g), two dosing intervals (8 and 12 h), four infusion times (0.5, 1, 2, and 3 h), various degrees of renal function, and various MICs.

4. Discussion

This study presents the PK properties of meropenem in critically ill Korean adult patients, including those undergoing ECMO. The PK of meropenem was best described by a two-compartment model, in which the glomerular filtration rate (GFR) was estimated using the CKD-EPI equation and identified as a significant covariate for CL. The final PK model demonstrated good predictive performance, while using ECMO did not affect meropenem PK. The results of Monte Carlo simulations to achieve more than 90% PTA at 40%$fT_{>MIC}$ suggest that the current dosage regimen of meropenem using i.v. infusion over 30 min is sufficient to treat *P. aeruginosa* at MIC $\leq$ 4 mg/L in the case of patients with a CL_{CR} of 50–90 mL/min/1.73 m². Prolonged i.v. infusion of meropenem over at least 2 h could attain a 90% PTA when the MIC is 4 mg/L for patients with augmented renal clearance (eGFR values of 130–170 mL/min/1.73 m²). However, to achieve PTA > 90% at 100%$fT_{>MIC}$ or 100%$fT_{>4\times MIC}$, prolonged infusion over 3 h or a high-dosage regimen of 2 g every 8 h should be considered, particularly for MIC > 2 mg/L or in patients with an eGFR of 130–170 mL/min/1.73 m^2.

Prescribing an antibiotic with a narrow therapeutic range is one of the most challenging concerns in the treatment of critically ill patients with time-varying and highly variable PK. The current paucity of knowledge about PK regarding ECMO use in critically ill patients makes it more difficult to adjust dosage regimens. Regardless of ECMO support, PTA for achieving 100%$fT_{>MIC}$ and 100%$fT_{>4\times MIC}$ in the present study was low when meropenem was used following the currently recommended dosage regimen to treat even susceptible *P. aeruginosa* (MIC ≤ 2 mg/L) in patients with normal renal clearance. These results are consistent with those of previous studies that performed population PK model-based simulations in critically ill patients, including those on ECMO support [10–12]. We postulate that prolonged infusion of meropenem over 3 h or a high-dosage regimen of 6 g/day should be considered, particularly for treating critically ill patients with increased renal clearance and those infected with less susceptible pathogens, to provide appropriate meropenem concentrations to them and those on ECMO support. Real-time therapeutic drug monitoring (TDM)-guided dosing optimization of meropenem using dosing software could further help clinicians to improve clinical outcomes and reduce toxicity in critically ill patients [14–16]. Evaluating the influence of TDM of meropenem on clinical outcomes in ECMO patients is warranted, since the use of inappropriate meropenem concentrations is possible, especially when using the standard-dose regimen [17].

Regarding poor clinical outcomes associated with elevated meropenem MIC [18–20], the development of guidance for appropriate meropenem dosage optimization for empirical treatment should be considered to overcome antimicrobial resistance in the ICU [21]. High-dosage regimens of meropenem using prolonged infusion over 3 h could be considered for the empirical treatment in critically ill patients [22–25], which is supported by our simulation results revealing the low PTA of empirical therapy using the current dosing regimen. Previous studies have reported the positive impact of prolonged meropenem infusion on clinical outcomes such as hospital mortality in critically ill patients [26,27]. Providing patients with ECMO support may help to better evaluate the influence of prolonged infusion or high-dosage regimen on clinical outcomes in critically ill patients.

The PK profile of meropenem in our study was well described by a two-compartment model. Model-predicted typical values of CL and steady-state volume of distribution ($V_{SS} = V_C + V_P$) for meropenem were 6.37 L/h and 17.0 L, respectively. These values were consistent with the results of previous population PK studies including patients with mild to severe renal impairment (CL, 2.0–7.7 L/h; V_{SS} 14.2–26.7 L) [28,29] or patients on ECMO (CL, 2.79–14.7 L/h; V_{SS}, 15.3–33.6 L) [10–12]. The mean (s.d.) CL and V_{SS} of individual estimates for patients without ECMO support were 5.90 (3.60) L/h and 17.8 (5.47) L, respectively, while those for patients on ECMO support were 6.55 (2.14) L/h and 17.0 (2.70) L, respectively. There were no differences between the two groups when independent *t*-tests for CL ($p = 0.5782$) and V_{SS} ($p = 0.6140$) were performed after the Shapiro–Wilk normality test, which was consistent with the results of three population PK studies involving ECMO patients that found no effect of ECMO on meropenem PK [10–12]. In these three studies, which included 10 to 14 patients on ECMO, the presence or absence of ECMO was not selected as a covariate affecting PK parameters, and ECMO factors such as VA/VV types, flow rate, or pump speed were not included as covariates in the pharmacokinetic model [10–12]. Shekar et al. compared the results of a population PK analysis of 11 ECMO patients with previously published data from 10 non-ECMO patients and found that ECMO patients demonstrated reduced meropenem CL and an increased V_{SS} when compared with controls, but these changes were not statistically significant [10]. Gijsen et al. compared 14 ECMO patients with 11 non-ECMO patients in one study and found no PK alteration by ECMO use [12]. We believe that variations in meropenem PK among critically ill patients of different races, regardless of ECMO support, are limited because the renal clearance of meropenem is largely dependent on the passive process of glomerular filtration [30–32].

We tested the effect of renal function on meropenem clearance. When renal function was estimated using Cockcroft–Gault (CG), Modification of Diet in Renal Disease (MDRD), modified MDRD, CKD-EPI, and CKD-EPI equations on the basic PK model, the OFV decreased by 24.512, 24.948, 22.202, 27.933, and 24.270, respectively. Therefore, the eGFR estimated using the CKD-EPI equation was considered the best covariate explaining the individual variation in CL. In previous population PK studies of meropenem, renal function calculated by CG equation [10,11,28,33–35], CKD-EPI formula [12], or MDRD [29,36] formula was selected as a covariate affecting CL. The difference in the reduction of OFV was not substantial in our study; there would have been no significant differences in the predictive performance of the model even if other formulas for renal function were used. In our study, only GFR estimated by the CKD-EPI equation was included as a covariate affecting CL, while a recently developed model included body weight and eGFR as covariates [12]. However, since the coefficients of body weight were fixed, only eGFR was the covariate selected by the modeling process.

The predictive performance of the final PK model was evaluated using an external validation dataset. Predictive errors of 203% and 564% were observed in two patients. The two samples were collected immediately prior to dosing but were recorded as being collected after initiating dosing; it was more likely to be an error in the documentation than an error in the conduct of the clinical trial. However, since the exact cause could not be identified, we analyzed all data and had poor predictive performance. When the two subjects were excluded, rBias and rRMSE decreased from 17.5% to 1.59% and from 91.5% to 29.4%, respectively, showing that our model has good predictive ability. The range of rBias and rRMSE of the tobramycin model that showed good performance ranged from 4.9% to 29.4% and from 47.8% to 66.9%, respectively [37].

Our study has some limitations. First, the number of patients on ECMO support ($n = 8$) was too small to accurately detect the effect of ECMO on meropenem PK parameters, although the total number of patients ($n = 26$) was sufficient to construct a population PK model. Given the physicochemical properties of meropenem, ECMO therapy may not significantly affect its PK. Second, only one covariate was included in the final PK model; hence, it is difficult to directly use this model for personalized treatments of patients. It is necessary to improve the model through follow-up studies. Third, the predictive performance of the final PK model for 26 patients was not good. The number of blood samples used for external validation was small and substantially affected by two extreme values. However, our model could accurately predict most meropenem concentrations for validation. Fourth, we did not validate our results of PK/PD analysis by evaluating clinical outcomes. Despite these limitations, our study is valuable because it is, to the best of our knowledge, the first population PK analysis of meropenem using model-based simulations in critically ill Korean patients, including those on ECMO support. We believe that the present study has important clinical implications for future research to develop the optimal dose recommendation for such important populations.

5. Conclusions

Our model shows that ECMO use does not affect meropenem PK in critically ill patients. Our simulation results suggest that the current dosing regimen of meropenem using i.v. infusion over 30 min may be related to a suboptimal concentration for empirical treatment in ICU. Therefore, prolonged i.v. infusion over 3 h or a high-dosage regimen of 2 g every 8 h should be considered, particularly at MIC > 2 mg/L or in patients with augmented renal clearance. Further studies are warranted to validate our model-based regimen, such as assessing the clinical outcomes and evaluating the influence of TDM on clinical outcomes in critically ill patients, including those on ECMO support.

Supplementary Materials: The following are available online at https://www.mdpi.com/article/10.3390/pharmaceutics13111861/s1, Figure S1: Individual fit plots. Closed circle, observed concentration; solid line, individual-predicted concentrations; dotted line, population-predicted concentrations, Figure S2: Relative prediction errors vs observations for the final population pharmacokinetic model of meropenem: (a) plots for all subjects ($n = 26$), (b) plots excluding the two patients with extreme values ($n = 24$).

Author Contributions: Conceptualization and methodology, D.-H.L., H.-S.K. and Y.-K.K.; Data curation, H.-S.K., S.P., H.-i.K., S.-H.L. and Y.-K.K.; Writing—Original draft preparation and formal analysis, D.-H.L., H.-S.K. and Y.-K.K.; Writing—Review and editing, D.-H.L., H.-S.K. and Y.-K.K. All authors have read and agreed to the published version of the manuscript.

Funding: This research was funded by the National Research Foundation of Korea (NRF), the Korea government Ministry of Science and ICT (MSIT) (grant number: NRF-2019R1F1A1062319).

Institutional Review Board Statement: The study protocol was reviewed and approved by the Institutional Review Board of the Hallym University Sacred Heart Hospital (approval cod: IRB No. 2019-05-034, approval date: 08 August 2020) and performed in agreement with the Declaration of Helsinki and Good Clinical Practice. A written informed consent form was signed by each patient or each patient's legally authorized representative before enrollment.

Informed Consent Statement: Informed consent was obtained from all subjects or subject's legally authorized representative.

Data Availability Statement: The datasets generated and/or analyzed during the current study are available from the corresponding author on reasonable request.

Conflicts of Interest: All authors declare no conflict of interest.

References

1. Roberts, J.A.; Abdul-Aziz, M.H.; Lipman, J.; Mouton, J.W.; Vinks, A.A.; Felton, T.W.; Hope, W.W.; Farkas, A.; Neely, M.N.; Schentag, J.J.; et al. International society of anti-infective pharmacology and the pharmacokinetics and pharmacodynamics study group of the European Society of Clinical Microbiology and infectious diseases. Individualised antibiotic dosing for patients who are critically ill: Challenges and potential solutions. *Lancet Infect. Dis.* **2014**, *14*, 498–509. [PubMed]
2. Blot, S.I.; Pea, F.; Lipman, J. The effect of pathophysiology on pharmacokinetics in the critically ill patient—Concepts appraised by the example of antimicrobial agents. *Adv. Drug Deliv. Rev.* **2014**, *77*, 3–11. [CrossRef] [PubMed]
3. Goncalves-Pereira, J.; Povoa, P. Antibiotics in critically ill patients: A systematic review of the pharmacokinetics of β-lactams. *Crit. Care* **2011**, *15*, R206. [CrossRef] [PubMed]
4. Mouton, J.W.; van den Anker, J.N. Meropenem clinical pharmacokinetics. *Clin. Pharmacokinet.* **1995**, *28*, 275–286. [CrossRef]
5. Baldwin, C.M.; Lyseng-Williamson, K.A.; Keam, S.J. Meropenem: A review of its use in the treatment of serious bacterial infections. *Drugs* **2008**, *68*, 803–838. [CrossRef] [PubMed]
6. De Rosa, F.G.; Corcione, S.; Pagani, N.; Stella, M.L.; Urbino, R.; Di Perri, G.; Raschke, R.A. High rate of respiratory MDR gram-negative bacteria in H1N1-ARDS treated with ECMO. *Intensive Care Med.* **2013**, *39*, 1880–1881. [CrossRef]
7. Aubron, C.; Cheng, A.C.; Pilcher, D.; Leong, T.; Magrin, G.; Cooper, D.J.; Scheinkestel, C.D.; Pellegrino, V. Infections acquired by adults who receive extracorporeal membrane oxygenation: Risk factors and outcome. *Infect. Control Hosp. Epidemiol.* **2013**, *34*, 24–30. [CrossRef]
8. Shekar, K.; Fraser, J.F.; Smith, M.T.; Roberts, J.A. Pharmacokinetic changes in patients receiving extracorporeal membrane oxygenation. *J. Crit. Care* **2012**, *27*, 741.e9–741.e18. [CrossRef]
9. Ha, M.A.; Sieg, A.C. Evaluation of altered drug pharmacokinetics in critically ill adults receiving extracorporeal membrane oxygenation. *Pharmacotherapy* **2017**, *32*, 221–235. [CrossRef] [PubMed]
10. Shekar, K.; Fraser, J.F.; Taccone, F.S.; Welch, S.; Wallis, S.C.; Mullany, D.V.; Lipman, J.; Roberts, J.A.; ASAP ECMO Study Investigators. The combined effects of extracorporeal membrane oxygenation and renal replacement therapy on meropenem pharmacokinetics: A matched cohort study. *Crit. Care* **2014**, *18*, 565. [CrossRef]
11. Hanberg, P.; Obrink-Hansen, K.; Thorsted, A.; Bue, M.; Tottrup, M.; Friberg, L.E.; Hardlei, T.F.; Søballe, K.; Gjedsted, J. Population pharmacokinetics of meropenem in plasma and subcutis from patients on extracorporeal membrane oxygenation treatment. *Antimicrob. Agents Chemother.* **2018**, *62*, e02390-17. [CrossRef] [PubMed]
12. Gijsen, M.; Dreesen, E.; Annaert, P.; Nicolai, J.; Debaveye, Y.; Wauters, J.; Spriet, I. Meropenem pharmacokinetics and target attainment in critically ill patients are not affected by extracorporeal membrane oxygenation: A matched cohort analysis. *Microorganisms* **2021**, *9*, 1310. [CrossRef]
13. Dosne, A.G.; Bergstrand, M.; Karlsson, M.O. A strategy for residual error modeling incorporating scedasticity of variance and distribution shape. *J. Pharmacokinet. Pharmacodyn.* **2016**, *43*, 137–151. [CrossRef] [PubMed]

14. Pea, F.; Della Siega, P.; Cojutti, P.; Sartor, A.; Crapis, M.; Scarparo, C.; Bassetti, M. Might real-time pharmacokinetic/pharmacodynamic optimisation of high-dose continuous-infusion meropenem improve clinical cure in infections caused by KPC-producing *Klebsiella pneumoniae*? *Int. J. Antimicrob. Agents* **2017**, *49*, 255–258. [CrossRef]
15. Heil, E.L.; Nicolau, D.P.; Farkas, A.; Roberts, J.A.; Thom, K.A. Pharmacodynamic target attainment for cefepime, meropenem, and piperacillin-tazobactam using a pharmacokinetic/pharmacodynamic-based dosing calculator in critically ill patients. *Antimicrob. Agents Chemother.* **2018**, *62*, e01008-18. [CrossRef] [PubMed]
16. Liebchen, U.; Klose, M.; Paal, M.; Vogeser, M.; Zoller, M.; Schroeder, I.; Schmitt, L.; Huisinga, W.; Michelet, R.; Zander, J.; et al. Evaluation of the MeroRisk calculator, a use-friendly tool to predict the risk of meropenem target non-attainment in critically ill patients. *Antibiotics* **2021**, *10*, 468. [CrossRef] [PubMed]
17. Kühn, D.; Metz, C.; Seiler, F.; Wehrfritz, H.; Roth, S.; Alqudrah, M.; Becker, A.; Bracht, H.; Wagenpfeil, S.; Hoffmann, M.; et al. Antibiotic therapeutic drug monitoring in intensive care patients treated with different modalities of extracorporeal membrane oxygenation (ECMO) and renal replacement therapy: A prospective, observational single-center study. *Crit. Care* **2020**, *24*, 664. [CrossRef]
18. Patel, T.S.; Nagel, J.L. Clinical outcomes of *Enterobacteriaceae* infections stratified by carbapenem MICs. *J. Clin. Microbiol.* **2015**, *53*, 201–205. [CrossRef]
19. Esterly, J.S.; Wagner, J.; McLaughlin, M.M.; Postelnick, M.J.; Qi, C.; Scheetz, M.H. Evaluation of clinical outcomes in patients with bloodstream infections due to Gram-negative bacteria according to carbapenem MIC stratification. *Antimicrob. Agents Chemother.* **2012**, *56*, 4885–4890. [CrossRef] [PubMed]
20. O'Donnell, J.N.; Rhodes, N.J.; Biehle, L.R.; Esterly, J.S.; Patel, T.S.; McLaughlin, M.M.; Hirsch, E.B. Assessment of mortality stratified by meropenem minimum inhibitory concentration in patients with Enterobacteriaceae bacteremia: A patient-level analysis of published data. *Int. J. Antimicrob. Agents* **2020**, *55*, 105849. [CrossRef]
21. De Waele, J.J.; Akova, M.; Antonelli, M.; Canton, R.; Carlet, J.; De Backer, D.; Dimopoulos, G.; Garnacho-Montero, J.; Kesecioglu, J.; Lipman, J.; et al. Antimicrobial resistance and antibiotic stewardship programs in the ICU: Insistence and persistence in the fight against resistance. A position statement from ESICM/ESCMID/WAAAR round table on multi-drug resistance. *Intensive Care Med.* **2018**, *44*, 189–196. [CrossRef] [PubMed]
22. Sjövall, F.; Alobaid, A.S.; Wallis, S.C.; Perner, A.; Lipman, J.; Roberts, J.A. Maximally effective dosing regimens of meropenem in patients with septic shock. *J. Antimicrob. Chemother.* **2018**, *73*, 191–198. [CrossRef] [PubMed]
23. Lertwattanachai, T.; Montakantikul, P.; Tangsujaritvijit, V.; Sanguanwit, P.; Sueajai, J.; Auparakkitanon, S.; Dilokpattanamongkol, P. Clinical outcomes of empirical high-dose meropenem in critically ill patients with sepsis and septic shock: A randomized controlled trial. *J. Intensive Care* **2020**, *8*, 26. [CrossRef]
24. Kothekar, A.T.; Divatia, J.V.; Myatra, S.N.; Patil, A.; Krishnamurthy, M.N.; Maheshwarappa, H.M.; Siddiqui, S.S.; Gurjar, M.; Biswas, S.; Gota, V. Clinical pharmacokinetics of 3-h extended infusion of meropenem in adult patients with severe sepsis and septic shock: Implications for empirical therapy against Gram-negative bacteria. *Ann. Intensive Care* **2020**, *10*, 4. [CrossRef] [PubMed]
25. Eisert, A.; Lanckohr, C.; Frey, J.; Frey, O.; Wicha, S.G.; Horn, D.; Ellger, B.; Schuerholzi, T.; Marx, G.; Simond, T.-P. Comparison of two empirical prolonged infusion dosing regimens for meropenem in patients with septic shock: A two-center pilot study. *Int. J. Antimicrob. Agents* **2021**, *57*, 106289. [CrossRef] [PubMed]
26. Ahmed, N.; Jen, S.P.; Altshuler, D.; Papadopoulos, J.; Pham, V.P.; Dubrovskaya, Y. Evaluation of meropenem extended versus intermittent infusion dosing protocol in critically ill patients. *J. Intensive Care Med.* **2020**, *35*, 763–771. [CrossRef]
27. Roberts, J.A.; Abdul-Aziz, M.H.; Davis, J.S.; Dulhunty, J.M.; Cotta, M.O.; Myburgh, J.; Bellomo, R.; Lipman, J. Continuous versus intermittent beta-lactam infusion in severe sepsis. A meta-analysis of individual patient data from randomized trials. *Am. J. Respir. Crit. Care Med.* **2016**, *194*, 681–691. [CrossRef] [PubMed]
28. Roberts, J.A.; Kirkpatrick, C.M.; Roberts, M.S.; Robertson, T.A.; Dalley, A.J.; Lipman, J. Meropenem dosing in critically ill patients with sepsis and without renal dysfunction: Intermittent bolus versus continuous administration? Monte Carlo dosing simulations and subcutaneous tissue distribution. *J. Antimicrob. Chemother.* **2009**, *64*, 142–150. [CrossRef]
29. Jaruratanasirikul, S.; Thengyai, S.; Wongpoowarak, W.; Wattanavijitkul, T.; Tangkitwanitjaroen, K.; Sukarnjanaset, W.; Jullangkoon, M.; Samaeng, M. Population pharmacokinetics and Monte Carlo dosing simulations of meropenem during the early phase of severe sepsis and septic shock in critically ill patients in intensive care units. *Antimicrob. Agents Chemother.* **2015**, *59*, 2995–3001. [CrossRef]
30. Kim, Y.K.; Lee, D.H.; Jeon, J.; Jang, H.J.; Kim, H.K.; Jin, K.; Lim, S.-N.; Lee, S.S.; Park, B.S.; Kim, W.; et al. Population pharmacokinetic analysis of meropenem after intravenous infusion in Korean patients with acute infections. *Clin. Ther.* **2018**, *40*, 1384–1395. [CrossRef]
31. Tsai, D.; Jamal, J.A.; Davis, J.S.; Lipman, J.; Roberts, J.A. Interethnic differences in pharmacokinetics of antibacterials. *Clin. Pharmacokinet.* **2015**, *54*, 243–260. [CrossRef]
32. Kim, K.; Johnson, J.A.; Derendorf, H. Differences in drug pharmacokinetics between East Asians and Caucasians and the role of genetic polymorphisms. *J. Clin. Pharmacol.* **2004**, *44*, 1083–1105. [CrossRef]
33. Isla, A.; Rodriguez-Gascon, A.; Troconiz, I.F.; Bueno, L.; Solinis, M.A.; Maynar, J.; Izquierdo, J.A.; Pedraz, J.L. Population pharmacokinetics of meropenem in critically ill patients undergoing continuous renal replacement therapy. *Clin. Pharmacokinet.* **2008**, *47*, 173–180. [CrossRef] [PubMed]

34. Chung, E.K.; Cheatham, S.C.; Fleming, M.R.; Healy, D.P.; Kays, M.B. Population pharmacokinetics and pharmacodynamics of meropenem in nonobese, obese, and morbidly obese patients. *J. Clin. Pharmacol.* **2017**, *57*, 356–368. [CrossRef]
35. Ehmann, L.; Zoller, M.; Minichmayr, I.K.; Scharf, C.; Huisinga, W.; Zander, J.; Kloft, C. Development of a dosing algorithm for meropenem in critically ill patients based on a population pharmacokinetic/pharmacodynamic analysis. *Int. J. Antimicrob. Agents* **2019**, *54*, 309–317. [CrossRef] [PubMed]
36. Frippiat, F.; Musuamba, F.T.; Seidel, L.; Albert, A.; Denooz, R.; Charlier, C.; Van Bambeke, F.; Wallemacq, P.; Descy, J.; Lambermont, B.; et al. Modelled target attainment after meropenem infusion in patients with severe nosocomial pneumonia: The PROMESSE study. *J. Antimicrob. Chemother.* **2015**, *70*, 207–216. [CrossRef] [PubMed]
37. Bloomfield, C.; Staatz, C.E.; Unwin, S.; Hennig, S. Assessing predictive performance of published population pharmacokinetic models of intravenous tobramycin in pediatric patients. *Antimicrob. Agents Chemother.* **2016**, *60*, 3407–3414. [CrossRef]

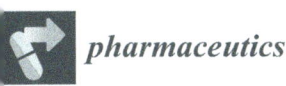

Article

In Vitro Pharmacokinetic/Pharmacodynamic Modelling and Simulation of Amphotericin B against *Candida auris*

Unai Caballero [1], Elena Eraso [2], Javier Pemán [3,4], Guillermo Quindós [2], Valvanera Vozmediano [5], Stephan Schmidt [5] and Nerea Jauregizar [1,*]

1. Department of Pharmacology, Faculty of Medicine and Nursing, University of the Basque Country (UPV/EHU), 48940 Leioa, Spain; unai.caballero@ehu.eus
2. Department of Immunology, Microbiology and Parasitology, Faculty of Medicine and Nursing, University of the Basque Country (UPV/EHU), 48940 Leioa, Spain; elena.eraso@ehu.eus (E.E.); guillermo.quindos@ehu.eus (G.Q.)
3. Microbiology Department, Hospital Universitario y Politécnico de La Fe, 46026 Valencia, Spain; javier.peman@gmail.com
4. Severe Infection Research Group, Health Research Institute Hospital La Fe, 46026 Valencia, Spain
5. Center for Pharmacometrics and Systems Pharmacology, Department of Pharmaceutics, College of Pharmacy, University of Florida, Orlando, FL 32627, USA; valva@cop.ufl.edu (V.V.); SSchmidt@cop.ufl.edu (S.S.)
* Correspondence: nerea.jauregizar@ehu.eus

Abstract: The aims of this study were to characterize the antifungal activity of amphotericin B against *Candida auris* in a static in vitro system and to evaluate different dosing schedules and MIC scenarios by means of semi-mechanistic pharmacokinetic/pharmacodynamic (PK/PD) modelling and simulation. A two-compartment model consisting of a drug-susceptible and a drug-resistant subpopulation successfully characterized the time-kill data and a modified E_{max} sigmoidal model best described the effect of the drug. The model incorporated growth rate constants for both subpopulations, a death rate constant and a transfer constant between both compartments. Additionally, the model included a parameter to account for the delay in growth in the absence or presence of the drug. Amphotericin B displayed a concentration-dependent fungicidal activity. The developed PK/PD model was able to characterize properly the antifungal activity of amphotericin B against *C. auris*. Finally, simulation analysis revealed that none of the simulated standard dosing scenarios of 0.6, 1 and 1.5 mg/kg/day over a week treatment showed successful activity against *C. auris* infection. Simulations also pointed out that an MIC of 1 mg/L would be linked to treatment failure for *C. auris* invasive infections and therefore, the resistance rate to amphotericin B may be higher than previously reported.

Keywords: *Candida auris*; PK/PD model; amphotericin B; time-kill curves

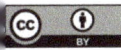

1. Introduction

Candida auris is a multidrug-resistant fungal pathogen that has emerged globally as a cause of different infections, such as severe cases of fungemia [1,2]. Candidemia due to this pathogen is associated with a high rate of mortality, especially in immunocompromised patients. Other risk factors for *C. auris* candidemia include previous exposure to antibiotics and underlying diseases such as diabetes, cardiovascular diseases or COVID-19 [3,4].

Additionally, the virulence and pathogenic capacity of *C. auris* and the decreased susceptibility to antifungal drugs is greatly worrying. Tentative epidemiological breakpoints for available antifungal drugs have recently been published. Those reports highlight that *C. auris* has high MIC values for polyenes, azoles, echinocandins and nucleoside analogues [5,6]. However, MIC related susceptibility categorization of *C. auris* isolates should be cautiously interpreted, since species-specific clinical breakpoints have not yet been defined [7]. *C. auris* is resistant to fluconazole and both intrinsic and acquired resistance has been reported [5,8]. Reduced susceptibility to the other azoles, including the newest isavuconazole, has also been described [8]. Echinocandins are the first line treatment to treat *C. auris* infections [9], but resistance to these drugs or therapeutic failures can emerge rapidly in *C. auris* [10].

Regarding amphotericin B, a wide range of MIC values has been reported, with resistance rates ranging from 0 to 30% using 1 mg/L as cut-off [7,11–15]. Recently, amphotericin B was described as the only in vitro fungicidal agent against *C. auris*, unlike echinocandins [16]. These facts, alongside with the fact that amphotericin B is the first alternative to echinocandins for *C. auris* infections [17,18], make it an interesting drug whose activity against this pathogen needs to be studied in deep.

In the current worrying scenario of reduced effective treatments to deal with *C. auris* infections, in vitro studies that use time–kill (T-K) curve experiments and pharmacokinetic/pharmacodynamic (PK/PD) models to simulate different dosing schedules and activity profiles, offer an attractive tool to describe the observed antifungal activity and to predict the efficacy of the studied drugs. There are few PK/PD models from in vitro kinetic data developed for antifungal drugs and *Candida*: caspofungin and fluconazole against *Candida albicans* [19]; voriconazole against *Candida* spp. [20]; and recently, anidulafungin against *Candida* spp. [21]. However, despite the relevance of *C. auris*, PK/PD modelling of antifungal drugs for this emergent species is still lacking.

The aim of this study was to develop a semi-mechanistic PK/PD model for amphotericin B against *C. auris* that can (a) describe the in vitro T-K experiment of clinical isolates of *C. auris* exposed to amphotericin B and (b) simulate the expected T-K curves for different dosing regimens and MIC scenarios.

2. Materials and Methods

Six *C. auris* blood isolates from the outbreak in Hospital Universitario y Politécnico La Fe (Valencia, Spain) were included in this study [22]. The MIC, defined as the minimum concentration producing ≥90% growth reduction, was determined following EUCAST guidelines [23]. The MIC of amphotericin B for the six isolates was 1 mg/L.

Amphotericin B was obtained from Sigma-Aldrich (Madrid, Spain) as a powder. Stock solutions were prepared with DMSO as solvent and stored at −80 °C until use.

Static T-K curve experiments were carried out on flat-bottomed microtitre plates in RPMI medium (Sigma-Aldrich), with a final volume of 200 μL per well at 37 °C for 48 h. *C. auris* blood isolates were grown at 37 °C for 24 h prior to the start of the experiment to obtain fungal cultures in early logarithmic phase growth. Cells were suspended in sterile distilled water to achieve a starting inoculum size of 1–5 × 10^5 colony forming units (CFU)/mL and added to the microtitre plate containing amphotericin B at concentrations 0.25, 0.5, 1, 2 and 4 times the MIC. Growth control was also measured by adding the inoculum to wells containing RPMI medium without amphotericin B. Sample for viable counts were taken at 0, 2, 4, 6, 8, 24 and 48 h, plated in triplicate onto Sabouraud dextrose agar (SDA) and incubated for 24–48 h at 37 °C. Depending on drug concentration, samples were either first diluted in PBS or plated directly. When it was expected a sterilizing activity, the whole well was sampled onto an SDA plate. Experiments were performed in duplicate for each isolate on different days. The lower limit of detection was 5 CFU/mL. However, due to the well-known sterilizing activity of amphotericin B, all the samples that showed no growth at all were considered to be 0 CFU/mL. Carryover effect was determined as previously described [24].

The basis of the semi-mechanistic model included two fungal stages in the PD part of the model, consisting of a drug-susceptible fungal subpopulation (S) and a drug-resistant subpopulation (R) [25]. This two-subpopulation model accounted for the biphasic killing behaviour observed in the individual isolate static T-K curves (individual plots not shown).

First-rate order constants that defined both populations were the natural growth rate (k_{growth}), natural death rate (k_{death}) and the transfer constant from S into R (k_{SR}). The equation that described S subpopulation in the absence of drug was as follows:

$$dS/dt = k_{growthS} \times S \times (1 - e^{-\alpha t}) - k_{death} \times S - k_{SR} \times S \qquad (1)$$

where dS/dt is the change in the number of the S subpopulation as a function of time.

It was not possible to perform a simultaneous estimation of both $k_{growthS}$ and k_{death} in this experimental setting. Hence, in an initial fit, $k_{growthS}$ was estimated by fitting a single-stage model [19] to the control data. Based on this estimation of k_{growth} (0.118 h^{-1}) and on previous analysis, k_{death} was then fixed to 0.01 h^{-1} for final parameter estimation in the two-stage model. Parameter α accounted for the delay in growth observed due to experimental settings.

A specific k_{growth} was estimated for the R subpopulation ($k_{growthR}$) to account for the regrowth observed at certain concentrations from 24 to 48 h. The k_{death} parameter was negligible in the final equation describing R subpopulation, hence it was not considered in the following equation:

$$dR/dt = k_{growthR} \times R + k_{SR} \times S \qquad (2)$$

As previously mentioned, k_{SR} is the parameter that described the transfer of fungal cells from a susceptible state into a resistant one. It was defined as follows:

$$k_{SR} = \frac{\left(k_{growth} - k_{death}\right) \times (S + R)}{N_{max}} \qquad (3)$$

where S and R are the compartments with susceptible and resistant fungal populations, respectively, and N_{max} is the maximum total density of fungal population in the stationary phase (in log CFU/mL).

The effect of amphotericin B on the fungal killing of the susceptible subpopulation was modelled using an E_{max} sigmoidal equation:

$$\text{Drug effect} = \frac{E_{max} \times C^h}{EC_{50}^h + C^h} \qquad (4)$$

where E_{max} is the maximum achievable drug-induced fungal killing-rate constant, EC_{50} is the drug concentration necessary to achieve half the maximum effect, C is the drug concentration and h is a Hill factor or sigmoidicity factor that modifies the steepness of the slope and smoothens the curve.

The final model for the S and R subpopulations were described according to Equations (2) and (5):

$$dS/dt = k_{growthS} \times S \times (1 - e^{-\alpha t}) - \text{Drug effect} \times S - k_{death} \times S - k_{SR} \times S \qquad (5)$$

$$dR/dt = k_{growthR} \times R + k_{SR} \times S$$

All T-K data were transformed into log CFU/mL and simultaneously analysed in NONMEM v7.4 with ADVAN13 subroutine and first-order conditional estimation method (FOCE). Residual variability was estimated by using an additive model. As six clinical isolates were analysed, inter-individual variability (IIV) was checked. Additionally, inter-occasion variability (IOV) was also investigated to account for the variability that might have arisen either from each experimental day or from microtitre plate batch preparation. Model performance was assessed by precision of parameter estimates, changes in objective function value (OFV) and evaluation of diagnostic plots. Final model selection was also assisted by the performance of visual predictive checks (VPCs) and non-parametric bootstrap. VPCs were performed and graphically represented with NONMEM and S-PLUS software, stratified by concentration, with the experimental plots overlaid by the median and 95% prediction interval of a simulated virtual population of 1000 individuals. Non-parametric bootstrap was conducted by resampling 1000 datasets using Perl speaks NONMEM (PsN).

In vivo PK parameters for amphotericin B deoxycholate were extracted from a tricompartmental model previously described in the literature, V_1 = 0.136 L/kg; V_2 = 0.275 L/kg; V_3 = 1.4 L/kg; Cl = 0.013 L/h/kg; Q_{12} = 0.35 L/h/kg; and Q_{13} = 0.026 L/h/kg [26]. The effect of treatments with standard clinical doses of 0.6, 1 and 1.5 mg/kg/day were simulated for a virtual population of 1000 patients, considering free drug plasma concentrations for a typical unbound fraction of 0.045 [27]. Additional simulations were performed to test scenarios where amphotericin B MICs for *C. auris* were 0.06–0.5 mg/L, according to the following equation [28]:

$$\text{MIC} = \left(\frac{d}{E_{max} - d}\right)^{1/h} \times EC_{50} \qquad (6)$$

where d is a drug-independent constant and h is the Hill factor. The EC_{50} value for each MIC scenario was then included in the PK/PD model and simulations were performed similarly. All simulations were conducted with NONMEM and S-PLUS.

3. Results

3.1. Time-Kill Experiments

Graphical representation of mean T-K curves for all isolates and replicates is shown in Figure 1. No antifungal carryover was observed. Amphotericin B showed concentration-dependent fungicidal activity. Fungicidal effect (3 log reduction compared to initial inoculum) was rapidly achieved, at 2 and 4 h, for concentrations of 4 mg/L and 2 mg/L, respectively. At concentrations of 1 mg/mL (equal to MIC), the effect was fungistatic overall, with a biphasic killing kinetic trend that showed fungal regrowth by the end of the experiment in some clinical isolates.

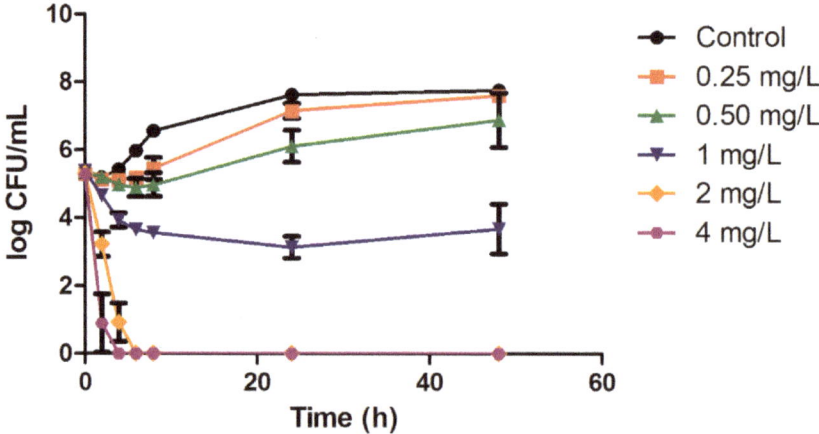

Figure 1. Mean time–kill curves for amphotericin B against *C. auris*. Each data point represents the mean result ± standard deviation (error bars) of the six isolates and replicates.

3.2. Semi-Mechanistic PK/PD Modelling

The developed model was able to describe successfully the effect of amphotericin B against the studied *C. auris* clinical isolates. This model could characterize the initial and higher killing rate at the higher amphotericin B concentrations, 2 and 4 mg/L, as well as the biphasic trend or regrowth observed in most experiments with the concentration of 1 mg/L. A schematic illustration of the final model is shown in Scheme 1.

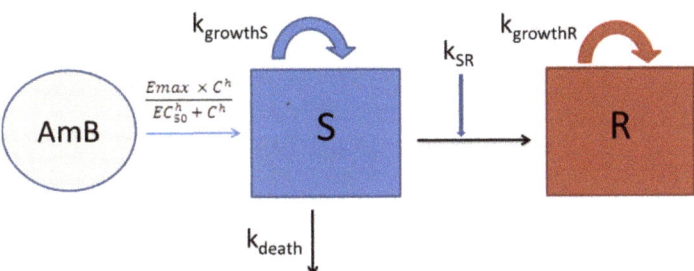

Scheme 1. Schematic illustration of the final PK/PD model. The total fungal population consists of two different subpopulations (S + R), with a first-rate order constant (k_{SR}) that describes the transfer of fungal cells from a susceptible state (S) to a resistant one (R). Amphotericin B (AMB) exerts its effect on the susceptible subpopulation. $k_{growthS}$: growth-rate of susceptible subpopulation; $k_{growthR}$: growth-rate of resistant subpopulation. k_{death}: death-rate constant of the susceptible subpopulation.

Final model parameters and the standard error of the estimates, alongside bootstrap estimations are presented in Table 1. Considering the standard errors and the bootstrap results, the parameters of the model were properly estimated. *Candida* related parameters were $k_{growthS}$ and k_{death} for S subpopulation (0.111 h^{-1} and 0.01 h^{-1}, respectively) and $k_{growthR}$ for R subpopulation (0.01 h^{-1}). k_{death} and $k_{growthR}$ were fixed whereas $k_{growthS}$ was allowed to be estimated. When the model incorporated different values of α (delay in growth) for the absence or presence of the drug, a better fit was achieved. A modified E_{max} sigmoidal model best described the effect of the drug; E_{max} was equal to 0.784 h^{-1} and EC_{50} was equal to 1.88 mg/L (1.88 times bigger than the MIC). Hill factor was fixed to enable a proper estimation of the PD parameters. Variability in the response was best captured by IOV on EC_{50} rather than IIV, where each occasion (four in total) was defined as each prepared batch of microtitre plates. Model appropriateness was supported by the VPCs depicted in Figure 2.

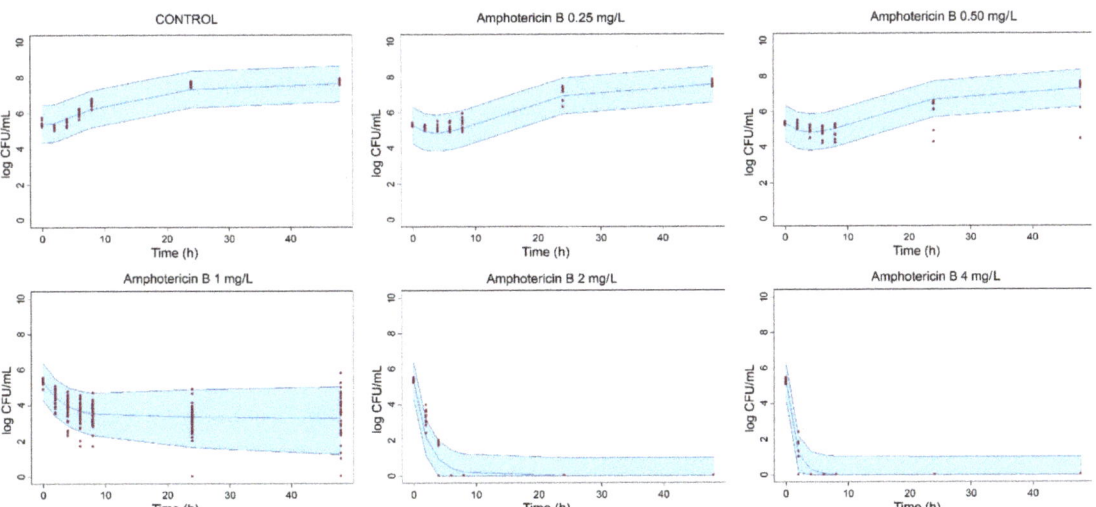

Figure 2. Visual predictive check (VPC) for the final model, with the observed fungal counts (full circles), the mean prediction (solid line) and 95% model prediction interval (shaded area) of the simulations.

Table 1. Parameter estimates (typical values and relative standard error –RSE– as CV %) and bootstrap estimates (mean and 95% CI) of the PK/PD model.

Parameter	Description	Model Estimate and RSE (CV %)	Bootstrap Estimate (Mean and 95% CI)
$k_{growthS}$ (h^{-1})	Fungal growth rate constant of the S subpopulation	0.111 (3%)	0.111 (0.101–0.116)
$k_{growthR}$ (h^{-1})	Fungal growth rate constant of the R subpopulation	0.01 (fixed)	-
k_{death} (h^{-1})	Fungal death rate constant	0.01 (fixed)	-
E_{max} (h^{-1})	Maximum kill rate constant of amphotericin B	0.784 (12%)	0.795 (0.635–1.04)
EC_{50} (mg/L)	Concentration of amphotericin B at which 50% of the E_{max} is achieved	1.88 (3%)	1.89 (1.78–2.05)
h	Hill factor that that modifies the steepness of the slope and smoothens the curve	4 (fixed)	-
α (control)	Delay in fungal growth in the absence of drug	0.748 (3%)	0.754 (0.664–0.882)
α (drug)	Delay in fungal growth in the presence of drug	0.231 (10%)	0.233 (0.193–0.274)
N_{max} (log CFU/mL)	Maximum fungal density	7.66 (1%)	7.67 (7.47–7.87)
σ (log CFU/mL)	Residual error	0.271 (14%)	0.270 (0.190–0.327)
$π_1$ (%CV)	Occasion 1	0 (fixed)	-
$π_2$ (%CV)	Occasion 2	9.5 (35%)	9.22 (2.45–15.34)
$π_3$ (%CV)	Occasion 3	18.4 (24%)	18.76 (10.07–28.12)
$π_4$ (%CV)	Occasion 4	7.5 (37%)	7.13 (2.75–13.19)

3.3. Simulation of Standard Treatments Using Human PK Data

The simulated total and unbound concentrations of amphotericin B for typical intravenous dosing regimens of 0.6, 1 and 1.5 mg/kg/day and their expected activity on *C. auris* after a one-week treatment are shown in Figure 3. None of the simulated standard dosing scenarios showed successful activity against *C. auris*.

Additional simulations with MIC scenarios of 0.06, 0.125, 0.25 and 0.5 mg/L (with EC_{50} of 0.12, 0.24, 0.47 and 0.94 mg/L, respectively) for a 1-week period are presented in Figure 4.

Simulations with the lowest dose, 0.6 mg/kg/day, showed that a fungistatic activity would be achieved at the 5th day of treatment for MIC values of amphotericin B of 0.06 mg/L. The next simulated dose, 1 mg/kg/day, resulted in fungicidal activity from the second day onwards and fungistatic with the first administration. Finally, the highest dose of 1.5 mg/kg/day led to a fungicidal endpoint immediately after the first administration. Additionally, for an MIC of 0.125 mg/L a fungistatic effect would be achieved at the 3rd day, and fungicidal at the 5th day at this highest dose level.

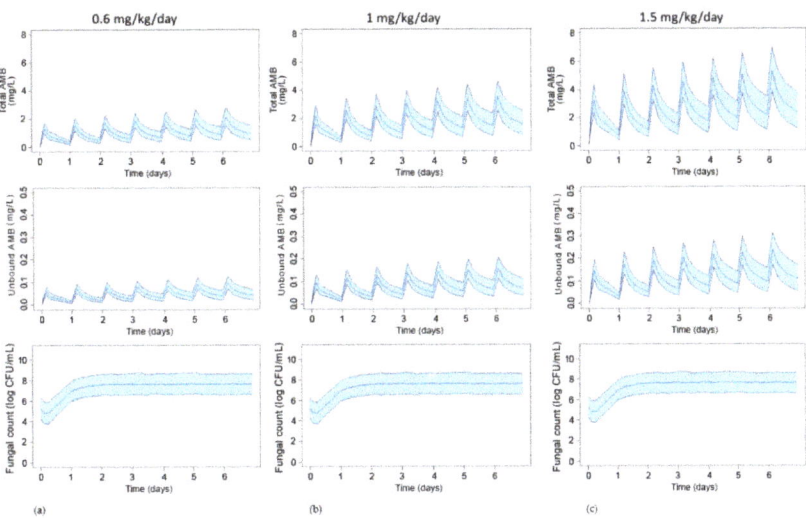

Figure 3. Predicted total (top row) and unbound (mid row) plasma concentrations of amphotericin B (D-AMB) and the effect on fungal burden (bottom row) for the treatment of 0.6 mg/kg/day (**a**), 1 mg/kg/day (**b**) and 1.5 mg/kg/day (**c**) of amphotericin B. The mean (solid line) and 95% prediction interval (coloured space) are represented.

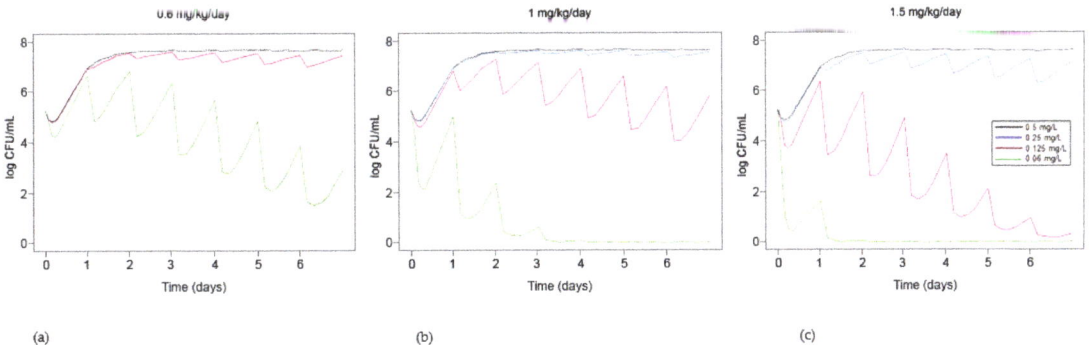

Figure 4. Simulations of the effect of amphotericin B on fungal burden by MIC and by dosing regimens of 0.6 mg/kg/day (**a**), 1 mg/kg/day (**b**) and 1.5 mg/kg/day (**c**). Black line: MIC of 0.5 mg/L; blue line: MIC of 0.25 mg/L; purple line: MIC of 0.125 mg/L; green line: MIC of 0.06 mg/L.

4. Discussion

C. auris is an emergent fungal pathogen with reduced susceptibility to first-line antifungal agents. Amphotericin B is an antifungal drug with proven efficacy against invasive candidiasis and a low resistance-rate despite more than six decades of use; a correct and thorough knowledge about the activity of this drug against *C. auris* is necessary. To date, most susceptibility studies on this pathogen have focused on the determination of the MIC. The MIC is the standard PD parameter used as a marker of fungal susceptibility and antimicrobial efficacy, yet it possesses some limitations. The antimicrobial activity of drugs is a dynamic process, while MIC is a threshold value. Concentrations below or above the MIC are ignored and thus, a more precise and quantitative information about the concentration-effect profile of the drug is often missing [29]. It is also noteworthy that even for the same microbial species, same MIC values among different isolates can result in different killing kinetics [24]. Thus, studies that characterize the antimicrobial activity beyond the measurement of MIC are needed. In vitro time–kill curves allow obtaining more information about the effect of different drug concentrations on microbial population over a time period. In combination with PK/PD M&S, these time–kill curve experiments provide an interesting tool to predict and simulate untested scenarios that may help in decision-making and design of further studies.

As determined for other species of *Candida* [30,31], in the present study amphotericin B showed concentration-dependent activity against *C. auris* in T-K experiments. Fungicidal activity was achieved at concentrations $\geq$2 mg/L and in less than 2 h. These results are in agreement with the only published work based on T-K curve methodology against *C. auris*, in which MIC values of amphotericin B were also 1 mg/L [16]. Additionally, this killing kinetic pattern has also been described for other species of *Candida* that have been regarded as resistant to amphotericin B treatment [31,32].

Few PK/PD models are available for antifungal agents [19–21]. To our knowledge, the present study is the first work that used a semi-mechanistic approach to model the antifungal activity of amphotericin B against *C. auris*. The static T-K experiments performed showed fungal regrowth or a biphasic trend, and therefore, a semi-mechanistic model that included two fungal subpopulations with different susceptibility to the drug best captured this behaviour. This approach has been extensively applied to successfully model antibiotic activity [25,33]. In the model of the present study, the emergence of resistance is triggered by a high microbial count, with the susceptible population switching to a resistant one, a process described by a first-order rate constant that also accounted for the self-limiting growth rate, as it has been previously proposed by other authors [25,34]. The model best fitted the data when a different growth rate constant for the resistant subpopulation was defined ($k_{growthR}$); this parameter was estimated to be 10 times lower than the growth rate constant for the susceptible subpopulation ($k_{growthS}$), which is in agreement with the 'fitness cost' observed in some species of *Candida* when they develop resistance mechanisms [35]. Moreover, phenotypic switching during treatment with amphotericin B has been described for *Candida lusitaniae* [36], a closely related species of *C. auris*. Nevertheless, the main goal of model building was to accurately describe the antimicrobial activity and perform simulations rather than to provide insight into resistance mechanisms, for which specific microbiological and molecular procedures would be needed. On the other hand, the lack of similar PK/PD models reports for *C. auris* or amphotericin B in the literature has precluded comparisons.

A three-compartment model for amphotericin B deoxycholate [26] was implemented for the simulation of plasma concentrations of the drug in human patients for dosing regimens of 0.6, 1 and 1.5 mg/kg/day. The latter is more commonly used for invasive aspergillosis rather than for candidemia [37], but we considered this dosing schedule for simulation purposes too due to the low susceptibility profile of *C. auris* and the concentration-dependent PD of amphotericin B shown in the present study, in concordance with other in vitro and in vivo results [16,38]. Higher doses were not considered due to the toxicity of the drug. Amphotericin B, as many antifungal agents, is highly bounded to plasma proteins, around 95% at clinically achievable concentrations [27], and this feature was taken into account in the PK/PD simulations.

With regard to the different pharmaceutical formulations available, liposomal amphotericin B (L-AMB) is the current first choice due to its improved safety profile and comparable efficacy to conventional amphotericin B deoxycholate. However, the cost can be too high for healthcare systems in developing countries, which makes the conventional formulation still relevant and listed as essential drug [39]. On the other hand, it is still not clear which fraction of the total plasma concentration of L-AMB is active, as protein binding is not applicable for this formulation [40], which makes the bridging between in vitro experiments and in vivo simulations harder to perform. Therefore, the simulations were carried out for the deoxycholate formulation. Nevertheless, studies in animal models of invasive candidiasis and clinical trials have shown similar efficacy for both formulations [40]. This may reflect a comparable exposition of the fungal population to free drug and therefore conclusions driven by PK/PD simulations may be applicable for L-AMB too. In fact, EUCAST susceptibility breakpoints are based on adult standard dosages of both formulations [41].

As previously mentioned, an approach solely based on the MIC of antimicrobials provides limited information. Conversely, PD parameters derived from the analysis of T-K curves, such as E_{max} and EC_{50}, give more detailed information on the activity of the drug. However, obtaining these data in the clinical setting is time-consuming, laborious and usually not feasible. This drawback can be overcome by employing mathematical relationship between the MIC and EC_{50}, as it has been demonstrated in the present study, since it is possible to link the results of the PK/PD modelling and simulation of T-K curves with the MIC of the drug [28].

Simulations of standard dosages of amphotericin B deoxycholate pointed out that the treatment would not be effective against the clinical isolates tested in this study. Additionally, other possible treatment outcomes were tested by simulating different susceptibility scenarios, with MICs below 1 mg/L. Standard treatments of 0.6 and 1 mg/kg/day would only be effective against *C. auris* isolates for an MIC of 0.06 mg/L. However, a higher dosage of 1.5 mg/kg/day would also be effective for an MIC up to 0.125 mg/L. Therefore, contrary to expectations [7], susceptibility breakpoint of amphotericin B for *C. auris* might be lower than 1 mg/L. Similar threshold values for amphotericin B have been reported for other species of *Candida* and filamentous fungi, such as *Aspergillus*. In a murine model of invasive candidiasis caused by *Candida krusei*, a daily dose of 1 mg/kg of amphotericin B was effective in reducing the kidney fungal burden when the MIC of the drug was of 0.125 mg/L, but ineffective when MIC was of 0.5 mg/L [42]. In another murine model study, doses of 1.5 mg/kg/day of amphotericin B resulted in a 15-day survival percentage of >50% for *Candida glabrata* and <25% for *Candida tropicalis*, the MIC being 1 mg/L for both species [43]. In an in vitro dynamic system that mimicked human PK of unbound amphotericin B against *Aspergillus*, those species considered resistant to amphotericin B had a probability of target attainment (PTA) of 0% when the MIC was 1 mg/L; for a PTA of 80% an MIC of 0.25 mg/L was needed [44]. On the other hand, a work that analysed the effect of antifungal drugs against *C. auris* infection in a murine model of invasive candidiasis concluded that the MIC cut-off for amphotericin B was 1.5 mg/L [38]. However, variability between strains was high and the 50% effective dose (ED_{50}) was as high as 5 mg/kg/day, a dose that can be lethal [45].

The results obtained in this study should be cautiously interpreted, as in vitro-in vivo correlation studies for amphotericin B against *C. auris* are lacking. Even though T-K curve methodology is a more complex technique that provides further information than MIC determination, it is still an in vitro approximation to the much more complex in vivo reality. Factors such as host immunity status and drug tissue distribution are overlooked, whereas fungal burden may be overestimated, as growth rate is much faster in the rich environment of the microbiological broth culture than in the human infection sites [46]. Nevertheless, the developed model and simulation results may help in the design of future preclinical and clinical studies, providing a useful tool for dosing regimen selection. It would also be of interest to further confirm in a murine candidiasis model if the MIC of 1 mg/L is linked to treatment failure.

5. Conclusions

In conclusion, the developed PK/PD model was able to properly characterize the antifungal activity of amphotericin B against *C. auris*. The simulations highlighted that an MIC of 1 mg/L would be linked to treatment failure and in consequence, the amphotericin B resistance rate in this fungal species may be higher than previously reported [1]. These results may be extrapolated to *C. auris* clinical isolates with similar EC_{50}/MIC ratio. Nevertheless, further studies are needed to fully characterize the susceptibility profile of *C. auris* and optimize antifungal therapy.

Author Contributions: Conceptualization, U.C., N.J., E.E. and G.Q.; methodology, U.C., E.E., J.P., V.V., S.S. and N.J.; software, U.C., V.V., S.S. and N.J.; validation, U.C. and V.V.; formal analysis, U.C. and N.J.; investigation, U.C., S.S., G.Q. and N.J.; resources, N.J., G.Q. and E.E.; data curation, U.C.; writing—original draft preparation, U.C., V.V. and N.J.; writing—review and editing, U.C., E.E., G.Q., V.V., S.S. and N.J.; visualization, U.C., E.E., G.Q., J.P., V.V., S.S. and N.J.; supervision, N.J. and G.Q.; project administration, N.J., E.E., J.P. and G.Q.; and funding acquisition, J.P., G.Q., E.E. and N.J. All authors have read and agreed to the published version of the manuscript.

Funding: This research was funded by Consejería de Educación, Universidades e Investigación of Gobierno Vasco-Eusko Jaurlaritza, GIC15/78 IT-990-16 and by FIS, Spain, PI17/01538. U.C. was funded by a Ph.D. grant from the University of the Basque Country, PIF 17/266.

Institutional Review Board Statement: Not applicable.

Informed Consent Statement: Not applicable.

Conflicts of Interest: The authors declare no conflict of interest.

References

1. Chowdhary, A.; Sharma, C.; Meis, J.F. *Candida auris*: A rapidly emerging cause of hospital-acquired multidrug-resistant fungal infections globally. *PLoS Pathog.* **2017**, *13*, e1006290. [CrossRef] [PubMed]
2. Quindós, G.; Marcos-Arias, C.; San-Millán, R.; Mateo, E.; Eraso, E. The continuous changes in the aetiology and epidemiology of invasive candidiasis: From familiar Candida albicans to multiresistant *Candida auris. Int. Microbiol.* **2018**, *21*, 107–119. [CrossRef]
3. Sekyere, J.O. *Candida auris*: A systematic review and meta-analysis of current updates on an emerging multidrug-resistant pathogen. *Microbiology* **2018**, *7*, e00578. [CrossRef] [PubMed]
4. Pemán, J.; Ruiz-Gaitán, A.; García-Vidal, C.; Salavert, M.; Ramírez, P.; Puchades, F.; García-Hita, M.; Alastruey-Izquierdo, A.; Quindós, G. Fungal co-infection in COVID-19 patients: Should we be concerned? *Rev. Iberoam. Micol.* **2020**, *37*, 41–46. [CrossRef]
5. Arendrup, M.C.; Prakash, A.; Meletiadis, J.; Sharma, C.; Chowdhary, A. Comparison of EUCAST and CLSI reference microdilution MICs of eight antifungal compounds for *Candida auris* and associated tentative epidemiological cutoff values. *Antimicrob. Agents Chemother.* **2017**, *61*, e00485-17. [CrossRef]
6. Chaabane, F.; Graf, A.; Jequier, L.; Coste, A.T. Review on Antifungal Resistance Mechanisms in the Emerging Pathogen *Candida auris. Front. Microbiol.* **2019**, *10*, 2788. [CrossRef]
7. Lockhart, S.R. *Candida auris* and multidrug resistance: Defining the new normal. *Fungal Genet. Biol.* **2019**, *131*, 103243. [CrossRef]
8. Chowdhary, A.; Prakash, A.; Sharma, C.; Kordalewska, M.; Kumar, A.; Sarma, S.; Tarai, B.; Singh, A.; Upadhyaya, G.; Upadhyay, S.; et al. A multicentre study of antifungal susceptibility patterns among 350 *Candida auris* isolates (2009–2017) in India: Role of the ERG11 and FKS1 genes in azole and echinocandin resistance. *J. Antimicrob. Chemother.* **2018**, *73*, 891–899. [CrossRef]
9. Kenters, N.; Kiernan, M.; Chowdhary, A.; Denning, D.W.; Pemán, J.; Saris, K.; Schelenz, S.; Tartari, E.; Widmer, A.; Meis, J.F.; et al. Control of *Candida auris* in healthcare institutions: Outcome of an International Society for Antimicrobial Chemotherapy expert meeting. *Int. J. Antimicrob. Agents* **2019**, *54*, 400–406. [CrossRef]
10. Biagi, M.J.; Wiederhold, N.P.; Gibas, C.; Wickes, B.; Lozano, V.; Bleasdale, S.C.; Danziger, L. Development of High-Level Echinocandin Resistance in a Patient with Recurrent *Candida auris* Candidemia Secondary to Chronic Candiduria. *Open Forum Infect. Dis.* **2019**, *6*, ofz262. [CrossRef] [PubMed]
11. Shin, J.H.; Kim, M.-N.; Jang, S.J.; Ju, M.Y.; Kim, S.H.; Shin, M.G.; Suh, S.P.; Ryang, D.W. Detection of Amphotericin B Resistance in Candida haemulonii and Closely Related Species by Use of the Etest, Vitek-2 Yeast Susceptibility System, and CLSI and EUCAST Broth Microdilution Methods. *J. Clin. Microbiol.* **2012**, *50*, 1852–1855. [CrossRef]
12. Morales, S.; Giraldo, C.M.P.; Garzón, A.C.; Martínez, H.P.; Rodríguez, G.J.; Moreno, C.A.A.; Rodriguez, J.Y. Invasive Infections with Multidrug-Resistant Yeast *Candida auris*, Colombia. *Emerg. Infect. Dis.* **2017**, *23*, 162–164. [CrossRef] [PubMed]
13. Chowdhary, A.; Sharma, C.; Duggal, S.; Agarwal, K.; Prakash, A.; Singh, P.K.; Jain, S.; Kathuria, S.; Randhawa, H.S.; Hagen, F.; et al. New Clonal Strain of *Candida auris*, Delhi, India. *Emerg. Infect. Dis.* **2013**, *19*, 1670–1673. [CrossRef]
14. Calvo, B.; Melo, A.S.A.; Perozo-Mena, A.; Hernandez, M.; Francisco, E.C.; Hagen, F.; Meis, J.F.; Colombo, A.L. First report of *Candida auris* in America: Clinical and microbiological aspects of 18 episodes of candidemia. *J. Infect.* **2016**, *73*, 369–374. [CrossRef]
15. Schelenz, S.; Hagen, F.; Rhodes, J.L.; Abdolrasouli, A.; Chowdhary, A.; Hall, A.; Ryan, L.; Shackleton, J.; Trimlett, R.; Meis, J.F.; et al. First hospital outbreak of the globally emerging *Candida auris* in a European hospital. *Antimicrob. Resist. Infect. Control.* **2016**, *5*, 1–7. [CrossRef]
16. Dudiuk, C.; Berrio, I.; Leonardelli, F.; Morales-Lopez, S.; Theill, L.; Macedo, D.; Rodriguez, J.Y.; Salcedo, S.; Marin, A.; Gamarra, S.; et al. Antifungal activity and killing kinetics of anidulafungin, caspofungin and amphotericin B against *Candida auris*. *J. Antimicrob. Chemother.* **2019**, *74*, 2295–2302. [CrossRef] [PubMed]
17. Spivak, E.S.; Hanson, K.E. *Candida auris*: An Emerging Fungal Pathogen. *J. Clin. Microbiol.* **2018**, *56*, e01588-17. [CrossRef] [PubMed]

18. Alastruey-Izquierdo, A.; Asensio, A.; Besoli, A.; Calabuig, E.; Fernández-Ruiz, M.; Garcia-Vidal, C.; Gasch, O.; Guinea, J.; Martín-Gomez, M.T.; Paño, J.R. GEMICOMED/GEIRAS-SEIMC recommendations for the management of *Candida auris* infection and colonization. *Rev. Iberoam. Micol.* **2019**, *36*, 109–114. [CrossRef]
19. Venisse, N.; Grégoire, N.; Marliat, M.; Couet, W. Mechanism-Based Pharmacokinetic-Pharmacodynamic Models of In Vitro Fungistatic and Fungicidal Effects against Candida albicans. *Antimicrob. Agents Chemother.* **2008**, *52*, 937–943. [CrossRef] [PubMed]
20. Li, Y.; Nguyen, M.H.; Cheng, S.; Schmidt, S.; Zhong, L.; Derendorf, H.; Clancy, C.J. A pharmacokinetic/pharmacodynamic mathematical model accurately describes the activity of voriconazole against *Candida* spp. in vitro. *Int. J. Antimicrob. Agents* **2008**, *31*, 369–374. [CrossRef]
21. Gil-Alonso, S.; Jauregizar, N.; Ortega, I.; Eraso, E.; Suarez, E.; Quindós, G. In vitro pharmacodynamic modelling of anidulafungin against *Candida* spp. *Int. J. Antimicrob. Agents* **2016**, *47*, 178–183. [CrossRef]
22. Ruiz-Gaitán, A.; Moret, A.M.; Tasias-Pitarch, M.; Aleixandre-López, A.I.; Morel, H.M.; Calabuig, E.; Salavert-Lletí, M.; Ramírez, P.; López-Hontangas, J.L.; Hagen, F.; et al. An outbreak due to *Candida auris* with prolonged colonisation and candidaemia in a tertiary care European hospital. *Mycoses* **2018**, *61*, 498–505. [CrossRef]
23. EUCAST. The European Committee for Antimicrobial Susceptibility Testing. Method for the Determination of Broth Dilution Minimum Inhibitory Concentrations of Antifungal Agents for Yeasts. EUCAST Definitive Document E.def 7.3.2. 2020. Available online: https://www.eucast.org/fileadmin/src/media/PDFs/EUCAST_files/AFST/Files/EUCAST_E_Def_7.3.2_Yeast_testing_definitive_revised_2020.pdf (accessed on 8 March 2021).
24. Gil-Alonso, S.; Jauregizar, N.; Canton, E.; Eraso, E.; Quindos, G. In vitro fungicidal activities of anidulafungin, caspofungin, and micafungin against *Candida glabrata*, *Candida bracarensis*, and *Candida nivariensis* evaluated by time-kill studies. *Antimicrob. Agents Chemother.* **2015**, *59*, 3615–3618. [CrossRef]
25. Nielsen, E.I.; Friberg, L.E. Pharmacokinetic-Pharmacodynamic Modeling of Antibacterial Drugs. *Pharmacol. Rev.* **2013**, *65*, 1053–1090. [CrossRef]
26. Bekersky, I.; Fielding, R.; Dressler, D.E.; Lee, J.W.; Buell, D.N.; Walsh, T.J. Pharmacokinetics, Excretion, and Mass Balance of Liposomal Amphotericin B (AmBisome) and Amphotericin B Deoxycholate in Humans. *Antimicrob. Agents Chemother.* **2002**, *46*, 828–833. [CrossRef] [PubMed]
27. Bekersky, I.; Fielding, R.; Dressler, D.E.; Lee, J.W.; Buell, D.N.; Walsh, T.J. Plasma Protein Binding of Amphotericin B and Pharmacokinetics of Bound versus Unbound Amphotericin B after Administration of Intravenous Liposomal Amphotericin B (AmBisome) and Amphotericin B Deoxycholate. *Antimicrob. Agents Chemother.* **2002**, *46*, 834–840. [CrossRef]
28. Schmidt, S.; Schuck, E.; Kumar, V.; Burkhardt, O.; Derendorf, H. Integration of pharmacokinetic/pharmacodynamic modeling and simulation in the development of new anti-infective agents—Minimum inhibitory concentration versus time-kill curves. *Expert Opin. Drug Discov.* **2007**, *2*, 849–860. [CrossRef]
29. Mueller, M.; de la Peña, A.; Derendorf, H. Issues in Pharmacokinetics and Pharmacodynamics of Anti-Infective Agents: Kill Curves versus MIC. *Antimicrob. Agents Chemother.* **2004**, *48*, 369–377. [CrossRef] [PubMed]
30. Klepser, M.E.; Wolfe, E.J.; Jones, R.N.; Nightingale, C.H.; Pfaller, M.A. Antifungal pharmacodynamic characteristics of fluconazole and amphotericin B tested against Candida albicans. *Antimicrob. Agents Chemother.* **1997**, *41*, 1392–1395. [CrossRef] [PubMed]
31. Cantón, E.; Pemán, J.; Gobernado, M.; Viudes, A.; Espinel-Ingroff, A. Patterns of Amphotericin B Killing Kinetics against Seven Candida Species. *Antimicrob. Agents Chemother.* **2004**, *48*, 2477–2482. [CrossRef] [PubMed]
32. Canton, E.; Peman, J.; Sastre, M.; Romero, M.; Espinel-Ingroff, A. Killing kinetics of caspofungin, micafungin, and ampho-tericin B against Candida guilliermondii. *Antimicrob. Agents Chemother.* **2006**, *50*, 2829–2832. [CrossRef]
33. Brill, M.; Kristoffersson, A.; Zhao, C.; Nielsen, E.; Friberg, L. Semi-mechanistic pharmacokinetic–pharmacodynamic modelling of antibiotic drug combinations. *Clin. Microbiol. Infect.* **2018**, *24*, 697–706. [CrossRef]
34. Nielsen, E.I.; Viberg, A.; Lowdin, E.; Cars, O.; Karlsson, M.O.; Sandstrom, M. Semimechanistic pharmacokinet-ic/pharmacodynamic model for assessment of activity of antibacterial agents from time-kill curve experiments. *Antimicrob. Agents Chemother.* **2007**, *51*, 128–136. [CrossRef]
35. Sasse, C.; Dunkel, N.; Schäfer, T.; Schneider, S.; Dierolf, F.; Ohlsen, K.; Morschhäuser, J. The stepwise acquisition of fluconazole resistance mutations causes a gradual loss of fitness inCandida albicans. *Mol. Microbiol.* **2012**, *86*, 539–556. [CrossRef]
36. Asner, S.; Giulieri, S.; Diezi, M.; Marchetti, O.; Sanglard, D. Acquired Multidrug Antifungal Resistance in Candida lusitaniae During Therapy. *Open Forum Infect. Dis.* **2015**, *59*, 7715–7722. [CrossRef]
37. European Committee on Antimicrobial Susceptibility Testing. Amphotericin B: Rationale for the Clinical Breakpoints, Version 2.0. 2020. Available online: http://www.eucast.org (accessed on 25 February 2021).
38. Lepak, A.J.; Zhao, M.; Berkow, E.L.; Lockhart, S.R.; Andes, D.R. Pharmacodynamic Optimization for Treatment of Invasive *Candida auris* Infection. *Antimicrob. Agents Chemother.* **2017**, *61*, 00791-17. [CrossRef]
39. World Health Organization Model List of Essential Medicines, 21st List, 2019. World Health Organization: Geneva, Switzerland, 2019. Available online: https://www.who.int/medicines/publications/essentialmedicines/en/ (accessed on 8 March 2021).
40. Groll, A.H.; Rijnders, B.; Walsh, T.J.; Adler-Moore, J.; Lewis, R.E.; Brüggemann, R.J.M. Clinical Pharmacokinetics, Pharmacodynamics, Safety and Efficacy of Liposomal Amphotericin B. *Clin. Infect. Dis.* **2019**, *68*, S260–S274. [CrossRef]

41. Arendrup, M.; Friberg, N.; Mares, M.; Kahlmeter, G.; Meletiadis, J.; Guinea, J.; Andersen, C.; Arikan-Akdagli, S.; Barchiesi, F.; Chryssanthou, E.; et al. How to interpret MICs of antifungal compounds according to the revised clinical breakpoints v. 10.0 European committee on antimicrobial susceptibility testing (EUCAST). *Clin. Microbiol. Infect.* **2020**, *26*, 1464–1472. [CrossRef]
42. Kardos, T.; Kovács, R.; Kardos, G.; Varga, I.; Bozó, A.; Tóth, Z.; Nagy, F.; Majoros, L. Poor in vivo efficacy of caspofungin, micafungin and amphotericin B against wild-type Candida krusei clinical isolates does not correlate with in vitro susceptibility results. *J. Chemother.* **2018**, *30*, 233–239. [CrossRef]
43. Mariné, M.; Espada, R.; Torrado, J.; Pastor, F.J.; Guarro, J. Efficacy of a new formulation of amphotericin B in murine disseminated infections by Candida glabrata or Candida tropicalis. *Int. J. Antimicrob. Agents* **2009**, *34*, 566–569. [CrossRef]
44. Elefanti, A.; Mouton, J.W.; Verweij, P.E.; Zerva, L.; Meletiadis, J. Susceptibility Breakpoints for Amphotericin B and Aspergillus Species in anIn VitroPharmacokinetic-Pharmacodynamic Model Simulating Free-Drug Concentrations in Human Serum. *Antimicrob. Agents Chemother.* **2014**, *58*, 2356–2362. [CrossRef]
45. Mohr, J.F.; Hall, A.C.; Ericsson, C.D.; Ostrosky-Zeichner, L. Fatal Amphotericin B Overdose Due to Administration of Nonlipid Formulation Instead of Lipid Formulation. *Pharmacother. J. Hum. Pharmacol. Drug Ther.* **2005**, *25*, 426–428. [CrossRef]
46. De la Peña, A.; Gräbe, A.; Rand, K.H.; Rehak, E.; Gross, J.; Thyroff-Friesinger, U.; Müller, M.; Derendorf, H. PK–PD modelling of the effect of cefaclor on four different bacterial strains. *Int. J. Antimicrob. Agents* **2004**, *23*, 218–225. [CrossRef]

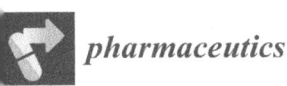

Article

Pharmacokinetic/Pharmacodynamic Model of Neutropenia in Real-Life Palbociclib-Treated Patients

Alexandre Le Marouille [1], Emma Petit [1], Courèche Kaderbhaï [2], Isabelle Desmoulins [2], Audrey Hennequin [2], Didier Mayeur [2], Jean-David Fumet [1,2], Sylvain Ladoire [1,2], Zoé Tharin [2], Siavoshe Ayati [2], Silvia Ilie [2], Bernard Royer [3,4] and Antonin Schmitt [1,5,*]

1. INSERM U1231, School of Medicine and Pharmacy, University of Burgundy Franche-Comté, 21000 Dijon, France; alemarouille@cgfl.fr (A.L.M.); emma.petit@edu.univ-fcomte.fr (E.P.); jdfumet@cgfl.fr (J.-D.F.); sladoire@cgfl.fr (S.L.)
2. Centre Georges-François Leclerc, Oncology Department, 21000 Dijon, France; cgkaderbhai@cgfl.fr (C.K.); idesmoulins@cgfl.fr (I.D.); ahennequin@cgfl.fr (A.H.); dmayeur@cgfl.fr (D.M.); ztharin@cgfl.fr (Z.T.); sayati@cgfl.fr (S.A.); silie@cgfl.fr (S.I.)
3. Laboratoire de Pharmacologie Clinique et Toxicologie, CHU Besançon, 25000 Besançon, France; broyer@chu-besancon.fr
4. INSERM, EFS BFC, UMR1098, RIGHT, Interactions Greffon-Hôte-Tumeur/Ingénierie Cellulaire et Génique, School of Medicine and Pharmacy, University of Bourgogne Franche-Comté, 25000 Besançon, France
5. Centre Georges-François Leclerc, Pharmacy Department, 21000 Dijon, France
* Correspondence: aschmitt@cgfl.fr

Abstract: Palbociclib is an oral CDK4/6 inhibitor indicated in HR+/HER2- advanced or metastatic breast cancer in combination with hormonotherapy. Its main toxicity is neutropenia. The aim of our study was to describe the kinetics of circulating neutrophils from real-life palbociclib-treated patients. A population pharmacokinetic (popPK) model was first constructed to describe palbociclib pharmacokinetic (PK). Individual PK parameters obtained were then used in the pharmacokinetic/pharmacodynamic (PK/PD) model to depict the relation between palbociclib concentrations and absolute neutrophil counts (ANC). The models were built with a population of 143 patients. Palbociclib samples were routinely collected during therapeutic drug monitoring, whereas ANC were retrospectively retrieved from the patient files. The optimal popPK model was a mono-compartmental model with a first-order absorption constant of 0.187 h^{-1} and an apparent clearance Cl/F of 57.09 L (32.8% of inter individuality variability (IIV)). The apparent volume of distribution (1580 L) and the lag-time (T_{lag}: 0.658 h) were fixed to values from the literature. An increase in creatinine clearance and a decrease in alkaline phosphatase led to an increase in palbociclib Cl/F. To describe ANC kinetics during treatment, Friberg's PK/PD model, with linear drug effect, was used. Parameters estimated were Base (2.92 G/L; 29.6% IIV), Slope (0.0011 L/μg; 28.8% IIV), Mean Transit Time (MTT; 5.29 days; 17.9% IIV) and γ (0.102). The only significant covariate was age on the initial ANC (Base), with lower ANC in younger patients. PK/PD model-based simulations show that the higher the estimated $C_{ress}SS$ (trough concentration at steady state), the higher the risk of developing neutropenia. In order to present a risk lower than 20% to developing a grade 4 neutropenia, the patient should show an estimated $C_{ress}SS$ lower than 100 μg/L.

Keywords: palbociclib; neutropenia; pharmacokinetic/pharmacodynamic

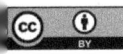

Citation: Marouille, A.L.; Petit, E.; Kaderbhaï, C.; Desmoulins, I.; Hennequin, A.; Mayeur, D.; Fumet, J.-D.; Ladoire, S.; Tharin, Z.; Ayati, S.; et al. Pharmacokinetic/ Pharmacodynamic Model of Neutropenia in Real-Life Palbociclib-Treated Patients. *Pharmaceutics* **2021**, *13*, 1708. https:// doi.org/10.3390/pharmaceutics13101708

Academic Editors: Jonás Samuel Pérez-Blanco and José Martínez Lanao

Received: 8 September 2021
Accepted: 14 October 2021
Published: 16 October 2021

Publisher's Note: MDPI stays neutral with regard to jurisdictional claims in published maps and institutional affiliations.

Copyright: © 2021 by the authors. Licensee MDPI, Basel, Switzerland. This article is an open access article distributed under the terms and conditions of the Creative Commons Attribution (CC BY) license (https:// creativecommons.org/licenses/by/ 4.0/).

1. Introduction

Palbociclib is an oral inhibitor of cyclin 4 and 6 dependent kinases (CDK4/6) used in HR+/HER2- breast cancer [1–5]. An absolute gain of 10.3 and 5.4 months in progression-free survival was observed, respectively, in patients treated with palbociclib and letrozole compared to letrozole alone, and in patients treated with palbociclib and fulvestrant compared to fulvestrant alone in patients previously treated with hormone therapy. The recommended dose of palbociclib is 125 mg per os once daily for 21 days out of 28.

Treatment continues until progression or serious adverse events. Dosage adjustments are made based on the occurrence of adverse events [3,5]. The most common adverse event is neutropenia [1–7]. To avoid complications, at the beginning of treatment with palbociclib and at the beginning of each cycle, as well as on day 15 of the first two treatment cycles, a blood count is performed. An absolute neutrophil count (ANC) $\geq 1000/\text{mm}^3$ (N: 1700 to $7500/\text{mm}^3$) is recommended to start/continue the treatment [3,5].

Two pharmacokinetic/pharmacodynamic (PK/PD) models describe the relationship between palbociclib and ANC kinetics. The first model developed by Sun et al. [8] is a population PK/PD model based on palbociclib phase II and III data. This model, derived from PK/PD models used for cytotoxic drugs (i.e., Friberg's model [9]), is the first PK/PD model applied to palbociclib in humans. It showed the impact of age, weight, and food effect on the pharmacokinetics (PK) of palbociclib and the impact of gender and albuminemia level on ANC kinetics. The second model, developed by Chen et al. [10], is a preclinical PK/PD model, constructed from in vitro data and using PK/PD data from endogenous G-CSF (granulocyte colony stimulating factor) studies. The authors used several concentrations of palbociclib on cell cultures to describe the effect of palbociclib on granulocyte stem cells. An inhibitory effect (i.e., by an inhibition effect of stem cells entering the S phase and a stimulation effect of stem cells entering the G0 phase) is modeled in order to mimic the palbociclib effect on the proliferation of the bone marrow stem cells.

The aim of the present work was to describe the PK of palbociclib and to model the PK/PD relationship between long-term kinetics of ANC and palbociclib concentrations, in the general population, based on data from real-life follow-up. Additionally, based on those models, simulations were conducted to determine the optimal exposure that limits the risk of neutropenia to a reasonable one.

2. Materials and Methods

2.1. Patients and Sampling

All consecutive patients included in the study from 28 October 2018 to 15 March 2021 received palbociclib as breast cancer (RH+/HER2- or HER2+ non-amplified) treatment in our institution. Patients with incomplete dosing history or insufficient ANC at the period of the study were not included in the PKPD part of the study (minimum of 3 ANC's samples per patient). Patient data were retrieved retrospectively from the patient record management software. Palbociclib therapeutic drug monitoring is routinely performed in our institution. Thus, blood samples to quantify patient palbociclib exposure were available. Additionally, ANC were extracted from biology reports completed during treatment as required by the marketing authorization or during any patients' hospitalizations, if deemed appropriate, during the first treatment year.

No specific informed consent was required, as samples were regular. However, a general consent was signed by patients stipulating that its data may anonymously be used for research purposes. Thus, data used in this manuscript were recorded in such a manner that confidentiality was ensured following these guidelines. Additionally, our protocol of analyses was approved by our Institutional Review Board and was in accordance with the Declaration of Helsinki.

2.2. Analytical Methods of Palbociclib

Palbociclib blood samples were analyzed by liquid chromatography-mass spectrometry using the method described by Jolibois et al. [11] which allows the simultaneous measurement of palbociclib, olaparib, cabozantinib, pazopanib, sorafenib, sunitinib and desethyl-sunitinib. After blood collection, samples were rapidly centrifuged and frozen until the analysis. Sample extraction was performed as follows: 150 µL of human plasma and 100 µL of NaOH were added to 10 µL of an internal standard solution (containing isotopic palbociclib, olaparib, cabozantinib, pazopanib, sorafenib and sunitinib). Samples were vortexed for a few seconds, then 700 µL of ethyl acetate was added. After being vortexed for 30 s, the samples were centrifuged at 10,000 RPM for 5 min. In an extraction tube, 600 µL of supernatant were collected and evaporated under nitrogen flow. The dried samples were reconstituted with 150 µL of a mixture of 55% of methanol/45% of solvent A (ammonium acetate 1 M in water, pH adjusted to 3.2 with formic acid). The samples were vortexed for 30 s and filtrated using Captiva ND Lipids plates and assayed with an LC-MS/MS device. With this method, the lower limit of quantification (LLOQ) of palbociclib was 6 ng/mL, and the between-run and within-run accuracy and precision were lower than 13.3% and 12.9% for the lowest level control, 7.5% and 10.0% for the medium level control and 2.8% and 5.0% for the highest level control, respectively.

2.3. Population Pharmacokinetic Model

Several population pharmacokinetic (popPK) models have been tested. The base model was a 1-compartmental model with first-order absorption and elimination clearance. Other models were tested such as with an absorption lag-time or a 2-compartmental model. Residual error was described either with an additive, a proportional or a combined error model.

2.4. Pharmacokinetic/Pharmacodynamic Model

The aim of this PK/PD model is to describe the relationship between the plasma concentrations of palbociclib and the ANC kinetic during the first year of treatment. Individual pharmacokinetic parameters were estimated with the popPK model and used as individual constants (regressors in Monolix®) in the model in order to compute palbociclib concentrations.

The structural model used as base is the one initially developed by Friberg et al. [9] to describe cytotoxic-induced neutropenia. This model is a semi-mechanistic model mimicking neutropoiesis (Figure 1).

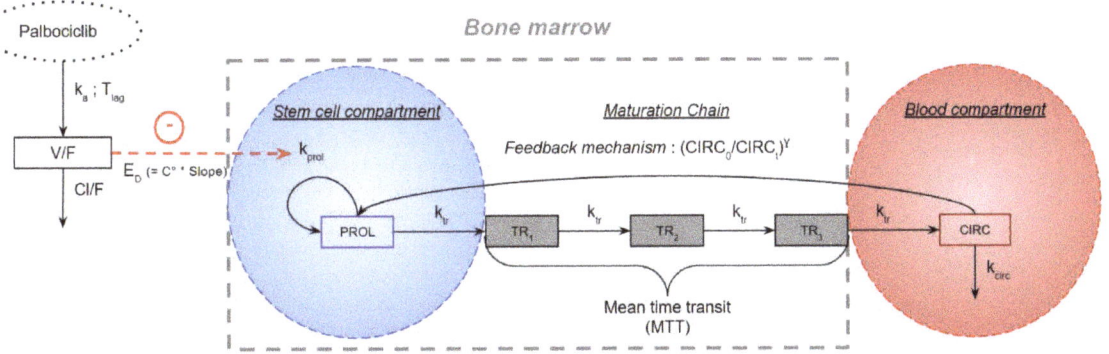

Figure 1. Pharmacokinetic/pharmacodynamic model. C°: concentration of palbociclib; CIRC: compartment corresponding to the circulating neutrophils; $CIRC_0$: ANC at time 0 in CIRC compartment; $CIRC_t$: ANC at time t in CIRC compartment; Cl/F: palbociclib apparent clearance; E_D: drug effect; γ: feedback mechanism; k_a: palbociclib absorption constant; k_{circ}: rate of elimination of neutrophils from the systemic circulation; k_{prol}: rate of stem cell proliferation; k_{tr}: maturation rate; MTT: mean transit time; PROL: proliferation compartment; Slope: sensitivity to palbociclib-induced neutropenia; T_{lag}: palbociclib absorption lag time; TR_X: transit compartments; V/F: palbociclib apparent volume of distribution.

This model is composed of five compartments. First, a PROL compartment, which is assumed to contain stem cells that will become neutrophils after maturation via three transit compartments (TR_1, TR_2 and TR_3). Lastly, a CIRC compartment corresponding to the circulating neutrophils.

The endogenous effect of G-CSF is represented by a feedback mechanism γ. The drug effect (E_D) is a linear proportionality constant relating palbociclib concentration to its effect on stem cells in the PROL compartment. It represents individual sensitivity to palbociclib-induced neutropenia. The mean transit time (MTT) is the average time it takes for a stem cell to reach the CIRC compartment. k_{tr} is equal to the number of compartments plus one (i.e., 3 + 1) divided by MTT. The rate of stem cell proliferation is k_{prol}. The rate of elimination of neutrophils from the systemic circulation is k_{circ}. In most applications of Friberg's model, it is assumed that the transfer constant (k_{tr}) is equal to the proliferation constant (k_{prol}) which is equal to the elimination constant of circulating neutrophils (k_{circ}). This simplifies the calculations and reduces the analysis time. At baseline, compartments PROL, TR_1, TR_2, TR_3 and CIRC are equal to the same value: Base. The ANC were log-transformed to facilitate the estimation of parameters. An additive residual error was used on log-transformed values (i.e., corresponding to a proportional error model on non-log-transformed data).

Patients without ANC samples or with incomplete follow-up history were not included in the analyses.

2.5. Estimation of Model Parameters and Software Used

To develop the popPK and the PK/PD model, a nonlinear mixed effects regression approach was used. For this step, the Monolix® software version 2020R1 was used (Lixoft SAS, Antony, France). The estimation of the population parameters was performed using the SAEM (Stochastic Approximation Expectation-Maximization) algorithm. The interindividual variability (IIV) was coded as $Param_i = Param_{pop} \times e^{\eta}$ with $Param_i$ the individual parameter value, $Param_{pop}$ the typical population value, and η the random effect that follows a normal distribution centered on 0 and of standard deviation ω. The result of this random effect is given as the coefficient of variation (CV in %) which is equal to: $CV = \sqrt{e^{\omega^2} - 1}$.

2.6. Covariate

For population PK analysis, covariates were selected based on routinely available data and physiological considerations. Continuous covariates selected for the popPK model were age, weight, creatininemia, creatinine clearance (Clcr) according to the Cockcroft–Gault formula, aspartate aminotransferase (ASAT), alanine aminotransferase (ALAT), γ-glutamyltranspeptidase (γ-GT), lactate dehydrogenase, total bilirubinemia, alkaline phosphatase (ALP) and albuminemia, whereas concurrent hormonotherapy (fulvestrant/letrozole/others/NK (not known)) was the only categorical covariate.

For PK/PD analysis, covariates were selected based on previous knowledge [8,9,12]. Continuous selected covariates for the PK/PD model were age and albuminemia. Selected categorical covariates were long-term hormonotherapy (yes/no/NK), previous radiotherapy (yes/no/NK), presence of metastases (yes/no/NK), concurrent hormonotherapy (fulvestrant/letrozole/others/NK), and the number of previous lines of chemotherapy.

Missing covariates were replaced by the median value in our population.

The selection of covariates was undertaken in the same way for the popPK and the PK/PD model. Covariates were plotted against random effect from the base models (i.e., models without covariates) in order to search for any tendency. Additionally, Wald tests were performed. If the Wald test was significant ($p < 0.05$) or if the graphical approach shows a relationship between the random effect and a covariate, a forward/backward approach was conducted [13]. Significant covariates were then included independently in the model. A covariate was considered relevant if a decrease in the objective function value (OFV) of 3.84 points (significant at 0.05) was observed. All covariates leading to an improvement in the OFV were then added to the model, leading to a full covariate model. Covariates were then excluded one by one and change in OFV was monitored. A covariate was considered relevant if an increase in the OFV of 6.64 points (significant at 0.01) was observed after its removal. The final model is the one with all covariates considered relevant after forward/backward steps.

The effect of continuous covariates was defined as follows:

$$Param_i = Param_{pop} \times \left(\frac{COV_i}{COV_{med}}\right)^{\beta_{cov}} \quad (1)$$

With $Param_i$ the individual parameter, $Param_{pop}$ the typical value of the population parameter, COV_{med} the median value of the covariate in the population, COV_i the value of the individual covariate, β_{cov} the impact of the covariate.

For categorical covariates, one class will be considered the reference class:

$$Param_i = Param_{pop} \times e^{\beta * cov_i} \quad (2)$$

With $Param_i$ the individual parameter, $Param_{pop}$ the typical value of the population parameter, Cov_i the covariate coded as 0 (reference class) and 1 and β the impact of the covariate.

2.7. Model Evaluation

Final model selection was based on comparison of the models' OFV, the relative standard error (RSE%, i.e., precision) of the parameter estimates, the ability of Monolix® to converge a parameter to a typical population value (i.e., if the model estimates the same parameter value after several runs), and graphical diagnostics plots, including observations versus individual predictions plots, and residual errors plots (individual residuals versus time or observed concentrations). The control of normalized prediction distribution errors (NDPE), numerical predictive checks and corrected visual checks were also performed.

Observations versus individual predictions plot visualizes the fit of the model to the data used. The RSE allow for judgement of the stability of the final model.

2.8. Simulation

Using Simulx2020R1® software, the impact of covariates on ANC kinetics was explored using simulation of the final PK/PD model. The simulations were run over 100 days with 28-day cycles (21 days with 125 mg palbociclib daily followed by 7 days off). Each covariate was set to either its median value or its minimum and maximum. IIV were not considered.

In addition, 5,000 ANC time courses were computed according to each C_{resSS}. The proportion of patients with at least grade 3 and the proportion of patients with grade 4 neutropenia was then calculated.

2.9. Palbociclib Exposure vs. Dose Reduction and Cut-Off Estimation

Trough palbociclib concentrations at steady state (C_{resSS}) during the first cycle were estimated via the final popPK model for each patient. Palbociclib areas under the curve of concentration time course (AUC in mg.h/L) for a single dose were computed according to the relation AUC = Dose/Cl (with the Dose, the dose at initiation in mg, Cl, the individual clearance estimated via the final popPK model in L/h). Percentage of patients with dose reduction was computed for 4 groups of patients according to their exposure metrics values (AUC or C_{resSS}). Only patients who started treatment at full dose (i.e., 125 mg/d) and with complete intake and follow-up history were included.

3. Results

3.1. Population Description

All of our patients were female and their characteristics are presented in Tables 1 and 2. In the construction of the popPK model, 181 samples from 143 unique patients were used. One hundred and eight patients had one PK sample taken, 32 patients had two different PK samples, and 3 patients had three different PK samples. Samples from the same patient were considered as independent.

Table 1. Patients' demographic and biological characteristics. ALP: alkaline phosphatase; ALAT: alanine aminotransferase; ASAT: aspartate aminotransferase; Cl_{cr}: creatinine clearance; γ-GT: γ-glutamyltranspeptidase; popPK: population pharmacokinetic; PK/PD: pharmacokinetic/pharmacodynamics.

	Population Used to Build the popPK Model (n = 143)		Population Used to Build the PK/PD Model (n = 128)	
	Median (min–max)	Number	Median (min–max)	Number
Age (years)	69 (40–92)		63 (40–92)	
Serum creatinine (µmol/L)	68.0 (31.0–301.8)		68.0 (31–169.7)	
Weight (kg)	67 (37–140)		66 (37–140)	
Clcr (according to Cockcroft–Gault formula) (mL/min)	71.6 (22.1–282.3)		73.5 (22.1–282.3)	
ALAT (UI/L)	18 (6–237)		17 (6–237)	
ASAT (UI/L)	23 (12–205)		22 (12–205)	
γ-GT (UI/L)	29 (9–1113)		28 (9–1113)	
ALP (UI/L)	89 (11–819)		81 (11–644)	
Lactate dehydrogenase (UI/L)	224 (85–675)		216 (85–675)	
Total bilirubin (mg/L)	5.0 (1.5–27.2)		4.7 (1.5–27.2)	
Albumin (g/L)	39.9 (20.0–48.0)		39.0 (20.0–48.0)	
Plasma protein (g/L)	70.6 (53.0–98.0)		69.0 (53.0–88.0)	

Table 2. Patients' treatment and disease characteristics. NK: not known; popPK: population pharmacokinetic; PK/PD: pharmacokinetic/pharmacodynamic.

	Population Used to Build the popPK Model (n = 143)		Population Used to Build the PK/PD Model (n = 128)	
	Median (min–max)	Number	Median (min–max)	Number
Number of previous chemotherapies	2 (0–12)		2 (0–12)	
Long-term hormonotherapy				
Yes		93 (65.0%)		90 (70.3%)
No		40 (28.0%)		38 (29.7%)
NK		10 (7.0%)		0 (0.0%)
Previous radiotherapy				
Yes		73 (51.0%)		73 (57.0%)
No		60 (42.0%)		55 (43.0%)
NK		10 (7.0%)		0.0 (0.0%)
Metastases				
Yes		108 (75.5%)		105 (82.0%)
No		25 (17.5%)		23 (18.0%)
NK		10 (7.0%)		0.0 (0.0%)
Concurrent hormonotherapy				
Fulvestrant		48 (33.6%)		45 (35.2%)
Letrozole		71 (49.6%)		69 (53.9%)
Others		14 (9.8%)		14 (10.9%)
NK		10 (7.0%)		0 (0.0%)

Palbociclib samples were collected between day 1 and 28 after the start of the cycle. Of these, 31 samples (18%) were collected during the first 8 days. The samples were collected between 0.9 and 197.25 h after the last administration of palbociclib. The mean concentration was 77 (±80.2) µg/L, while concentrations ranged from 6 (LLOQ) to 229 µg/L. No concentration was below the LLOQ. Doses administered during the PK evaluation were 75 mg (n = 16), 100 mg (n = 38), and 125 mg (n = 127) per day, 21 days out of 28.

3.2. Population Pharmacokinetic Model

The model that best described the PK data was a mono-compartmental model with an absorption lag-time (T_{lag}), an absorption rate (k_a), and an additive error model. The lack of early observations (4% of the samples were taken 2 h maximum after the last intake) did not allow us to estimate T_{lag} and V/F, so they were fixed to the values of a mono-compartmental model of palbociclib developed by Royer et al. [14]. IIV was added only on Cl/F, as when other IIV were added, the estimations were not sufficiently precise. Parameter values estimated by Monolix® are presented in Table 3. The RSE are below 40%, showing a good stability of the model.

Table 3. Estimated parameters of the final popPK model. ALP: alkaline phosphatase; Cl/F: palbociclib apparent oral clearance; CV: coefficient of variation; Cl_{cr}: creatinine clearance according to Cockcroft–Gault formula; IIV: inter individuality variability; k_a: Palbociclib absorption rate; med: median; RSE: relative standard error; T_{lag}: Palbociclib absorption lag time; V/F: palbociclib apparent volume of distribution.

	Population PK Model without Covariates		Final Population PK Model with Covariates		Bootstrap of the Final Population PK Model [a]		Consequences of Covariates
Objective Function Value	1775.75		1734.37				
	Parameter	RSE (%)	Parameter	RSE (%)	Parameter	2.5th 97.5th percentiles	
Cl/F (L/h)	57.42	3.2	57.13	2.8	57.21	[54.19–60.42]	
Cl_{cr} (med = 71.6 mL/mn) on Cl/F	.	.	0.44	15.1	0.46	[0.35–0.57]	Cl/F increase when Cl_{cr} increase
ALP (med = 88.6 UI/L) on Cl/F	.	.	−0.14	34.1	−0.15	[−0.24–−0.05]	Cl/F increase when ALP decrease
V/F (L)	1580	.	1580	.	.	.	
k_a (h^{-1})	0.187	21.2	0.187	22.2	0.18	[0.17–0.19]	
T_{lag} (h) (fix)	0.658	.	0.658	.	.	.	
Cl/F IIV (CV %)	41.4	6.5	32.6	9.3	30.7	[21.8–37.1]	
Additive error (µg/L)	10.12	19.6	13.84	20.5	14.70	[6.46–22.48]	

[a] Estimates are presented with the median and 2.5th–97.5th percentiles values of the bootstrap (n = 1000).

Construction of a bicompartmental model was not possible, as the model failed to converge on typical second-compartment population parameters (second-compartment volume and inter-compartment clearance).

Covariates tested according to graphical approach and/or Wald test were creatinine-mia, creatinine clearance (according to the Cockcroft–Gault formula), age, weight, and ALP concentration. Fourteen patients had missing covariates, so they had the median value for our population. Only two covariates significantly decreased OFV after forward/backward approach: Cl_{cr} and ALP concentration on apparent clearance (Cl/F). Their addition resulted in a decrease in OFV of 41.38 points and a decrease in Cl/F IIV of 8.8%.

The numerical predictive checks (Supplementary Figure S1) showed a good adequacy of the model with our data. The cumulative distribution function and the probability density function of the NDPE also showed a reasonable agreement (Supplementary Figures S2 and S3).

The Figure 2A,B shows a good fit of the final popPK model to the data. The population predictions versus observed concentration did not show any particular mismatch, whereas a slight under-prediction of high values and an over-prediction of low values is observed when individual predictions are compared to observed palbociclib concentrations.

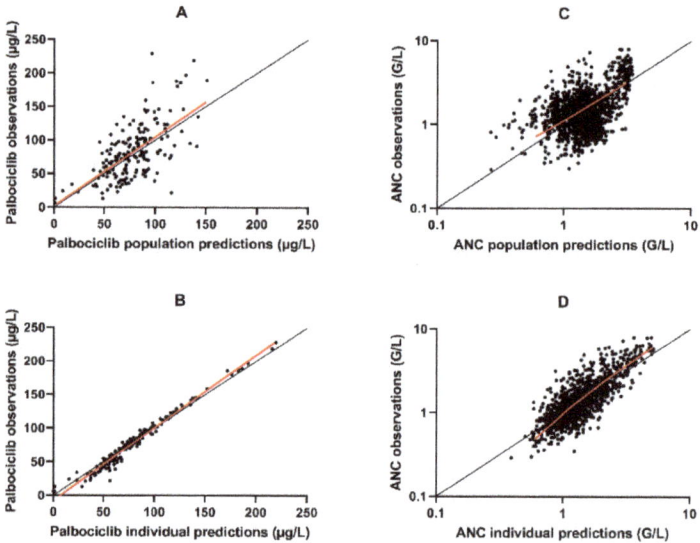

Figure 2. Observations versus population or individual predictions. (**A**) Palbociclib observations versus palbociclib population predictions of the popPK model. (**B**) Palbociclib observations versus palbociclib individual predictions of the popPK model. (**C**) ANC observations versus ANC population predictions of the PK/PD model (log scale). (**D**) ANC observations versus ANC individual predictions of the PK/PD model (log scale). The x-axis represents the population or individual predictions, and the y-axis represents the observations. The red line (solid line) represents the trend of the points. The black line represents the y = x line.

3.3. Pharmacokinetic/Pharmacodynamic Model

Of the 143 patients used for the popPK model, 15 patients could not be used for the PK/PD analysis: 10 patients without ANC samples in our database and 5 patients with incomplete intake and follow-up history (but not related to toxicity).

PK/PD patients' characteristics are presented in Tables 1 and 2. One thousand five hundred and eight ANC were recovered, i.e., an average of 11.8 ANC per patient with a minimum of 3 and a maximum of 41. The duration of follow-up ranged from 35 days to 1 year (13 cycles). ANC values ranged from 0.29 G/L to 8 G/L. One point six percent of samples had a value below 0.5 G/L, 25.7% between 0.5 and 1 G/L, 50.8% between 1 and 2 G/L and 21.9% above 2 G/L.

Several semi-mechanistic models were tested, such as Friberg's model with an E_{max} effect, a model with more complex G-CSF effect and a model with quiescent compartments of stem cells. The most relevant model was the one developed by Friberg with a linear drug effect. During the model building phases, Monolix® failed to converge to a value for gamma variability. By removing this variability, the OFV did not change significantly (<3.84), so this variability was removed. The parameters estimated by Monolix® are presented in Table 4. The RSE of the population parameters are less than 40% showing good model stability.

Table 4. Estimated parameters of the final PK/PD model. CV: coefficient of variation; IIV: inter individuality variability; med: median; MTT: mean transit time; RSE: relative standard error.

	Population PK/PD Model without Covariates		Final PK/PD Model with Covariates		Consequences of Covariates	Bootstrap Simulation	
Objective Function Value	2410.37		2400.90				
	Parameter	RSE (%)	Parameter	RSE (%)		Median Parameter [a]	2.5th–97.5th Percentiles
Base (G/L)	2.94	3.70	2.92	3.55		2.95	[2.75–3.16]
Slope (L/µg)	0.0011	6.60	0.0011	6.46		0.0011	[0.0009–0.0014]
MTT (days)	5.32	4.81	5.29	4.93		5.36	[4.61–6.30]
Gamma	0.109	7.52	0.103	7.01		0.104	[0.085–0.137]
Base IIV (CV %)	31.8	8.67	29.6	9.21		29.0	[24.6–33.1]
Age on Base (med = 63.7 years)			0.465	34.00	Base increases with age increase	0.51	[0.23–0.78]
Slope IIV (CV %)	26.4	12.80	28.8	11.70		28.0	[21.2–34.1]
MTT IIV (CV %)	18.1	21.00	17.9	21.10		19.0	[10.0–33.0]
Exponential error	0.34	2.40	0.34	2.02		0.33	[0.31–0.36]

[a] Estimates are presented with the median values of the bootstrap ($n = 100$).

Covariates significant in the forward step were age and albuminemia on Base, but only age was significant in the backward step. Age decreased the OFV of the final model by 9.47 points and the baseline IIV by 2.2%. The median parameters of the 100 bootstrap simulations are close to the parameters estimated in the final PK/PD model (Table 4).

The observations versus individual predictions plot (Figure 2C,D) comparing observations to predictions shows a slight underestimation of the highest values (> 2.5 G/L) and an overestimation of lowest values (< 0.6 G/L).

The corrected visual predictive checks (Supplementary Figure S4) showed that the model gave a good description of the ANC during the first year of treatment with palbociclib. The cumulative distribution function and the probability density function of the NDPE showed a good distribution of the empirical NDPE of the PK/PD model (Supplementary Figures S5 and S6).

3.4. Simulation

Looking at the different simulations of ANC kinetics as a function of covariates (Figure 3), we observe that a "median" patient (i.e., with median covariates) does not experience neutropenia. Decreased Cl_{cr} or increased ALP leads to an increase in plasma concentrations and therefore in the neutropenic effect. According to our model, the younger a patient, the lower her baseline ANC. Consequently, younger patients are more at risk of neutropenia.

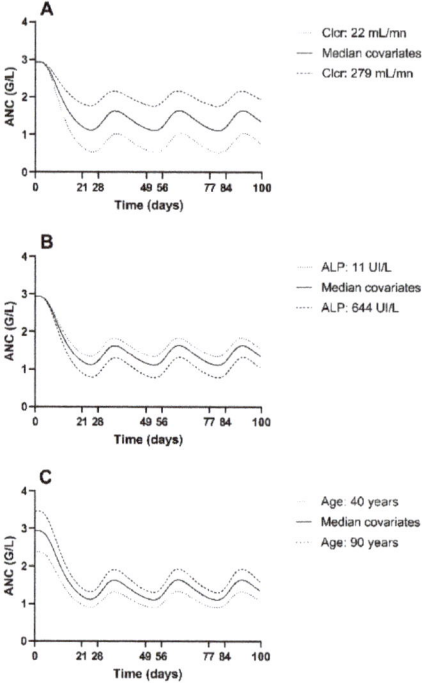

Figure 3. Simulation of the impact of different covariates' values on ANC time course. (**A**) Simulations of palbociclib treatment with median covariates except Cl_{cr}. (**B**) Simulations of palbociclib treatment with median covariates except ALP. (**C**) Simulations of palbociclib treatment with median covariates except age. Cycle of 21 days of treatment (125 mg of palbociclib per day), then 7 days of therapeutic pause. In each graph, only one covariate is changed, the others are fixed at the median value. The extreme values of the covariates in the population were selected for each simulation.

The risk of developing a grade 3 or 4 neutropenia at the nadir increases with estimated C_{resSS} (Figure 4). At an estimated C_{resSS} of 100 μg/L, a patient has an 18% risk of developing grade 4 neutropenia (Figure 4).

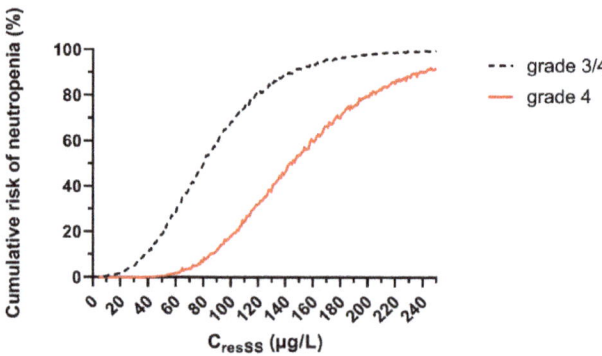

Figure 4. Risk of grade 3 or grade 3/4 neutropenia depending on the residual concentration at steady state. 5000 simulations of ANC kinetics were simulated at every C_{resSS} to 0 at 250 μg/L.

3.5. Palbociclib Exposure vs. Dose Reduction and Cut-Off Estimation

Of the 143 patients, 127 could be used to calculate the relation between palbociclib exposure and a dose reduction (10 patients without complete intake and follow-up history and 6 patients who began at dose lower than 125 mg/d). Of these 127 patients, 75 were not subject to a dose decrease during treatment.

For both the estimated AUC and estimated C_{resSS}, we observed that the proportion of patients with a dose reduction was more important in the highest exposure group (estimated AUC > 2.77 mg.h/L or estimated C_{resSS} > 95 µg/L): 75% to 78.1% of the most exposed patients had a dose decrease, compared to 25% to 32.3% in the other groups (Figure 5).

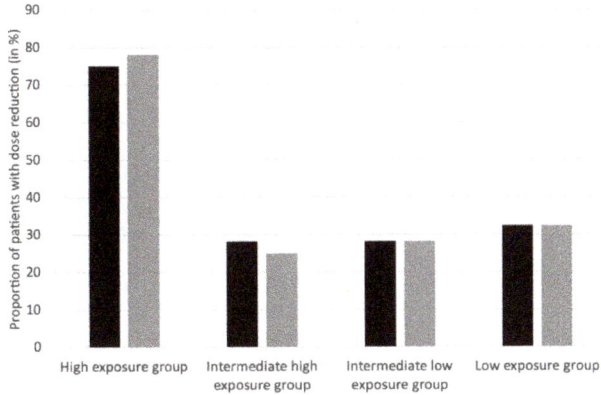

Figure 5. Proportion of patients with dose reduction. Black bars represent AUC (Area under the curve (in mg.h/L)) and gray bars represent C_{resSS} (Residual concentration at the steady state (in µg/L)). High exposure group (n = 32): 2.77 < AUC < 5.63 or 95 < C_{resSS} < 204, intermediate high exposure group (n = 32): 2.17 < AUC < 2.76 or 70 < C_{resSS} < 94, intermediate low exposure group (n = 32): 1.76 < AUC < 2.16 or 53 < C_{resSS} < 69, and low exposure group (n = 31): 1.12 < AUC < 1.75 or 27 < C_{resSS} < 52.

4. Discussion

Neutropenia is the most common adverse event during treatment with palbociclib [1–3,5,6,15]. In the event of grade 3 (ANC < 1 G/L) and grade 4 (ANC < 0.5 G/L) neutropenia, the treatment is interrupted, and the dose may be reduced [3,5]. Investigation of ANC kinetic during palbociclib treatment may provide a better understanding of the exposure-toxicity relationship and allow us to predict which patients are more at risk. This study is the first PK/PD model of ANC time-course in real-life patients treated by palbociclib during one year.

To our knowledge, the only popPK model of palbociclib built from rich data is the one developed by Sun [16]. This model was built with data from phase I and I/II clinical trials (183 patients with an average of 10.6 observations per patient). This model is a bicompartmental model with an absorption lag time and a first-order constant of absorption. With our data, the estimation of either lag time or bicompartmental model was impossible. Indeed, only 4% of the samples were taken before the 2nd hour after the last dose and 5.5% after the 30th hour after the last dose. This lack of early and late observations makes it impossible to estimate parameters associated with the second compartment. Moreover, in contrast to the model proposed by Royer [14], we were not able to estimate the value of the volume of distribution and the variability of the absorption constant. Nevertheless, we observed a good fit of the model to the data as shown in Figure 2B.

During the covariate step, in addition to ALP, age, weight, creatininemia and Cl_{cr} (according to the Cockcroft–Gault formula) were significantly linked to Cl/F IIV when added solely. However, during the backward step, only the Cl_{cr} (and ALP) showed a significant impact. This may be explained by the fact that Cl_{cr} considers all the other covariates. Although renal elimination is not the major elimination route of palbociclib, study showed a relationship between renal insufficiency (according to the Cl_{cr} calculated by the Cockcroft–Gault formula) and palbociclib AUC, which quantifies the exposure to palbociclib. A decrease in Cl_{cr} leads to an increase in the AUC as a consequence of a decrease in the elimination of palbociclib [17]. According to its main route of elimination (i.e., hepatic [3,5]), the model also showed a relationship between ALP and palbociclib elimination. The higher the ALP, the lower the elimination. An increase in ALP can be explained by liver damage secondary to breast cancer or during liver disease [18].

Parameters estimated to describe the ANC time course were Base (2.92 G/L; 29.6% IIV), Slope (0.0011 L/μg; 28.8% IIV), Mean Transit Time (MTT; 5.29 days; 17.9% IIV) and γ (0.102). They are close to most of the previous PK/PD models for other compounds, but also to the model by Sun [9,19,20]. The fact that a patient experiences metastases and/or has already had chemotherapy and/or long-term hormone therapy and/or radiotherapy could suggest that the patient suffers from an advanced disease and therefore a poorer general condition that could lead to a higher risk of neutropenia [21]. After modelling the ANC kinetic, these covariates did not show a significant impact in our PK/PD model, nor the type of concomitant hormone therapy. The fact that these covariates did not emerge as significant indicates that these characteristics are not of major interest in the choice of palbociclib dosage. This observation is in agreement with several other pre-existing models that did not show relationships between these covariates and ANC kinetics during cytotoxic dosing [9,19,20].

The only covariate that emerged as significant in the PK/PD model was the effect of age on the patient circulating neutrophils at baseline. The older the patient, the more circulating neutrophils at the beginning of treatment. In several existing models, a negative correlation between ANC at initiation and albuminemia was highlighted: the lower the albuminemia, the higher the ANC. According to Schmitt et al. [12], the relationship between albuminemia and circulating neutrophils can be explained by the fact that low albuminemia is a sign of inflammation and therefore of increased neutrophils synthesis. In the paper by Sun, the impact of albuminemia on ANC was also evidenced, with a parameter associated with baseline albuminemia of −1.03. In our data, albuminemia did not show a significant impact on ANC at initiation, whereas age did. In our population, there is a negative correlation between age and albuminemia (data not shown), which may explain why age has an impact on the parameter Base. Indeed albuminemia showed a significant impact in the forward step but not in the backward step. Part of the effect of albuminemia must be accounted for by age. Sun also showed the impact of gender on the Base value. Our study cannot evidence this correlation because all our patients were female. Nevertheless, Base value is lower than the one for women estimated by Sun (2.92 versus 3.63 G/L). Our study is based on real life patients and not on patients selected for clinical trials. Therefore, we may treat patients in poorer general condition and with lower ANC. Among other parameters independent of treatment intake, MTT and γ do not differ too much from pre-existing models [8,9,19,20].

Regarding the limitations of this work, we assume a good compliance of the patient, and an error-free completion of patients' information. However, as we conducted a retrospective study, some patient records did not include all the blood samples recommended by the French drug agency (ANSM). The poor estimation of the extreme values of our data can be explained by the low number of observations for patients with grade 3 (25.7%) and grade 4 (1.6%) neutropenia. The small number of patients may also be a limitation in the determination of covariates. A last limitation of our work is the absence of PK/efficacy analysis. A non-significant trend between mean trough concentrations and progression-free survival was highlighted [22]. Yet, our data were not mature enough to draw any firm conclusion for efficacy.

Because no formal target concentration exists for palbociclib, Mueller-Schoell et al. suggest using the mean trough concentration observed in the clinical trials (61 μg/L) as a target [23]. This concentration leads to a risk of grade 3 neutropenia of approximately 31%

and of grade 4 neutropenia of approximately 2%. As patients experiencing severe palbociclib-induced neutropenia are at low risk of infection [24], we have refined this therapeutic target to a higher value. Based on our simulations, in order to avoid a risk of grade 4 neutropenia greater than 20%, estimated C_{resSS} should not exceed 100 µg/L. This is confirmed, in real life, by the fact that patients with C_{resSS} > 95 µg/L benefit of nearly 3 times more dose reductions than patients with lower exposure (Figure 5). Thus, a C_{resSS} lower than 100 µg/L seems reasonable to avoid severe toxicity. It should be noted that, as not all measured concentrations were trough at steady-state, C_{resSS} was estimated for all patients. Thus, all our interpretations are based on C_{resSS} estimated from our popPK model.

5. Conclusions

A popPK model and a semi-mechanistic PK/PD model constructed from general population data were presented. Interindividual variability in Cl/F was partially explained by Cl_{cr} and ALP concentration. Interindividual variability in ANC at baseline was also partially explained by age (without any physiological explanation). Based on our simulations, an estimated palbociclib C_{resSS} below 100 µg/L would limit the risk of grade 4 neutropenia below 20% and should not be exceeded. In order to obtain a full target (i.e., a low boundary in addition to this high boundary), exposure/efficacy relationships should be investigated.

Supplementary Materials: The following are available online at https://www.mdpi.com/article/10.3390/pharmaceutics13101708/s1. Figure S1. Numerical predictive checks (NPC) of the palbociclib final population pharmacokinetic model. Figure S2. Cumulative distribution functions of the normalised prediction distribution errors (NPDE) of the final Palbociclib population pharmacokinetic model. Figure S3. Probability density function of the normalised prediction distribution errors (NPDE) of the final Palbociclib population pharmacokinetic model. Figure S4. Prediction corrected visual predictive checks (VPCc) of the final Palbociclib pharmacokinetic/pharmacodynamic model. Figure S5. Cumulative distribution functions of the normalised prediction distribution errors (NPDE) of the final Palbociclib pharmacokinetic/pharmacodynamic model. Figure S6. Probability density function of the normalised prediction distribution errors (NPDE) of the final Palbociclib pharmacokinetic/pharmacodynamic model.

Author Contributions: Conceptualization, B.R. and A.S.; methodology, A.L.M. and A.S.; formal analysis, A.L.M., E.P. and A.S.; investigation, C.K., J.-D.F., A.H., I.D., S.L., Z.T., S.A., D.M. and S.I.; resources, B.R.; data curation, A.L.M. and E.P.; writing—original draft preparation, A.L.M. and A.S.; writing—review and editing, A.L.M. and A.S.; supervision, A.S. All authors have read and agreed to the published version of the manuscript.

Funding: This research, as part of STARTER-BFC platform, was funded by "Agence Régionale de Santé Bourgogne-Franche-Comté" and "Omedit Bourgogne–Franche-Comté".

Institutional Review Board Statement: No specific informed consent was required, as samples were regular. However, a general consent was signed by patients stipulating that its data may anonymously be used for research purposes. Thus, data used in this manuscript were recorded in such a manner that confidentiality was ensured following these guidelines. Additionally, our protocol of analyses was approved by our Institutional Review Board and was in accordance with the Declaration of Helsinki.

Informed Consent Statement: No specific informed consent was required, as samples were regular. However, a general consent is signed by patients stipulating that its data may anonymously be used for research purposes. Thus, data used in this manuscript were recorded in such a manner that confidentiality was ensured.

Data Availability Statement: Data available on request.

Conflicts of Interest: The authors declare no conflict of interest.

References

1. Vilquin, P.; Cohen, P.; Maudelonde, T.; Tredan, O.; Treilleux, I.; Bachelot, T.; Heudel, P.E. New therapeutical strategies in metastatic hormone-dependent breast cancer. *Bull. Cancer* **2015**, *102*, 367–380. [CrossRef] [PubMed]

2. Mangini, N.S.; Wesolowski, R.; Ramaswamy, B.; Lustberg, M.B.; Berger, M.J. Palbociclib: A Novel Cyclin-Dependent Kinase Inhibitor for Hormone Receptor-Positive Advanced Breast Cancer. *Ann. Pharmacother.* **2015**, *49*, 1252–1260. [CrossRef] [PubMed]
3. Wu, Y.; Zhang, Y.; Pi, H.; Sheng, Y. Current Therapeutic Progress of CDK4/6 Inhibitors in Breast Cancer. *Cancer Manag. Res.* **2020**, *12*, 3477–3487. [CrossRef] [PubMed]
4. Beaver, J.A.; Amiri-Kordestani, L.; Charlab, R.; Chen, W.; Palmby, T.; Tilley, A.; Zirkelbach, J.F.; Yu, J.; Liu, Q.; Zhao, L.; et al. FDA Approval: Palbociclib for the Treatment of Postmenopausal Patients with Estrogen Receptor–Positive, HER2-Negative Metastatic Breast Cancer. *Clin. Cancer Res.* **2015**, *21*, 4760–4766. [CrossRef] [PubMed]
5. Dhillon, S. Palbociclib: First global approval. *Drugs* **2015**, *75*, 543–551. [CrossRef]
6. Iwata, H.; Im, S.-A.; Masuda, N.; Im, Y.-H.; Inoue, K.; Rai, Y.; Nakamura, R.; Kim, J.H.; Hoffman, J.T.; Zhang, K.; et al. PALOMA-3: Phase III Trial of Fulvestrant With or Without Palbociclib in Premenopausal and Postmenopausal Women with Hormone Receptor–Positive, Human Epidermal Growth Factor Receptor 2–Negative Metastatic Breast Cancer That Progressed on Prior Endocrine Therapy—Safety and Efficacy in Asian Patients. *J. Glob. Oncol.* **2017**, *3*, 289–303.
7. Finn, R.S.; Crown, J.P.; Lang, I.; Boer, K.; Bondarenko, I.M.; Kulyk, S.O.; Ettl, J.; Patel, R.; Pinter, T.; Schmidt, M.; et al. The cyclin-dependent kinase 4/6 inhibitor palbociclib in combination with letrozole versus letrozole alone as first-line treatment of oestrogen receptor-positive, HER2-negative, advanced breast cancer (PALOMA-1/TRIO-18): A randomised phase 2 study. *Lancet Oncol.* **2015**, *16*, 25–35. [CrossRef]
8. Sun, W.; O'Dwyer, P.J.; Finn, R.S.; Ruiz-Garcia, A.; Shapiro, G.I.; Schwartz, G.K.; DeMichele, A.; Wang, D. Characterization of Neutropenia in Advanced Cancer Patients Following Palbociclib Treatment Using a Population Pharmacokinetic-Pharmacodynamic Modeling and Simulation Approach. *J. Clin. Pharmacol.* **2017**, *57*, 1159–1173. [CrossRef]
9. Friberg, L.E.; Henningsson, A.; Maas, H.; Nguyen, L.; Karlsson, M.O. Model of Chemotherapy-Induced Myelosuppression with Parameter Consistency Across Drugs. *J. Clin. Oncol.* **2002**, *20*, 4713–4721. [CrossRef]
10. Chen, W.; Boras, B.; Sung, T.; Yu, Y.; Zheng, J.; Wang, D.; Hu, W.; Spilker, M.E.; D'Argenio, D.Z. A physiological model of granulopoiesis to predict clinical drug induced neutropenia from in vitro bone marrow studies: With application to a cell cycle inhibitor. *J. Pharmacokinet. Pharmacodyn.* **2020**, *47*, 163–182. [CrossRef]
11. Jolibois, J.; Schmitt, A.; Royer, B. A simple and fast LC-MS/MS method for the routine measurement of cabozantinib, olaparib, palbociclib, pazopanib, sorafenib, sunitinib and its main active metabolite in human plasma. *J. Chromatogr. B Analyt. Technol. Biomed. Life Sci.* **2019**, *1132*, 121844. [CrossRef]
12. Schmitt, A.; Gladieff, L.; Laffont, C.M.; Evrard, A.; Boyer, J.-C.; Lansiaux, A.; Bobin-Dubigeon, C.; Etienne-Grimaldi, M.-C.; Boisdron-Celle, M.; Mousseau, M.; et al. Factors for Hematopoietic Toxicity of Carboplatin: Refining the Targeting of Carboplatin Systemic Exposure. *J. Clin. Oncol.* **2010**, *28*, 4568–4574. [CrossRef] [PubMed]
13. Mould, D.R.; Upton, R.N. Basic concepts in population modeling, simulation, and model-based drug development-part 2: Introduction to pharmacokinetic modeling methods. *CPT Pharmacomet. Syst. Pharmacol.* **2013**, *2*, 1–14. [CrossRef] [PubMed]
14. Royer, B.; Kaderbhaï, C.; Fumet, J.-D.; Hennequin, A.; Desmoulins, I.; Ladoire, S.; Ayati, S.; Mayeur, D.; Ilie, S.; Schmitt, A. Population Pharmacokinetics of Palbociclib in aReal-World Situation. *Pharm. Basel Switz.* **2021**, *14*, 181.
15. Flaherty, K.T.; Lorusso, P.M.; Demichele, A.; Abramson, V.G.; Courtney, R.; Randolph, S.S.; Shaik, M.N.; Wilner, K.D.; O'Dwyer, P.J.; Schwartz, G.K. Phase I, dose-escalation trial of the oral cyclin-dependent kinase 4/6 inhibitor PD 0332991, administered using a 21-day schedule in patients with advanced cancer. *Clin. Cancer Res.* **2012**, *18*, 568–576. [CrossRef] [PubMed]
16. Sun, W.; Wang, D.D. 462P—A Population Pharmacokinetic (Pk) Analysis of Palbociclib (Pd-0332991) in Patients (Pts) with Advanced Solid Tumors. *Ann. Oncol.* **2014**, *25*, iv154. [CrossRef]
17. Yu, Y.; Hoffman, J.; Plotka, A.; O'Gorman, M.; Shi, H.; Wang, D. Palbociclib (PD-0332991) pharmacokinetics in subjects with impaired renal function. *Cancer Chemother. Pharmacol.* **2020**, *86*, 701–710. [CrossRef]
18. Siller, A.F.; Whyte, M.P. Alkaline Phosphatase: Discovery and Naming of Our Favorite Enzyme. *J. Bone Miner. Res.* **2018**, *33*, 362–364. [CrossRef]
19. Mangas-Sanjuan, V.; Buil-Bruna, N.; Garrido, M.J.; Soto, E.; Trocóniz, I.F. Semimechanistic Cell-Cycle Type–Based Pharmacokinetic/Pharmacodynamic Model of Chemotherapy-Induced Neutropenic Effects of Diflomotecan under Different Dosing Schedules. *J. Pharmacol. Exp. Ther.* **2015**, *354*, 55–64. [CrossRef]
20. Pastor, M.L.; Laffont, C.M.; Gladieff, L.; Schmitt, A.; Chatelut, E.; Concordet, D. Model-Based Approach to Describe G-CSF Effects in Carboplatin-Treated Cancer Patients. *Pharm. Res.* **2013**, *30*, 2795–2807. [CrossRef]
21. Lyman, G.H.; Lyman, C.H.; Agboola, O. Risk Models for Predicting Chemotherapy-Induced Neutropenia. *Oncologist* **2005**, *10*, 427–437. [CrossRef]
22. Food and Drug Administration. Center for Drug Evaluation and Research (2014) Palbociclib Clinical Pharmacology and Biopharmaceutics Review. Available online: https://www.accessdata.fda.gov/drugsatfda_docs/nda/2015/207103Orig1s000ClinPharmR.pdf (accessed on 6 August 2021).
23. Mueller-Schoell, A.; Groenland, S.L.; Scherf-Clavel, O.; van Dyk, M.; Huisinga, W.; Michelet, R.; Jaehde, U.; Steeghs, N.; Huitema, A.D.R.; Kloft, C. Therapeutic drug monitoring of oral targeted antineoplastic drugs. *Eur. J. Clin. Pharmacol.* **2021**, *77*, 441–464. [CrossRef]
24. Pramanik, R.; Sahoo, R.K.; Gogia, A. Neutropenia due to palbociclib: A word of caution? *Indian J. Med. Paediatr. Oncol.* **2016**, *37*, 206. [CrossRef] [PubMed]

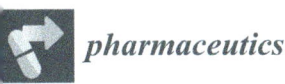

Article

Molecular Epidemiology, Antimicrobial Surveillance, and PK/PD Analysis to Guide the Treatment of *Neisseria gonorrhoeae* Infections

Rodrigo Alonso [1,2], Ainara Rodríguez-Achaerandio [2,3], Amaia Aguirre-Quiñonero [2,3], Aitor Artetxe [1,2], Ilargi Martínez-Ballesteros [1,2], Alicia Rodríguez-Gascón [2,4,*], Javier Garaizar [1,2] and Andrés Canut [2,3,*]

1. Department of Immunology, Microbiology and Parasitology, Faculty of Pharmacy, University of the Basque Country UPV/EHU, 01006 Vitoria-Gasteiz, Spain; rodrigo.alonso@ehu.eus (R.A.); a.artetxe.arrate@gmail.com (A.A.); ilargi.martinez@ehu.eus (I.M.-B.); javier.garaizar@ehu.eus (J.G.)
2. Bioaraba Microbiology, Infectious Disease, Antimicrobial Agents, and Gene Therapy Group, 01009 Vitoria-Gasteiz, Spain; ainara.rodriguezachaerandio@osakidetza.eus (A.R.-A.); amaia.aguirrequinonero@osakidetza.eus (A.A.-Q.)
3. Microbiology Service, Araba University Hospital, Osakidetza Basque Health Service, 01009 Vitoria-Gasteiz, Spain
4. Pharmacokinetic, Nanotechnology and Gene Therapy Group (PharmaNanoGene), Faculty of Pharmacy, University of the Basque Country UPV/EHU, 01006 Vitoria-Gasteiz, Spain
* Correspondence: alicia.rodriguez@ehu.eus (A.R.-G.); andres.canutblasco@osakidetza.eus (A.C.)

Citation: Alonso, R.; Rodríguez-Achaerandio, A.; Aguirre-Quiñonero, A.; Artetxe, A.; Martínez-Ballesteros, I.; Rodríguez-Gascón, A.; Garaizar, J.; Canut, A. Molecular Epidemiology, Antimicrobial Surveillance, and PK/PD Analysis to Guide the Treatment of *Neisseria gonorrhoeae* Infections. *Pharmaceutics* **2021**, *13*, 1699. https://doi.org/10.3390/pharmaceutics13101699

Academic Editors: José Martínez Lanao and Jonás Samuel Pérez-Blanco

Received: 31 August 2021
Accepted: 12 October 2021
Published: 15 October 2021

Publisher's Note: MDPI stays neutral with regard to jurisdictional claims in published maps and institutional affiliations.

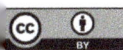

Copyright: © 2021 by the authors. Licensee MDPI, Basel, Switzerland. This article is an open access article distributed under the terms and conditions of the Creative Commons Attribution (CC BY) license (https://creativecommons.org/licenses/by/4.0/).

Abstract: The aim of this study was to apply molecular epidemiology, antimicrobial surveillance, and PK/PD analysis to guide the antimicrobial treatment of gonococci infections in a region of the north of Spain. Antibiotic susceptibility testing was performed on all isolates (2017 to 2019, n = 202). A subset of 35 isolates intermediate or resistant to at least two antimicrobials were selected to search for resistance genes and genotyping through WGS. By Monte Carlo simulation, we estimated the probability of target attainment (PTA) and the cumulative fraction of response (CFR) of the antimicrobials used to treat gonorrhea, both indicative of the probability of treatment success. In total, 2.0%, 6.4%, 5.4%, and 48.2% of the isolates were resistant to ceftriaxone, cefixime, azithromycin, and ciprofloxacin, respectively. Twenty sequence types were identified. Detected mutations were related to antibiotic resistance. PK/PD analysis showed high probability of treatment success of the cephalosporins. In conclusion, multiple populations of *N. gonorrhoeae* were identified. We can confirm that ceftriaxone (even at the lowest dose: 250 mg) and oral cefixime are good candidates to treat gonorrhea. For patients allergic to cephalosporins, ciprofloxacin should be only used if the MIC is known and ≤0.125 mg/L; this antimicrobial is not recommended for empirical treatment.

Keywords: *N. gonorrhoeae*; antibiotic resistance; cephalosporins; azithromycin; pharmacokinetic/pharmacodynamic (PK/PD) analysis; whole-genome sequencing (WGS)

1. Introduction

Sexually transmitted infections (STIs) are a serious global health problem [1]. The prevalence of gonorrhea has increased significantly in recent years. The World Health Organization (WHO) estimates that there are 87 million new cases of gonorrhea each year [2].

In recent years, the most frequently prescribed antibiotics for the treatment of gonorrhea have become less effective, in part due to the inexorable progression of gonococcal antimicrobial resistance [3,4]. In 2018, the WHO reported the expansion of multidrug-resistant strains of *N. gonorrhoeae* worldwide [5]. In Europe, the Euro-GASP (depending on the European Centre for Disease Prevention and Control) provides important data at the European level on antimicrobial resistance, which are used to inform treatment guidelines [6]. Thus, the determination of antimicrobial susceptibility to identify isolates with less susceptibility and resistance to antimicrobial agents, and monitoring of strain populations via molecular techniques to identify gonococcal clones that are important for driving the transmission of multidrug-resistant gonococci, become crucial. Additionally, ensuring effective empirical therapy is also essential.

Current guidelines—such as the European guidelines for the diagnosis and treatment of gonorrhea in adults [7], and the Center for Disease Control and Prevention (CDC) Treatment Guidelines for Gonococcal Infection [8], both from 2020—recommend a dual therapy with extended-spectrum cephalosporins (ESCs, such as ceftriaxone or cefixime) and azithromycin for the treatment of uncomplicated gonorrhea when the antimicrobial susceptibility is unknown. Some guidelines recommend fluoroquinolones as an alternative treatment of pharyngeal infections if the isolate is known to be fluoroquinolone-susceptible and there are indications against using ceftriaxone—for instance, history of severe hypersensitivity to cephalosporins [7,9].

Recently, improved methods for the evaluation of the effects of pharmacokinetics (PK) and pharmacodynamics (PD) on treatment outcomes have become available for a number of other infections. In this regard, better data and new research on PK contributors to gonorrhea treatment outcomes are needed [10]. PK/PD analysis integrates information about the concentration of the drug that reaches the infection site and induces the therapeutic response, and the susceptibility of the pathogen to the antibiotic, expressed as the minimum inhibitory concentration (MIC). This allows researchers or clinicians to select the optimal antibiotic and dosing regimen for each infectious process and patient in order to enhance the effect of the antibiotic, minimizing the incidence of side effects and the emergence of resistance [11].

The aim of this work was to apply molecular epidemiology—including whole-genome sequencing (WGS) information, antimicrobial surveillance data, and PK/PD analysis—to guide the antimicrobial treatment of gonococci infections.

2. Materials and Methods

2.1. N. gonorrhoeae Isolates

All isolates from 2017 to 2019 were collected at the Microbiology Service of the University Hospital of Araba (HUA). The hospital, located in the Basque Country (Spain), covers a population of ~400,000 inhabitants, and has 780 beds.

Non-duplicated *N. gonorrhoeae* isolates from patients attending to the Emergency, Infectious Disease, and Primary Care services were included in the study. Gonococcal isolation was performed on chocolate agar PolyViteX VCA and Chocolate agar PVX plates (bioMérieux, Marcy-l'Étoile, France). The suspected colonies were then identified by mass spectrometry using the MALDI-TOF MS (Microflex LT, Bruker-Daltonics, Bremen, Germany) methodology [12].

This study met the exemption criteria of the ethics committee of clinical research because the isolates analyzed were collected in routine practice, and did not allow the identification of patients.

2.2. Antibiotic Susceptibility Testing

Isolated strains were subjected to antibiotic susceptibility testing using the MIC gradient strip tests (Liofilchem, Roseto degli Abruzzi, Italy) according to the manufacturer's instructions. The minimum inhibitory concentrations (MICs) of tetracycline, penicillin, cefixime, ceftriaxone, ciprofloxacin, and azithromycin were determined. From the MIC distribution data of all of the isolates, the calculation of MIC50 and MIC90—i.e., the lowest concentration of the antimicrobial capable of inhibiting 50% and 90% of the isolates, respectively—was performed. Resistance rates were calculated with reference to the European Committee on Antimicrobial Susceptibility Testing (EUCAST) [13] and the Clinical and Laboratory Standards Institute (CLSI) [14]. The current EUCAST MIC breakpoints for penicillin are ≤ 0.06 mg/L (susceptible) and >1 mg/L (resistant); for ceftriaxone and cefixime, ≤ 0.125 mg/L (susceptible) and >0.125 mg/L (resistant); for ciprofloxacin, ≤ 0.03

mg/L (susceptible) and >0.06 mg/L (resistant); and for tetracycline, ≤0.5 mg/L (susceptible) and >1 mg/L (resistant). For azithromycin, the EUCAST epidemiological cutoff (ECOFF) of 1 mg/L was used to identify non-wild-type (WT) isolates. CLSI breakpoints were the following: for penicillin, ≤0.06 mg/L (susceptible), 0.12–1 mg/L (intermediate), and ≥2 mg/L (resistant); for ceftriaxone and cefixime, ≤0.25 mg/L (susceptible); for azithromycin, ≤1 mg/L (susceptible); for ciprofloxacin, ≤0.06 mg/L (susceptible), 0.12–0.5 mg/L (intermediate), and ≥1 mg/L (resistant); and for tetracycline, ≤0.25 mg/L (susceptible), 0.5–1 mg/L (intermediate), and ≥2 mg/L (resistant).

2.3. WGS Molecular Epidemiology and Antimicrobial Resistance Determinants

A subset of 35 strains intermediate or resistant to at least two of the antimicrobials tested were selected to search for resistance genes and genotyping through WGS. The DNA of the strains was extracted using the NucleoSpin Tissue Kit (Macherey-Nagel, Duren, Germany) and sequenced using the Illumina MiSeq platform with the Nextera DNA Flex Library Prep Kit (Illumina, San Diego, CA, USA). The genomic information was received as small nucleotide sequence reads, and longer sequences as contigs. These sequence data were submitted to GenBank under the BioProject accession number PRJNA684048 (https://www.ncbi.nlm.nih.gov/sra/PRJNA684048, accessed on 10 December 2020). Subsequently, the assembled genomes of the isolates were input to the ResFinder 3.2 tool on the CGE website (https://cge.cbs.dtu.dk, accessed on 10 December 2020) for the identification of acquired antimicrobial resistance genes and chromosomal mutations. Default thresholds of 90% identity and 60% gene coverage were employed. Additionally, the PubMLST tool was employed to detect antimicrobial resistance determinants (https://pubmlst.org/neisseria/, accessed on 10 December 2020). Multilocus sequence typing (MLST) and *N. gonorrhoeae* multi-antigen sequence typing (NG-MAST) were performed on the sequences produced by WGS, and they were compared with existing alleles on the Neisseria MLST website (http://pubmlst.org/neisseria/, accessed on 10 December 2020) and NG-MAST (http://www.ng-mast.net/, accessed on 10 December 2020) schemes for the determination of allele numbers and sequence types (STs). All new alleles or STs were submitted to the NG-MAST or MLST website curators to be assigned an allelic number and ST. The genomic epidemiology of the isolates was determined based on whole-genome analysis. An SNP phylogenetic tree, based on FASTQ files, was generated by using the default settings of the MINTyper 1.0 server, available at https://cge.cbs.dtu.dk/services/MINTyper/ (accessed on 10 December 2020). The complete genome of isolate FA1090 (NC_002946.2) was used as a reference. Furthermore, a genome-based clustering was also performed using the TYGS platform, accessible at https://tygs.dsmz.de/ (accessed on 10 December 2020).

2.4. Pharmacokinetic/Pharmacodynamic (PK/PD) Analysis

In order to predict the probability of PK/PD target attainment, different antibiotics and dosing regimens were evaluated (Table 1).

From the published pharmacokinetic parameters listed in Table 1 [15–19], and from the study sample MIC distribution, we estimated the probability of target attainment (PTA, defined as the probability that at least a specific value of a PK/PD index is achieved at a certain minimum inhibitory concentration) and calculated the cumulative fraction of response (CFR, defined as the expected population probability of target attainment for a specific drug dose and a specific population of microorganisms). PK/PD indices and values related to efficacy are also listed in Table 1. Five-thousand-subject Monte Carlo simulations with Oracle® Crystal Ball Fusion Edition v.11.1.2.3.500 (Oracle USA Inc., Redwood City, CA, USA) were used to estimate the PTA and CRF values, indicative of the probability of target success. PTA and CFR ≥ 80% but < 90% were associated with moderate probabilities of success, whereas a CFR ≥ 90% was considered optimal against that bacterial population. More detailed information about the PTA and CFR calculations is presented in the Supplementary Materials.

Table 1. Dose regimen, PK/PD index, and pharmacokinetic parameters used for simulations.

	Ciprofloxacin	Azithromycin	Ceftriaxone	Cefixime
Dose regimen	500 mg single dose, PO	1 g, 2 g single dose, PO	0.25, 0.5, 1 g single dose, IM; 2 g/day, IV	400 mg/day, PO
PK/PD index	$AUC_{0-\infty}/MIC \geq 125$	$AUC_{0-\infty}/MIC \geq 59.5$	$fT_{>MIC} \geq 20$ h (IM); $fT_{>MIC} \geq 60\%$ (IV)	$fT_{>MIC} \geq 60\%$
$AUC_{0-\infty}$ (mg h/L)	10.7 ± 2.6			
CL/F (L/h)		144 ± 39.5		
Ke (h^{-1})			0.082 ± 0.029	0.204 ± 0.02
Vd (L)			14.70 ± 4.93	19 ± 0.03
Fu			0.05	0.35
F			1	0.42 ± 0.045
Ka (h^{-1})			1	0.55
References	[15,16]	[17,18]	[19]	[19]

IM: intramuscular; IV: intravenous; PO: oral; $AUC_{0-\infty}$: area under the plasma concentration vs. time curve from 0 to infinity; CL: clearance; F: bioavailability; Fu: unbound fraction; Ka: absorption constant rate; Ke: elimination constant rate; Vd: volume of distribution.

3. Results

3.1. N. gonorrhoeae Isolates and Antibiotic Susceptibility Testing

A total of 202 isolates of *N. gonorrhoeae* were collected in the study period (2017–2019). Of these, 85% were collected from men, and 15% from women. In men, the urethral exudate was the most common sample (87%); other locations were anal exudate (11%) and pharyngeal exudate (2%). Endocervical (64%) and vaginal exudate (33%) were the most common among women, and anal exudate (1%) was also detected. The average age was 31 years (range 14–67) and 33 years (age range 16–61) for men and women, respectively. A total of 10 patients had *N. gonorrhoeae*-positive cultures in two anatomical sites (7 pharynx and rectum, 3 pharynx and urethra), but only one isolate per patient was included in the susceptibility study.

Table 2 shows the antimicrobial susceptibility of *N. gonorrhoeae* isolates. The higher resistance rates were obtained for ciprofloxacin and tetracycline. Eleven isolates were resistant to azithromycin (5.4% of the total), all of which were collected in 2019. Resistant isolates had MICs of 1.5 mg/L (*n* = 5), 2 mg/L (*n* = 5), and 16 mg/L (*n* = 1). The percentage of isolates resistant to cephalosporins varied depending on the EUCAST and CLSI clinical breakpoints: for cefixime, resistance rates were 6.4% (EUCAST) and 1.6% (CLSI), and for ceftriaxone they were 2.0% (EUCAST) and 0.5% (CLSI). The MIC distribution of the six antibiotics is presented in Figure S1.

Table 2. Antimicrobial susceptibility of 202 *N. gonorrhoeae* isolates collected in 2017–2019 (*n* = 202).

Antimicrobial	MIC Range (mg/L)	MIC$_{50}$ (mg/L)	MIC$_{90}$ (mg/L)	R (%) EUCAST	R (%) CLSI
Penicillin	0.002–64	0.19	3	12.6	12.6
Cefixime	0.008–0.75	0.008	0.047	6.4	1.6
Ceftriaxone	0.002–0.5	0.008	0.094	2.0	0.5
Azithromycin	0.016–16	0.19	0.75	5.4 [a]	5.4
Ciprofloxacin	0.015–64	0.012	8	48.2	45.2
Tetracycline	0.9->256	1	32	34.2	34.2

MIC: minimum inhibitory concentration; MIC50 and MIC90: minimum inhibitory concentration at which 50% and 90% of the isolates were inhibited, respectively; R: percentage of resistant isolates. [a]: According to the epidemiological cutoff (ECOFF) value.

3.2. Genotyping: MLST and NG-MAST

MLST genotyping identified multiple distinct populations of *N. gonorrhoeae* in the isolates of HUA in 2017–2019 (Table 3). Overall, a total of 20 MLST STs were identified among the 35 isolates analyzed, with ST-9363 being the most common (*n* = 8), followed by ST-7363 (*n* = 4) and ST-7822 (*n* = 3), while 14 STs were represented by a single isolate.

Two new MLST STs (ST-14274 and ST-14304) were previously unreported, and resulted from combinations of known alleles. NG-MAST further discriminated between strains with identical MLST-STs, and 27 different NG-MAST STs were observed among the 35 isolates analyzed. ST-6765 predominated ($n = 7$), ST-470 and ST-13070 were observed in two isolates, and the remaining STs were represented by single isolates. Additionally, six NG-MAST STs (17.1%) were previously unreported, and resulted from new combinations of known alleles.

Table 3. Genotypes, MICs, and antimicrobial resistance determinants for the 35 *Neisseria gonorrhoeae* isolates sequenced by WGS.

Isolate	Year	Genotype			Susceptibility (mg/L)					Acquired Gene	Chromosomal Mutations								
		MLST	NG-MAST	P	CRO	CFM	TET	CIP	AZM		PBP2	PBP1	PorB	GyrA	ParC	S10	mtrR Promoter [a]	MtrR	23S rRNA
2	2017	10,314	12,547	0.25	0.016	nd	0.5	3	0.125	-	Type V non-mosaic	L421P	-	S91F, D95A	S87R	V57M	-	A39T	-
3	2017	1588	3750	0.38	0.023	nd	64	8	0.125	tet(M)	Type XIX non-mosaic	L421P	G120K, A121G	S91F, D95A	S87R	V57M	-	A39T	-
6	2017	1596	19,728	0.125	0.008	nd	0.125	0.006	0.25	-	Type 81 semi Mosaic	-	-	-	-	-	-35A Del	-	-
9	2017	1583	19,729	0.125	0.006	nd	0.25	0.004	0.125	-	Type II non-mosaic	-	-	-	-	V57M	G	-	-
11	2017	14,274	587	0.19	0.008	nd	0.5	0.006	0.75	-	Type II non-mosaic	-	-	-	-	V57M	-	-	-
17	2017	1567	13,971	>32	0.012	nd	24	1.5	0.094	blaTEM-1B, tet(M)	Type XIV non-mosaic	-	-	-	D86N	V57M	-	-	-
19	2017	10,935	15,728	2	0.006	nd	24	0.003	0.032	blaTEM-1B, tet(M)	Type XIV non-mosaic	-	-	-	-	V57M	-	-	-
24	2017	8145	19,730	2	0.004	nd	0.5	0.004	0.125	blaTEM-1B	Type XIV non-mosaic	-	-	-	-	V57M	-	-	-
31	2017	7363	11,547	0.5	0.094	nd	1	>32	0.094	-	Type X mosaic	L421P	G120N, A121G	S91F, D95N	S87R, S88P	V57M	-	-	-
33	2017	7363	13,070	0.75	0.125	nd	1	>32	0.25	-	Type X mosaic	L421P	G120N, A121G	S91F, D95N	S87R, S88P	V57M	-	-	-
35	2017	8143	14,306	0.125	0.008	nd	1	8	0.125	-	Type II non-mosaic	L421P	-	S91F, D95A	S87R	V57M	-	A39T	-
50	2018	14,304	13,070	0.5	0.125	nd	1	>32	0.125	-	Type X mosaic	L421P	G120N, A121G	S91F, D95N	S87R, S88P	V57M	-	-	-
51	2018	7363	9184	0.38	0.064	0.016	1.5	8	0.25	-	Type IX mosaic	L421P	G120N, A121G	S91F, D95G	E91G	V57M	-35A Del	-	-
52	2018	1901	1407	0.75	0.25	-	3	>32	0.5	-	Type XXXIV mosaic	L421P	G120N, A121N	S91F, D95G	S87R	V57M	-35A Del	-	-
56	2018	10,890	1407	0.5	0.125	-	4	>32	0.5	-	Type XXXIV mosaic	L421P	G120N, A121N	S91F, D95G	S87R	V57M	-35A Del	-	-
58	2018	1901	19,111	0.5	0.125	-	2	>32	0.5	-	Type XXXIV mosaic	L421P	G120N, A121N	S91F, D95G	S87R	V57M	-35A Del	-	-
59	2018	1583	217	>32	0.006	nd	64	16	0.064	blaTEM-1B, tet(M)	Type II non-mosaic	-	G120N, A121D	S91F, D95G	D86N	V57M	-35A Del	G45D	-
61	2018	7363	15,198	0.25	0.064	nd	2	8	0.25	-	Type IX non-mosaic	L421P	G120N, A121N	S91F, D95G	E91G	V57M	-	-	-
7244	2018	11428	2992	0.025	0.008	0.016	0.25	0.016	0.75	-	Type II non-mosaic	-	G120K, A121N	-	-	V57M	G	A39T	-
8661	2018	15,573	17,371	0.125	0.012	0.016	2	0.016	1	-	Type II non-mosaic	-	G120K, A121N	-	-	V57M	G	-	-
293	2019	9363	6765	0.19	0.012	<0.016	2	0.012	1	-	Type II non-mosaic	-	A121N	-	-	V57M	G	-	-
1941	2019	1580	470	0.125	0.03	0.016	2	0.002	1.5	-	Type 93 semi Mosaic	-	A121S	-	-	V57M	G	-	-
1943	2019	1580	470	0.125	0.008	<0.016	2	0.002	1.5	-	Type 93 semi Mosaic	-	A121S	-	-	V57M	G	-	-
3023	2019	9363	6765	0.25	0.016	<0.016	1.5	0.008	2	-	Type II non-mosaic	-	G120K, A121N	-	-	V57M	G	-	C2599T
3526	2019	9363	6765	0.19	0.023	<0.016	3	0.008	0.75	-	Type II non-mosaic	-	G120K, A121N	-	-	V57M	G	-	C2599T
3569	2019	9363	6765	0.38	0.012	<0.016	2	0.016	2	-	Type II non-mosaic	-	G120K, A121N	-	-	V57M	G	A39T	-
3700	2019	11,706	17,972	0.19	0.003	<0.016	1.5	2	0.75	-	Type V non-mosaic	L421P	-	S91F, D95A	S87R	V57M	-	A39T	-
4458	2019	13,292	9208	0.094	0.004	nd	2	0.003	0.75	-	Type II non-mosaic	-	-	-	-	V57M	G	A39T	-
4315	2019	9363	6765	0.38	0.016	0.032	3	0.008	1.5	-	Type II non-mosaic	-	G120K, A121N	-	-	V57M	G	-	C2611T
4726	2019	9363	6765	0.19	0.016	<0.016	3	0.008	1	-	Type II non-mosaic	-	G120K, A121N	-	-	V57M	G	-	-
5903	2019	7822	14,994	0.25	0.023	<0.016	1	4	1	-	Type V non-mosaic	-	-	S91F, D95A	S87R	V57M	-	A39T	-
7079	2019	9363	6765	0.125	0.008	<0.016	1.5	0.012	1.5	-	Type II non-mosaic	-	G120K, A121N	-	-	V57M	G	-	-
7181	2019	9363	19,731	0.19	0.016	<0.016	3	0.004	1.5	-	Type II non-mosaic	-	G120K, A121N	-	-	V57M	G	-	-
7789	2019	7822	14,994	0.125	0.012	<0.016	0.75	2	1	-	Type V non-mosaic	L421P	-	S91F, D95A	S87R	V57M	G	A39T	-
9051	2019	7822	14,994	0.38	0.016	<0.016	1.5	6	1.5	-	Type V non-mosaic	L421P	-	S91F, D95A	S87R	V57M	G	A39T	-

P: penicillin; CRO: ceftriaxone; CFM: cefixime; TET: tetracycline; CIP: ciprofloxacin; AZ: azithromycin; nd: no data available; -: wild type. [a] G, deletion of one G (guanine), 20 nucleotides downstream of where the -35A deletion occurs.

3.3. Antimicrobial Resistance Determinants

Genomic markers associated with resistance to ciprofloxacin, tetracycline, β-lactams, and azithromycin were found (Table 3). All of the ciprofloxacin-resistant strains investigated presented two substitutions in GyrA and one or two substitutions in ParC. At GyrA, they presented substitutions in positions 91 (all presented an S91F) and 95 (D95A/G/N). The main amino acid substitution observed in ParC was S87R ($n = 13$), either alone, or associated with S88P. Other substitutions included D86N and E91G.

The *tetM* gene was detected in the four highly tetracycline-resistant strains (MIC $\geq$ 24 mg/L). The V57M substitution in the ribosomal protein S10 subunit encoded by the *rpsJ* gene was detected in 33/35 (94.3%) of the strains investigated, irrespective of their tetracycline susceptibility. Chromosomal mutations in the *porB* gene were also found in tetracycline-resistant strains. The G120K substitution was detected in 14 isolates, and was associated with A121G/N/D.

The only sequenced isolate resistant to ceftriaxone (MIC: 0.25 mg/L) presented the *penA* mosaic allele XXXIV associated with an L421P substitution in PBP1, a G120K/A121N in the PorB, and an adenine deletion (-35A Del) in the *mtrR* promoter.

Twenty-five isolates showed different degrees of penicillin resistance. The four high-level penicillin-resistant strains ($n = 4$; MIC $\geq$ 2 mg/L) carried the *bla*$_{TEM-1B}$ gene, which encodes the TEM-1 β-lactamase; these four strains were β-lactamase producers, as determined by the nitrocefin test. The remaining isolates ($n = 21$) presented an MIC range between 0.19 and 0.75 mg/L. Nineteen isolates were associated with non-mosaic *penA* alleles, with non-mosaic II being the most common ($n = 10$); the remaining six isolates were associated with mosaic *penA* alleles (mosaic X and XXXIV, $n = 3$ each). The major amino acid substitution observed in the PBP1 protein was Leu421Pro ($n = 13$), which was correlated with a degree of intermediate resistance. Simultaneous substitutions at amino acids G120 and A121 in the PorB porin—associated with decreased intake of several antimicrobials—were observed in 16 penicillin-resistant isolates, with the substitutions of G120K/A121N being the most common ($n = 10$).

The 13 isolates with an MIC of 1–2 mg/L against azithromycin were associated with mutations in the promoter region and coding sequence of the *mtrR* genes, and with mutations in the gene encoding the 23S rRNA. Two isolates presented the C2599T mutation in the 23S rRNA gene associated with a G45D substitution in the MtrR protein. A deletion of one guanine (G), 20 nucleotides downstream of the -35A deletion, was observed in the *mtrR* promoter of 11 isolates; their sequences showed a 98.48% identity with that of strain 38,194 (GenBank accession number KT954125), and 86.36% with strain FA1090 (GenBank accession number NC_002946). The -35A deletion in the repeated sequence of the *mtrR* promoter was not observed in the resistant isolates; however, it was observed in six susceptible isolates (MIC, <0.5 mg/L) as the only mechanism related to azithromycin resistance. In the MtrR protein, the amino acid substitutions of A39T ($n = 3$) and G45D ($n = 2$) were detected in azithromycin-resistant strains. The alignment of partial sequences is presented in Supplementary Figure S2.

Whole-genome SNP-based phylogenetic analysis of the 35 sequenced isolates revealed a great genetic dissimilarity between isolates, with differences ranging from 0 to 2378 SNPs; however, three clades involving non-azithromycin-susceptible isolates were identified (Figure 1). Clade 1 consisted of three isolates belonging to MLST ST-7822, with an Ala39Thr substitution in the *MtrR* gene and a deletion of one G, 20 nucleotides downstream of where the -35A deletion occurs; no SNP differences were observed. Clade 2 consisted of two isolates belonging to MLST ST-1580, with the C2599T mutation in the *23S rRNA* gene and a Gly45Thr substitution in the *MtrR* gene; no SNP differences were observed. Clade 3 consisted of eight closely related isolates belonging to MLST ST-9363, with a deletion of one G, 20 nucleotides downstream of where the -35A deletion occurs; differences between these isolates ranged from 0 to 20 SNPs. The same three clusters were obtained when the phylogenetic tree was constructed from the whole genome (data not shown).

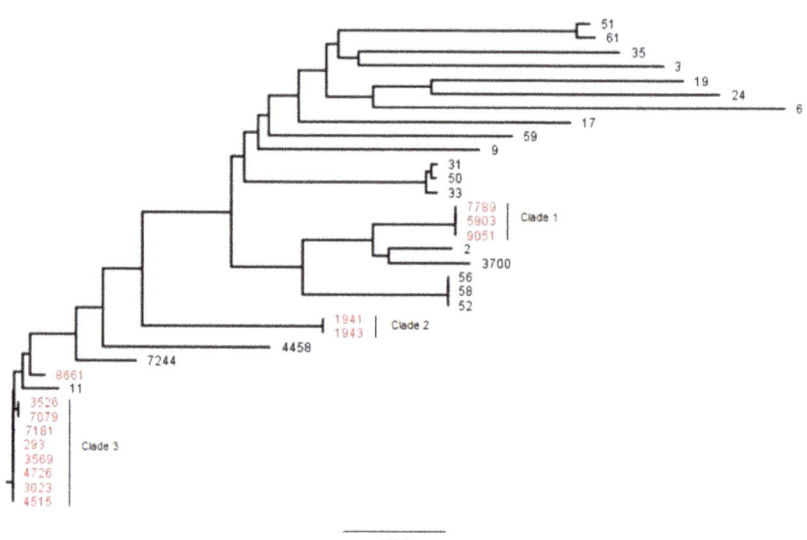

Figure 1. Clustering of the 35 *N. gonorrhoeae* sequences obtained by WGS, based on genome SNPs; red indicates non-azithromycin-susceptible isolates.

3.4. Pharmacokinetic/Pharmacodynamic (PK/PD) Analysis

Figure 2 shows the probability of target attainment (PTA) values of all of the antimicrobial agents studied, as well as their MIC distribution. On the basis of the simulation results, and taking into account the targets for the different antimicrobial agents, PTA values equal to or higher than 90% were achieved with (1) azithromycin at single doses of 1 g and 2 g, for MICs up to 0.064 and 0.125 mg/L, respectively; (2) ceftriaxone at 250, 500, and 1000 g, administered intramuscularly as single doses, for MICs up to 0.064, 0.125, and 0.25 mg/L, respectively, and for MICs equal to or lower than 1 mg/L for 2 g/day via the intravenous route; (3) cefixime at 400 mg/day by oral route, for MICs up to 0.125 mg/L; and (4) single oral doses of ciprofloxacin at 500 mg, for MICs up to 0.125 mg/L.

Table 4 features the CFR values obtained after the PK/PD analysis and Monte Carlo simulations. Values higher than 90% were only achieved with the two cephalosporins.

Table 4. Cumulative fraction of response (CFR) calculated for all antibiotics and dosing regimens.

Antibiotic	Dosing Regimen	CFR (%)
Ciprofloxacin	500 mg, single dose, PO	51
Azithromycin	1 g single dose, PO	33
	2 g single dose, PO	64
Ceftriaxone	1 g, single dose, IM	100
	500 mg, single dose, IM	98
	250 mg, single dose, IM	96
	2 g/day, IV	100
Cefixime	400 mg/day, PO	97

PO: oral administration; IM: intramuscular; IV: intravenous.

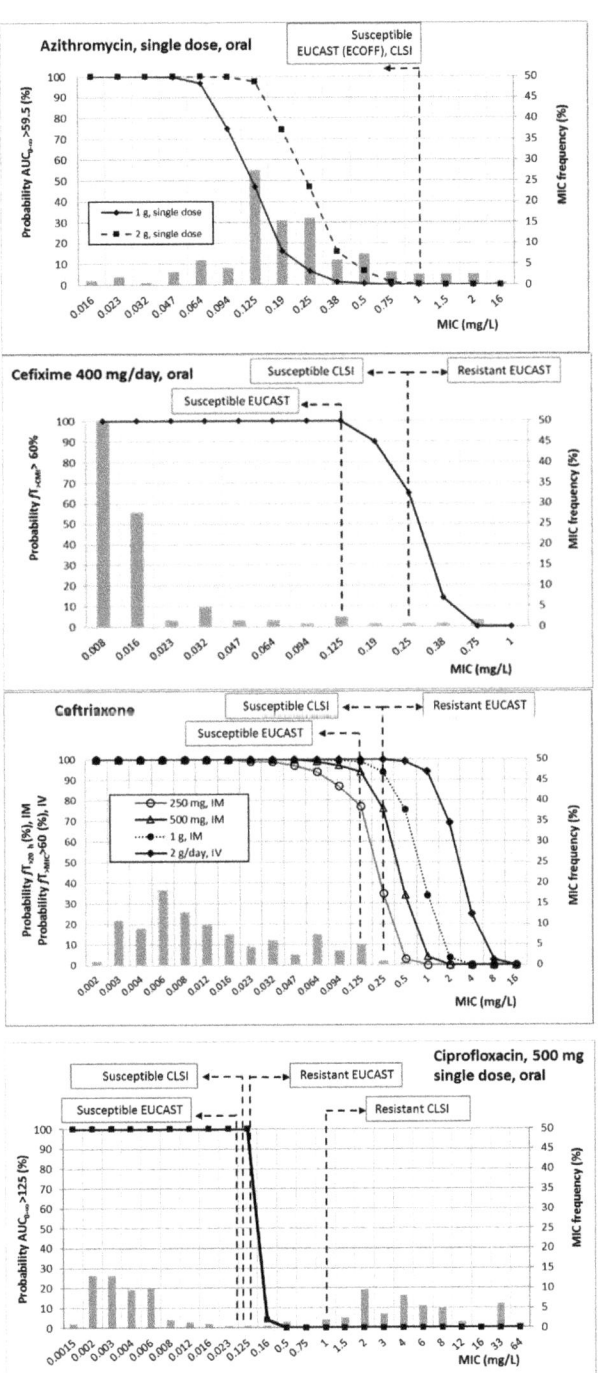

Figure 2. Probability of target attainment (PTA) of azithromycin, ceftriaxone, cefixime, and ciprofloxacin. Grey bars: MIC frequency.

In supplementary Tables S2–S9, the mean, median, and 2.5% and 97.5% confidence intervals of PTA and CFR for every antimicrobial and dosing regimen are presented.

4. Discussion

To address the antimicrobial resistance problem, more efficient means of evaluating therapies for gonorrhea are needed. Our purpose in this study was to apply molecular epidemiology—including whole-genome sequencing (WGS) information, antimicrobial surveillance data, and PK/PD analysis—to guide the antimicrobial treatment of gonococci infections in the Basque Country (Spain).

In this region of the north of Spain, the percentage of resistance was of the same order as recent data obtained from Madrid [20] and Barcelona [21,22], and also of those reported in other European countries [23]. As expected, the highest percentage of resistance was detected for ciprofloxacin (>45%). The historical resistance of gonococci to ciprofloxacin is very well known, and it has been related to the incidence of gonorrhea at the population level. In fact, ciprofloxacin is no longer recommended for treatment of this STI, except for pharyngeal infections if susceptibility has been proven or if the patient is allergic to β-lactams [9].

In spite of the differences in the resistance breakpoint between EUCAST [13] and CLSI [14] for ciprofloxacin (0.125 and 1 mg/L, respectively), the percentage resistance we obtained was similar, since very few isolates are affected by the discrepancies in the breakpoints (Figure 1). However, discrepancies in the clinical breakpoint for cephalosporins (0.25 mg/L from EUCAST and 0.5 mg/L from CLSI) justify the difference in the percentage resistance for cefixime (6.5% vs. 1.6%) and ceftriaxone (2.0% vs. 0.5%). Unlike the other antibiotics, all isolates resistant to azithromycin were collected in 2019 ($n = 11$). These data are consistent with the recent increase in the resistance of *N. gonorrhoeae* to azithromycin in Spain and worldwide [22,23]. Some studies support the notion that the selection/induction of azithromycin resistance in *N. gonorrhoeae* may be associated with the general use of azithromycin for the treatment of respiratory infections or non-gonococcal urethritis [24]. According to the susceptibility profile, azithromycin and cephalosporins are the most active antimicrobials. These results are in agreement with the European guidelines, which recommend the use of a dual therapy with ceftriaxone and azithromycin for all gonorrhea cases [7].

Antibiotic susceptibility data were consistent with those obtained through WGS, and the mutations detected were related to resistance to the studied antibiotics. The genomic study detected the main antimicrobial resistance determinants associated with resistance to β-lactams (*penA*, *porB*, *ponA*, *mtrR*, and *bla*$_{TEM1-B}$), ciprofloxacin (*gyrA* and *parC*), and tetracycline (*tetM* and *rpsJ*). All ciprofloxacin-resistant strains presented two substitutions in GyrA, together with substitutions in the ParC protein, while among the ciprofloxacin-susceptible isolates, no mutations in the *gyrA* and *parC* genes were detected, as previously reported [25]. Regarding ceftriaxone—and as expected—the mutations found in the analyzed resistant isolates were associated with reduced susceptibility or resistance to ESC [26]. Tetracycline resistance in *N. gonorrhoeae* may be related to the presence of the plasmid-mediated TetM protein (MIC, 16–64 mg/L), or to mutations in some chromosomal genes (MIC, 2–4 mg/L) [27,28]. In our study, the *tetM* gene was detected only in high-level resistant isolates; meanwhile, low-level resistant isolates only presented mutations in the chromosomal genes *penB* (PorB), *rpsJ* (S10), and *mtrR* and its promoter. These isolates presented at least two or three mutated genes, suggesting that more than one antimicrobial resistance determinant is needed to confer resistance.

Resistance to β-lactams, macrolides, and tetracycline may result from overexpression of the MtrCDE efflux pump related to mutations in the promoter and/or coding regions of the *mtrR* repressor, which causes not only resistance, but also an increase in the MIC [25]. The -35A deletion in the promoter sequence—the most common mutation—was detected only in isolates recovered in 2017 and 2018, but it was not observed in those from 2019. Several mutations—including insertions, deletions, or transversions—have been described in this promoter region [29]. Related to azithromycin resistance, a guanine (G) deletion in this promoter was observed in most of the azithromycin-resistant isolates, either alone or associated with the A39T substitution in MtrR repressor. In some isolates, this mutation was associated with substitutions in the MtrD protein (data not shown), so the exact contribution of this G deletion to antimicrobial resistance should be determined.

The majority of genotyped azithromycin-resistant isolates were MLST ST-9363. In a recent study carried out in Barcelona (Spain) [22], this genotype was associated with outbreaks of *N. gonorrhoeae* with high-level azithromycin resistance (MIC $\geq$ 256 mg/L) between 2016 and 2018. In that study, this genotype was found mainly in men who have sex with men. Contrary to Barcelona isolates, our ST-9363 isolates were not high-level azithromycin resistant, and their MIC values were 1 and 2 mg/L. The phylogenetic analysis of both the SNPs and the complete genome using the WGS showed similar results and, together with the application of the other epidemiological markers and antibiotic resistance, allowed the epidemiological characterization of the strains analyzed. The joint analysis of the data obtained from the WGS allowed the detection of three clusters that involved eight, three, and two non-azithromycin-susceptible isolates, respectively, all of them isolated in 2019 and with an MIC $\geq$ 1 mg/L to azithromycin.

Among the interventions to mitigate the current and future impact of antimicrobial resistance, the development of new generations of antimicrobials is one of the most accepted. Another recognized strategy to diminish antibiotic resistance is the optimization of the dosing regimen of available antimicrobials. PK/PD analysis and Monte Carlo simulation have shown to be very useful tools to select adequate antibiotic dosages, with the goal of increasing treatment efficacy and reducing the risk of multidrug-resistant pathogens [30]. Although integrated PK/PD analysis has been applied to identify changes in the antimicrobial activity of antibiotics [31,32], until now it has not been applied to gonorrhea for optimizing dosage and correlating exposure with clinical outcomes [33]. Therefore, by using Monte Carlo simulation, we evaluated the probability of PK/PD target attainment by MIC (PTA), as well as taking into account the MIC distribution (CFR), which is indicative of treatment success.

At EUCAST susceptibility breakpoints, all antibiotics except for azithromycin and the lowest dose of ceftriaxone provided high (>90%) probability of treatment success (Figure 2). Moreover, the highest doses of ceftriaxone also showed adequate results for higher MICs (1 g IM would cover an MIC of 0.25 mg/L, and 2 g/day IV would cover an MIC of 1 mg/L). Regarding azithromycin in monotherapy, 1 g would be an option only when the MIC is 0.064 mg/L or lower, and 2 g if the MIC is equal to or lower than 0.125 mg/L.

Empirical treatments with antimicrobial drugs (i.e., without susceptibility testing) provide progressive development of decreasing susceptibility, which threatens personal and public health. The estimation of CFR is a very useful tool to guide empirical treatments, since it allows us to know which antimicrobial and dose regimen would have the best likelihood of success to treat bacterial isolates from a particular hospital or geographical area. Considering the MIC distribution of our isolates, CFR values—indicative of the probability of empirical treatment success (Table 4)—allow us to confirm that ceftriaxone (even at the lowest dose: 250 mg) and oral cefixime are good candidates to empirically treat gonorrhea (CFR around 100%) in our geographical area. On the other hand, ciprofloxacin should not be used empirically. For both ESCs and ciprofloxacin, the probability of treatment success was correlated with the susceptibility rate. However, the susceptibility rate of azithromycin was much higher than the estimated CFR. This discrepancy may be explained in part by the fact that, in contrast to β-lactams—which do not accumulate within the cell (extracelluar: intracellular ratio of 1)—azithromycin achieves intracellular concentrations several-fold higher than in plasma and extracellular fluid [34]. Taking into account that *N. gonorrhoeae* presents intracellular localization, the treatment success of azithromycin may be underestimated.

Our results are consistent with the European guidelines for the diagnosis and treatment of gonorrhea in adults [7], and with the CDC [8], both of which recommend ceftriaxone monotherapy for the treatment of uncomplicated gonorrhoeae. Because *N. gonorrhoeae* remains highly susceptible to ceftriaxone, and azithromycin resistance is increasing, prudent use of antimicrobial agents supports limiting their use. In spite of that, continuous monitoring for the emergence of resistance to this cephalosporin is necessary in order to ensure the efficacy of the recommended regimens. In this sense, surveillance programs and health care provider reports of treatment failures are essential.

For empirical treatment, the WHO recommends that the selected gonorrhea treatment should have ≥95% probability of being effective—that is, 5% or fewer of gonococcal isolates are likely to be resistant to the antimicrobial used for first-line empirical treatment [35]. In our opinion, PK/PD analysis must be also considered; in this sense, the selection of the most adequate antibiotic and dosing regimen should be based on local epidemiology. Moreover, PK/PD analysis results are also beneficial when the MIC value is known, and in the case of ceftriaxone, would allow the selection of lower doses. In previous studies, PK/PD analysis has been shown to be a useful tool for the surveillance of antimicrobial activity, as a complement to the simple assessment of MIC values [32,36–38]. Thus, it could be applied to guide therapy along with surveillance programs of gonococcal resistance. In this sense, the surveillance of gonococcal antimicrobial resistance could be implemented with PK/PD analysis by using the susceptibility data collected by the Euro-GASP.

This study presents some limitations. First, PK/PD analysis was performed by using the mean and standard deviation of the PK parameters, without considering the potential influence of covariates on the PK profile; second, our simulations are based on plasma concentrations and, therefore, dosing recommendations may be more beneficial for gonococcal bacteremia than for extragenital infection.

In spite of these limitations, our study represents a good example of how to combine molecular epidemiology, antimicrobial surveillance, and PK/PD analysis to provide quality data to support treatment guidelines—especially empirical treatments.

5. Conclusions

In our geographical area, multiple distinct populations of *N. gonorrhoeae* were identified. We can confirm that ceftriaxone (even at the lowest dose: 250 mg) and oral cefixime are good candidates to treat gonorrhea. For patients allergic to β-lactam antibiotics, or with pharyngeal infections, ciprofloxacin should be only used if the MIC is known and is equal to or lower than 0.125 mg/L; this antimicrobial is not recommended to be used empirically.

Supplementary Materials: The following are available online at https://www.mdpi.com/article/10.3390/pharmaceutics13101699/s1, Figure S1: MIC frequency of all antimicrobials studie. Figure S2: Alignment of partial sequences of the *mtrR* promoter from *Neisseria gonorrhoeae* FA1090 (GenBank accession number NC_002946), *Neisseria gonorrhoeae* 38197 (GenBank accession number KT954125), and some *N. gonorrhoeae* isolates from this study. The -10 and -35 promoter sequences for the *mtrR* gene are shown in overlines. The 13-bp inverted repeat (IR) is underlined. Lowercase letters represent the single-base-pair deletion (-35A Del) within the IR. *—location of the single base-pair deletion (G) 20 nucleotides downstream of where the -35A deletion occurs; Table S1: Dose regimen, PK/PD index, and pharmacokinetic parameters used for simulations; Table S2: Probability of target attainment (PTA) and cumulative fraction of response (CFR) of ciprofloxacin, 500 mg, single dose, oral administration; Table S3: Probability of target attainment (PTA) and cumulative fraction of response (CFR) of azithromycin, 1 g, single dose, oral administration; Table S4: Probability of target attainment (PTA) and cumulative fraction of response (CFR) of azithromycin, 2 g, single dose, oral administration; Table S5: Probability of target attainment (PTA) and cumulative fraction of response (CFR) of ceftriaxone, 250 mg, single dose, intramuscular administration; Table S6: Probability of target attainment (PTA) and cumulative fraction of response (CFR) of ceftriaxone, 500 mg, single dose, intramuscular administration; Table S7: Probability of target attainment (PTA) and cumulative fraction of response (CFR) of ceftriaxone, 1 g, single dose, intramuscular administration; Table S8: Probability of target attainment (PTA) and cumulative fraction of response (CFR) of ceftriaxone, 2 g/day, intravenous administration; Table S9: Probability of target attainment (PTA) and cumulative fraction of response (CFR) of cefixime, 400 mg/day, oral administration.

Author Contributions: Conceptualization, R.A., A.R.-G., J.G. and A.C.; data curation, A.R.-A., A.A.-Q., A.A. and I.M.-B.; formal analysis, R.A., I.M.-B. and A.R.-G.; funding acquisition, A.R.-G. and J.G.; investigation, R.A., J.G. and A.C.; methodology, R.A., A.A.-Q., A.A. and I.M.-B.; project administration, A.C.; supervision, A.R.-G. and J.G.; validation, A.C.; writing—original draft, R.A., A.R.-G. and A.C.; writing—review and editing, R.A., A.R.-A., A.A.-Q., A.A., A.R.-G., I.M.-B., J.G. and A.C. All authors have read and agreed to the published version of the manuscript.

Funding: This research was funded by the University of the Basque Country UPV/EHU (GIU20/048; PA20/03), Spain.

Institutional Review Board Statement: Not applicable.

Informed Consent Statement: Not applicable.

Data Availability Statement: The data presented in this study are available in Supplementary Materials.

Acknowledgments: We thank Irati Miguel from SGIKER, UPV/EHU, Spain, and Javier Gamboa from Biogenetics, Spain, for their technical advice and the performance of the sequencing procedure.

Conflicts of Interest: The authors declare no conflict of interest in the interpretation of data, in the writing of the manuscript, or in the decision to publish the results.

References

1. Fasciana, T.; Capra, G.; Di Carlo, P.; Calà, C.; Vella, M.; Pistone, G.; Colomba, C.; Giammanco, A. Socio-Demographic Characteristics and Sexual Behavioral Factors of Patients with Sexually Transmitted Infections Attending a Hospital in Southern Italy. *Int. J. Environ. Res. Public Health* **2021**, *18*, 4722. [CrossRef]
2. World Health Organization, WHO. *Antimicrobial Resistance: Global Report on Surveillance*; World Health Organization: Geneva, Switzerland, 2014.
3. Chesson, H.W.; Kirkcaldy, R.D.; Gift, T.L.; Owusu-Edusei, K., Jr.; Weinstock, H.S. Ciprofloxacin resistance and gonorrhea incidence rates in 17 cities, United States, 1991–2006. *Emerg. Infect. Dis.* **2014**, *20*, 612–619. [CrossRef] [PubMed]
4. Hook, E.W., 3rd; Kirkcaldy, R.D. A Brief History of Evolving Diagnostics and Therapy for Gonorrhea: Lessons Learned. *Clin. Infect. Dis.* **2018**, *67*, 1294–1299. [CrossRef]
5. World Health Organization, WHO. *Report on Global Sexually Transmitted Infection Surveillance*; World Health Organization: Geneva, Switzerland, 2018; Available online: https://www.who.int/reproductivehealth/publications/stis-surveillance-2018/en/ (accessed on 3 August 2021).
6. Cole, M.J.; Quinten, C.; Jacobsson, S.; Amato-Gauci, A.J.; Woodford, N.; Spiteri, G.; Unemo, M.; Euro-GASP Network. The European gonococcal antimicrobial surveillance programme (Euro-GASP) appropriately reflects the antimicrobial resistance situation for *Neisseria gonorrhoeae* in the European Union/European Economic Area. *BMC Infect. Dis.* **2019**, *19*, 1040. [CrossRef] [PubMed]
7. Unemo, M.; Ross, J.; Serwin, A.B.; Gomberg, M.; Cusini, M.; Jensen, J.S. Background review for the '2020 European guideline for the diagnosis and treatment of gonorrhoea in adults'. *Int. J. STD AIDS* **2021**, *32*, 108–126. [CrossRef] [PubMed]
8. St Cyr, S.; Barbee, L.; Workowski, K.A.; Bachmann, L.H.; Pham, C.; Schlanger, K.; Torrone, E.; Weinstock, H.; Kersh, E.N.; Thorpe, P. Update to CDC's Treatment Guidelines for Gonococcal Infection, 2020. *MMWR Morb. Mortal. Wkly. Rep.* **2020**, *69*, 1911–1916. [CrossRef]
9. Unemo, M. Current and future antimicrobial treatment of gonorrhoea—The rapidly evolving *Neisseria gonorrhoeae* continues to challenge. *BMC Infect. Dis.* **2015**, *15*, 364. [CrossRef]
10. Hook, E.W.; Newman, L.; Drusano, G.; Evans, S.; Handsfield, H.H.; Jerse, A.E.; Kong, F.Y.S.; Lee, J.Y.; Taylor, S.N.; Deal, C. Development of New Antimicrobials for Urogenital Gonorrhea Therapy: Clinical Trial Design Considerations. *Clin. Infect Dis.* **2020**, *70*, 1495–1500. [CrossRef] [PubMed]
11. Asín-Prieto, E.; Rodríguez-Gascón, A.; Isla, A. Applications of the pharmacokinetic/pharmacodynamic (PK/PD) analysis of antimicrobial agents. *J. Infect. Chemother.* **2015**, *21*, 319–329. [CrossRef]
12. Caruso, G.; Giammanco, A.; Virruso, R.; Fasciana, T. Current and Future Trends in the Laboratory Diagnosis of Sexually Transmitted Infections. *Int. J. Environ. Res. Public Health* **2021**, *18*, 1038. [CrossRef]
13. The European Committee on Antimicrobial Susceptibility Testing. Breakpoint Tables for Interpretation of MICs and Zone Diameters. Version 10.0. 2020. Available online: http://www.eucast.org (accessed on 3 August 2021).
14. CLSI. *Performance Standards for Antimicrobial Susceptibility Testing*, 30th ed.; CLSI Supplement M100; Clinical and Laboratory Standards Institute: Wayne, PA, USA, 2020.
15. Lettieri, J.T.; Rogge, M.C.; Kaiser, L.; Echols, R.M.; Heller, A.H. Pharmacokinetic profiles of ciprofloxacin after single intravenous and oral doses. *Antimicrob. Agents Chemother.* **1992**, *36*, 993–996. [CrossRef]

16. Koomanachai, P.; Bulik, C.C.; Kuti, J.L.; Nicolau, D.P. Pharmacodynamic modeling of intravenous antibiotics against gram-negative bacteria collected in the United States. *Clin. Ther.* **2010**, *32*, 766–779. [CrossRef]
17. Dumitrescu, T.P.; Anic-Milic, T.; Oreskovic, K.; Padovan, J.; Brouwer, K.L.R.; Zuo, P.; Schmith, V.D. Development of a population pharmacokinetic model to describe azithromycin whole-blood and plasma concentrations over time in healthy subjects. *Antimicrob. Agents Chemother.* **2013**, *57*, 3194–3201. [CrossRef]
18. Soda, M.; Ito, S.; Matsumaru, N.; Matsumaru, N.; Nakamura, S.; Nagase, I.; Takahashi, H.; Ohno, Y.; Yasuda, M.; Yamamoto, M.; et al. Evaluation of the microbiological efficacy of a single 2-gram dose of extended-release azithromycin by population pharmacokinetics and simulation in japanese patients with gonococcal urethritis. *Antimicrob. Agents Chemother.* **2017**, *62*, e01409-17. [CrossRef]
19. Chisholm, S.A.; Mouton, J.W.; Lewis, D.A.; Nichols, T.; Ison, C.A.; Livermore, D.M. Cephalosporin MIC creep among gonococci: Time for a pharmacodynamic rethink? *J. Antimicrob. Chemother.* **2010**, *65*, 2141–2148. [CrossRef]
20. Guerrero-Torres, M.D.; Menéndez, M.B.; Guerras, C.S.; Tello, E.; Ballesteros, J.; Clavo, P.; Puerta, T.; Vera, M.; Ayerdi, O.; Carrio, J.C.; et al. Epidemiology, molecular characterisation and antimicrobial susceptibility of *Neisseria gonorrhoeae* isolates in Madrid, Spain, in 2016. *Epidemiol. Infect.* **2019**, *147*, e274. [CrossRef] [PubMed]
21. Salmerón, P.; Viñado, B.; El Ouazzani, R.; Hernández, M.; Barbera, M.J.; Alberny, M.; Jané, M.; Larrosa, N.; Pumarola, T.; Hoyos-Mallecot, Y. Antimicrobial susceptibility of *Neisseria gonorrhoeae* in Barcelona during a five-year period, 2013 to 2017. *Eur. Surveill.* **2020**, *25*, 1900576. [CrossRef]
22. Salmerón, P.; Moreno-Mingorance, A.; Trejo, J.; Amado, R.; Viñado, B.; Cornejo-Sanchez, T.; Alberny, M.; Barbera, M.J.; Arando, M.; Pumarola, T.; et al. Emergence and dissemination of three mild outbreaks of *Neisseria gonorrhoeae* with high-level resistance to azithromycin in Barcelona, 2016–2018. *J. Antimicrob. Chemother.* **2021**, *76*, 930–935. [CrossRef]
23. Unemo, M.; Lahra, M.M.; Cole, M.M.; Galarza, P.; Ndowa, F.; Martin, I.; Dillon, I.A.R.; Ramon-Pardo, P.; Bolan, G.; Ti, T.W. World Health Organization Global Gonococcal Antimicrobial Surveillance Program (WHO GASP): Review of new data and evidence to inform international collaborative actions and research efforts. *Sex Health* **2019**, *16*, 412–425. [CrossRef] [PubMed]
24. Unemo, M.; Workowski, K. Dual antimicrobial therapy for gonorrhoea: What is the role of azithromycin? *Lancet Infect. Dis.* **2018**, *18*, 486–488. [CrossRef]
25. Calado, J.; Castro, R.; Lopes, Â.; Campos, M.J.; Rocha, M.; Pereira, F. Antimicrobial resistance and molecular characteristics of *Neisseria gonorrhoeae* isolates from men who have sex with men. *Int. J. Infect. Dis.* **2019**, *79*, 116–122. [CrossRef] [PubMed]
26. Ryan, L.; Golparian, D.; Fennelly, N.; Rose, L.; Walsh, P.; Lawlor, B.; Mac Aogáin, M.; Unemo, M.; Crowley, B. Antimicrobial resistance and molecular epidemiology using whole-genome sequencing of *Neisseria gonorrhoeae* in Ireland, 2014–2016: Focus on extended-spectrum cephalosporins and azithromycin. *Eur. J. Clin. Microbiol. Infect. Dis.* **2018**, *37*, 1661–1672. [CrossRef]
27. Młynarczyk-Bonikowska, B.; Majewska, A.; Malejczyk, M.; Młynarczyk, G.; Majewski, S. Multiresistant *Neisseria gonorrhoeae*: A new threat in second decade of the XXI century. *Med. Microbiol. Immunol.* **2020**, *209*, 95–108. [CrossRef]
28. Low, N.; Unemo, M. Molecular tests for the detection of antimicrobial resistant *Neisseria gonorrhoeae*: When, where, and how to use? *Curr. Opin. Infect. Dis.* **2016**, *29*, 45–51. [CrossRef]
29. Ohneck, E.A.; Zalucki, Y.M.; Johnson, P.J.; Dhulipala, V.; Golparian, D.; Unemo, M.; Jerse, A.E.; Shafer, W.M. A novel mechanism of high-level, broad-spectrum antibiotic resistance caused by a single base pair change in *Neisseria gonorrhoeae*. *mBio* **2011**, *2*, e00187-11. [CrossRef]
30. Asín, E.; Isla, A.; Canut, A.; Rodríguez Gascón, A. Comparison of antimicrobial pharmacokinetic/pharmacodynamic breakpoints with EUCAST and CLSI clinical breakpoints for Gram-positive bacteria. *Int. J. Antimicrob. Agents* **2012**, *40*, 313–322. [CrossRef] [PubMed]
31. Valero, A.; Isla, A.; Rodríguez-Gascón, A.; Canut, A.; Solinís, M.A. Susceptibility of *Pseudomonas aeruginosa* and antimicrobial activity using PK/PD analysis: An 18-year surveillance study. *Enferm. Infecc. Microbiol. Clin.* **2019**, *37*, 626–633. [CrossRef] [PubMed]
32. Zelenitsky, S.A.; Rubinstein, E.; Ariano, R.E.; Zhanel, G.G.; Canadian Antimicrobial Resistance Alliance. Integrating pharmacokinetics, pharmacodynamics and MIC distributions to assess changing antimicrobial activity against clinical isolates of *Pseudomonas aeruginosa* causing infections in Canadian hospitals (CANWARD). *J. Antimicrob. Chemother.* **2013**, *68* (Suppl. S1), i67–i72. [CrossRef] [PubMed]
33. Theuretzbacher, U.; Barbee, L.; Connolly, K.; Drusano, G.; Fernandes, P.; Hook, E.; Jerse, A.; O'Donnell, J.; Unemo, M.; Van Bambeke, F.; et al. Pharmacokinetic/pharmacodynamic considerations for new and current therapeutic drugs for uncomplicated gonorrhoea-challenges and opportunities. *Clin. Microbiol. Infect.* **2020**, *26*, 1630–1635. [CrossRef] [PubMed]
34. Matzneller, P.; Krasniqi, S.; Kinzig, M.; Sörgel, F.; Hüttner, S.; Lackner, E.; Müller, M.; Zeitlinger, M. Blood, tissue, and intracellular concentrations of azithromycin during and after end of therapy. *Antimicrob. Agents Chemother.* **2013**, *57*, 1736–1742. [CrossRef]
35. Tapsall, J. *Antimicrobial Resistance in Neisseria Gonorrhoeae*; World Health Organization: Geneva, Switzerland, 2001; Available online: https://apps.who.int/iris/bitstream/handle/10665/66963/WHO_CDS_CSR_DRS_2001.3.pdf (accessed on 3 August 2021).
36. Ibar-Bariain, M.; Isla, A.; Solinís, M.Á.; Sanz-Moreno, J.C.; Canut, A.; Rodríguez-Gascón, A. Pharmacokinetic/pharmacodynamic evaluation of the antimicrobial therapy of pneumococcal invasive disease in adults in post-PCV13 vaccine period in Madrid, Spain. *Eur. J. Clin. Microbiol. Infect. Dis.* **2021**, *40*, 2145–2152. [CrossRef] [PubMed]

37. Valero, A.; Isla, A.; Rodríguez-Gascón, A.; Calvo, B.; Canut, A.; Solinís, M.Á. Pharmacokinetic/pharmacodynamic analysis as a tool for surveillance of the activity of antimicrobials against *Pseudomonas aeruginosa* strains isolated in critically ill patients. *Enferm. Infecc. Microbiol. Clin.* **2019**, *37*, 380–386. [CrossRef] [PubMed]
38. Rodríguez-Gascón, A.; Solinís, M.Á.; Isla, A. The Role of PK/PD Analysis in the Development and Evaluation of Antimicrobials. *Pharmaceutics* **2021**, *13*, 833. [CrossRef] [PubMed]

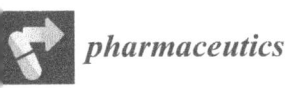

Article

Population Pharmacokinetics of Levetiracetam and Dosing Evaluation in Critically Ill Patients with Normal or Augmented Renal Function

Idoia Bilbao-Meseguer [1,2], Helena Barrasa [3,4], Eduardo Asín-Prieto [5,†], Ana Alarcia-Lacalle [2,6], Alicia Rodríguez-Gascón [2,6], Javier Maynar [3,4], José Ángel Sánchez-Izquierdo [7], Goiatz Balziskueta [3,4], María Sánchez-Bayton Griffith [7], Nerea Quilez Trasobares [7], María Ángeles Solinís [2,6,*] and Arantxa Isla [2,6,*]

1. Department of Pharmacy, Cruces University Hospital, Plaza de Cruces 12, 48903 Barakaldo, Spain; idoia.bilbaomeseguer@osakidetza.eus
2. Pharmacokinetic, Nanotechnology and Gene Therapy Group (PharmaNanoGene), Faculty of Pharmacy, Centro de Investigación Lascaray Ikergunea, University of the Basque Country UPV/EHU, Paseo de la Universidad 7, 01006 Vitoria-Gasteiz, Spain; ana.alarcia@ehu.eus (A.A.-L.); alicia.rodriguez@ehu.eus (A.R.-G.)
3. Instituto de Investigación Sanitaria Bioaraba, 01009 Vitoria-Gasteiz, Spain; helena.barrasagonzalez@osakidetza.eus (H.B.); FRANCISCOJAVIER.MAYNARMOLINER@osakidetza.eus (J.M.); goiatz.baltziskuetaflorez@osakidetza.eus (G.B.)
4. Intensive Care Unit, Araba University Hospital, Osakidetza Basque Health Service, 01009 Vitoria-Gasteiz, Spain
5. Inserm U1070: Pharmacologie des Anti-Infectieux, Pôle Biologie Santé, Université de Poitiers, Bâtiment B36, 1 Rue Georges Bonnet, 86022 Poitiers, France; eduardo.asin.prieto@gmail.com
6. Instituto de Investigación Sanitaria Bioaraba, Microbiology, Infectious Disease, Antimicrobial Agents, and Gene Therapy, 01006 Vitoria-Gasteiz, Spain
7. Intensive Care Unit, Doce de Octubre Hospital, Avda de Córdoba, s/n, 28041 Madrid, Spain; jasiruci@gmail.com (J.Á.S.-I.); mariabayton@hotmail.com (M.S.-B.G.); nerida.mia@gmail.com (N.Q.T.)
* Correspondence: marian.solinis@ehu.eus (M.Á.S.); arantxa.isla@ehu.eus (A.I.)
† Present address: Pharma Mar S.A., Avda. de los Reyes, 1, Pol. Ind. La Mina, 28770 Colmenar Viejo, Spain.

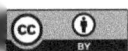

Abstract: Levetiracetam is a broad-spectrum antiepileptic drug commonly used in intensive care units (ICUs). The objective of this study is to evaluate the adequacy of levetiracetam dosing in patients with normal or augmented renal clearance (ARC) admitted to the ICU by population modelling and simulation. A multicentre prospective study including twenty-seven critically ill patients with urinary creatinine clearance (CrCl) > 50 mL/min and treated with levetiracetam was developed. Levetiracetam plasma concentrations were best described by a two-compartment model. The parameter estimates and relative standard errors (%) were clearance (CL) 3.5 L/h (9%), central volume of distribution (V1) 20.7 L (18%), intercompartmental clearance 31.9 L/h (22%), and peripheral volume of distribution 33.5 L (13%). Interindividual variability estimates were, for the CL, 32.7% (21%) and, for V1, 56.1% (29%). The CrCl showed significant influence over CL. Simulations showed that the administration of at least 500 mg every 8 h or 1000 mg every 12 h are needed in patients with normal renal function. Higher doses (1500 or 2000 mg, every 8 h) are needed in patients with ARC. Critically ill patients with normal or ARC treated with levetiracetam could be at high risk of being underdosed.

Keywords: levetiracetam; augmented renal clearance; intensive care; critically ill patients; population pharmacokinetic; modelling; Monte Carlo simulations; seizure

1. Introduction

Levetiracetam is a broad-spectrum antiepileptic drug with proven efficacy in treating multiple seizure types, in both the adult and paediatric population. Because of its improved safety profile and ease of use compared to other conventional antiepileptic drugs such as phenytoin, it is frequently used in the treatment of status epilepticus and in seizure prophylaxis after a neurologic injury, being a commonly used treatment in intensive care units (ICUs) [1–3].

Levetiracetam has a linear pharmacokinetic profile. It is rapidly and almost completely absorbed when administered orally, with a time to reach the peak concentration (Tmax) of 1–2 h and a high bioavailability (>95%). Its apparent volume of distribution is 0.5–0.7 L/kg with non-significant plasma protein binding (<3%). Renal clearance represents the main elimination mechanism with a 66% of the dose excreted unchanged in urine, which leads to a good correlation between levetiracetam clearance and a patient's creatinine clearance (CrCl). Additionally, a fraction of the dose (24%) is eliminated by metabolism through enzymatic hydrolysis of the acetamide group, carried out by a type B esterase, mainly in blood. Clinically relevant interactions are not expected, as this metabolic pathway is only responsible for the metabolism of a small part of the administered dose. Additionally, levetiracetam does not induce or inhibit CYP enzymes resulting in minimal drug-drug interactions. The metabolites have no known pharmacological activity and are renally excreted [1,4,5].

There is no clear correlation between levetiracetam serum concentration and efficacy or tolerability. The current reference range for trough concentrations is 12–46 mg/L [6], although some authors have proposed a more modest target range of 6–20 mg/L [7]. The favourable pharmacokinetic profile together with the absence of major drug interactions and broad therapeutic window makes routine therapeutic drug monitoring (TDM) unnecessary. However, TDM, as a way to ensure effective and safe exposures, may be indicated in certain circumstances, such as in patients with altered levetiracetam clearance. This is the case of elderly patients, children, pregnant women, patients with renal insufficiency or critically ill patients [8,9].

In fact, the pharmacokinetic behaviour of levetiracetam has been poorly studied in critically ill patients with augmented renal clearance (ARC). The ARC, defined as a CrCl > 130 mL/min/1.73 m^2, is present in 20–65% of critically ill patients, being more common in certain conditions, such as traumatic brain injury (TBI) (85%) or subarachnoid haemorrhage (SAH) (100%). Although the physiological mechanism responsible for ARC in critically ill patients is not well-defined, the combination of systemic inflammation coupled with a greater renal functional reserve and together with intensive fluid therapy and the administration of inotropic and vasopressor drugs could explain this phenomenon. The presence of ARC could lead to faster elimination of renally excreted drugs, such as levetiracetam, potentially resulting in subtherapeutic concentrations and poorer clinical outcomes [10–13].

In this regard, the aim of this study is to evaluate the adequacy of levetiracetam dosing for the achievement of therapeutic levels in patients with normal or high renal clearance admitted to the ICU by the characterization of the levetiracetam pharmacokinetics by population modelling and simulation.

2. Materials and Methods

2.1. Study Design and Patient Population

A multicentric open-label prospective study was conducted in critically ill patients admitted to the ICUs of Araba University Hospital (Vitoria-Gasteiz, Spain) and Doce de Octubre Hospital (Madrid, Spain). Patients were recruited during 2019 and 2020 following a protocol previously approved by the Basque Clinical Research Ethics Committee (EPA2018019 (SP)). The study was carried out in accordance with ICH Guidelines for Good Clinical Practice. Samples and data from patients were provided by the Basque Biobank (www.biobancovasco.org) and were processed following standard operation procedures with appropriate ethical approval. ICU patients were eligible if they were treated with levetiracetam and had a CrCl > 50 mL/min measured in urine. The exclusion criteria were age less than 18 years, pregnancy or hypersensitivity to the active substance or to any of the excipients.

2.2. Drug Administration, Sampling Procedure and Analytical Method

Each patient received a dose of 500, 1000 or 1500 mg of levetiracetam every 12 h, as a 30-min intravenous infusion. For each patient, blood samples (3 mL) were taken at 0 h (pre-dose), at the end of the infusion (0.5 h) and at the end of the dosing interval (12 h). Moreover, one sample was taken within the intervals of 1–2 h, 3–5 h and 6–8 h after drug administration. Each sample was immediately centrifuged at 3000 rpm for 10 min to collect the plasma, which was immediately frozen at $-20\ °C$. Within the following week, samples were stored at $-80\ °C$ until analysis.

Plasma concentrations of levetiracetam were quantified with a high-performance liquid chromatography (HPLC) assay with ultraviolet detection at a wavelength of 205 nm. The method was validated following the US Food and Drug Administration (FDA) (2018) and the European Medicines Agency (EMA) (2012) guidelines. Separation was performed on a Symmetry® C18 (4.6 mm × 150 mm × 5 μm) column (Waters, Milford, Massachusetts, United States) eluted with ammonium phosphate and acetonitrile (95:5, v:v) mobile phase and it was delivered at 1.2 mL/min. Sample preparation consisted of protein precipitation with acetonitrile and centrifugation for 10 min at $15,000 \times g$. The supernatants were then injected into the HPLC system.

The assay was linear over the concentration range from 2 to 100 mg/L. Specificity was assessed using six blank standards and lower limit of quantification (LLOQ) level samples. The chromatograms were checked for interference, with no interference peaks detected at the retention time of levetiracetam. Intra–batch and inter–batch accuracy and precision were evaluated at four different concentration levels (LLOQ and low, middle, and high quality control) in six replicates. The intra–day and inter–day coefficients of variation (CV) and bias were never above 15%. Stock solution stability, the stability of levetiracetam in storage conditions (at $-20\ °C$ for one month and at $-80\ °C$ for one year), freeze–thaw stability of the analyte in the matrix from freezer storage conditions to room temperature, and auto-sampler rack stability were also evaluated and confirmed. Levetiracetam substance for standards and quality controls was a reference standard, United States Pharmacopoeia, USP.

2.3. Noncompartmental Analysis

PK parameters for levetiracetam were initially explored by noncompartmental analysis using Phoenix 64 (Build 8.3.0.5005, Certara, Princeton, NJ, USA). The following PK parameters were provided for levetiracetam: the area under the concentration-time curve within the dosing interval (AUC_{12}), peak plasma concentration (Cmax), apparent systemic clearance (CL), elimination half-life ($t_{1/2}$) and apparent volume of distribution (Vz). Area under the concentration-time curve was calculated using the linear-log trapezoidal rule. Afterwards, the correlation between clearance and CrCl at an individual level was explored.

Statistical analysis was performed with IBM® SPSS® Statistics for Windows, Version 26. Student t tests were used to compare the pharmacokinetic parameters of levetiracetam between patients in different groups. Statistical significance was assessed at $p < 0.05$.

2.4. Pharmacometric Modelling

Nonlinear mixed-effects modelling was implemented in NONMEM (v.7.4), using first-order conditional estimation method with interaction (FOCE+I). On the basis of visual exploration of the data and a review of the literature, one- and two-compartment models were considered to describe the levetiracetam concentration-time data. Regarding the variability model, interindividual variability (IIV) associated with the structural pharmacokinetic parameters was modelled exponentially, whereas the residual variability was tested as either proportional, additive or combined error model. The significance of the off-diagonal elements of the Ω variance–covariance matrix was also explored.

Selection between models was based on the following criteria. First, biological plausibility. Second, a significant reduction in the objective function value (OFV = $-2 \times$ log-likelihood). Third, the precision of the parameter estimation expressed as the relative standard error (RSE [%]) and calculated as the ratio between the standard error and the parameter estimate. Fourth, visual inspection of the goodness-of-fit (GOF) plots, including the observed versus individual and population predicted concentration and the residuals plots.

The covariates assessed at baseline evaluated in the analysis included demographic factors (sex, age, height and serum albumin), CrCl (measured in urine), blood chemistry (glucose, albumin, total bilirubin, haemoglobin and leukocytes), acute physiology and chronic health evaluation (APACHE II) and diagnosis. Random effects associated with parameters of interest were plotted versus covariates to explore potential relationships and the Stepwise Covariate Model building tool of Perl speaks NONMEM (v.4.8) was performed as a preliminary selection of covariates. Categorical covariates were modelled as a shift in the typical value for the least common categories, whereas continuous covariates were modelled using linear, exponential or power functions after centring on the median. CrCl was explored as a continuous covariate, but it was also dichotomized into two groups, CrCl < 130mL/min or CrCl $\geq$ 130 mL/min. Covariates were retained in the model if their inclusion produced a significant decrease of the OFV $\geq$ 3.84 units (equivalent to $p < 0.05$ for one degree of freedom) in comparison with the previous model without the covariate. This forward inclusion approach was followed by its reverse (backward elimination) removing those covariates, whose elimination did not produce a significant increase of the OFV $\leq$ 6.63 (equivalent to $p > 0.01$ for one degree of freedom). Therefore, when all the statistically significant covariates were added to the model, each of them was individually removed. If the removal of a covariate was found not to be significant it was dropped in favour of the simpler model.

2.5. Final Model Evaluation

GOF plots were used as the first indicator of goodness-of-fit, including the plotting of model-based individual predictions (IPRED) and population predictions (PRED) versus the observed concentrations (DV), conditional weighted residual errors (CWRES) vs time after dose (TAD) and the CWRES vs PRED. The parameter precision was evaluated by running a 2000 sample bootstrap (PsN v.4.8). Finally, a simulation-based model diagnostic to study the performance of the final model, a prediction-corrected Visual Predictive Check (pcVPC), was constructed by replicating 1000 studies with the same design as the original clinical study and representing the 10th, 50th, and 90th percentiles of the observed data and the 95% confidence intervals for the mentioned predicted percentiles, based on the simulated data sets.

2.6. Dosing Simulations

Using the same dosing regimens administered to patients, 1000 subjects with different CrCl were simulated (80, 120, 160, 200 and 240 mL/min) to evaluate the impact of the covariate on the levetiracetam clearance. Moreover, stochastic simulations were performed to predict levetiracetam plasma minimum concentrations (Cmin) under various dosing regimens (doses from 500 mg to 2000 mg given at either 12- or 8-h intervals, as a 30-min intravenous infusion) and to estimate the probability of target attainment. The target trough concentrations were 12 to 46 mg/L at steady state as recommended by the International League Against Epilepsy (ILAE). A lower target trough range (>6 mg/L) was also investigated. Simulations with the final model were performed with 1000 virtual subjects with CrCl values within the range from 80 to 240 mL/min. CrCl cut-off values were selected based on the observed distribution of CrCl values of the population included in the study and on the summary of product characteristics of levetiracetam, where dosage adjustments are recommended for CrCl below 80 mL/min, but not above this threshold [1].

Simulations extending infusion time to 2 h were performed in those situations in which target attainment with a minimum probability of 80% was not reached.

3. Results

3.1. Patient Demographics

Twenty-seven critically ill patients were included in the study. The main diagnoses were haemorrhagic strokes ($n = 10$), trauma ($n = 8$) or other diagnostics such as meningitis, space occupying lesions, convulsive crisis, encephalopathy, arteriovenous malformations or low level of consciousness. Subject characteristics are described in Table 1. A total of 158 plasma samples were analysed, with a median of six, and a minimum of five, plasma samples per patient. Most of the patients (18 out of 27) were treated with 500 mg/12 h of levetiracetam and 10 presented ARC. Levetiracetam was well tolerated, as no evidence of adverse events was recorded, even with the highest dose. Concentration versus time profile of levetiracetam in all the patients is represented in Figure 1.

Table 1. Characteristics of the population included in the study.

Covariate	N (%)	Median (Range)
Sex:		
• Male	18 (67)	-
• Female	9 (33)	-
ARC (CrCl > 130 mL/min):		
• Yes	10 (37)	
• No	17 (63)	
Diagnostic:		
• Haemorrhagic strokes	10 (37)	-
• Trauma	8 (30)	-
• Others	9 (33)	-
Age (years)	-	60 (23–81)
Weight (kg)	-	80 (58–115)
Height (cm)	-	168 (148–189)
BSA (m^2) [1]	-	1.9 (1.59–2.33)
APACHE II	-	18 (5–35)
CrCl (mL/min) [2]	-	117 (54–239)
Glucose (mg/dL)	-	142 (91–337)
Albumin (g/dL)	-	3.4 (2.1–3.9)
Total bilirubin (mg/dL)	-	0.6 (0.2–2.1)
Hemoglobin (g/dL)	-	11.6 (6.7–14.5)
Leukocytes (10^9/L)	-	10.4 (3–24.6)

APACHE: acute physiology and chronic health evaluation; ARC: Augmented renal clearance; BSA: Body Surface Area; CrCl: creatinine clearance. [1] Body surface area (Du Bois method) = $0.007184 \times \text{Height}^{0.725} \times \text{Weight}^{0.425}$. [2] Creatinine clearance = [Urine creatinine (mg/dL) × Volume of urine per minute (mL/min)]/Creatinine plasma level (mg/dL).

3.2. Noncompartmental Analysis

Pharmacokinetic parameters obtained with noncompartmental analysis are summarized in Table 2. The dose-normalized Cmax and CL were significantly higher in patients with ARC than in those with normal CrCl ($p > 0.05$). Figure 2 shows the correlation between CrCl and levetiracetam clearance calculated by noncompartmental analysis.

3.3. Population Pharmacokinetic Modelling

Plasma concentrations were best described by a two-compartment linear model, characterized by drug total body clearance (CL), central volume of distribution (V1), peripheral volume of distribution (V2) and intercompartmental clearance (Q). IIV was exponentially included for CL and V1, and no correlation was detected between the random effects associated with the pharmacokinetic parameters. Residual variability was proportionally modelled. The goodness of fit of the base model was verified by GOF plots.

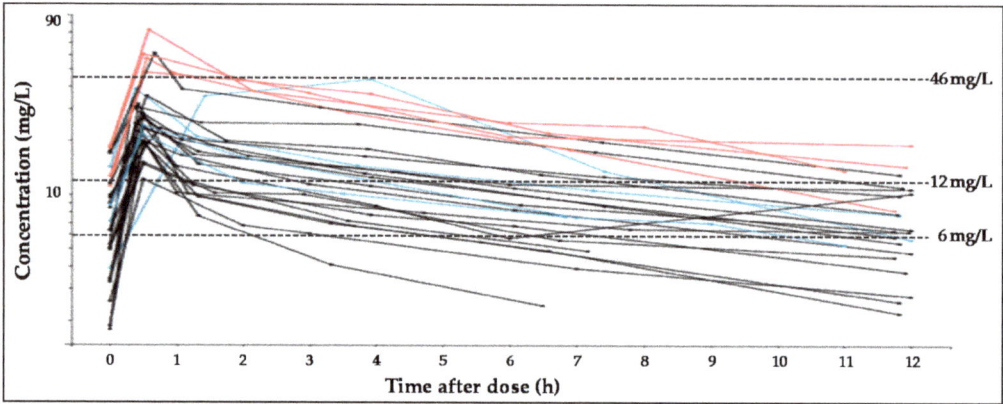

Figure 1. Spaghetti plots for plasma levetiracetam concentration-time profiles, according to dose received by each subject. In black, lines represent profiles after dose of 500 mg, blue lines, 1000 mg and red lines, 1500 mg. Dashed lines represent the target concentration values (6 mg/L, 12 mg/L or 46 mg/L).

Table 2. Levetiracetam pharmacokinetic parameters (mean and standard deviation) at steady state following intravenous administration of 500–1500 mg every 12 h to critically ill patients.

	Cmax (mg/L)	Cmax/D (L^{-1})	AUC_{12} (mg·h/L)	AUC_{12}/D (h/L)	$t_{1/2}$ (h)	CL (L/h)	Vz (L)
No ARC	36.36 (17.93)	0.053 (0.032)	186.49 (97.79)	0.267 (0.118)	8.86 (6.13)	4.28 (1.40)	54.41 (42.79)
ARC	24.25 (12.41)	0.036 (0.011) *	121.05 (66.08)	0.182 (0.081)	7.25 (4.11)	6.51 (2.65) *	61.09 (25.07)

ARC: Augmented renal clearance; Cmax: peak plasma concentration; D: dose; AUC_{12}: area under the concentration-time curve within the dosing interval, $t_{1/2}$: elimination half-life; CL: apparent systemic clearance; Vz: apparent volume of distribution; * statistically significant differences between patient with or without ARC ($p < 0.05$).

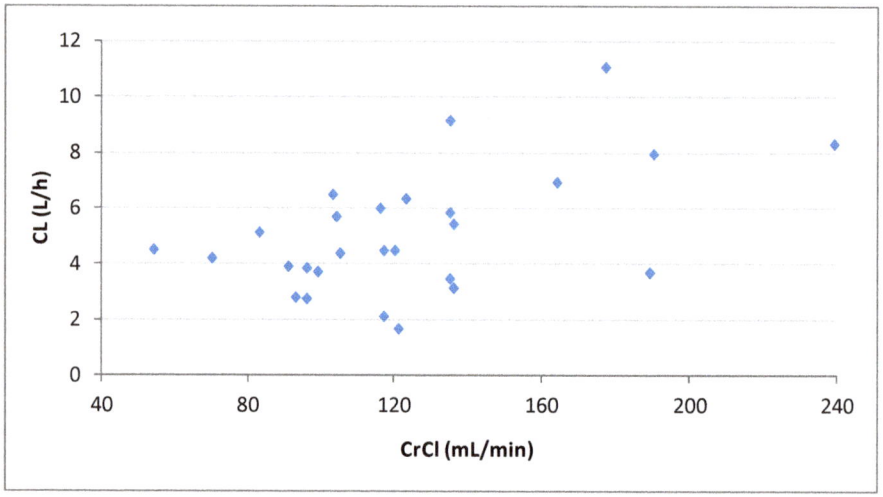

Figure 2. Plot of the individual levetiracetam clearances (CL) calculated by noncompartmental analysis vs. creatinine clearances (CrCl) for the 27 patients.

Both the CrCl, as a continuous variable, and the ARC, as a categorical covariate showed significant influence over CL. CrCl was selected for the final model since the reduction in IIV was greater than with the categorical variable (5.6% vs 3.9%). trauma vs non-trauma diagnosis and APACHE II also showed influence over V1. However, they were eventually excluded from the final model since their individual deletion did not significantly increase the OFV. Therefore, the final model only considered the CrCl as a covariate of the total clearance.

The final model equations were:

$$CL(L/h) = \left(3.5 + \left(\frac{CrCl}{120}\right)^{2.5}\right) \times e^{\eta 1}$$

$$V1(L) = 20.7 \times e^{\eta 2}$$

where CL is clearance, CrCl is urinary creatinine clearance, V1 is central volume of distribution, η1 and η2 represent the interindividual variability for CL, and V1, respectively, which followed normal distributions with a mean of 0.

Inclusion of the CrCl on the CL decreased the unexplained IIV of CL from 38.3% in the base model to 32.7% in the final model and a statistically significant drop of the OFV was obtained with respect to the base model (ΔOFV > 6.63). The population PK model and the results of the bootstrap analysis are shown in Table 3. The residual standard errors revealed that all parameters were precisely estimated. Moreover, the estimates of the parameters were very similar to the median values obtained from the bootstrap analysis. Figure 3 displays the GOF plots for the final model. Figure 4 shows the correlation found between CrCl and levetiracetam clearance. The pcVPC, provided in Figure 5, confirmed that the model appropriately predicts both central tendency and variability of the observed concentrations.

Table 3. Base and final population pharmacokinetic models estimates, shrinkage [a] values and bootstrap results.

Parameter	Base Model Estimate (RSE (%))	Final Model Estimate (RSE (%))	Bootstrap Median (95% CI)
CL (L/h) = θnr + (CrCl/120)^θr	4.6 (8)	-	
θnr	-	3.5 (9)	3.5 (2.8–4.1)
θr	-	2.5 (17)	2.5 (0.9–3.9)
V1 (L)	20.8 (18)	20.7 (18)	20.8 (13.4–27.7)
Q (L/h)	31.4 (21)	31.9 (22)	30.9 (22.5–47.8)
V2 (L)	34.1 (14)	33.5 (13)	34.2 (19.9–45.4)
IIV_CL (%)	38.3 (19)	32.7 (21)	30.7 (20.2–48.3)
IIV_V1 (%)	54.4 (29)	56.1 (29)	58.0 (22.6–114.0)
RE_proportional (%)	22.3 (15)	22.3 (15)	21.5 (15.7–27.7)

CL, clearance; CrCl, creatinine clearance; V1, central volume of distribution; Q, intercompartmental clearance; V2, peripheral volume of distribution; IIV, inter-individual variability; RE, Residual error; RSE, Relative standard errors; CI, Confidence interval. [a] CL ηsh = 2%; V1 ηsh = 23%; εsh = 12%.

3.4. Dosing Simulations

Tables 4 and 5 show the probability of target attainment for simulated patients with different CrCl, calculated as the percentage of virtual subjects (n = 1000) who had levetiracetam trough concentrations above the previously defined values. Considering the target of trough concentrations higher than 12 mg/L, with the twice daily dosing regimen, probabilities higher than 80% were only obtained in patients with no ARC and with the highest doses. More specifically, doses of 1500 mg and 2000 mg every 12 h would be needed for patients with CrCl of 80 and 120 mL/min, respectively. In patients with CrCl of 160 and 200 mL/min, dosing schedules with 8-h interval would be needed (doses of 1500 and 2000 mg, respectively). With those dosing regimens, the probability of Cmin to exceed the value of 46 mg/L is low (<5%) in the respective group of patients. Notably, in patients with CrCl of 240 mL/min the targeted minimum concentration of 12 mg/L was not reached even with doses of 2000 mg every 8 h. Extending the infusion time of the 2000 mg dose to 2 h in this group, did not increase enough the probability of reaching the targeted minimum concentration of 12 mg/L (from 59% to 67%).

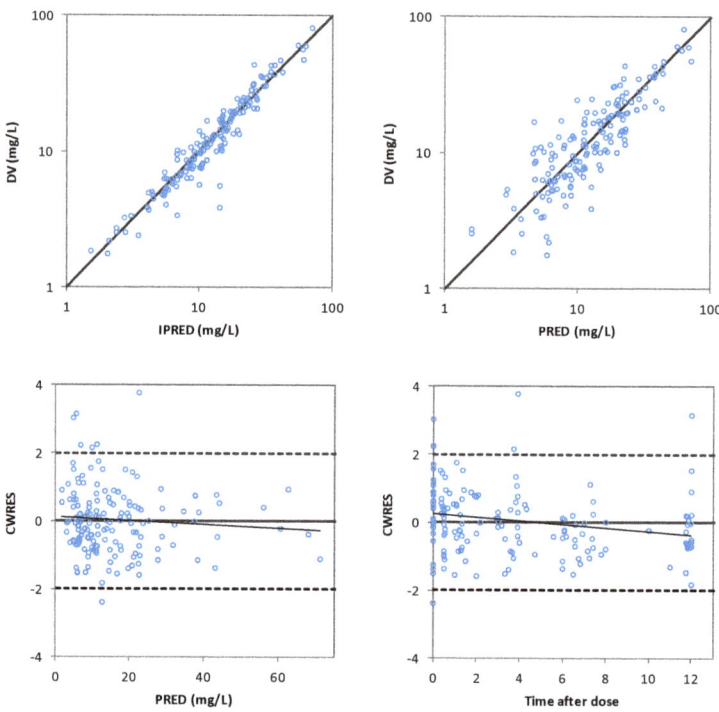

Figure 3. The goodness of fit plots of individual predicted (IPRED) versus the observed (DV) levetiracetam concentrations (**top-left**), population predicted (PRED) versus DV levetiracetam concentrations (**top-right**), conditional weighted residuals (CWRES) versus PRED (**bottom-left**) and CWRES versus time after dose (**bottom-right**) of the final model.

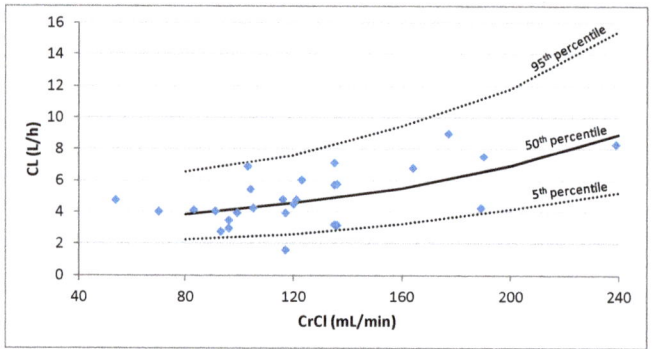

Figure 4. Plot of the individual predicted levetiracetam clearances (CL) estimated by population PK analysis vs. creatinine clearance (CrCl) for the 27 patients. Lines represent the 5th, 50th, and 95th percentiles of 1000 simulations performed at CrCl values of 80, 160, 200, and 240 mL/min.

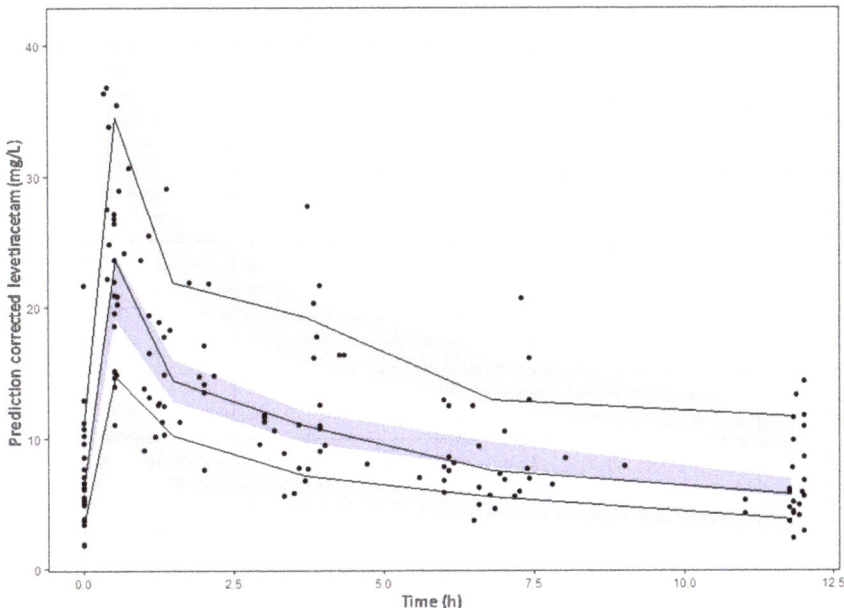

Figure 5. Prediction-corrected visual predictive check of the final model. The dots represent the prediction–corrected concentrations (mg/L). The continuous line represents the 10th, 50th and 90th observed percentiles. Simulation-based 95% confidence intervals for the median and the 10th and 90th percentiles are displayed by dark and light grey shading, respectively.

Table 4. Probability of target attainment based on simulations of the final population model with different doses administered every 12 h. In bold are represented those probabilities ≥80%.

CrCl (mL/min)	Dose (mg)	Perfusion Duration (min)	Daily Dose (mg)	Probability of Cmin (%)		
				>6 mg/L	>12 mg/L	>46 mg/L
			Twice Daily (Tau = 12 h)			
80	500	30	1000	62	12	0
	1000	30	2000	**93**	60	0
	1500	30	3000	**99**	**85**	3
	2000	30	4000	**100**	**94**	14
120	500	30	1000	43	6	0
	1000	30	2000	**86**	43	0
	1500	30	3000	**95**	72	2
	2000	30	4000	**98**	**85**	6
160	500	30	1000	22	1	0
	1000	30	2000	67	22	0
	1500	30	3000	**87**	51	0
	2000	30	4000	**94**	69	2
200	1000	30	2000	39	6	0
	1500	30	3000	68	25	0
	2000	30	4000	**80**	42	0
240	1500	30	3000	37	7	0
	2000	30	4000	55	15	0

Cmin, Minimum levetiracetam concentration; CrCl, creatinine clearance; Tau, dosing interval.

Table 5. Probability of target attainment based on simulations of the final population model with different doses administered every 8 h. In bold are represented those probabilities ≥80%.

CrCl (mL/min)	Dose (mg)	Perfusion Duration (min)	Daily Dose (mg)	Probability of Cmin (%) >6 mg/L	>12 mg/L	>46 mg/L
Three Times Daily (Tau = 8 h)						
80	500	30	1500	**94**	51	0
	1000	30	3000	**100**	**93**	5
	1500	30	4500	**100**	**99**	31
120	500	30	1500	**84**	33	0
	1000	30	3000	**99**	**84**	2
	1500	30	4500	**100**	**96**	17
160	500	30	1500	65	12	0
	1000	30	3000	**94**	65	0
	1500	30	4500	**99**	**89**	5
	2000	30	6000	**100**	**97**	17
200	500	30	1500	38	4	0
	1000	30	3000	**83**	39	0
	1500	30	4500	**95**	69	1
	2000	30	6000	**98**	**84**	5
240	1000	30	3000	61	15	0
	1500	30	4500	**80**	38	0
	2000	30	6000	**89**	59	1
	2000	120	6000	**94**	67	1

Cmin, Minimum levetiracetam concentration; CrCl, creatinine clearance; Tau, dosing interval.

When considering the lower target trough concentrations of >6 mg/L twice daily dosing regimens were able to reach the therapeutic interval with a probability greater than 80%, except in patients with CrCl of 240 mL/min, in which dosing every 8 h seemed mandatory. In detail, 1000 mg every 12 h would be suitable for patients with normal renal function, 1500 mg every 12 h for patients with CrCl of 160 mL/min, 2000 mg every 12 h for patients with CrCl of 200 mL/min and 1500 mg every 8 h for patients with CrCl of 240 mL/min.

4. Discussion

In this study, a population pharmacokinetic model of levetiracetam in critically ill patients was developed, for a better selection or optimization of the dose regimen, with special focus on ARC condition. ICU patients commonly show altered pharmacokinetics due to their intrinsic heterogeneity and the disease status that can lead to suboptimal drug concentrations. In fact, the high variability observed in levetiracetam concentrations, partially explained by patients' renal function, suggested the need for dosing optimization in patients with ARC and Monte Carlo simulations revealed the need of high doses to attain the target concentrations.

The ARC condition has recently drawn attention due to its prevalence (present in 20–65% of the patients [10,14] in the intensive care setting), and its potential impact on the elimination of the drugs, especially those primarily eliminated by renal excretion. Pharmacokinetics of renally excreted antimicrobials, such as vancomycin, β-lactams or linezolid, have demonstrated to be significantly modified in patients with ARC [15–19], leading to sub-therapeutic concentrations. In this regard, clinicians should routinely assess the renal function of critically ill patients, by measuring urinary CrCl, not only with the aim of detecting renal impairment, but also, to detect ARC, in order to adjust drug doses.

Levetiracetam is a widely used drug in ICUs, both in treatment and in prophylaxis of seizures, and is mainly excreted unchanged in urine (66%) making it vulnerable to suffer from increased elimination in patients who display ARC. Nevertheless, the effect of ARC on levetiracetam serum concentrations has been poorly investigated. In a case report, Cook et al. described a 22-year-old girl with severe TBI who displayed ARC. The patient presented a higher than usual systemic clearance of levetiracetam and required significantly higher dose [20].

In a study published by Spencer et al. [21], in 12 neurocritical care patients requiring seizure prophylaxis who received 500 mg twice daily, they found a higher levetiracetam clearance and a shorter half-life, compared with previously published results in healthy volunteers. ARC was not present in their population, but there was a statistically significant relationship between the systemic clearance of levetiracetam and estimated CrCl. Just one patient with renal impairment (CrCl 42 mL/min), achieved a steady-state trough concentration greater than 6 mg/L. Recently, two population pharmacokinetic models of levetiracetam in neurocritical patients have been published [22,23]. Sime et al. [22] developed a population pharmacokinetics model in 30 critically ill patients with TBI or SAH without renal disfunction. ARC (urinary CrCl > 130 mL/min/1.73 m^2) was present in 70% of the patients. Urinary CrCl was found as a covariate that significantly influences levetiracetam clearance, whereas body surface area (BSA) was found to influence levetiracetam clearance, volume of distribution and the absorption rate constant. For every 40 mL/min/1.73 m^2 increase in urinary CrCl, levetiracetam clearance increased by 50% and the median trough concentrations were reduced by 50%. They performed dosing simulations with dosages ranging from 1000 mg every 12 h to 2000 mg every 8 h and concluded that for urinary CrCl greater than 120 mL/min/1.73 m^2, none of the simulated regimens had a probability of 80% or above of achieving trough concentrations higher than 12 mg/L. Similarly, Ong et al. [23] have recently developed a population pharmacokinetics model in 20 neurosurgical patients with TBI, SAH or brain tumour resection. ARC (estimated CrCl > 150 mL/min/1.73 m^2) was present in 30% of the patients. In this study, no covariates were found to significantly influenced levetiracetam pharmacokinetic parameters. They also performed Monte Carlo simulations showing a low probability of reaching trough concentrations > 6 mg/L with the 500 mg twice daily dosing regimen. A dose of 1000 mg twice daily was required to achieve a probability of 80%.

In our study, the pharmacokinetics of levetiracetam were best described by a two-compartment model, agreeing with that reported by Sime et al. [22] and Ong et al. [23]. None of the variables analysed had a significant influence on V1. Trauma diagnosis showed statistical significance at a level of $p < 0.05$, but not at the level of $p < 0.01$, probably because of the scarce number of patients presenting this diagnosis ($n = 10$), and thereby; was not retained in the final model. Other authors have found significant influence of BSA [22,24] or body weight [25] in levetiracetam V1 and/or CL. In a systematic review about levetiracetam pharmacokinetics [25] in paediatric population, healthy subjects or non-critically ill adults, great differences in the volume of distribution, with values from 33 L to 69.9 L (calculated for a 75 kg subject), were reported. In our study, the total volume of distribution was 54.9 L, in the range of most studies, although higher than that observed by Sime et al. (32 L) and Ong et al. (37.2 L) [22,23].

In our model, the levetiracetam CL was only dependent on CrCl, which had a great influence on patients with ARC (mean levetiracetam CL increased from 4.5 L/h to 9.2 L/h in patients with CrCl from 120 to 240 mL/min). Sime et al. [22] also included CrCl as a covariate for CL. However, for similar values of CrCl, their model estimates higher levetiracetam clearance. The discrepancies observed between both models could, in part, be due to the differences among the recruited subjects; Sime et al. [22] included only TBI and SAH patients, whereas our population was more heterogeneous according to diagnosis, and also, to age, body weight and CrCl. Ong et al. [23] found similar levetiracetam clearance to that found in our study (3.6 vs. 4.1 L/h for a mean CrCl of 100 mL/min), however, they could not include CrCl as a covariate. This may be, in part, because the subjects included in their study had a narrower range of CrCl than our patients. Moreover, it has to be considered that their patients' renal function was estimated according to equations, instead of being based on CrCl measured in urine.

Despite the differences in the in the PK parameters, all studies bring out the risk of not achieving the target concentrations in ARC patients. Currently, the most accepted target is to achieve trough concentrations between 12 and 46 mg/L, proposed by ILAE [6], although other authors have proposed lower values. This is the case of the Norwegian Association of Clinical Pharmacology, which recommends target trough concentrations of 5 to 41 mg/L [26]. While ILAE recommendations are based on a retrospective database study that only included the highest doses used by each patient [3], the latter also considered other studies (globally 45% of all samples were below 12 mg/L, and 80% of all samples were between 5 and 25 mg/L) [26]. Moreover, other authors also propose a target trough range of 6–20 mg/L based on typical concentrations values reached with doses ranging from 500 to 1500 mg every 12 h [7].

In our study, a dose of 500 mg every 12 h has shown to be insufficient in critical patients with normal or augmented renal function. In fact, 100% and 67% of these patients had at least one sub-therapeutic level considering the threshold of 12 mg/L or 6 mg/L, respectively. Our results corroborate the need for dose optimization, as the risk for under dosing is highly variable and dependent on the dosing regimen and the renal function of the patients.

Monte Carlo simulations showed that the maximum dose approved in the summary of product characteristics (1500 mg every 12 h) only guarantees to achieve trough concentration of 12 mg/L in critically ill patients with CrCl $\leq$ 80 mL/min. In fact, the probability to achieve target trough concentrations higher than 12 mg/L is very low in ARC patients receiving levetiracetam in a twice daily dosing. Doses of 1500 mg and 2000 mg every 8 h are needed to achieve probabilities >80% for individuals with CrCl $\geq$ 160 and 200 mL/min, respectively, while in patients with CrCl of 240 mL/min, or higher this objective was not reached, even with 2000 mg every 8 h. Several studies have proposed prolonged or continuous infusion to ensure therapeutic concentrations of drugs in patients with ARC [19,27]. We evaluated in patients with CrCl $\geq$ 240 mL/min if the probability of achieving Cmin target would improve by prolonging the infusion time to 2 h. Monte Carlo simulation showed only a mild improvement. Longer infusions were not studied due to concerns about the stability of levetiracetam solutions at room temperature beyond 4 h [28]. When considering the target trough concentrations of 6 mg/L, probabilities greater than 80% were obtained with 1500 mg every 12 h only for patients with CrCl up to 160 mL/min. Sime et al. [22] reported worse results in their population, as they concluded that even with doses as high as 6 g of levetiracetam per day, trough concentrations within the currently accepted target range were not guaranteed. Therefore, further studies are needed in order to better elucidate the optimal dosing regimen in this population. Moreover, although the role of TDM of levetiracetam has not yet been established, its use in ascertaining compliance and managing patients that are at risk of being over- or under-dosed, such as critically ill patients, would be surely helpful. In addition, it is important to bear in mind that ARC is a dynamic a temporary situation [10], and accordingly, the renal function of the patients should be daily evaluated in order to adjust dosing regimens if needed.

This study has several limitations. Firstly, this study enrolled a relatively small number of patients, leading to a lack of external validation of the population PK model and limited statistical power. Previous studies were also carried out with a similar number of patients (20–30 patients) [22,23], but a larger sample could allow including any other covariates able to explain some of the remaining variability. In any case, accurate and precise estimates of all parameters were obtained, since a rich sampling strategy was followed in our study. Finally, the lack of consensus about the trough concentration target is a point to address. It would be advisable to determine a well-defined and universally accepted therapeutic range, although it is difficult to establish a correlation between drug concentration and clinical efficacy when levetiracetam is administered prophylactically to prevent seizures.

5. Conclusions

A population pharmacokinetic model has been developed for levetiracetam in critically ill patients with normal or ARC. The pharmacokinetics of the drug were best described by a two-compartment model and CrCl was found to have a significant effect on levetiracetam clearance, which can lead to a high risk of under-exposure, especially in patients with ARC. According to our results, the administration of 500 mg every 12 h could not be enough to achieve the target plasma concentration in the studied population. At least 500 mg every 8 h or 1000 mg every 12 h could be needed in patients with normal renal function. Even the maximum dose approved in the summary of product characteristics (1500 mg every 12 h) could be insufficient in the presence of ARC. However, further studies with a greater number of patients are necessary to determine effective and safety dose regimens in ARC patients.

Author Contributions: Conceptualization, I.B.-M., H.B., M.Á.S. and A.I.; methodology, I.B.-M., H.B., E.A.-P., A.A.-L., J.M., J.Á.S.-I., G.B., M.S.-B.G. and N.Q.T.; formal analysis, I.B.-M.; investigation, I.B.-M., H.B., E.A.-P., A.A.-L., A.R.-G., J.M., J.Á.S.-I., G.B., M.S.-B.G., N.Q.T., M.Á.S., A.I.; writing—original draft preparation, I.B.-M.; writing—review and editing, H.B., E.A.-P., A.A.-L., A.R.-G., J.M., J.Á.S.-I., G.B., M.S.-B.G., N.Q.T., M.Á.S., A.I.; supervision, H.B., A.R.-G., M.Á.S. and A.I.; project administration, M.Á.S. and A.I.; funding acquisition, A.R.-G. and A.I. All authors have read and agreed to the published version of the manuscript.

Funding: This research was funded by Department of Education of the Basque Government, grant number PIBA 2019-57; and by the University of the Basque Country UPV/EHU, grant number GIU20/048. A.A.-L. thanks the University of the Basque Country UPV/EHU for her research grant, number PIFG19/23.

Institutional Review Board Statement: The study was conducted according to the guidelines of the Declaration of Helsinki and ICH Guidelines for Good Clinical Practice, and approved by the Basque Clinical Research Ethics Committee (protocol code EPA2018019 and date of approval 15 May 2018).

Informed Consent Statement: Informed consent was obtained from all subjects involved in the study.

Acknowledgments: Authors want to particularly acknowledge the patients enrolled in this study for their participation and the Basque Biobank for its collaboration.

Conflicts of Interest: The authors declare no conflict of interest.

References

1. European Medicines Agency. Keppra 100 mg/mL Concentrate for Solution for Infusion-Summary of Product Characteristics (SPC). 2021. Available online: https://www.ema.europa.eu/en/documents/product-information/keppra-epar-product-information_en.pdf (accessed on 7 April 2021).
2. Glauser, T.; Shinnar, S.; Gloss, D.; Alldredge, B.; Arya, R.; Bainbridge, J.; Bare, M.; Bleck, T.; Dodson, W.E.; Garrity, L.; et al. Evidence-based guideline: Treatment of convulsive status epilepticus in children and adults: Report of the Guideline Committee of the American Epilepsy Society. *Epilepsy Curr.* **2016**, *16*, 48–61. [CrossRef]
3. Szaflarski, J.P.; Sangha, K.S.; Lindsell, C.J.; Shutter, L.A. Prospective, randomized, single-blinded comparative trial of intravenous levetiracetam versus phenytoin for seizure prophylaxis. *Neurocrit. Care* **2010**, *12*, 165–172. [CrossRef] [PubMed]
4. Patsalos, P.N.; Spencer, E.P.; Berry, D.J. Therapeutic drug monitoring of antiepileptic drugs in epilepsy: A 2018 update. *Drug Monit.* **2018**, *40*, 526–548. [CrossRef]
5. Patsalos, P.N. Clinical pharmacokinetics of levetiracetam. *Clin. Pharmacokinet.* **2004**, *43*, 707–724. [CrossRef] [PubMed]
6. Patsalos, P.N.; Berry, D.J.; Bourgeois, B.F.D.; Cloyd, J.C.; Glauser, T.A.; Johannessen, S.I.; Leppik, I.E.; Tomson, T.; Perucca, E. Antiepileptic drug-best practice guidelines for therapeutic drug monitoring, ILAE commission on therapeutic strategies. *Epilepsia* **2008**, *49*, 1239–1276. [CrossRef] [PubMed]
7. Johannessen, S.I.; Battino, D.; Berry, D.J.; Bialer, M.; Krämer, G.; Tomson, T.; Patsalos, P.N. Therapeutic drug monitoring of the newer antiepileptic drugs. *Ther. Drug Monit.* **2003**, *25*, 347–363. [CrossRef]
8. Sourbron, J.; Chan, H.; van der Heijdenb, E.A.M.; Klarenbeek, P.; Wijnen, B.F.M.; de Haan, G.-J.; van der Kuy, H.; Evers, S.; Majoie, M. Review on the relevance of therapeutic drug monitoring of levetiracetam. *Seizure* **2018**, *62*, 131–135. [CrossRef]
9. Jarvie, D.; Mahmoud, S.H. Therapeutic Drug Monitoring of Levetiracetam in Select Populations. *J. Pharm. Pharm. Sci.* **2018**, *21*, 149–176. [CrossRef]
10. Bilbao-Meseguer, I.; Rodríguez-Gascón, A.; Barrasa, H.; Isla, A.; Solinis, M.A. Augmented Renal Clearance in Critically Ill Patients: A Systematic Review. *Clin. Pharmacokinet.* **2018**, *57*, 1107–1121. [CrossRef]

11. Cook, A.M.; Hatton-Kolpek, J. Augmented Renal Clearance. *Pharmacotherapy* **2019**, *39*, 346–354. [CrossRef]
12. Atkinson, A.J., Jr. Augmented renal clearance. *Transl. Clin. Pharmacol.* **2018**, *26*, 111–114. [CrossRef]
13. Mahmoud, S.H.; Shen, C. Augmented Renal Clearance in Critical Illness: An Important Consideration in Drug Dosing. *Pharmaceutics* **2017**, *9*, 36. [CrossRef]
14. Jamal, J.A.; Roger, C.; Roberts, J.A. Understanding the impact of pathophysiological alterations during critical illness on drug pharmacokinetics. *Anaesth. Crit. Care Pain Med.* **2018**, *37*, 515–517. [CrossRef]
15. Campassi, M.L.; Gonzalez, M.C.; Masevicius, F.D.; Vazquez, A.R.; Moseinco, M.; Navarro, N.C.; Previgliano, L.; Rubatto, N.P.; Benites, M.H.; Estenssoro, E.; et al. Augmented renal clearance in critically ill patients: Incidence, associated factors and effects on vancomycin treatment. *Rev. Bras. Ter. Intensiva* **2014**, *26*, 13–20. [CrossRef]
16. Carlier, M.; Carrette, S.; Roberts, J.A.; Stove, V.; Verstraete, A.; Hoste, E.; Depuydt, P.; Decruyenaere, J.; Lipman, J.; Wallis, S.C. Meropenem and piperacillin/tazobactam prescribing in critically ill patients: Does augmented renal clearance affect pharmacokinetic/pharmacodynamic target attainment when extended infusions are used? *Crit. Care* **2013**, *17*, R84. [CrossRef]
17. Udy, A.A.; Varghese, J.M.; Altukroni, M.; Briscoe, S.; McWhinney, B.C.; Ungerer, J.P.; Lipman, J.; Roberts, J.A. Subtherapeutic initial beta-lactam concentrations in select critically Ill patients: Association between augmented renal clearance and low trough drug concentrations. *Chest* **2012**, *142*, 30–39. [CrossRef] [PubMed]
18. Baptista, J.P.; Sousa, E.; Martins, P.J.; Pimentel, J.M. Augmented renal clearance in septic patients and implications for vancomycin optimisation. *Int. J. Antimicrob. Agents* **2012**, *39*, 420–423. [CrossRef] [PubMed]
19. Barrasa, H.; Soraluce, A.; Usón, E.; Sainz, J.; Martín, A.; Sánchez-Izquierdo, J.Á.; Maynar, J.; Rodríguez-Gascón, A.; Isla, A. Impact of augmented renal clearance on the pharmacokinetics of linezolid: Advantages of continuous infusion from a pharmacokinetic/pharmacodynamic perspective. *Int. J. Infect. Dis.* **2020**, *93*, 329–338. [CrossRef] [PubMed]
20. Cook, A.M.; Arora, S.; Davis, J.; Pittman, T. Augmented Renal Clearance of Vancomycin and Levetiracetam in a Traumatic Brain Injury Patient. *Neurocrit. Care* **2013**, *19*, 210–214. [CrossRef] [PubMed]
21. Spencer, D.D.; Jacobi, J.; Juenke, J.M.; Fleck, J.D.; Kays, M.B. Steady-state pharmacokinetics of intravenous levetiracetam in neurocritical care patients. *Pharmacotherapy* **2011**, *31*, 934–941. [CrossRef]
22. Sime, F.B.; Roberts, J.A.; Jeffree, R.L.; Pandey, S.; Adiraju, S.; Livermore, A. Population Pharmacokinetics of Levetiracetam in Patients with Traumatic Brain Injury and Subarachnoid Hemorrhage Exhibiting Augmented Renal Clearance. *Clin. Pharmacokinet.* **2021**. [CrossRef] [PubMed]
23. Ong, C.L.J.; Goh, P.S.J.; Teo, M.M.; Lim, T.P.; Goh, K.K.K.; Ang, X.Y.; Lim, L.J.K.; Jamaludin, N.H.B.; Ang, B.T.; Kwa, L.H.A. Pharmacokinetics of levetiracetam in neurosurgical ICU patients. *J. Crit. Care* **2021**, *64*, 255–261. [CrossRef] [PubMed]
24. Hernandez-Mitre, M.P.; Medellín-Garibay, S.E.; Rodriguez-Leyva, I.; Rodriguez-Pinal, C.J.; Zarazúa, S.; Jung-Cook, H.H.; Roberts, J.A.; Romano-Moreno, S.; Milán-Segovia, R.D.C. Population pharmacokinetics and dosing recommendations of levetiracetam in adult and elderly patients with epilepsy. *J. Pharm. Sci.* **2020**, *109*, 2070–2078. [CrossRef] [PubMed]
25. Methaneethorn, J.; Leelakanok, N. Population Pharmacokinetics of Levetiracetam: A Systematic Review. *Curr. Clin. Pharmacol.* **2021**. Epub Ahead of Print. [CrossRef] [PubMed]
26. Reimers, A.; Berg, J.A.; Burns, M.L.; Brodtkorb, E.; Johannessen, S.I.; Landmark, C.J. Reference ranges for antiepileptic drugs revisited: A practical approach to establish national guidelines. *Drug Des. Dev. Ther.* **2018**, *12*, 271–280. [CrossRef] [PubMed]
27. Roberts, J.A.; Lipman, J. Optimal doripenem dosing simulations in critically ill nosocomial pneumonia patients with obesity, augmented renal clearance, and decreased bacterial susceptibility. *Crit. Care Med.* **2013**, *41*, 489–495. [CrossRef]
28. Food and Drug Administration. KEPPRA® (Levetiracetam) Injection, for Intravenous Use-Summary of Product Characteristics. 2020. Available online: https://www.accessdata.fda.gov/drugsatfda_docs/label/2020/021872s029lbl.pdf (accessed on 7 May 2021).

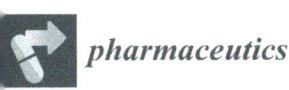

Article

Model-Informed Precision Dosing during Infliximab Induction Therapy Reduces Variability in Exposure and Endoscopic Improvement between Patients with Ulcerative Colitis

Ruben Faelens [1], Zhigang Wang [1], Thomas Bouillon [1,†], Paul Declerck [1], Marc Ferrante [2,3], Séverine Vermeire [2,3] and Erwin Dreesen [1,*]

1. Department of Pharmaceutical and Pharmacological Sciences, Katholieke Universiteit Leuven, 3000 Leuven, Belgium; ruben.faelens@kuleuven.be (R.F.); zhigang.wang@kuleuven.be (Z.W.); thomas.bouillon@bionotus.com (T.B.); paul.declerck@kuleuven.be (P.D.)
2. Department of Gastroenterology and Hepatology, University Hospitals Leuven, 3000 Leuven, Belgium; marc.ferrante@uzleuven.be (M.F.); severine.vermeire@uzleuven.be (S.V.)
3. Department of Chronic Diseases and Metabolism, Katholieke Universiteit Leuven, 3000 Leuven, Belgium
* Correspondence: erwin.dreesen@kuleuven.be; Tel.: +32-16-37-27-53
† Current Address: BioNotus, 2845 Niel, Belgium.

Abstract: Model-informed precision dosing (MIPD) may be a solution to therapeutic failure of infliximab for patients with ulcerative colitis (UC), as underexposure could be avoided, and the probability of endoscopic improvement (pEI; Mayo endoscopic subscore $\leq$ 1) could be optimized. To investigate in silico whether this claim has merit, four induction dosing regimens were simulated: 5 mg/kg (label dosing), 10 mg/kg, covariate-based MIPD (fat-free mass, corticosteroid use, and presence of extensive colitis at baseline), and concentration-based MIPD (based on the trough concentration at day 14). Covariate- and concentration-based MIPD were chosen to target the same median area under the infliximab concentration-time curve up to endoscopy at day 84 (AUC_{d84}), as was predicted from 10 mg/kg dosing. Dosing at 5 mg/kg resulted in a mean $\pm$ standard deviation pEI of 55.7 $\pm$ 9.0%. Increasing the dose to 10 mg/kg was predicted to improve pEI to 65.1 $\pm$ 6.1%. Covariate-based MIPD reduced variability in exposure and pEI (65.1 $\pm$ 5.5%). Concentration-based MIPD decreased variability further (66.0 $\pm$ 3.9%) but did so at an increased average dose of 2293 mg per patient, as compared to 2168 mg for 10 mg/kg dosing. Mean pEI remained unchanged between 10 mg/kg dosing and MIPD, since the same median AUC_{d84} was targeted. In conclusion, quantitative simulations predict MIPD will reduce variability in exposure and pEI between patients with UC during infliximab induction therapy.

Keywords: infliximab; monoclonal antibody; ulcerative colitis; inflammatory bowel disease; endoscopy; population pharmacokinetics-pharmacodynamics; simulations; therapeutic drug monitoring; model-informed precision dosing

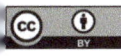

1. Introduction

Infliximab is a monoclonal antibody that binds and neutralizes the functional activity of tumor necrosis factor-alpha (TNFα). Based on the results of the landmark Active Ulcerative Colitis Trials (ACT) 1 and 2, infliximab was approved for inducing and maintaining remission in patients with moderate-to-severe ulcerative colitis (UC) [1]. In these studies, endoscopic improvement (defined as a Mayo endoscopic subscore $\leq$ 1) was achieved in about 60% of patients after administration of three infliximab infusions (5 mg/kg body weight, at weeks 0, 2, and 6; endoscopy at week 8). In post-marketing studies, endoscopic improvement rates were lower (e.g., 47% in Brandse et al. [2]), making unpredictable outcomes of infliximab induction therapy a challenge [2–5].

Dose finding in ACT 1 and 2 failed to show a consistent benefit of 10 mg/kg dosing over 5 mg/kg dosing [1]. However, higher infliximab serum concentrations during induction therapy were found to correlate with short-term endoscopic improvement, as well as long-term relapse-free and colectomy-free survival [6]. To date, the infliximab exposure-response relationship in patients with UC has been well-established [4,7–9]. Consequently, it has been hypothesized that targeting infliximab to a predefined "optimal" exposure has the potential to improve the response rate and identify primary non-responders (defined as non-response despite optimal infliximab exposure) [2,10,11]. To date, most therapeutic drug monitoring (TDM) studies of infliximab focus on maintenance therapy, whereas induction therapy is relatively unexplored. Moreover, the utility of TDM of infliximab in patients with UC remains controversial because of poor evidence from prospective TDM studies [10,12–14]. One potential reason for the weak evidence can be the use of inefficient TDM algorithms (analogous flowcharts and decision trees) in these TDM studies [15]. Therefore, model-informed precision dosing (MIPD), a more efficient and precise dose optimization strategy as compared to analogous TDM, has been suggested as a way out of this dilemma [15,16].

MIPD can be implemented through either a priori or a posteriori dose optimization, both utilizing a population pharmacokinetic (popPK) model that serves as a prior. A priori dose optimization is done by involving patient's covariates/characteristics that explain between- and within-subject variability, while a posteriori dose optimization (Bayesian forecasting) is based on previous infliximab serum concentration measurements [17]. Through these two approaches, the MIPD software tool can recommend a dose that facilitates attainment of the therapeutic target exposure. Patient covariates such as C-reactive protein (CRP), serum albumin, antibodies to infliximab (ATI), body weight or fat-free mass, and fecal calprotectin have previously been identified in popPK modeling studies [9,18].

In a previous popPK and exposure-response modeling analysis, we identified the relation between the area under the infliximab concentration-time curve up to endoscopy at day 84 (AUC_{d84}) and the probability of endoscopic improvement at day 84 [18]. Based on these results, we suggested that increased exposures would result in better clinical outcomes. We further suggested that any increased drug consumption may be offset through the use of MIPD. In the present work, we investigated these claims further by performing population simulations of these different dosing scenarios and comparing exposures, probability of endoscopic improvement, and average drug consumption.

2. Materials and Methods

2.1. Population Pharmacokinetic and Exposure-Response Models

A previously published one-compartment popPK model with interindividual and interoccasion variability was used to simulate infliximab exposure [18]. This model was built on a total of 583 samples from 204 patients with UC, and included C-reactive protein (CRP), serum albumin, and fat-free mass (FFM) as time-varying covariates, and Mayo endoscopic subscore, presence of extensive colitis, and corticosteroid use as baseline covariates.

Even though dose proportionality applies, when administering a higher dose of infliximab (*cf.* Section 2.3. *Dosing Scenarios*), a more positive disease evolution is expected, thereby influencing the time-course of CRP and serum albumin, both acute phase proteins, and possibly fat-free mass as well. Since the original dataset used for popPK model building did not include patients on higher infliximab doses (*cf.* Section 2.2 *Virtual Population*), and to avoid bias in the scenarios with higher dosing, we chose to re-estimate the model without these covariates. In theory, this should increase the unexplained interoccasion variability and residual error instead.

The logistic regression exposure–response model was adapted as well. The model was built on a subset of 159 patients and fitted the original data well [18]. However, this model predicted an ever-increasing probability of endoscopic improvement with increasing infliximab exposure. This could not be reconciled with the current line of thinking for infliximab treatment in UC, which assumes the existence of intrinsic non-responders [19]. The model was adapted to introduce maximum transition probabilities $E_{max,3\to2}$ and $E_{max,2\to1/0}$ for transitioning from a severe disease state (Mayo endoscopic subscore 3) to a moderate disease state (Mayo endoscopic subscore 2) and from a moderate disease state to endoscopic improvement (Mayo endoscopic subscore 1 or 0), respectively. Likelihood profiling was performed to identify the confidence bound for these parameters [20]. These E_{max} parameters were varied across a wide range of values and the associated $AUC_{50}s$ (i.e., the infliximab exposures required to achieve half-maximal transition probabilities) were estimated, yielding a log-likelihood (LL) estimate for each parameter set. Estimates with $\Delta 2LL = 3.84$ showed the lower 95% confidence bound for the exposure–response model. These parameter estimates were then used for subsequent simulations.

2.2. Virtual Population

To construct the virtual population for the dosing simulations, the original clinical dataset was used [7]. Only patients with a baseline Mayo endoscopic subscore of 2 or 3 were included, resulting in a source dataset of 194 patients. This dataset was expanded through Monte Carlo sampling of interindividual variability (200 samples per individual patient), yielding a total of 38,800 virtual patients.

Baseline covariates were collected in a study conducted in accordance with the principles of good clinical practice and the Declaration of Helsinki. All patients provided written informed consent prior to participation in the Ethics Committee-approved IBD Biobank [B322201213950/S53684], whereby patients' characteristics and samples were collected prospectively on a series of predefined time points.

2.3. Dosing Scenarios

Four distinct dosing scenarios were evaluated. First, a standard dosing regimen of 5 mg/kg at days 0, 14, and 42 was applied to all virtual patients. Based on the exposure–response analysis of the original dataset, there was support for a higher dose [18]. Therefore, 10 mg/kg was evaluated as a second dosing scenario.

We aimed for covariate-based and concentration-based MIPD to result in the same mean predicted probability of endoscopic improvement as in the 10 mg/kg dosing scenario. Therefore, MIPD scenarios were designed to target the same median AUC_{d84} as was predicted from the 10 mg/kg dosing scenario. The third dosing scenario was purely based on the covariates (a priori MIPD). The popPK model was used to determine the covariate-based dose required to hit the exposure target associated with the predefined probability of endoscopic improvement.

Finally, Bayesian forecasting (a posteriori MIPD) was evaluated as a fourth dosing scenario. The first dose was the same as in the covariate-based MIPD scenario. The sampled interindividual variability was used to simulate the trough concentration on day 14 resulting from the covariate-based first dose. Residual error was sampled and added to this concentration. This simulated concentration was subsequently used to perform an empirical Bayesian estimation of the patient's individual PK parameters. These individual estimates were then used to adapt the subsequent doses at days 14 and 42. Both doses were adapted to the same value, predicted to result in an AUC_{d84} exposure metric resulting in the target probability of endoscopic improvement.

2.4. Evaluation of Dosing Scenarios

The mean dose per patient and resulting exposures (AUC_{d84}) in each scenario were evaluated graphically as density plots. To quantify efficacy, the mean probability of endoscopic improvement was evaluated, as this reflects the expected fraction of patients attaining endoscopic improvement. Additionally, the mean overall dose per patient was evaluated. Finally, a robustness analysis was performed to determine whether our conclusions hold for other E_{max} parameter values.

2.5. Software

The adapted popPK and exposure–response models were estimated using NONMEM (version 7.4.3; Icon Development Solutions, Gaithersburg, MD, USA). Simulation of the dosing scenarios was performed using R (version 4.0.2; R Foundation for Statistical Computing, R Core Team, Vienna, Austria) with RxODE [21] and *tdmore*. The *tdmore* R package was developed at KU Leuven to perform simulation and evaluation of MIPD. It is available as open-source at github.com/tdmore-dev/tdmore (accessed on 27 August 2021). The NONMEM code and *tdmore* R code are provided in the Supplementary File.

3. Results

3.1. Population Pharmacokinetic and Exposure-Response Models

The popPK model was adapted to include only covariates at baseline. As expected, the interindividual variability on the elimination rate constant and the proportional residual error increased (Table S1, Supplementary Material). A visual predictive check of the updated popPK model is available in Figure S1.

Likelihood profiling of the exposure–response model showed a wide range of probable $E_{max,3\to2}$–$E_{max,2\to1/0}$ pairs. In Figure S2, the likelihood profile is shown for different parameter combinations. The $\Delta 2LL = 3.84$ contour line in red shows parameter combinations limits for $E_{max,3\to2}$–$E_{max,2\to1/0}$ of either 92.6–100% or 100–78.4%. Figure 1 shows the simulated PD model at parameter estimates with associated $\Delta 2LL = 3.84$. Based on this plot, $E_{max,2\to1/0} = 78.4\%$/$E_{max,3\to2} = 100\%$ was selected for further simulations, as the most "pessimistic" scenario. The remainder of the possible parameter values were explored in the sensitivity analysis.

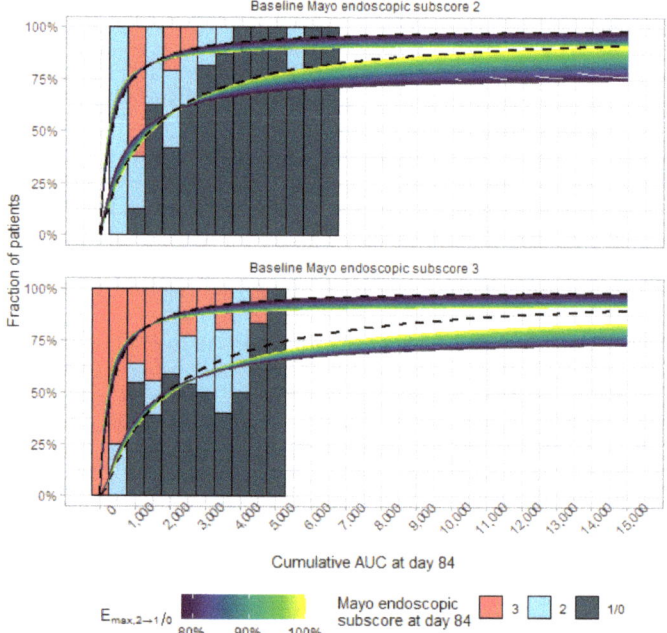

Figure 1. Exposure–response dataset (bars), binned per cumulative area under the curve (AUC) at day 84 and categorized according to Mayo endoscopic subscore at day 84, and corresponding simulated exposure–response models (lines representing the fraction of patients achieving a Mayo endoscopic subscore ≤ 1 [lower line] and ≤ 2 [upper line]). The original exposure–response model of Dreesen et al. [18] is shown as a black dashed line ($E_{max,3\to2}$ and $E_{max,2\to0/1}$ are both 100%). Colored lines represent models at $\Delta 2LL = 3.84$ with $E_{max,3\to2}$ 93% and different $E_{max,2\to1/0}$ values. All presented models fit the exposure–response dataset equally well (at $\alpha = 0.05$) but have different predictions outside the observed exposure range.

3.2. Dosing Simulations: Exposure and Efficacy

Simulation results are summarized in Table 1 and will be presented hereafter as median [95% prediction interval] for exposure (AUC_{d84}) and mean ± standard deviation for probability of endoscopic improvement. As exposure and efficacy targets differ depending on the baseline endoscopic disease severity, results are reported for baseline Mayo endoscopic subscores of 2 (moderate disease severity; reported first) and 3 (high disease severity; reported second), separately. Exposures and associated probabilities of endoscopic improvement are shown in Figures 2 and 3.

Table 1. Summary of the simulation results.

Baseline Mayo Endoscopic Subscore	Dosing scenario	AUC_{d84} (mg/L × Day)		pEI (%)		Cumulative Dose (mg)	
		median	[90%PI]	mean	±sd	mean	±sd
2	5 mg/kg	2455	[1215–4805]	61.2	±5.51	1090	±196
	10 mg/kg	4910	[2431–9609]	68.6	±3.60	2181	±393
	Covariate-based MIPD	4895	[2661–8522]	68.7	±3.08	2166	±443
	Concentration-based MIPD	5095	[3683–6879]	69.3	±1.67	2298	±613
3	5 mg/kg	1979	[953–3990]	50.3	±8.36	1078	±214
	10 mg/kg	3958	[1906–7981]	61.6	±6.05	2155	±428
	Covariate-based MIPD	3933	[2123–7045]	61.7	±5.06	2137	±417
	Concentration-based MIPD	4125	[3056–5431]	62.8	±2.51	2287	±643
Combined (2:3; 49%:51%)	5 mg/kg	2210	[1049–4448]	55.7	±8.96	1084	±205
	10 mg/kg	4419	[2098–8895]	65.1	±6.11	2168	±411
	Covariate-based MIPD	4372	[2302–7940]	65.1	±5.46	2151	±431
	Concentration-based MIPD	4561	[3209–6516]	66.0	±3.91	2293	±628

The systematically lower exposure at a baseline Mayo endoscopic subscore of 3 (severely active ulcerative colitis), as compared to a baseline Mayo endoscopic subscore of 2 (moderately active ulcerative colitis), may mechanistically be explained by a higher target load (target-mediated drug disposition) and protein-losing enteropathy (fecal drug loss). AUC_{d84}, the area under the infliximab concentration-time curve from baseline up to endoscopy at day 84 (week 12); MIPD, model-informed precision dosing; pEI, probability of endoscopic improvement; PI, prediction interval; q, quantile; sd, standard deviation.

The 5 mg/kg dosing scenario resulted in an AUC_{d84} of 2455 [1215–4805] mg × day/L and 1979 [953–3990] mg × day/L, for baseline Mayo endoscopic subscore 2 and 3, respectively. This resulted in a predicted probability of endoscopic improvement of 61.2 ± 5.5% and 50.3 ± 8.4%. By increasing the dose to 10 mg/kg, exposure doubled to 4910 [2431–9609] mg × day/L and 3958 [1906–7981] mg × day/L. Probabilities of endoscopic improvement also increased to 68.6 ± 3.6% and 61.6 ± 6.1%.

Adapting the dose based on relevant covariates allowed more precise dosing, as between-population-variability can be taken into account. As can be seen in Figure 2, covariate-based MIPD resulted in the same median exposure as 10 mg/kg dosing, at a reduced variability (4895 [2661–8522] mg × day/L and 3933 [2123–7045] mg × day/L, for baseline Mayo endoscopic subscore 2 and 3, respectively). Dose adaptation based on the trough concentration measured at day 14 (Bayesian forecasting) further reduced this variability (5095 [3683–6879] mg × day/L and 4125 [3056–5431] mg × day/L). The probability of endoscopic improvement followed a similar pattern, with similar mean probabilities across 10 mg/kg dosing, covariate-based MIPD, and concentration-based MIPD.

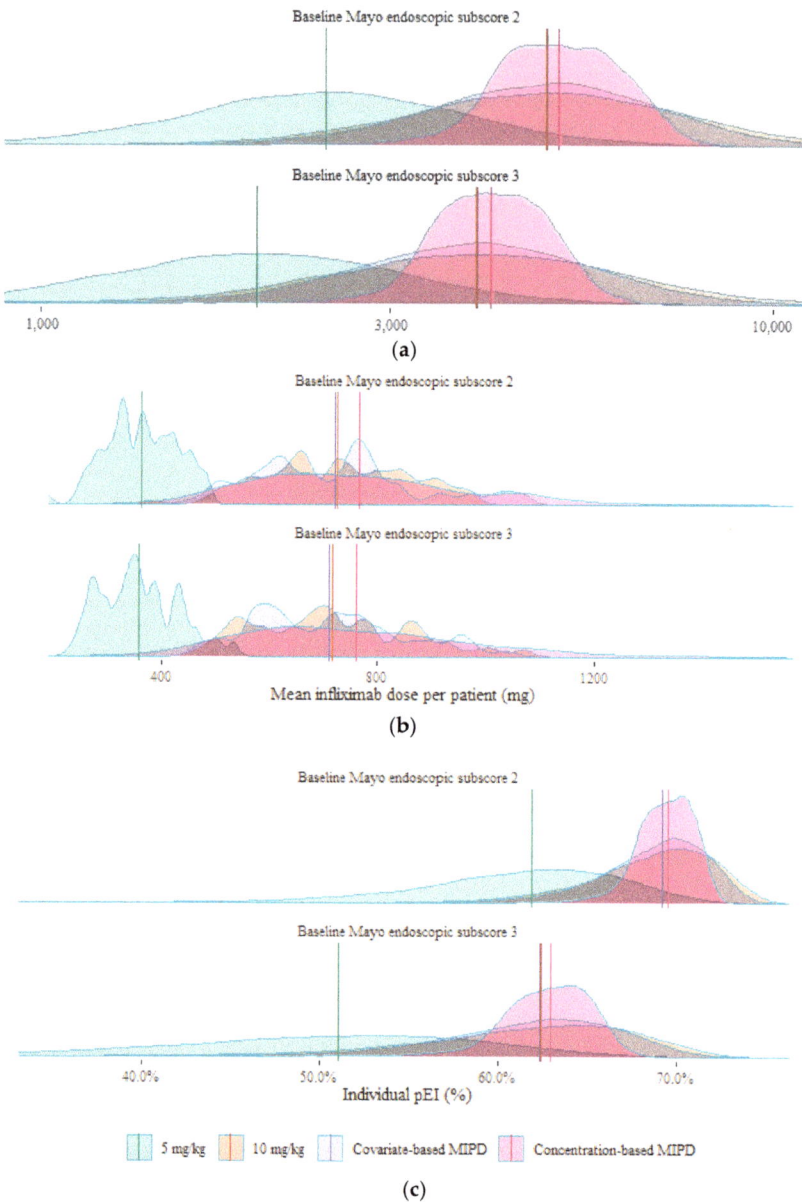

Figure 2. (**a**) Density plots of exposure in each of the four dosing scenarios, per baseline Mayo endoscopic subscore. Vertical lines show median exposure per scenario. (**b**) Density plots of the mean doses in each of the four dosing scenarios, per baseline Mayo endoscopic subscore. Vertical lines show overall mean dose per scenario. (**c**) Density plots of the individual probability of endoscopic improvement in each of the four dosing scenarios, per baseline Mayo endoscopic subscore. Vertical lines show overall mean pEI per scenario. CAUC, cumulative area under the curve; MIPD, model-informed precision dosing; pEI, probability of endoscopic improvement.

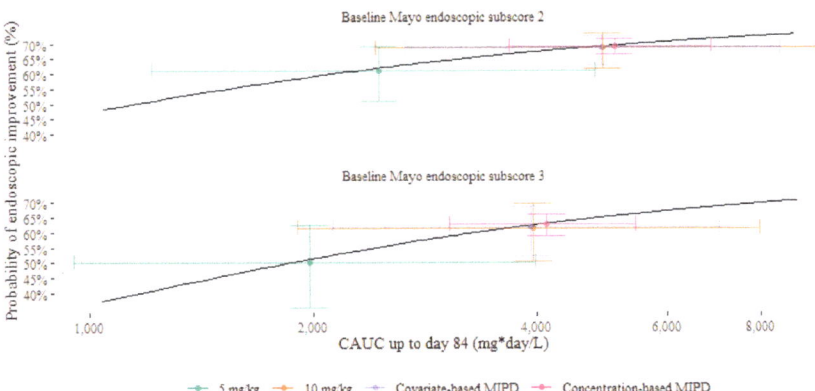

Figure 3. Predicted mean probability of endoscopic improvement versus median exposure, with 90% prediction interval in each scenario, per baseline Mayo endoscopic subscore. Black lines show model-predicted response. CAUC, cumulative area under the curve; MIPD, model-informed precision dosing.

3.3. Dosing Simulations: Drug Consumption

Looking at the average infliximab dose used per patient (see also Figure 2), 5 mg/kg dosing resulted in 1084 mg per patient, and 10 mg/kg dosing doubled the dose usage to 2168 mg per patient. Covariate-based MIPD used an average of 2151 mg per patient. Concentration-based MIPD used, at average, 2293 mg per patient.

3.4. Sensitivity Analysis

The analysis presented above assumed an E_{max} plateau of 78% for the probability of transitioning from a Mayo endoscopic subscore of 2 (moderate disease severity) to a Mayo endoscopic subscore of 0 or 1 (endoscopic improvement). This plateau benefited MIPD, as overexposed patients were dose-reduced without significantly reducing the probability of endoscopic improvement, while underexposed patients were dose-increased, thereby significantly increasing the probability of endoscopic improvement.

Repeating our simulation study with higher values for $E_{max,2\to1/0}$ decreased this benefit, further favoring 10 mg/kg dosing, as is illustrated in Figure 2. Other parameter combinations at $\Delta 2LL = 3.84$, as well as for the base model ($\Delta 2LL = 0$), consistently showed less favorable results for MIPD.

At $E_{max,3\to2}$–$E_{max,2\to1/0}$ of 92.6–100%, the probability of endoscopic improvement for 10 mg/kg dosing was 77.0% [62.7–86.5%] and 65% [48.1–76.7%], for baseline Mayo endoscopic subscore 2 and 3, respectively, at an average drug consumption of 2168 mg per patient. Bayesian forecasting resulted in a probability of endoscopic improvement of 77.6% [71.7–82.3%] and 65.8% [59.4–70.9%], for baseline Mayo endoscopic subscore 2 and 3, at an average drug consumption of 2293 mg per patient.

4. Discussion

In this study, we compared four possible dosing scenarios for infliximab induction therapy in patients with UC: 5 mg/kg weight-based dosing (label dosing), and three dosing strategies with increased exposure: 10 mg/kg weight-based dosing, covariate-based MIPD, and concentration-based MIPD, all with unchanged timing of the infusions (day 0, 14, and 42). The 10 mg/kg dosing scenario was predicted to significantly improve endoscopic outcomes as compared to 5 mg/kg dosing. By design, MIPD (based on either covariates or the day 14 trough concentration) resulted in the same median exposure (AUC_{d84}) and, consequently, the same mean probability of endoscopic improvement as observed in the 10 mg/kg dosing scenario. MIPD was predicted to successfully adapt individual patient doses, reducing the interindividual variability in infliximab exposure and, with it, the probability of endoscopic improvement, thereby providing "more equal" chances of endoscopic remission to all patients. Surprisingly, it did so at a higher average drug consumption per patient. Underexposed patients indeed received a relative dose increase, while overexposed patients received a relative dose decrease. However, this is a non-zero sum, as, e.g., 10 mg × 2 + 10 mg × 0.5 > 10 mg + 10 mg. Therefore, our simulation study showed improved outcomes under 10 mg/kg dosing as compared to 5 mg/kg dosing and showed additional benefit of MIPD over 10 mg/kg for reducing variability in exposure and efficacy between patients; however, at a higher direct drug cost. Performing MIPD may thus require a willingness to "pay for equality" amongst patients [22]. Consequently, we may consider shifting focus from outcome rates at the population level (the traditional industry perspective) to outcome chances at the individual patient level. It is at the individual patient level that MIPD may show value. Since the majority of patients attain the target under empirical dosing, it is important that future MIPD studies are restricted to vulnerable populations, such as patients with acute severe ulcerative colitis [23].

The simulations described in this work were based on a previously established popPK model and exposure–response model of infliximab [18]. These models described the relation between the infliximab dose and exposure, and the AUC_{d84} and the probability of endoscopic improvement at day 84, respectively. The models were established on a dataset of 204 patients with moderate-to-severe UC. Since the majority of the infliximab doses in the original cohort were 5 mg/kg (approximately 90%), and only about 10% of the doses were 10 mg/kg, it should be noted that the exposure–response model was built on a relatively limited range of exposures. The exposures simulated in the present work exceed this range. However, this weakness was mitigated by a thorough analysis of exposure–response model parameter confidence intervals and likelihood profiling, and a sensitivity analysis. Our findings hold throughout the full range of probable model parameter values.

The exposure–response model assumes a causal effect between exposure and response. Previous clinical studies have indeed found a correlation between low trough concentrations and primary nonresponse to anti-TNFα therapy [24]. However, the causality assumed in our exposure–response model was never established in clinical studies. In light of this, time-varying disease-related covariates may instead be simulated in a joint model, avoiding potential underestimation of exposure at higher doses and reduced disease severity. Further research is needed to definitively establish whether non-response at low trough concentrations is due to mechanistic failure (pharmacodynamic [PD] failure) or underexposure (PK failure), as others have attempted to model this distinction [25,26]. Underexposure can be resolved through dose increase, while the mechanistic failure suggests switching to a different drug with another mechanism of action. A more fine-grained model of continuous endpoints may distinguish between PK and PD failure.

High exposure to infliximab may pose safety concerns. The 10 mg/kg dosing may result in very high exposures, which were predicted in the present study to be beneficial to patients. In reality, these highly exposed patients may present with adverse drug reactions such as infections, especially in the elderly, and MIPD may benefit these patients by reducing toxicity [27–29].

Our findings seemingly contradict the pivotal ACT 1 and 2 trials [1], which showed no significant difference between 5 mg/kg and 10 mg/kg in endoscopic improvement rates on day 56 of therapy. Nevertheless, in the post-hoc PK-PD analysis of ACT 1 and 2, the exposure–response relationship has been established [6]. It would be worthwhile to repeat the presented modeling and simulation exercise, including the data from these pivotal trials. Notwithstanding these results, clinical trials are currently underway, evaluating an intensified induction regimen of 10 mg/kg [30].

MIPD of infliximab has been implemented in clinical practice mainly in tertiary care centers, however, even there, the confidence in MIPD is crumbling as the results of the landmark TAXIT, TAILORIX, and NOR-DRUM trials do not live up to expectations [12,14,31]. Our research showed that in silico simulations are a low-cost alternative to these clinical studies. Nevertheless, the translation of findings from a virtual trial into the real world may be challenged by noise due to, for example, sampling and measurement errors, rounding of doses and dosing intervals, etc. [32].

MIPD is classically used to improve the probability of target attainment, with the target window defined by efficacy and toxicity. In this context, efficacy is ever-increasing with higher exposures, while a dose increase is largely limited by cost rather than toxicity. It may be interesting to quantify the effect of infliximab as quality-adjusted life years (QALY) instead, allowing a direct comparison to increased cost and a straightforward optimization of QALY/cost.

In summary, we performed simulations to illustrate and predict the impact of three dosing strategies for increasing infliximab exposure during induction therapy as compared to 5 mg/kg weight-based label dosing, thereby improving the probability of endoscopic improvement. The use of 10 mg/kg dosing was indeed predicted to improve the probability of endoscopic improvement to 65.1% at an average drug consumption of 2168 mg per patient during induction therapy. Individualized dose adaptation could maintain the same mean probability of endoscopic improvement while reducing variability between individual patients. Although MIPD showed benefit for reducing variability in exposure and efficacy between patients, this comes at a higher direct drug cost as compared to 10 mg/kg weight-based dosing.

Supplementary Materials: The following are available online at https://www.mdpi.com/article/10.3390/pharmaceutics13101623/s1, Figure S1: Prediction-corrected visual predictive check of the original population pharmacokinetic model, Figure S2. Log-likelihood surface for the exposure-response model, Table S1. Parameter estimates of the original and adapted population pharmacokinetic models.

Author Contributions: Conceptualization, R.F., T.B. and E.D.; Data curation, P.D., M.F., S.V. and E.D.; Formal analysis, R.F. and Z.W.; Funding acquisition, E.D.; Investigation, R.F., Z.W. and E.D.; Methodology, R.F., Z.W. and E.D.; Project administration, E.D.; Resources, P.D., M.F., S.V. and E.D.; Software, R.F.; Supervision, T.B. and E.D.; Validation, R.F., T.B. and E.D.; Visualization, R.F., Z.W. and E.D.; Writing—original draft, R.F., Z.W. and E.D.; Writing—review & editing, T.B., P.D., M.F. and S.V. All authors have read and agreed to the published version of the manuscript.

Funding: This research was funded by the Research Foundation—Flanders (FWO), Belgium: T.B. received a TBM grant (grant number T003117N), P.D. received a TBM grant (grant number T003716N), M.F. is a Senior Clinical Investigator, and E.D. is a postdoctoral research fellow (grant number: 12X9420N).

Institutional Review Board Statement: The study was conducted according to the guidelines of the Declaration of Helsinki and approved by the Ethics Committee Research of UZ/KU Leuven (3000, IBD Biobank; B322201213950/S53684)."

Informed Consent Statement: Informed consent was obtained from all subjects involved in the study.

Data Availability Statement: The data presented in this study are available in the research article and supplementary material here.

Acknowledgments: We acknowledge Vera Ballet for an excellent job in maintaining the Leuven IBD patient database; Griet Compernolle, Sophie Tops, Els Brouwers, and Miet Peeters for performing the infliximab serum concentration measurements; and Pieter Annaert for the guidance and management of student R.F.

Conflicts of Interest: R.F. performed consulting work for Janssen Pharmaceutica on compounds not related to Remicade in the employ of SGS Exprimo NV. T.B. is a paid employer of BioNotus. M.F. received research grant from AbbVie, Amgen, Biogen, Janssen, Pfizer, and Takeda; speakers fee from Abbvie, Amgen, Biogen, Boehringer-Ingelheim, Falk, Ferring, Janssen, Lamepro, MSD, Mylan, Pfizer, Sandoz, Takeda and Truvion Healthcare; consultancy fee from Abbvie, Boehringer-Ingelheim, Celltrion, Janssen, Lilly, Medtronic, MSD, Pfizer, Sandoz, Takeda and Thermo Fisher. S.V. received financial support for research from AbbVie, J&J, Pfizer, and Takeda; consulting and/or speaking fees from AbbVie, Arena Pharmaceuticals, Avaxia, Boehringer Ingelheim, Celgene, Falk Pharma, Ferring, Galapagos, Genentech-Roche, Gilead, Hospira, Janssen, Mundipharma, MSD, Pfizer, Prodigest, Progenity, Prometheus, Robarts Clinical Trials, Second Genome, Shire, Takeda, Theravance, and

Tillots Pharma AG. E.D. received consultancy fees from argenx and Janssen (all fees paid to the University). Z.W. and P.D. declare no conflict of interest. The funders had no role in the design of the study; in the collection, analyses, or interpretation of data; in the writing of the manuscript, or in the decision to publish the results.

References

1. Rutgeerts, P.; Sandborn, W.J.; Feagan, B.G.; Reinisch, W.; Olson, A.; Johanns, J.; Travers, S.; Rachmilewitz, D.; Hanauer, S.B.; Lichtenstein, G.R.; et al. Infliximab for Induction and Maintenance Therapy for Ulcerative Colitis. *N. Engl. J. Med.* **2005**, *353*, 2462–2476. [CrossRef]
2. Brandse, J.F.; Mathôt, R.A.; van der Kleij, D.; Rispens, T.; Ashruf, Y.; Jansen, J.M.; Rietdijk, S.; Löwenberg, M.; Ponsioen, C.Y.; Singh, S.; et al. Pharmacokinetic Features and Presence of Antidrug Antibodies Associate With Response to Infliximab Induction Therapy in Patients With Moderate to Severe Ulcerative Colitis. *Clin. Gastroenterol. Hepatol.* **2016**, *14*, 251–258.e2. [CrossRef] [PubMed]
3. Seow, C.H.; Newman, A.; Irwin, S.P.; Steinhart, A.H.; Silverberg, M.S.; Greenberg, G.R. Trough serum infliximab: A predictive factor of clinical outcome for infliximab treatment in acute ulcerative colitis. *Gut* **2010**, *59*, 49–54. [CrossRef]
4. Papamichael, K.; Van Stappen, T.; Vande Casteele, N.; Gils, A.; Billiet, T.; Tops, S.; Claes, K.; Van Assche, G.; Rutgeerts, P.; Vermeire, S.; et al. Infliximab Concentration Thresholds During Induction Therapy Are Associated With Short-term Mucosal Healing in Patients With Ulcerative Colitis. *Clin. Gastroenterol. Hepatol.* **2016**, *14*, 543–549. [CrossRef] [PubMed]
5. Farkas, K.; Rutka, M.; Golovics, P.A.; Végh, Z.; Lovász, B.D.; Nyári, T.; Gecse, K.B.; Kolar, M.; Bortlik, M.; Duricova, D.; et al. Efficacy of infliximab biosimilar CT-P13 induction therapy on mucosal healing in ulcerative colitis. *J. Crohns Colitis* **2016**, *10*, 1273–1278. [CrossRef] [PubMed]
6. Adedokun, O.J.; Sandborn, W.J.; Feagan, B.G.; Rutgeerts, P.; Xu, Z.; Marano, C.W.; Johanns, J.; Zhou, H.; Davis, H.M.; Cornillie, F.; et al. Association between serum concentration of infliximab and efficacy in adult patients with ulcerative colitis. *Gastroenterology* **2014**, *147*, 1296–1307.e5. [CrossRef]
7. Arias, M.T.; Vande Casteele, N.; Vermeire, S.; de Buck van Overstraeten, A.; Billiet, T.; Baert, F.; Wolthuis, A.; Van Assche, G.; Noman, M.; Hoffman, I.; et al. A panel to predict long-term outcome of infliximab therapy for patients with ulcerative colitis. *Clin. Gastroenterol. Hepatol.* **2015**, *13*, 531–538. [CrossRef]
8. Kobayashi, T.; Suzuki, Y.; Motoya, S.; Hirai, F.; Ogata, H.; Ito, H.; Sato, N.; Ozaki, K.; Watanabe, M.; Hibi, T. First trough level of infliximab at week 2 predicts future outcomes of induction therapy in ulcerative colitis—results from a multicenter prospective randomized controlled trial and its post hoc analysis. *J. Gastroenterol.* **2016**, *51*, 241–251. [CrossRef]
9. Vande Casteele, N.; Jeyarajah, J.; Jairath, V.; Feagan, B.G.; Sandborn, W.J. Infliximab Exposure-Response Relationship and Thresholds Associated With Endoscopic Healing in Patients With Ulcerative Colitis. *Clin. Gastroenterol. Hepatol.* **2019**, *17*, 1814–1821. [CrossRef]
10. Vande Casteele, N.; Herfarth, H.; Katz, J.; Falck-Ytter, Y.; Singh, S. American Gastroenterological Association Institute Technical Review on the Role of Therapeutic Drug Monitoring in the Management of Inflammatory Bowel Diseases. *Gastroenterology* **2017**, *153*, 835–857. [CrossRef]
11. Harbord, M.; Eliakim, R.; Bettenworth, D.; Karmiris, K.; Katsanos, K.; Kopylov, U.; Kucharzik, T.; Molnár, T.; Raine, T.; Sebastian, S.; et al. Third European evidence-based consensus on diagnosis and management of ulcerative colitis. Part 2: Current management. *J. Crohns Colitis* **2017**. [CrossRef]
12. Vande Casteele, N.; Ferrante, M.; Van Assche, G.; Ballet, V.; Compernolle, G.; Van Steen, K.; Simoens, S.; Rutgeerts, P.; Gils, A.; Vermeire, S. Trough concentrations of infliximab guide dosing for patients with inflammatory bowel disease. *Gastroenterology* **2015**, *148*, 1320–1329. [CrossRef] [PubMed]
13. Mitrev, N.; Vande Casteele, N.; Seow, C.H.; Andrews, J.M.; Connor, S.J.; Moore, G.T.; Barclay, M.; Begun, J.; Bryant, R.; Chan, W.; et al. Review article: Consensus statements on therapeutic drug monitoring of anti-tumour necrosis factor therapy in inflammatory bowel diseases. *Aliment. Pharmacol. Ther.* **2017**, *46*, 1037–1053. [CrossRef] [PubMed]
14. Syversen, S.W.; Goll, G.L.; Jørgensen, K.K.; Sandanger, Ø.; Sexton, J.; Olsen, I.C.; Gehin, J.E.; Warren, D.J.; Brun, M.K.; Klaasen, R.A.; et al. Effect of Therapeutic Drug Monitoring vs Standard Therapy During Infliximab Induction on Disease Remission in Patients With Chronic Immune-Mediated Inflammatory Diseases: A Randomized Clinical Trial. *JAMA* **2021**, *325*, 1744–1754. [CrossRef] [PubMed]
15. Wang, Z.; Dreesen, E. Therapeutic drug monitoring of anti-tumor necrosis factor agents: Lessons learned and remaining issues. *Curr. Opin. Pharmacol.* **2020**, *55*, 53–59. [CrossRef]
16. Keizer, R.J.; ter Heine, R.; Frymoyer, A.; Lesko, L.J.; Mangat, R.; Goswami, S. Model-Informed Precision Dosing at the Bedside: Scientific Challenges and Opportunities. *CPT Pharmacomet. Syst. Pharmacol.* **2018**, *7*, 785–787. [CrossRef] [PubMed]
17. Vermeire, S.; Dreesen, E.; Papamichael, K.; Dubinsky, M.C. How, When, and for Whom Should We Perform Therapeutic Drug Monitoring? *Clin. Gastroenterol. Hepatol.* **2019**. [CrossRef]
18. Dreesen, E.; Faelens, R.; Van Assche, G.; Ferrante, M.; Vermeire, S.; Gils, A.; Bouillon, T. Optimising infliximab induction dosing for patients with ulcerative colitis. *Br. J. Clin. Pharmacol.* **2019**, *85*, 782–795. [CrossRef]
19. Ben-Horin, S.; Kopylov, U.; Chowers, Y. Optimizing anti-TNF treatments in inflammatory bowel disease. *Autoimmun. Rev.* **2014**, *13*, 24–30. [CrossRef]

20. Sheiner, L.B. Analysis of pharmacokinetic data using parametric models. III. Hypothesis tests and confidence intervals. *J. Pharmacokinet. Biopharm.* **1986**, *14*, 539–555. [CrossRef]
21. Fidler, M.L.; Hallow, M.; Wilkins, J.; Wang, W. RxODE: Facilities for Simulating from ODE-Based Models 2021. R package version 1.1.0. Available online: https://CRAN.R-project.org/package=RxODE (accessed on 20 August 2021).
22. Dreesen, E. New Tools for Therapeutic Drug Monitoring: Making Big Things out of Small Pieces. *J. Crohns Colitis* **2021**. [CrossRef] [PubMed]
23. Battat, R.; Hemperly, A.; Truong, S.; Whitmire, N.; Boland, B.S.; Dulai, P.S.; Holmer, A.K.; Nguyen, N.H.; Singh, S.; Vande Casteele, N.; et al. Baseline Clearance of Infliximab Is Associated With Requirement for Colectomy in Patients With Acute Severe Ulcerative Colitis. *Clin. Gastroenterol. Hepatol.* **2021**, *19*, 511–518.e6. [CrossRef] [PubMed]
24. Ding, N.S.; Hart, A.; De Cruz, P. Systematic review: Predicting and optimising response to anti-TNF therapy in Crohn's disease-Algorithm for practical management. *Aliment. Pharmacol. Ther.* **2016**, *43*, 30–51. [CrossRef]
25. Dreesen, E.; Berends, S.; Laharie, D.; D'Haens, G.; Vermeire, S.; Gils, A.; Mathôt, R. Modelling of the relationship between infliximab exposure, faecal calprotectin and endoscopic remission in patients with Crohn's disease. *Br. J. Clin. Pharmacol.* **2020**, *87*, 106–118. [CrossRef] [PubMed]
26. Brekkan, A.; Lopez-Lazaro, L.; Yngman, G.; Plan, E.L.; Acharya, C.; Hooker, A.C.; Kankanwadi, S.; Karlsson, M.O. A Population Pharmacokinetic-Pharmacodynamic Model of Pegfilgrastim. *AAPS J.* **2018**, *20*, 91. [CrossRef]
27. Kantasiripitak, W.; Verstockt, B.; Alsoud, D.; Lobatón, T.; Thomas, D.; Gils, A.; Vermeire, S.; Ferrante, M.; Dreesen, E. The effect of aging on infliximab exposure and response in patients with inflammatory bowel diseases. *Br. J. Clin. Pharmacol.* **2021**. [CrossRef]
28. Bejan-Angoulvant, T.; Ternant, D.; Daoued, F.; Medina, F.; Bernard, L.; Mammou, S.; Paintaud, G.; Mulleman, D. Brief Report: Relationship Between Serum Infliximab Concentrations and Risk of Infections in Patients Treated for Spondyloarthritis. *Arthritis Rheumatol.* **2017**, *69*, 108–113. [CrossRef]
29. Landemaine, A.; Petitcollin, A.; Brochard, C.; Miard, C.; Dewitte, M.; Le, E.; Grainville, T.; Bellissant, E.; Siproudhis, L.; Bouguen, G. Cumulative Exposure to Infliximab, But Not Trough Concentrations, Correlate With Rate of Infection. *Clin. Gastroenterol. Hepatol.* **2020**. [CrossRef] [PubMed]
30. NIH U.S. Natial Library of Medicine ClinicalTrials.gov. Optimising Infliximab Induction Therapy for Acute Severe Ulcerative Colitis (PREDICT-UC). Available online: https://clinicaltrials.gov/ct2/show/NCT02770040 (accessed on 16 July 2021).
31. D'Haens, G.; Vermeire, S.; Lambrecht, G.; Baert, F.; Bossuyt, P.; Pariente, B.; Buisson, A.; Bouhnik, Y.; Filippi, J.; vander Woude, J., et al. Increasing Infliximab Dose Based on Symptoms, Biomarkers, and Serum Drug Concentrations Does Not Increase Clinical, Endoscopic, and Corticosteroid-Free Remission in Patients With Active Luminal Crohn's Disease. *Gastroenterology* **2018**, *154*, 1343–1351.e1. [CrossRef] [PubMed]
32. Alihodzic, D.; Broeker, A.; Baehr, M.; Kluge, S.; Langebrake, C.; Wicha, S.G. Impact of Inaccurate Documentation of Sampling and Infusion Time in Model-Informed Precision Dosing. *Front. Pharmacol.* **2020**, *11*, 1–12. [CrossRef]

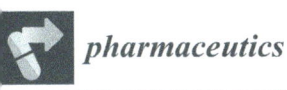

Article

Ustekinumab Dosing Individualization in Crohn's Disease Guided by a Population Pharmacokinetic–Pharmacodynamic Model

Jurij Aguiar Zdovc [1,†], Jurij Hanžel [2,3,†], Tina Kurent [2], Nejc Sever [2], Matic Koželj [2], Nataša Smrekar [2], Gregor Novak [2], Borut Štabuc [2,3], Erwin Dreesen [4,5], Debby Thomas [4], Tomaž Vovk [1], Barbara Ostanek [6], David Drobne [2,3] and Iztok Grabnar [1,*]

1. Department of Biopharmaceutics and Pharmacokinetics, Faculty of Pharmacy, University of Ljubljana, 1000 Ljubljana, Slovenia; jurij.aguiar.zdovc@ffa.uni-lj.si (J.A.Z.); tomaz.vovk@ffa.uni-lj.si (T.V.)
2. Department of Gastroenterology, University Medical Centre Ljubljana, 1000 Ljubljana, Slovenia; jurij.hanzel@gmail.com (J.H.); tina.kurent@gmail.com (T.K.); nejc.sever@gmail.com (N.S.); kozelj.matic@gmail.com (M.K.); nsmreki@gmail.com (N.S.); grega84@gmail.com (G.N.); borut.stabuc@gmail.com (B.Š.); david.drobne@gmail.com (D.D.)
3. Department of Internal Medicine, Medical Faculty, University of Ljubljana, 1000 Ljubljana, Slovenia
4. Department of Pharmaceutical and Pharmacological Sciences, KU Leuven, 3000 Leuven, Belgium; erwin.dreesen@kuleuven.be (E.D.); debby.thomas@kuleuven.be (D.T.)
5. Department of Pharmacy, Uppsala University, 751 23 Uppsala, Sweden
6. Department of Clinical Biochemistry, Faculty of Pharmacy, University of Ljubljana, 1000 Ljubljana, Slovenia; barbara.ostanek@ffa.uni-lj.si
* Correspondence: iztok.grabnar@ffa.uni-lj.si; Tel.: +386-1-4769-543
† These authors contributed equally.

Abstract: Ustekinumab is a monoclonal antibody used in Crohn's disease (CD). Dose optimization in case of non-response and the role of pharmacokinetic–pharmacodynamic (PK-PD) monitoring remain unresolved dilemmas in clinical practice. We aimed to develop a population PK-PD model for ustekinumab in CD and simulate efficacy of alternative dosing regimens. We included 57 patients and recorded their characteristics during 32 weeks after starting with ustekinumab therapy. Serum ustekinumab concentration was prospectively measured and fecal calprotectin (FC) concentration was used to monitor the disease activity. Ustekinumab PK-PD was described by a two-compartment target-mediated drug disposition model linked to an indirect response model. Lower fat-free mass, higher serum albumin, previous non-exposure to biologics, *FCGR3A*-158 V/V variant and lower C-reactive protein were associated with higher ustekinumab exposure. Model-based simulation suggested that 41.9% of patients receiving standard dosing achieve biochemical remission at week 32. In patients not achieving remission with standard dosing at week 16, transition to 4-weekly subcutaneous maintenance dosing with or without intravenous reinduction resulted in comparably higher remission rates at week 32 (51.1% vs. 49.2%, respectively). Our findings could be used to guide stratified ustekinumab treatment in CD, particularly in patients with unfavorable characteristics, who might benefit from early transition to 4-weekly maintenance dosing.

Keywords: ustekinumab; inflammatory bowel disease; fecal calprotectin; pharmacokinetics-pharmacodynamics; therapeutic drug monitoring

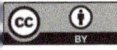

1. Introduction

Crohn's disease (CD) is a debilitating, relapsing-remitting, incurable inflammatory disease of the digestive tract [1]. Treatment goals have shifted from symptomatic improvement to a combination of endoscopic and clinical remission [2]. Biomarker remission was identified as an adjunct treatment goal with fecal calprotectin (FC) being sensitive for endoscopic disease activity [3,4].

Ustekinumab is an IgG1κ monoclonal antibody that binds with high affinity to the p40 subunit shared by interleukin 12 (IL12) and interleukin 23 (IL23) [5]. Standard dosing with weight-based intravenous induction followed by 90 mg subcutaneous injections every 8 weeks is not effective for all patients, with real-world studies reporting that only up to one half of the patients achieve clinical remission, and up to 25% of patients achieve endoscopic remission [6–11]. The exposure–response relationship between peak ustekinumab serum concentration after the induction dose and endoscopic remission at 24 weeks suggests that a subset of patients not responding to conventional dosing may benefit from dose escalation [11]. Recent real-world studies assessing off-label intensified maintenance therapy with 90 mg administered every four weeks in patients with insufficient response have shown favorable rates of clinical, biochemical and endoscopic remission [12–15].

It remains unclear which patients are best suited for dose optimization, what is the most suitable dosing strategy (intravenous re-induction or dosing interval shortening for subcutaneous therapy) and how pharmacokinetic–pharmacodynamic (PK-PD) monitoring could improve the effectiveness of ustekinumab. Moreover, clinical PK studies of ustekinumab in CD are scarce and data on how demographic, pathophysiological, and genetic factors impact the drug's PK and PD, are limited.

Our objective was to develop a population PK-PD model linking ustekinumab dosing regimen to the time course of FC concentrations. Through model-based simulations, which integrate both PK and PD data, we aimed to explore different dosing strategies, which are increasingly used in daily clinical practice.

2. Materials and Methods

2.1. Patients and Study Design

This was a prospective observational study in patients with CD starting treatment with ustekinumab at a single tertiary referral center. The study design and clinical results have partially been reported elsewhere [11]. Briefly, consecutive patients aged ≥18 years with CD who started treatment with ustekinumab between October 2017 and June 2019 were screened for eligibility and included in the current study, regardless of baseline endoscopic disease activity. They received a weight-based intravenous induction dose (≤55 kg: 260 mg; 55–85 kg: 390 mg; >85 kg: 520 mg) infused over one hour at baseline, followed by a fixed subcutaneous maintenance dose of 90 mg every 8 weeks. The duration of follow-up was 32 weeks.

2.2. Pharmacokinetic and Pharmacodynamic Data

Serum samples for the PK analysis were prospectively collected at baseline, 1 h after the end of the intravenous infusion (peak), and subsequently at weeks 2, 4, 8, 9, 10, 12, 16, 20, 24, and 32. Fecal samples of the first morning bowel movement were collected for the PD analysis at baseline, and subsequently at weeks 8, 16, 24, and 32. Ileocolonoscopies were performed within 2 months before starting ustekinumab to determine the presence of mucosal ulcerations to define endoscopically active luminal disease at baseline. Blood samples for genotyping analyses were collected at baseline.

Serum unbound ustekinumab concentration (hereafter referred to as ustekinumab concentration) was measured with a validated enzyme-linked immunosorbent assay (ELISA, ImmunoGuide®, AybayTech Biotechnology, Ankara, Turkey), with a lower limit of quantification (LOQ) at 0.35 µg/mL [11]. Antibodies to ustekinumab were measured with a drug-tolerant ELISA in serum samples with ustekinumab concentration <1 µg/mL [10]. FC was measured with a Calprest ELISA assay (Eurospital, Triest, Italy) with a measurement range of 15.6–500 mg/kg.

Genomic DNA was isolated from whole blood collected in EDTA tubes by using a FlexiGene DNA kit (Qiagen, Hilden, Germany). The concentration and purity of DNA were measured on NanoDrop™ One/OneC Microvolume UV-Vis Spectrophotometer (Thermo Fischer Scientific, Waltham, MA, USA). Genotyping of single nucleotide polymorphisms (SNPs) was performed by TaqMan® Pre-Designed SNP Genotyping Assays (Thermo Fischer

Scientific, Waltham, MA, USA) on a LightCycler 480II real-time polymerase chain reaction instrument (Roche, Basel, Switzerland) according to manufacturer's recommendations. SNPs were selected based on previously identified associations with ustekinumab treatment outcomes in psoriasis or a possible role in the mediation of IgG clearance [16–18]. The analyzed SNPs and the specific assays used were: *IL12B* (rs3212227, assay ID: C_2084293_10; rs3213094, assay ID: C_29927086_10; and rs6887695, assay ID: C_1994992_10), *FCGR2A* (rs1801274, assay ID: C_9077561_20) and *FCGR3A* (rs396991, assay ID: C_25815666_10). To validate our results, 20% of the samples were re-genotyped for each SNP, and the results were found to be reproducible with no discrepancies noted.

Demographic characteristics (age, weight, height, sex), clinical data (co-morbidities, disease history and disease location, concomitant and previous treatment) and biochemical markers (C-reactive protein (CRP), serum albumin) were recorded. Fat-free mass (FFM) was determined using the Janmahasatian model [19].

2.3. Statistical Analysis and Pharmacokinetic–Pharmacodynamic Modeling

Descriptive statistics were used to present the data as non-normally distributed with medians and inter-quartile ranges (IQR). The nonlinear mixed-effects methodology and NONMEM® software (version 7.3, Icon Development Solutions, Ellicott City, MD, USA) was used to analyze the PK and PD data and develop a population PK-PD model, linking ustekinumab concentrations, patients' characteristics and FC at all time points.

A population PK model was developed using the ustekinumab concentrations converted to nanomolar concentration, assuming its molecular weight of 149 kDa. A linear one- and two-compartment models, and approximations of the target mediated drug disposition (TMDD) model were tested [20–23]. First-order absorption of ustekinumab was assumed after the subcutaneous dosing. Considering the concentration of ustekinumab target (p40 subunit of IL12 and IL23) was not measured, it was modeled as a latent variable in TMDD models. The PK studies in monkeys report a bi-exponential decline of the cytokines containing the p40 subunit (IL12 and IL23) [24,25]. Therefore, the PK data were extracted from these studies and PK parameters for the IL12 and IL23 were estimated and allometrically scaled to human. These estimates were used as initial estimates of the PK parameters of the target disposition in the TMDD models. One- and two-compartment models were tested to describe the distribution of the target.

Additive, proportional and combination (additive + proportional) error models were tested for residual variability. The logit transformation was used to describe the interindividual variability (IIV) of fraction of absorbed ustekinumab and the exponential model was used to describe the IIV of other parameters. The model with the lowest Akaike information criterion (AIC) was used as a base PK model (Table S1), for the subsequent covariate model building.

To explain the estimated IIV in the PK parameters, the candidate parameter–covariate relationships were selected based on scientific plausibility, previously reported relationships, and trends in correlation plots between individual PK parameters and covariates. Stepwise covariate procedure ($p < 0.05$ in the forward inclusion, $p < 0.01$ in the backward elimination) was used to test the significance of parameter–covariate relationships. To estimate the effect of the body size, FFM was chosen over total body weight, considering the distribution of monoclonal antibodies is predominantly limited to extracellular fluids. The evaluated continuous covariates were: disease duration, FFM, baseline serum CRP concentration and serum albumin concentration. The evaluated categorical covariates were: previous biological therapy (bio-naïve), smoking, and SNPs in *IL12B* (rs3212227, rs3213094, rs6887695), *FCGR2A* (rs1801274) and *FCGR3A* (rs396991). Linear and power model were tested for continuous covariates and dominant and recessive grouping combinations were tested for SNPs.

The individual PK parameters obtained from the final PK model were used for the subsequent PD analysis [26], to describe the relationship between ustekinumab PK, target disposition and FC concentration. The bio-phase distribution model, indirect response model and signal transduction (transit compartment indirect response) model were tested to describe the delay between ustekinumab PK and PD [27]. Exponential model, as well as Box-Cox transformation were tested to describe the IIV of baseline FC concentration (FC_0).

Laplacian estimation with interaction was used for parameter estimation. The M3 method was used for data below the lower or above the upper LOQ [28]. AIC was used for model comparison. The model was internally validated with a visual predictive check (VPC, n = 2000) and parameter uncertainty was assessed with bootstrap with replacement method (n = 2000).

2.4. Model Based Simulations

The final PK-PD model and NONMEM® were used for simulation of various treatment regimens and scenarios of PK and PD monitoring. The proportion of patients achieving biochemical remission (FC < 100 mg/kg) at week 8, week 16, week 24 and week 32 after the first dose was estimated for every treatment regimen, to compare the efficacy. This cut-off was chosen based on test characteristics identified by meta-analyses [29], with emphasis on studies using the same assay as our center, considering the large inter-assay variability [30].

First, a virtual population of 10,000 CD patients was created, which resembled the observed cohort regarding the distributions and correlations of patients' characteristics. Subsequently, several clinically relevant scenarios were simulated, as follows:

(a). All patients received standard ustekinumab treatment, with weight-based induction dose at baseline, followed by fixed 90 mg maintenance doses every eight weeks (standard treatment);
(b). All patients received weight-based induction dose at baseline followed by fixed 90 mg maintenance doses every four weeks;
(c). All patients received weight-based induction doses every eight weeks;
(d). Patients receiving standard treatment who were not in remission at week 16, switched to maintenance doses every four weeks from week 20;
(e). Patients receiving standard treatment who were not in remission at week 16 received a weight-based reinduction dose at week 16, and continued with maintenance doses every eight weeks;
(f). Patients receiving standard treatment who were not in remission at week 16 received a weight-based reinduction dose at week 16 and switched to maintenance doses every four weeks from week 20.

R software, version 4.0.2 (R Development Core Team, Vienna, Austria), RStudio version 1.3.1073 (RStudio Team, PBC, Boston, MA, USA) and packages mvtnorm, plyr, dplyr, reshape2 and ggplot2 were used for creating the virtual patient population, data wrangling and visualizations.

3. Results

3.1. Baseline Patient Characteristics

The study included 57 patients: the median disease duration was 14 years (IQR 7–22), 66.7% (38/57) had been previously exposed to biological therapy, and 77.2% (44/57) had endoscopically active disease at baseline (Table 1). All patients completed the study.

Table 1. Patients' characteristics at baseline (n = 57).

Characteristic	Value
Women, n (%)	32 (56)
Age at UST initiation, years, median (IQR)	49 (32–56)
Weight, kg, median (IQR)	70 (59–84)
Fat-free mass [a], median (IQR)	45 (39–62)
Height, cm, median (IQR)	169 (163–179)
Intravenous ustekinumab dose, n (%)	
260 mg	9 (15.8)
390 mg	35 (61.4)
520 mg	13 (22.8)
Disease duration, years, median (IQR)	14 (7–22)
Disease location, n (%)	
ileal (L1)	17 (29.8)
colonic (L2)	4 (7)
ileocolonic (L3)	36 (63.2)
upper gastrointestinal involvement (L4)	6 (10.5)
Fistulizing perianal disease, n (%)	10 (17.5)
History of CD-related surgery, n (%)	34 (59.6)
Smoking status, n (%)	
active smoking	10 (17.5)
previously smoking	12 (21.1)
never smoked	35 (61.4)
Previous biological therapy, n (%)	38 (66.7)
previous anti-TNF exposure	38 (66.7)
previous vedolizumab exposure	10 (17.5)
previous anti-TNF and vedolizumab exposure	9 (15.8)
Systemic steroids at baseline, n (%)	9 (15.8)
Topical steroids at baseline, n (%)	3 (5.3)
Immunomodulators at baseline, n (%)	5 (8.8)
azathioprine	4 (7)
methotrexate	1 (1.8)
Harvey–Bradshaw score, median (IQR)	6 (3–10)
Fecal calprotectin, mg/kg, median (IQR)	134 (53–213)
C-reactive protein, mg/L, median (IQR)	3 (3–11)
Serum albumin, g/L, median (IQR)	43 (41–44)
Endoscopically active disease at baseline, n (%)	44 (77.2)
Samples available (ustekinumab measurement), n	574
Samples available (Fecal calprotectin), n	224
Samples with fecal calprotectin below the limit of quantification, n (%)	15 (6.8)
Samples with fecal calprotectin above the limit of quantification, n (%)	11 (5)
Genotype frequencies	
IL12B rs3212227, n (%)	
A/A	37 (64.9)
A/C	17 (29.8)
C/C	3 (5.3)
IL12B rs3213094, n (%)	
C/C	37 (64.9)
C/T	17 (29.8)
T/T	3 (5.3)
IL12B rs6887695, n (%)	
G/G	22 (38.6)
C/G	25 (43.9)
C/C	10 (17.5)
FcGR2A rs1801274, n (%)	
A/A	21 (36.8)
A/G	29 (50.9)
G/G	7 (12.3)

Table 1. Cont.

Characteristic	Value
FcGR3A rs396991, n (%)	
A/A	21 (36.8)
A/C	31 (54.4)
C/C	5 (8.8)

CD—Crohn's disease; IQR—interquartile range; TNF—tumor necrosis factor; UST—ustekinumab. [a] The fat-free mass was predicted using the semi-mechanistic model developed by Janmahasatian et al. [19].

3.2. Pharmacokinetic and Pharmacodynamic Data

A total of 574 serum samples was available for ustekinumab measurement. Five samples had an ustekinumab concentration below the lower LOQ, and none of the analyzed samples had measurable antibodies to ustekinumab. SNPs were analyzed for all patients, and all genotype frequencies were in Hardy–Weinberg equilibrium (Table 1). A total of 224 samples was available for FC measurement. There were 15 samples with FC concentration below the lower LOQ and 11 samples above the upper LOQ.

3.3. Pharmacokinetic–Pharmacodynamic Model

A quasi-equilibrium approximation of the TMDD model [23] best described the time profile of the ustekinumab concentration (Table S1). The model (Figure 1) assumes rapid binding of ustekinumab to the target antigen and was extended with distribution of the unbound ustekinumab and unbound target into a peripheral compartment since it resulted in an improved fit (Table S1). The binding was assumed in the central compartment. Estimated parameters comprised linear ustekinumab PK, linear target PK and parameters related to the binding of ustekinumab to the target (Table 2). The terminal half-life of ustekinumab after the induction dose in a typical patient was estimated at 17 days and the volume of distribution was low, with volumes of central and peripheral compartment of ustekinumab estimated at 3.57 L and 3.30 L, respectively. There was a high IIV of the rate constant of target synthesis (K_{syn}), with the coefficient of variation estimated at 99.5%.

Table 2. Base and final pharmacokinetic model parameter estimates.

Parameter (Units)	Base Model	Final Model	
	Estimate	Estimate	Bootstrap Median (95% CI)
Ustekinumab pharmacokinetics			
K_a (day^{-1})	0.518	0.381	0.380 (0.341–0.422)
CL (L/day) [a]	0.264	0.277	0.275 (0.259–0.294)
FFM on CL	/	0.598	0.596 (0.539–0.673)
bio-naïve on CL	/	-0.227	-0.232 (-0.280–-0.192)
Serum albumin on CL	/	-0.0165	-0.0170 (-0.0224–-0.0127)
V_c (L) [b]	2.18	3.57	3.56 (3.41–3.70)
FFM on V_c	/	0.590	0.587 (0.534–0.644)
Q (L/day)	20.1	1.89	1.88 (1.69–2.11)
V_p (L) [c]	5.04	3.30	3.27 (3.01–3.52)
FFM on V_p	/	0.586	0.581 (0.512–0.660)
Fraction absorbed, F (%)	71.7	/	/
FCGR3A-158 V/V	/	88.8	88.8 (86.1–92.4)
FCGR3A-158 V/F, F/F	/	71.0	70.8 (65.3–75.8)
Target pharmacokinetics			
K_{syn} (nmol/L × day^{-1}) [d]	1.65×10^{-8}	9.86×10^{-9}	9.85×10^{-9} (8.75×10^{-9}–1.09×10^{-8})
Serum CRP on K_{syn}	/	0.0846	0.0843 (0.0772–0.0883)
K_{deg} (day^{-1})	1.85×10^{-10}	9.26×10^{-10}	9.26×10^{-10} (8.53×10^{-10}–1.06×10^{-9})
$V_{c-target}$ (L)	18.8	2.44	2.44 (2.27–2.81)
Q_{target} (L/d)	0.752	0.493	0.488 (0.440–0.539)
$V_{p-target}$ (L)	22.6	11.0	10.9 (9.87–12.0)

Table 2. Cont.

Parameter (Units)	Base Model	Final Model	
	Estimate	Estimate	Bootstrap Median (95% CI)
Binding			
K_{int} (day^{-1})	1.71×10^{-7}	2.83×10^{-6}	2.82×10^{-6} (2.56×10^{-6}–3.15×10^{-6})
K_d (nmol/L)	0.350	0.168	0.168 (0.154–0.196)
Interindividual variability			
IIV CL (%, CV) [e]	27.9 (13)	18.0 (16)	18.0 (16.0–20.1)
IIV V_c (%, CV) [e]	32.9 (16)	9.79 (22)	9.79 (8.88–10.8)
IIV V_p (%, CV) [e]	21.5 (23)	24.1 (24)	23.6 (19.7–26.0)
IIV F (%, SD) [e]	16.6 (21)	17.3 (22)	17.4 (15.8–20.2)
IIV K_{syn} (%, CV) [e]	105 (25)	99.2 (27)	98.4 (83.4–110)
Residual variability			
Additive RUV (nmol/L) [e]	4.46 (18)	4.55 (17)	4.58 (4.09–5.86)
Proportional RUV (%) [e]	7.84 (18)	7.77 (17)	7.74 (6.94–8.55)

CI—confidence interval; K_a—ustekinumab absorption rate constant after subcutaneous administration; CL—clearance of ustekinumab; FFM—fat-free mass; V_c—volume of distribution in central compartment; Q—intercompartmental clearance; V_p—volume of distribution in peripheral compartment; F—fraction of absorbed ustekinumab after subcutaneous administration; K_{syn}—rate constant of target synthesis; CRP—C-reactive protein; K_{deg}—rate constant of target degradation; K_{int}—elimination rate constant due to binding; K_d—equilibrium constant; IIV—interindividual variability; CV—coefficient of variation; SD—standard deviation; RUV—residual unexplained variability. [a] $CL\left(\frac{L}{day}\right) = 0.277 \times \left(\frac{FFM}{45}\right)^{0.598} \times (1 - 0.0165 \times (Serum\ albumin - 43)) \times (1 - 0.227 \times bio - naïve)$. [b] $V_c(L) = 3.57 \times \left(\frac{FFM}{45}\right)^{0.590}$. [c] $V_p(L) = 3.30 \times \left(\frac{FFM}{45}\right)^{0.586}$. [d] $K_{syn}\left(\frac{nmol}{L} \times day^{-1}\right) = 9.86 \times 10^{-9} \times (1 + 0.0846 \times (CRP - 3))$. [e] For variability terms % shrinkage is presented in brackets.

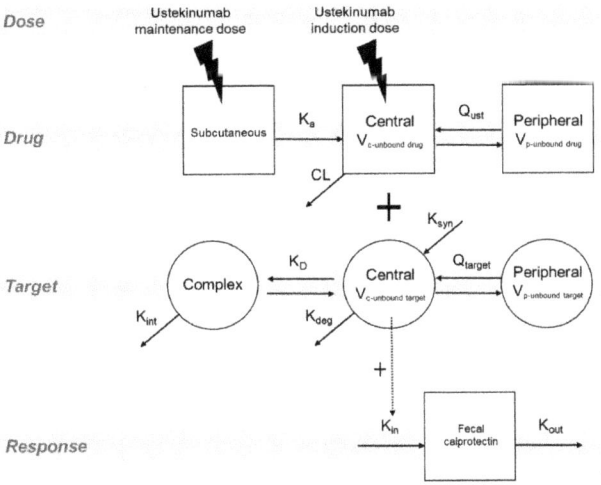

Figure 1. Schematic of the population pharmacokinetic–pharmacodynamic model. A first-order absorption of ustekinumab (drug) is assumed after the subcutaneous administration. The distribution of the unbound drug and unbound target is described with the two-compartment models. The binding is assumed in the central compartment and is described with the quasi-equilibrium approximation of the target-mediated drug disposition model. The stimulating effect of the unbound target on the fecal calprotectin is described with the indirect response model. Ka: ustekinumab absorption rate constant after the subcutaneous administration; V_c: volume of distribution in the central compartment; V_p: volume of distribution in the peripheral compartment; Q_{UST}: intercompartmental clearance of unbound ustekinumab; CL: clearance of unbound ustekinumab; K_{syn}: rate constant of target synthesis; K_{deg}: rate constant of target degradation; K_D: constant of the equilibrium between unbound drug, unbound target and drug-target complex; K_{int}: rate constant of internalization of the drug-target complex into the cells; Q_{target}: intercompartmental clearance of unbound target; K_{in}: rate constant of calprotectin production; K_{out}: rate constant of fecal calprotectin degradation.

Covariates associated with PK parameters were as follows: ustekinumab clearance was higher with increasing FFM, decreasing serum albumin, and in patients with previous exposure to biologics (Table 2). A power model described the increase of volumes of the central and peripheral compartment of ustekinumab with increasing FFM (Table 2). The fraction of absorbed ustekinumab was higher in valine homozygous (V/V) patients of rs396991 *FCGR3A* polymorphism, compared to phenylalanine homozygotes (F/F) and heterozygotes (V/F) combined (Table 2, Figure S1). Additionally, K_{syn} increased with increasing baseline CRP (Table 2).

The concentration of the unbound target was linked to the FC concentration via the indirect response model, which best described the stimulating effect of the unbound target on the FC production (Table 3). Thus, the model explains the ustekinumab effect on the decrease in FC concentration via the intermediate target layer (Figure 1). The initial concentration of the target and FC were modelled as K_{syn}/K_{deg} and FC_0, respectively. In the absence of ustekinumab, steady concentration of the target and FC is assumed. In contrast, when ustekinumab is administered and bound to the target, the unbound target concentration decreases, which inhibits the FC production. Exponential model best described the IIV on FC_0 and patients who started ustekinumab due to endoscopically active disease, had higher baseline FC concentration, which was accounted for in the PD model as a binary covariate on FC_0 (Table 3). There was a good agreement between model predictions and the observed data (Figure 2 and Figure S2).

Table 3. Final pharmacodynamic model [a] parameter estimates.

Parameter (Units)	Estimate	Bootstrap Median (95% CI)
K_{out} (day^{-1})	0.0581	0.0641 (0.0249–0.110)
FC_0 (mg/kg)		
Patients without ulcers at baseline	102	105 (54.4–188)
Patients with ulcers at baseline	213	214 (157–287)
E_{max} (%)	219	227 (128–442)
C_{50} (nmol/L)	2.46	2.56 (0.413–13.9)
Interindividual variability		
IIV FC_0 (%) [b]	99.0 (2)	98.0 (75.0–128)
Residual variability		
Proportional RUV (%) [b]	57.3 (17)	56.4 (48.8–65.0)

CI—confidence interval; K_{out}—fecal calprotectin degradation rate constant; FC_0—baseline fecal calprotectin concentration; E_{max}—maximum effect; C_{50}—target concentration at half-maximum effect; IIV—interindividual variability; RUV—residual unexplained variability. [a.] $\frac{dFC}{dt} = \frac{FC_0 \times K_{out}}{1 + \frac{E_{max} \times \frac{K_{syn}}{K_{deg}}}{C_{50} + \frac{K_{syn}}{K_{deg}}}} \times \left(1 + \frac{E_{max} \times unbound\ target\ concentration}{C_{50} + unbound\ target\ concentration}\right) - K_{out} \times FC.$ [b.] For variability terms % shrinkage is presented in brackets.

3.4. Simulations

The simulation of patients receiving standard ustekinumab regimen demonstrates that patients with weight ≤55 kg have lower ustekinumab concentration in the induction phase, and higher ustekinumab concentration in the maintenance phase, compared to patients with weight >55 kg. In addition, patients in the lowest weight group had higher unbound p40 and FC concentrations during the induction phase (Figure S3).

After the first ustekinumab administration, the unbound target rapidly decreases. A subsequent increase in the target concentration is observed, due to the constant target synthesis. A faster increase in the target concentration in patients with weight >55 kg is observed, compared to patients with weight ≤55 kg, because of the fixed 90 mg subcutaneous dose in the maintenance phase and thus higher exposure to ustekinumab of patients with weight ≤55 kg (Figure S3). In addition, initial target concentration influences the peak ustekinumab concentration. A patient with the 10-fold higher K_{syn} compared to the typical value, would have approximately 15 µg/mL lower peak ustekinumab concentration (Figure S4).

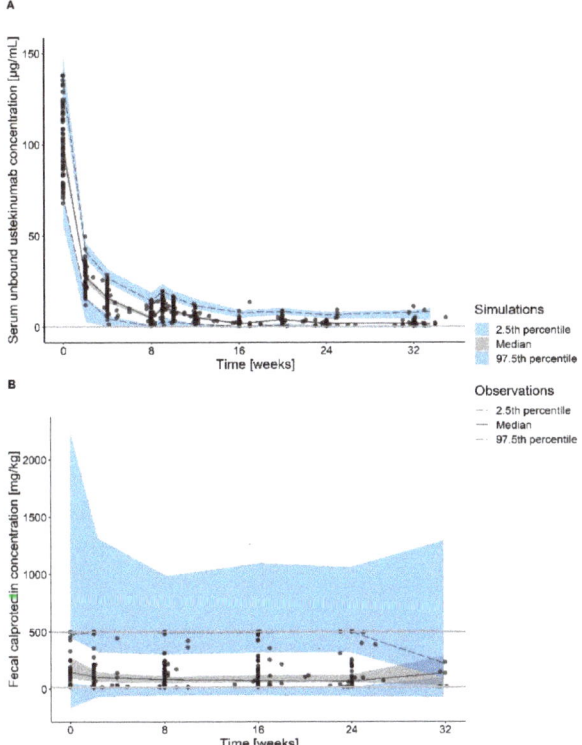

Figure 2. Visual predictive check (n = 2000) of the final pharmacokinetic (**A**) and final pharmacodynamic (**B**) models. Observations (points), medians (black lines), 5th and 95th percentiles (dashed black lines), 95% confidence intervals of the simulated medians (grey shaded areas), 2.5th and 97.5th percentiles (blue shaded areas).

The dynamics of the FC are similar across the weight groups, with faster increase of the FC concentration in higher weight groups (Figure S3). Patients with the endoscopically active disease at baseline had higher FC concentration, and only these patients were considered for the rest of simulations.

The proportions of patients in remission at week 32 receiving standard treatment with maintenance dosing every 8 weeks, treatment with initial induction and subsequent maintenance dosing every four weeks from week 4 or treatment with induction dosing every eight weeks are 41.9%, 52.2% and 56.0%, respectively (Figure 3). In patients not achieving remission with standard treatment at week 16, transition to subcutaneous maintenance dosing every 4 weeks with or without intravenous reinduction resulted in similar biochemical remission at week 32 (51.1% vs. 49.2%, respectively), while reinduction and continuation with maintenance dosing every 8 weeks was comparable to standard dosing (Figure 4).

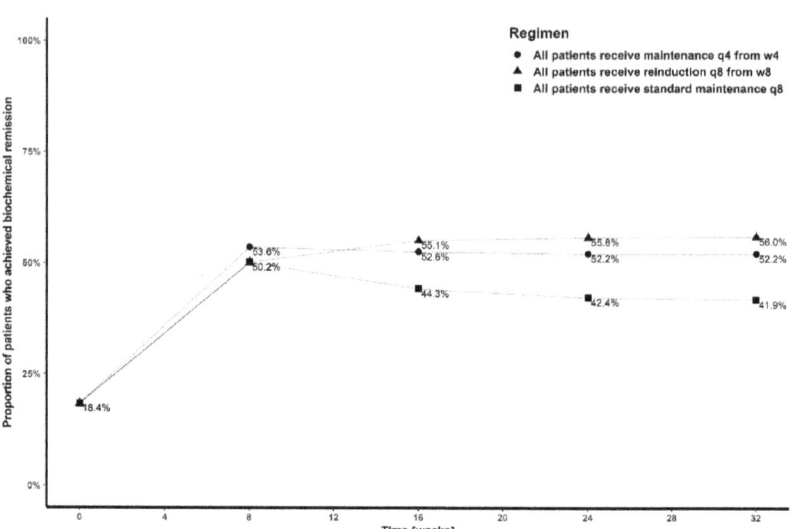

Figure 3. Proportion of patients achieving biochemical remission at weeks 8, 16, 24 and 32, with standard treatment (■), treatment with initial induction, followed by maintenance dosing every four weeks from week 4 (●) and induction dosing every eight weeks (▲).

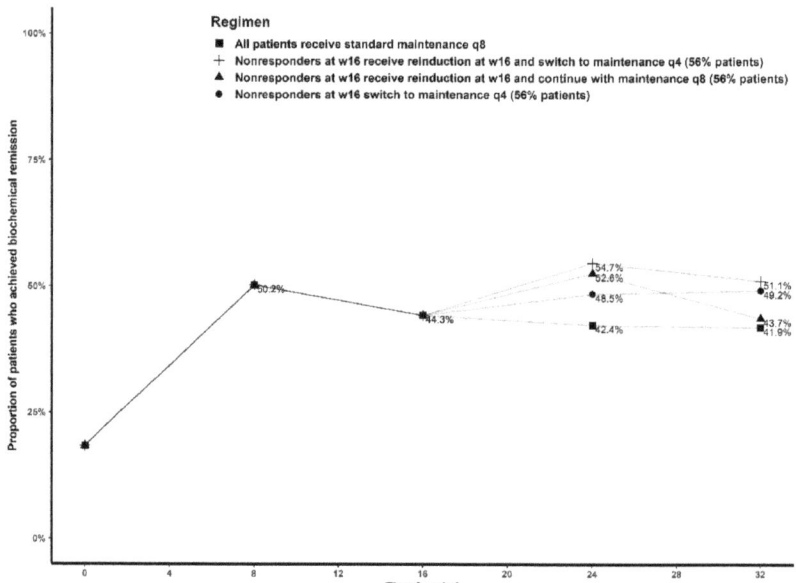

Figure 4. Proportion of patients who achieved biochemical remission at weeks 8, 16, 24 and 32, with standard treatment (■), treatment where patients not in remission at week 16 received maintenance dosing every four weeks from week 20 (●), treatment where patients not in remission at week 16 received intravenous reinduction at week 16 and continued with maintenance dosing every eight weeks (▲), and treatment where patients not in remission at week 16 received intravenous reinduction at week 16, followed by maintenance dosing every four weeks from week 20 (+).

4. Discussion

Clinical PK studies of ustekinumab are relatively scarce, and there is currently no consensus on the optimal management of inadequate response to treatment. To our knowledge, this is the first study to present a semi-mechanistic PK-PD model linking ustekinumab PK, CD patients' clinical characteristics, binding to p40 subunit and FC dynamics. Additionally, we are the first to evaluate the influence of genetic factors on ustekinumab PK-PD in CD. Model-based simulations suggest the possibility of achieving better outcomes with intensified dosing and provide further insight into managing patients with insufficient response at week 16.

Building on previous work identifying an exposure–response relationship for ustekinumab for biochemical and endoscopic outcomes [8,10,11,31], our PK-PD model suggests that rates of biochemical remission could be improved by using intensified dosing regimens to increase ustekinumab exposure (Figure 4). A subgroup of patients at risk of insufficient exposure to ustekinumab (albumin < 43 g/L, previously exposed to biological treatment, V/F or F/F genotype of rs396991, CRP > 5 mg/L) were predicted to benefit the most from dosing escalation. These patients could also be considered for potential proactive dosing escalation in future studies (Figures S5 and S6). The proportion of patients achieving biochemical remission decreased with an increasing number of unfavorable covariates, and this trend was attenuated by dosing escalation (Figure S6).

Different approaches have been used in patients not responding or losing response to standard dosing of ustekinumab: dosing interval shortening [12–15], intravenous reinduction [32] or a combination of both [32,33]. These modifications were made at week 16 of treatment or later. Clinical remission, defined as a Harvey–Bradshaw Index ≤ 4, was reported in 28–40% of patients after interval shortening to every 4 weeks [12–14], CRP normalization occurred in 22% of patients [12]. The interpretation of endoscopic remission rates around 35% (4/11, 14/39) is confounded by low numbers and potential selection bias where patients with biochemically active disease did not undergo endoscopic assessment [12,14]. None of the studies conducted so far were designed and powered to compare the efficacy of different strategies. Simulations based on our model showed that switching to maintenance dosing every 4 weeks from week 16 leads to similar rates of biochemical remission at week 32 regardless of an additional intravenous reinduction dose. A single additional reinduction dose followed by maintenance every 8 weeks is expected to provide only transient benefit (Figure 4). This is broadly concordant with the findings of a retrospective real-world series, where 15/18 patients responded clinically to an additional intravenous infusion and 10/15 required escalated subcutaneous dosing in ongoing maintenance [32]. Even patients already on maximized subcutaneous dosing may benefit from an additional intravenous infusion, although none of these studies included PK assessment [33].

Our findings should be compared with the recently reported results of the STARDUST trial (NCT03107793) evaluating the efficacy of a treat-to-target (T2T) approach to guide treatment escalation decisions compared to standard of care (SOC) [34]. Clinical responders at week 16 underwent randomization, dosing in the T2T arm was first determined based on the change in endoscopic score from baseline and subsequently on combined clinical and biomarker (CRP, FC) monitoring. At week 48, endoscopic response (T2T: 37.7%; SOC: 29.9%) and remission (T2T: 11.4%; SOC: 14.5%) were not significantly different between the two groups. Notably, only 17% of patients in the T2T arm were on four-weekly dosing at week 48, although this percentage is also affected by the 20% discontinuation rate in this arm as patients not achieving treatment targets within four weeks of starting four-weekly dosing discontinued the study. It also remains to be seen what proportion of discontinuations was driven by clinical disease activity despite biochemical remission, as both were required to meet the target. Despite these results, dose escalation may still hold added benefit, particularly if applied early after induction to a selected subpopulation of patients unlikely to respond to standard dosing due to low drug exposure.

The estimated terminal half-life in our study is in accordance with PK studies in psoriasis, psoriatic arthritis, and IBD [35–38], reporting half-life between 19 and 22 days. The distribution of ustekinumab into tissues was limited, which is consistent with its high molecular weight and hydrophilic properties. Ustekinumab linear clearance was in range of reported clearance values in other studies in IBD [37–39], and the TMDD PK model is consistent with the recent findings of the TNF-mediated PK of infliximab in ulcerative colitis [40]. Notably, the elimination of ustekinumab in our model was captured in two catabolic pathways, distinct for IgG antibodies [41]: a linear, non-specific clearance, and a nonlinear, specific clearance, mediated by the binding of the antibody to its target. Therefore, a higher concentration of the target reflecting increased inflammatory burden may lead to accelerated ustekinumab clearance and lower ustekinumab concentration. In CD, the concentration of the p40 subunit is related to the disease activity, although the reported serum concentrations of IL12 and IL23 are highly variable [42,43].

The PK model additionally includes a bi-exponential decline of the concentration of the target, which reflects the possible distribution of the target to other tissues and is in line with the in vivo studies of IL12 and IL23 [24,25]. Thus, the initial binding of ustekinumab to the target in the serum may explain the influence of the target on the peak ustekinumab concentration and volume of distribution (Figure S4). The subsequent redistribution of the target from other tissues into the serum, as well as the constant target synthesis, may explain the target-mediated ustekinumab clearance.

We have identified similar factors influencing ustekinumab PK compared to other studies [35–38]. Ustekinumab exposure was found to increase with decreasing FFM. However, dosing regimens seemed similarly efficient in patients stratified by the weight according to the induction dose (Figure S6). This indicates that the weight is not related with ustekinumab efficacy and is in line with the recent post hoc analysis of IM-UNITI study, assessing the impact of body mass index on clinical efficacy [44]. The exposure increased with increasing serum albumin, as well. A more severe disease may result in a leakage of the albumin and drug into the bowel. The correlation may additionally be explained by the role of FcRn in homeostatic regulation of both, IgG and albumin [45]. Moreover, ustekinumab exposure was higher in bio-naïve patients. Presumably, these patients are less likely to have a more severe type of disease compared to those who have previously failed therapy with other biologics. Therefore, bio-naïve patients may express lower target concentrations, which leads to lower ustekinumab clearance and higher exposure.

We also observed higher fraction of absorbed ustekinumab, and higher exposure related with V/V variant of the rs396991 polymorphism, otherwise known as *FCGR3A*-158 V/F (Figure S1, Table 2). This is a functionally significant polymorphism in *FCGR3A* gene, which encodes the FcγRIIIa receptor. Our finding is highly interesting, since it mirrors the studies reporting association between the V/V genotype and better outcomes of CD treatment with infliximab [46,47]. The V variant is presumably related with higher affinity between FcγRIIIa and the IgG antibodies, compared to the F variant, which may result in altered binding at the absorption site and lead to a variable response to treatment in IBD [48]. However, further studies are necessary to clarify the clinical relevance and the mechanistic involvement of *FCGR3A*-158 polymorphism in ustekinumab PK-PD.

The indirect response PD model for FC has been previously used in a PK-PD studies of infliximab and ustekinumab in CD [38,49]. Notably, the rates of FC degradation are similar, which may additionally account for the different FC measurement assays. In our study, all patients regardless of the endoscopic disease activity were included, and the presence of mucosal ulcerations at baseline was associated with higher baseline FC and CRP, indicating a higher inflammatory burden in patients with confirmed active luminal disease. Antibodies to ustekinumab were not detected in any of the tested samples, which is consistent with the low observed rates of immunogenicity in registration studies [50–52].

Specifically, our PK-PD model is in line with the recent study by Wang et al. [38], who reported a PK-PD model linking ustekinumab, FC and endoscopic outcomes, based on the sparse data from an exposure-response study by Verstockt et al. [10]. Notably, the estimated ustekinumab linear CL is similar (Wang et al.: 0.235 L/day; our study: 0.277 L/day), both models assumed the disposition of ustekinumab into the peripheral compartment and included similar covariates affecting the PK (Wang et al.: serum albumin, body weight; vs. our study: serum albumin, FFM, bio-naïve, *FCGR3A*-158, CRP). The difference in the percent of bio-naïve patients (Wang et al.: 5%; vs. our study: 33%) and the testing of the genetic data in our study may in part explain the different covariate model structure. The simulated median trough steady state ustekinumab concentration for standard regimen (Wang et al.: 1.3 μg/mL; vs. our study: 1.5 μg/mL) and regimen with maintenance dosing every 4 weeks (Wang et al.: 5.3 μg/mL vs. our study: 5.1 μg/mL) were similar, as well.

Additionally, both studies used indirect response PD models with comparable K_{out} estimate for FC (Wang et al.: 0.0416 day^{-1}; vs. our study: 0.0581 day^{-1}), although there was a large observed difference in the average FC concentration due to the different assay [53], and in our model the FC concentration was linked to the latent target instead of the ustekinumab. The residual unexplained PD variability was relatively high in both studies, at more than 55%. Nevertheless, both studies suggested the potential benefit of the shorter interval of the maintenance dosing.

Our findings should be interpreted in the context of the study's limitations. The model was developed in a small cohort of patients and the target concentration was not measured. Despite the plausibility of covariates explaining the PK of ustekinumab, which overlap with findings from other immune-mediated inflammatory diseases and models for other monoclonal antibodies in IBD, the model should be further validated in an independent cohort. Notwithstanding the correlation between endoscopic outcomes and FC concentrations, normalization of the latter is neither an independent treatment goal nor does its normalization guarantee endoscopic remission as observed in the STARDUST trial. Finally, outcomes of simulations based on our model should be regarded as hypothesis-generating for future study design and not used to inform clinical practice here and now.

In conclusion, this article presents a semi-mechanistic population PK-PD model for ustekinumab in CD, and the findings could be used to guide future attempts to personalize treatment with ustekinumab in CD. Especially patients with low serum albumin, previous failure of biological therapy, *FCGR3A*-158 V/F or F/F variant and high CRP might benefit from early optimization of ustekinumab therapy to 4-weekly maintenance dosing.

Supplementary Materials: The following are available online at https://www.mdpi.com/article/10.3390/pharmaceutics13101587/s1, Figure S1: Fraction of absorbed ustekinumab after subcutaneous administration according to *FCGR3A* rs396991 polymorphism, Figure S2: Diagnostic plots of the final pharmacokinetic and pharmacodynamic model, Figure S3: A population simulation using the final pharmacokinetic–pharmacodynamic model and representative virtual patient population, Figure S4: Serum unbound ustekinumab concentration time-profile in a patient with high, typical, or low target synthesis rate constant, Figure S5: Simulated ustekinumab and fecal calprotectin concentration time-profile of a typical patient according to ustekinumab exposure and target synthesis, Figure S6: Proportion of patients who achieved biochemical remission at week 32 stratified by each covariate, Table S1: Comparison of the tested base pharmacokinetic models, Supplementary information S1: NONMEM control stream for the population PK and PD model.

Author Contributions: Conceptualization, J.A.Z., J.H., D.D. and I.G.; methodology, J.A.Z., J.H., D.D. and I.G.; software, J.A.Z. and I.G.; formal analysis, J.A.Z., J.H. and I.G.; investigation, J.A.Z., J.H., N.S. (Nejc Sever), B.O., D.T. and T.V.; data curation, J.A.Z., J.H., D.D. and I.G.; writing—original draft preparation, J.A.Z., J.H., D.D. and I.G.; writing—review and editing, J.A.Z., J.H., T.K., N.S. (Nejc Sever), M.K., N.S. (Nataša Smrekar), G.N., B.Š., E.D., D.T., T.V., B.O., D.D. and I.G.; visualization, J.A.Z.; supervision, D.D. and I.G.; project administration, D.D. and I.G.; funding acquisition, T.V. and I.G. All authors have read and agreed to the published version of the manuscript.

Funding: This work was financially supported by the Slovenian Research Agency (ARRS Grant P1-0189).

Institutional Review Board Statement: The study was conducted according to the guidelines of the Declaration of Helsinki and approved by the Slovenian National Committee of Medical Ethics (0120-013/2016-2; KME 18 January 2016).

Informed Consent Statement: Informed consent was obtained from all subjects involved in the study.

Data Availability Statement: The data presented in this study are available upon reasonable request from the corresponding author.

Acknowledgments: We would like to thank Carmen Bobnar Sekulić and Tadeja Polanc for collecting the samples and providing administrative support.

Conflicts of Interest: J.H. reports lecture fees from Janssen and Takeda outside the submitted work. N.Sm. reports lecture fees from Takeda outside the submitted work. M.K. reports lecture fees from Takeda and Biogen. G.N. reports lecture and consultant fees from Takeda, MSD, Abbvie and Janssen. B.Š. reports lecture and consultant fees from Krka, Bayer, Takeda, Janssen and grants from Krka outside the submitted work. E.D. is a postdoctoral research fellow of the Research Foundation—Flanders (FWO), Belgium (grant number 12X9420N) and received consultancy fees from argenx and Janssen (all honoraria/fees paid to the University). D.D. reports speaker and consultant fees from Abbvie, Dr. Falk Pharma, Ferring, Janssen, Krka, Lek, MSD, Novartis, Pfizer, Roche, and Takeda, all of which were outside of the submitted work. All other authors declare no conflict of interest.

References

1. Torres, J.; Mehandru, S.; Colombel, J.-F.; Peyrin-Biroulet, L. Crohn's disease. *Lancet* **2017**, *389*, 1741–1755. [CrossRef]
2. Peyrin-Biroulet, L.; Sandborn, W.; Sands, B.E.; Reinisch, W.; Bemelman, W.; Bryant, R.V.; D'Haens, G.; Dotan, I.; Dubinsky, M.; Feagan, B.; et al. Selecting Therapeutic Targets in Inflammatory Bowel Disease (STRIDE): Determining Therapeutic Goals for Treat-to-Target. *Am. J. Gastroenterol.* **2015**, *110*, 1324–1338. [CrossRef]
3. D'Haens, G.; Ferrante, M.; Vermeire, S.; Baert, F.; Noman, M.; Moortgat, L.; Geens, P.; Iwens, D.; Aerden, I.; Van Assche, G.; et al. Fecal calprotectin is a surrogate marker for endoscopic lesions in inflammatory bowel disease. *Inflamm. Bowel Dis.* **2012**, *18*, 2218–2224. [CrossRef]
4. Mosli, M.H.; Zou, G.; Garg, S.K.; Feagan, S.G.; MacDonald, J.K.; Chande, N.; Sandborn, W.J.; Feagan, B.G. C-Reactive Protein, Fecal Calprotectin, and Stool Lactoferrin for Detection of Endoscopic Activity in Symptomatic Inflammatory Bowel Disease Patients: A Systematic Review and Meta-Analysis. *Am. J. Gastroenterol.* **2015**, *110*, 802–819. [CrossRef]
5. Moschen, A.R.; Tilg, H.; Raine, T. IL-12, IL-23 and IL-17 in IBD: Immunobiology and therapeutic targeting. *Nat. Rev. Gastroenterol. Hepatol.* **2019**, *16*, 185–196. [CrossRef] [PubMed]
6. Iborra, M.; Beltrán, B.; Fernández-Clotet, A.; Gutiérrez, A.; Antolín, B.; Huguet, J.M.; De Francisco, R.; Merino, O.; Carpio, D.; García-López, S.; et al. Real-world short-term effectiveness of ustekinumab in 305 patients with Crohn's disease: Results from the ENEIDA registry. *Aliment. Pharmacol. Ther.* **2019**, *50*, 278–288. [CrossRef] [PubMed]
7. Biemans, V.B.C.; van der Meulen-de Jong, A.E.; van der Woude, C.J.; Löwenberg, M.; Dijkstra, G.; Oldenburg, B.; de Boer, N.K.H.; van der Marel, S.; Bodelier, A.G.L.; Jansen, J.M.; et al. Ustekinumab for Crohn's Disease: Results of the ICC Registry, a Nationwide Prospective Observational Cohort Study. *J. Crohn's Colitis* **2019**, *14*, jjz119. [CrossRef] [PubMed]
8. Battat, R.; Kopylov, U.; Bessissow, T.; Bitton, A.; Cohen, A.; Jain, A.; Martel, M.; Seidman, E.; Afif, W. Association Between Ustekinumab Trough Concentrations and Clinical, Biomarker, and Endoscopic Outcomes in Patients With Crohn's Disease. *Clin. Gastroenterol. Hepatol.* **2017**, *15*, 1427–1434.e2. [CrossRef]
9. Ma, C.; Fedorak, R.N.; Kaplan, G.G.; Dieleman, L.A.; Devlin, S.M.; Stern, N.; Kroeker, K.I.; Seow, C.H.; Leung, Y.; Novak, K.L.; et al. Clinical, endoscopic and radiographic outcomes with ustekinumab in medically-refractory Crohn's disease: Real world experience from a multicentre cohort. *Aliment. Pharmacol. Ther.* **2017**, *45*, 1232–1243. [CrossRef] [PubMed]
10. Verstockt, B.; Dreesen, E.; Noman, M.; Outtier, A.; Van den Berghe, N.; Aerden, I.; Compernolle, G.; Van Assche, G.; Gils, A.; Vermeire, S.; et al. Ustekinumab Exposure-outcome Analysis in Crohn's Disease Only in Part Explains Limited Endoscopic Remission Rates. *J. Crohn's Colitis* **2019**, *13*, 864–872. [CrossRef]
11. Hanžel, J.; Zdovc, J.; Kurent, T.; Sever, N.; Javornik, K.; Tuta, K.; Koželj, M.; Smrekar, N.; Novak, G.; Štabuc, B.; et al. Peak Concentrations of Ustekinumab After Intravenous Induction Therapy Identify Patients With Crohn's Disease Likely to Achieve Endoscopic and Biochemical Remission. *Clin. Gastroenterol. Hepatol.* **2021**, *19*, 111–118.e10. [CrossRef] [PubMed]
12. Ollech, J.E.; Normatov, I.; Peleg, N.; Wang, J.; Patel, S.A.; Rai, V.; Yi, Y.; Singer, J.; Dalal, S.R.; Sakuraba, A.; et al. Effectiveness of Ustekinumab Dose Escalation in Patients With Crohn's Disease. *Clin. Gastroenterol. Hepatol.* **2020**, *19*, 104–110. [CrossRef] [PubMed]
13. Kopylov, U.; Hanzel, J.; Liefferinckx, C.; De Marco, D.; Imperatore, N.; Plevris, N.; Baston-Rey, I.; Harris, R.J.; Truyens, M.; Domislovic, V.; et al. Effectiveness of ustekinumab dose escalation in Crohn's disease patients with insufficient response to standard-dose subcutaneous maintenance therapy. *Aliment. Pharmacol. Ther.* **2020**, *52*, 135–142. [CrossRef] [PubMed]

14. Fumery, M.; Peyrin-Biroulet, L.; Nancey, S.; Altwegg, R.; Gilletta, C.; Veyrard, P.; Bouguen, G.; Viennot, S.; Poullenot, F.; Filippi, J.; et al. Effectiveness And Safety Of Ustekinumab Intensification At 90 Mg Every Four Weeks In Crohn's Disease: A Multicenter Study. *J. Crohn's Colitis* **2020**, *15*, 222–227. [CrossRef] [PubMed]
15. Hanžel, J.; Koželj, M.; Špes Hlastec, A.; Kurent, T.; Sever, N.; Zdovc, J.; Smrekar, N.; Novak, G.; Štabuc, B.; Grabnar, I.; et al. Ustekinumab concentrations shortly after escalation to monthly dosing may identify endoscopic remission in refractory Crohn's disease. *Eur. J. Gastroenterol. Hepatol.* **2021**. [CrossRef]
16. Van den Reek, J.M.P.A.; Coenen, M.J.H.; van de L'Isle Arias, M.; Zweegers, J.; Rodijk-Olthuis, D.; Schalkwijk, J.; Vermeulen, S.H.; Joosten, I.; van de Kerkhof, P.C.M.; Seyger, M.M.B.; et al. Polymorphisms in CD84, IL12B and TNFAIP3 are associated with response to biologics in patients with psoriasis. *Br. J. Dermatol.* **2017**, *176*, 1288–1296. [CrossRef]
17. Galluzzo, M.; Boca, A.N.; Botti, E.; Potenza, C.; Malara, G.; Malagoli, P.; Vesa, S.; Chimenti, S.; Buzoianu, A.D.; Talamonti, M.; et al. IL12B (p40) Gene Polymorphisms Contribute to Ustekinumab Response Prediction in Psoriasis. *Dermatology* **2016**, *232*, 230–236. [CrossRef]
18. Rožman, S.; Novaković, S.; Grabnar, I.; Cerkovnik, P.; Novaković, B.J. The impact of FcγRIIa and FcγRIIIa gene polymorphisms on responses to RCHOP chemotherapy in diffuse large B-cell lymphoma patients. *Oncol. Lett.* **2016**, *11*, 3332–3336. [CrossRef]
19. Janmahasatian, S.; Duffull, S.B.; Ash, S.; Ward, L.C.; Byrne, N.M.; Green, B. Quantification of lean bodyweight. *Clin. Pharmacokinet.* **2005**, *44*, 1051–1065. [CrossRef]
20. Mager, D.E.; Jusko, W.J. General pharmacokinetic model for drugs exhibiting target-mediated drug disposition. *J. Pharmacokinet. Pharmacodyn.* **2001**, *28*, 507–532. [CrossRef]
21. Gibiansky, L.; Gibiansky, E. Target-mediated drug disposition model: Approximations, identifiability of model parameters and applications to the population pharmacokinetic–pharmacodynamic modeling of biologics. *Expert Opin. Drug Metab. Toxicol.* **2009**, *5*, 803–812. [CrossRef] [PubMed]
22. Ternant, D.; Monjanel, H.; Venel, Y.; Prunier-Aesch, C.; Arbion, F.; Colombat, P.; Paintaud, G.; Gyan, E. Nonlinear pharmacokinetics of rituximab in non-Hodgkin lymphomas: A pilot study. *Br. J. Clin. Pharmacol.* **2019**, *85*, 2002–2010. [CrossRef] [PubMed]
23. Mager, D.E.; Krzyzanski, W. Quasi-equilibrium pharmacokinetic model for drugs exhibiting target-mediated drug disposition. *Pharm. Res.* **2005**, *22*, 1589–1596. [CrossRef] [PubMed]
24. Nadeau, R.R.; Ostrowski, C.; Ni-Wu, G.; Liberato, D.J. Pharmacokinetics and pharmacodynamics of recombinant human interleukin-12 in male rhesus monkeys. *J. Pharmacol. Exp. Ther.* **1995**, *274*, 78–83.
25. Zhang, T.T.; Ma, J.; Durbin, K.R.; Montavon, T.; Lacy, S.E.; Jenkins, G.J.; Doktor, S.; Kalvass, J.C. Determination of IL-23 Pharmacokinetics by Highly Sensitive Accelerator Mass Spectrometry and Subsequent Modeling to Project IL-23 Suppression in Psoriasis Patients Treated with Anti-IL-23 Antibodies. *AAPS J.* **2019**, *21*, 1–11. [CrossRef]
26. Zhang, L.; Beal, S.L.; Sheiner, L.B. Simultaneous vs. Sequential Analysis for Population PK/PD Data I: Best-case Performance. *Simulation* **2003**, *30*, 387–404. [CrossRef]
27. Felmlee, M.A.; Morris, M.E.; Mager, D.E. Mechanism-Based Pharmacodynamic Modeling. In *Computational Toxicology*; Humana Press: Totowa, NJ, USA, 2012; pp. 583–600. [CrossRef]
28. Bergstrand, M.; Karlsson, M.O. Handling data below the limit of quantification in mixed effect models. *AAPS J.* **2009**, *11*, 371–380. [CrossRef]
29. Lin, J.-F.; Chen, J.-M.; Zuo, J.-H.; Yu, A.; Xiao, Z.-J.; Deng, F.-H.; Nie, B.; Jiang, B. Meta-analysis: Fecal Calprotectin for Assessment of Inflammatory Bowel Disease Activity. *Inflamm. Bowel Dis.* **2014**, *20*, 1407–1415. [CrossRef]
30. Guidi, L.; Marzo, M.; Andrisani, G.; Felice, C.; Pugliese, D.; Mocci, G.; Nardone, O.; De Vitis, I.; Papa, A.; Rapaccini, G.; et al. Faecal calprotectin assay after induction with anti-Tumour Necrosis Factor α agents in inflammatory bowel disease: Prediction of clinical response and mucosal healing at one year. *Dig. Liver Dis.* **2014**, *46*, 974–979. [CrossRef]
31. Adedokun, O.J.; Xu, Z.; Gasink, C.; Jacobstein, D.; Szapary, P.; Johanns, J.; Gao, L.-L.L.; Davis, H.M.; Hanauer, S.B.S.; Feagan, B.G.; et al. Pharmacokinetics and Exposure Response Relationships of Ustekinumab in Patients With Crohn's Disease. *Gastroenterology* **2018**, *154*, 1660–1671. [CrossRef]
32. Hudson, J.; Herfarth, H.; Barnes, E. Letter: Optimising response to ustekinumab therapy for patients with Crohn's disease. *Aliment. Pharmacol. Ther.* **2020**, *52*, 906. [CrossRef] [PubMed]
33. Sedano, R.; Guizzetti, L.; McDonald, C.; Jairath, V. Intravenous Ustekinumab Reinduction Is Effective in Prior Biologic Failure Crohn's Disease Patients Already on Every-4-Week Dosing. *Clin. Gastroenterol. Hepatol.* **2020**, *19*, 1497–1498. [CrossRef] [PubMed]
34. Danese, S.; Vermeire, S.; D'Haens, G.; Panés, J.; Dignass, A.; Magro, F.; Nazar, M.; Le Bars, M.; Sloan, S.; Lahaye, M.; et al. DOP13 Clinical and endoscopic response to ustekinumab in Crohn's disease: Week 16 interim analysis of the STARDUST trial. *J. Crohn's Colitis* **2020**, *14*, S049–S052. [CrossRef]
35. Zhu, Y.; Hu, C.; Lu, M.; Liao, S.; Marini, J.C.; Yohrling, J.; Yeilding, N.; Davis, H.M.; Zhou, H. Population pharmacokinetic modeling of ustekinumab, a human monoclonal antibody targeting IL-12/23p40, in patients with moderate to severe plaque psoriasis. *J. Clin. Pharmacol.* **2009**, *49*, 162–175. [CrossRef] [PubMed]
36. Zhu, Y.W.; Mendelsohn, A.; Pendley, C.; Davis, H.M.; Zhou, H. Population pharmacokinetics of ustekinumab in patients with active psoriatic arthritis. *Int. J. Clin. Pharmacol. Ther.* **2010**, *48*, 830–846. [CrossRef]
37. Xu, Y.; Hu, C.; Chen, Y.; Miao, X.; Adedokun, O.J.; Xu, Z.; Sharma, A.; Zhou, H. Population Pharmacokinetics and Exposure-Response Modeling Analyses of Ustekinumab in Adults With Moderately to Severely Active Ulcerative Colitis. *J. Clin. Pharmacol.* **2020**, *60*, 889–902. [CrossRef]

38. Wang, Z.; Verstockt, B.; Sabino, J.; Vermeire, S.; Ferrante, M.; Declerck, P.; Dreesen, E. Population pharmacokinetic-pharmacodynamic model-based exploration of alternative ustekinumab dosage regimens for patients with Crohn's disease. *Br. J. Clin. Pharmacol.* **2021**, 1–13. [CrossRef]
39. Hu, C.; Adedokun, O.J.; Chen, Y.; Szapary, P.O.; Gasink, C.; Sharma, A.; Zhou, H. Challenges in longitudinal exposure-response modeling of data from complex study designs: A case study of modeling CDAI score for ustekinumab in patients with Crohn's disease. *J. Pharmacokinet. Pharmacodyn.* **2017**, *44*, 425–436. [CrossRef]
40. Berends, S.E.; van Steeg, T.J.; Ahsman, M.J.; Singh, S.; Brandse, J.F.; D'Haens, G.R.A.M.; Mathôt, R.A.A. Tumor necrosis factor-mediated disposition of infliximab in ulcerative colitis patients. *J. Pharmacokinet. Pharmacodyn.* **2019**, *46*, 543–551. [CrossRef]
41. Dirks, N.L.; Meibohm, B. Population Pharmacokinetics of Therapeutic Monoclonal Antibodies. *Clin. Pharmacokinet.* **2010**, *49*, 633–659. [CrossRef]
42. Ogawa, K.; Matsumoto, T.; Esaki, M.; Torisu, T.; Iida, M. Profiles of circulating cytokines in patients with Crohn's disease under maintenance therapy with infliximab. *J. Crohn's Colitis* **2012**, *6*, 529–535. [CrossRef] [PubMed]
43. Lucaciu, L.; Ilies, M.; Iuga, C.; Seicean, A. P136 Serum IL-17 and IL-23 levels can distinguish between severe and non-severe inflammatory bowel disease. *J. Crohn's Colitis* **2018**, *12*, S163. [CrossRef]
44. Wong, E.C.L.; Marshall, J.K.; Reinisch, W.; Narula, N. Body Mass Index Does Not Impact Clinical Efficacy of Ustekinumab in Crohn's Disease: A Post Hoc Analysis of the IM-UNITI Trial. *Inflamm. Bowel Dis.* **2020**, *27*, 848–854. [CrossRef] [PubMed]
45. Sand, K.M.K.; Bern, M.; Nilsen, J.; Noordzij, H.T.; Sandlie, I.; Andersen, J.T. Unraveling the Interaction between FcRn and Albumin: Opportunities for Design of Albumin-Based Therapeutics. *Front. Immunol.* **2015**, *5*, 682. [CrossRef] [PubMed]
46. Moroi, R.; Endo, K.; Kinouchi, Y.; Shiga, H.; Kakuta, Y.; Kuroha, M.; Kanazawa, Y.; Shimodaira, Y.; Horiuchi, T.; Takahashi, S.; et al. FCGR3A-158 polymorphism influences the biological response to infliximab in Crohn's disease through affecting the ADCC activity. *Immunogenetics* **2013**, *65*, 265–271. [CrossRef] [PubMed]
47. Louis, E.; El Ghoul, Z.; Vermeire, S.; Dall'Ozzo, S.; Rutgeerts, P.; Paintaud, G.; Belaiche, J.; De Vos, M.; Van Gossum, A.; Colombel, J.-F.; et al. Association between polymorphism in IgG Fc receptor IIIa coding gene and biological response to infliximab in Crohn's disease. *Aliment. Pharmacol. Ther.* **2004**, *19*, 511–519. [CrossRef]
48. Castro-Dopico, T.; Clatworthy, M.R. IgG and Fcγ receptors in intestinal immunity and inflammation. *Front. Immunol.* **2019**, *10*, 805. [CrossRef]
49. Dreesen, E.; Berends, S.; Laharie, D.; D'Haens, G.; Vermeire, S.; Gils, A.; Mathôt, R. Modelling of the relationship between infliximab exposure, faecal calprotectin and endoscopic remission in patients with Crohn's disease. *Br. J. Clin. Pharmacol.* **2020**, 1–13. [CrossRef]
50. Feagan, B.G.; Sandborn, W.J.; Gasink, C.; Jacobstein, D.; Lang, Y.; Friedman, J.R.; Blank, M.A.; Johanns, J.; Gao, L.L.; Miao, Y.; et al. Ustekinumab as induction and maintenance therapy for Crohn's disease. *N. Engl. J. Med.* **2016**, *375*, 1946–1960. [CrossRef]
51. Hanauer, S.B.; Sandborn, W.J.; Feagan, B.G.; Gasink, C.; Jacobstein, D.; Zou, B.; Johanns, J.; Adedokun, O.J.; Sands, B.E.; Rutgeerts, P.; et al. IM-UNITI: Three-year efficacy, safety, and immunogenicity of ustekinumab treatment of Crohn's disease. *J. Crohn's Colitis* **2020**, *14*, 23–32. [CrossRef]
52. Sands, B.E.; Sandborn, W.J.; Panaccione, R.; O'Brien, C.D.; Zhang, H.; Johanns, J.; Adedokun, O.J.; Li, K.; Peyrin-Biroulet, L.; Van Assche, G.; et al. Ustekinumab as Induction and Maintenance Therapy for Ulcerative Colitis. *N. Engl. J. Med.* **2019**, *381*, 1201–1214. [CrossRef]
53. Labaere, D.; Smismans, A.; Van Olmen, A.; Christiaens, P.; D'Haens, G.; Moons, V.; Cuyle, P.-J.; Frans, J.; Bossuyt, P. Comparison of six different calprotectin assays for the assessment of inflammatory bowel disease. *United Eur. Gastroenterol. J.* **2014**, *2*, 30–37. [CrossRef] [PubMed]

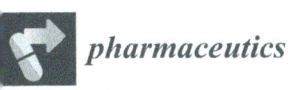

Article

External Model Performance Evaluation of Twelve Infliximab Population Pharmacokinetic Models in Patients with Inflammatory Bowel Disease

Christina Schräpel [1,2], Lukas Kovar [1], Dominik Selzer [1], Ute Hofmann [2], Florian Tran [3,4], Walter Reinisch [5], Matthias Schwab [2,6] and Thorsten Lehr [1,*]

1. Clinical Pharmacy, Saarland University, 66123 Saarbrücken, Germany; christina.schraepel@uni-saarland.de (C.S.); lukas.kovar@uni-saarland.de (L.K.); dominik.selzer@uni-saarland.de (D.S.)
2. Dr. Margarete Fischer-Bosch-Institute of Clinical Pharmacology, University of Tübingen, 70376 Stuttgart, Germany; ute.hofmann@ikp-stuttgart.de (U.H.); matthias.schwab@ikp-stuttgart.de (M.S.)
3. Institute of Clinical Molecular Biology, Kiel University and University Medical Center Schleswig-Holstein, 24105 Kiel, Germany; f.tran@ikmb.uni-kiel.de
4. Department of Internal Medicine I, University Medical Center Schleswig-Holstein, 24105 Kiel, Germany
5. Department of Internal Medicine III, Medical University of Vienna, 1090 Vienna, Austria; walter.reinisch@meduniwien.ac.at
6. Departments of Clinical Pharmacology, Pharmacy and Biochemistry, University of Tübingen, 72076 Tübingen, Germany
* Correspondence: thorsten.lehr@mx.uni-saarland.de; Tel.: +49-681-302-70255

Abstract: Infliximab is approved for treatment of various chronic inflammatory diseases including inflammatory bowel disease (IBD). However, high variability in infliximab trough levels has been associated with diverse response rates. Model-informed precision dosing (MIPD) with population pharmacokinetic models could help to individualize infliximab dosing regimens and improve therapy. The aim of this study was to evaluate the predictive performance of published infliximab population pharmacokinetic models for IBD patients with an external data set. The data set consisted of 105 IBD patients with 336 infliximab concentrations. Literature review identified 12 published models eligible for external evaluation. Model performance was evaluated with goodness-of-fit plots, prediction- and variability-corrected visual predictive checks (pvcVPCs) and quantitative measures. For anti-drug antibody (ADA)-negative patients, model accuracy decreased for predictions > 6 months, while bias did not increase. In general, predictions for patients developing ADA were less accurate for all models investigated. Two models with the highest classification accuracy identified necessary dose escalations (for trough concentrations < 5 µg/mL) in 88% of cases. In summary, population pharmacokinetic modeling can be used to individualize infliximab dosing and thereby help to prevent infliximab trough concentrations dropping below the target trough concentration. However, predictions of infliximab concentrations for patients developing ADA remain challenging.

Keywords: infliximab; population pharmacokinetics; inflammatory bowel disease; model-informed precision dosing; dose individualization

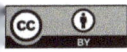

1. Introduction

Infliximab is an intravenously administered recombinant chimeric monoclonal antibody that inhibits both soluble and membrane-bound tumor necrosis factor alpha (TNF-α) [1]. Infliximab is approved for treatment of various chronic inflammatory diseases including the inflammatory bowel diseases (IBD) Crohn's disease (CD) and ulcerative colitis (UC) [2,3]. After its approval in 1999 by the European Medicines Agency (EMA), infliximab revolutionized the treatment of CD and UC because of its ability to induce long-term remission, reduce hospitalizations, and restore quality of life [4,5]. Today, infliximab is still widely used and available as different biosimilars [3].

Infliximab exhibits linear pharmacokinetic behavior, while low trough concentrations are associated with impaired or even loss of response to infliximab therapy [6–9]. UC patients with detectable serum infliximab trough concentrations showed a 4 times higher probability and CD patients even a 13 times higher probability of being in clinical remission, making serum infliximab levels a predictor of clinical response [6,9–12]. According to a recent guideline from the American Gastroenterological Association Institute, infliximab should be dosed to achieve target trough concentrations of ≥ 5 µg/mL in order to improve therapy outcome [13]. However, a high inter-individual variability in infliximab trough levels has been observed contributing to a high rate of treatment failure [9,12–14]. About 10–40% of patients fail to respond to induction therapy (primary non-response) [15], and subsequently, 13% of patients lose response annually after initially responding (secondary non-response) [16]. One of the reasons for primary and secondary non-response is the formation of anti-drug antibodies (ADAs) against infliximab, leading to an increased infliximab clearance (CL) [9,17,18].

A good understanding of the high variability in infliximab trough levels is essential for dose individualization strategies [4,19–22]. In the past, several efforts have been made to characterize infliximab pharmacokinetics (PK), including the quantification and explanation of inter-individual variability, and to develop population pharmacokinetic models for dose individualization [21,23–27]. While these analyses identified various covariates (e.g., albumin levels, sex, weight, ADA development, and use of concomitant immunomodulators) that influence infliximab CL and volume of distribution (V_d), the covariates could only partly explain the observed inter-individual and inter-occasion variability (IOV) [23,24,26,27].

Thus, population pharmacokinetic models combined with data from therapeutic drug monitoring could help to optimize drug dosing regimens in individual patients via model-informed precision dosing (MIPD) [28–32]. Infliximab models have recently been used to simulate dosing regimens for different patient populations or for evaluation of individualized dose adjustments and incidences of loss of response [31,33,34]. However, a comprehensive external evaluation of the different infliximab population pharmacokinetic modeling approaches including assessment of accuracy and bias of model predictions over time as well as the ability to predict the need for dose escalation is still pending. Hence, the aim of this work was to provide an overview of published infliximab population pharmacokinetic models for patients with IBD as well as to evaluate and compare model performance with a focus on differences between ADA-negative and ADA-positive subpopulations in a Bayesian forecasting setting using an external data set.

2. Materials and Methods
2.1. External Evaluation Data Set

For predictive external model evaluation, data originated from a previously published observational study that was reviewed and approved by the institutional review board of the Medical University of Vienna [35]. All participating patients had signed an informed consent form.

Patients with an established diagnosis of CD and UC were enrolled in the study. All participants had previously responded to induction therapy, receiving three infusions at weeks zero, two, and six, and were assigned to a maintenance dosing regimen. Serum samples of patients (median 2, range 1–12 samples) were collected during infliximab therapy at both midpoint and trough times of a dosing interval while exact time points were not specified in the protocol. Laboratory and demographic data were collected, including serum infliximab concentrations, ADA levels, serum albumin concentrations, C-reactive protein levels, weight, use of concomitant immunomodulators, Harvey–Bradshaw index (HBI), and smoking status.

Serum infliximab concentrations used in this analysis were measured with a commercially available enzyme-linked immunosorbent assay (ELISA) method (Immundiagnostik Germany, Bensheim, Germany) with a lower limit of quantification (LLOQ) of

2.68 ng/mL [36]. ADA concentrations were determined using the homogeneous mobility shift assay (HMSA) from Prometheus Labs Inc., San Diego, CA, USA with an LLOQ of 3.13 U/mL [37]. Patients were assigned to the ADA-positive patient cohort if any measured ADA concentration was above the threshold of 6.6 U/mL [37,38].

2.2. Population Pharmacokinetic Models and Software

A comprehensive and systematic literature search in PubMed was performed for infliximab population pharmacokinetic analyses in patients with IBD. The search terms were "infliximab" AND "population" AND "pharmacokinetics" and reference lists of identified articles were manually screened for further eligible studies. Subsequently, modeling and study information was collected, including model structure, population pharmacokinetic parameter values, covariates, inter-individual variability, residual variability, information on patient cohorts, disease type, number of patients, number of collected blood samples, and ADA immunogenicity rate. The population pharmacokinetic models described in the gathered studies were implemented and evaluated using the nonlinear mixed effects modeling software NONMEM® version 7.4 (Icon Development Solutions, Ellicott City, MD, USA). Computations for prediction- and variability-corrected visual predictive checks (pvcVPCs) were generated with the PsN (version 4.9.0) tool "vpc" [39,40]. Data management, graphics, and quantitative model diagnostics were carried out using the R programming language version 3.6.3 (R Foundation for Statistical Computing, Vienna, Austria) and R Studio® version 1.2.5019 (R Studio, Inc., Boston, MA, USA).

2.3. Model Performance Evaluation

For the implemented population pharmacokinetic models, all parameters (fixed and random effects) were set to published values of the respective study. To assess the potential applications in a clinical setting, model performances to predict serum infliximab concentrations with a Bayesian approach were evaluated with the external data set. Here, the first measured serum infliximab concentration of each patient (C_{MAP}) was used for maximum a posteriori (MAP) estimation of individual pharmacokinetic parameters (empirical Bayes pharmacokinetic parameter estimates [EBEs]) considering interaction between inter-individual variability and residual variability for prediction of subsequent serum infliximab concentrations (Bayesian forecasting). As recommended by Abrantes and coworkers, IOV was included in the estimation of EBEs but excluded in the calculation of individual pharmacokinetic parameters used for predictions [41]. For prospective predictions, individual patient covariates for times after C_{MAP} were imputed using last observation carried forward.

Visual and quantitative methods were applied for the evaluation of predictive model performances. Goodness-of-fit plots of individual predicted infliximab concentrations vs. observed infliximab concentrations were generated for visual evaluation. Moreover, two quantitative measures were calculated, including the median symmetric accuracy (ζ, Equation (1)) and the symmetric signed percentage bias (SSPB, Equation (2)) to evaluate the model regarding prediction accuracy and prediction bias.

$$\zeta = 100 \times \left[e^{\left(\text{median}\left(\left|\ln\left(\frac{y_i}{x_i}\right)\right|\right)\right)} - 1 \right], \tag{1}$$

$$\text{SSPB} = 100 \times \left[\text{sign}\left(\text{median}\left(\ln\left(\frac{y_i}{x_i}\right)\right)\right) \right] \times \left[e^{\left(\left|\text{median}\left(\ln\left(\frac{y_i}{x_i}\right)\right)\right|\right)} - 1 \right]. \tag{2}$$

In Equations (1) and (2) x_i represents the ith observed infliximab serum concentration and y_i the corresponding predicted serum concentration.

ζ represents the typical absolute percentage error with 50% of absolute percentage errors below ζ [42]. The SSPB, a measure of bias, estimates the central tendency of the error penalizing underprediction and overprediction equally as illustrated by Morley and coworkers [42].

As mentioned before, dose escalation can be beneficial in patients with trough concentrations below the target threshold of 5 µg/mL. Hence, a model's ability to correctly predict the need for dose escalation was further investigated. For that, observed and predicted trough concentrations were split into two categories: C_{trough} < 5 µg/mL (dose escalation needed) and $C_{trough} \geq$ 5 µg/mL (no dose escalation needed). Correct predictions of need for dose escalation are referred to as "true positive" while correct predictions of no need for dose escalation are referred to as "true negative". Model accuracy, i.e., the fraction of observed and corresponding predicted trough concentrations, both <5 µg/mL or both $\geq$ 5 µg/mL, were calculated for all models. Here, model classification performance was evaluated for trough samples in which ADA status was negative and for trough samples in which ADA status was positive individually.

In addition, pvcVPCs were performed with multiple replicates (n = 1000) of the study population. The simulated concentrations (median, 5th, and 95th percentiles), the corresponding 95% confidence intervals as well as prediction- and variability-corrected observed concentrations (with median, 5th, and 95th percentiles) were plotted against time after dose.

3. Results

3.1. Characteristics of Published Population Pharmacokinetic Models of Infliximab in Patients with IBD

The comprehensive literature search in PubMed for population pharmacokinetic analyses of infliximab in patients with IBD revealed 25 population pharmacokinetic models, which are listed in Table 1 together with the respective model characteristics. The models partially differ both in base model structure as well as tested and integrated covariates. The majority of the studies used a 2-compartment model (n = 18) with first-order elimination, while seven models implemented a 1-compartment model. Yet, five out of seven studies that used a 1-compartment base model were developed with sparse data including only infliximab trough samples in the model building process.

Integrated covariates on infliximab CL and central volume of distribution (V_c) include patient characteristics (sex, weight, and age), clinical characteristics (albumin levels, HBI, ADA status, etc.) as well as concomitant medication of immunomodulators (IMM).

Of the 25 models, 14 included albumin concentrations, 14 weight, and four sex as a covariate on CL. Moreover, four models included an IOV for the CL parameter. Eighteen models integrated ADA as a covariate (sixteen as binary, one as ordinal, and one as continuous covariate), two models implemented a risk function of developing ADA, and three did not include ADA status in the model since only a small fraction of patients in the respective model building data set were ADA positive ($\leq$3%). Two studies did not include ADA-positive patients for the model building process (see Table 1).

Furthermore, model building data sets vastly differed in patient and sample numbers, patient cohort (patients with CD/UC; adult/pediatric patients) as well as sampling times (see Table 1). Eleven models used data from both patients with CD and UC, eleven from patients with CD, and three from patients with UC. The majority of models were developed with data from adult patients (19/25), three with data from both adult and pediatric patients, and three with data from pediatric patients only.

3.2. Eligible Population Pharmacokinetic Models for Evaluation

Twelve out of 25 population pharmacokinetic models (entries marked with an asterisk in Table 1) were eligible for model performance evaluation with the external data set. From Fasanmade et al., 2011, two of three models that were developed using a data set of adult patients and a data set of both pediatric and adult patients, respectively, were included in the analysis [24]. Edlund et al. published three different approaches for handling the ADA covariate [43]. All three models based on ADA measurements by HMSA were included in the analysis and are, hereafter, referred to as I (ADA covariate on the patient level), II (ADA covariate on sample level), and III (ADA concentrations as a continuous covariate). Eleven out of 25 models (Ternant et al., 2008 [44], Dotan et al., 2014 [45], Ternant et al., 2015 [46], Brandse et al., 2017 [47], Kevans et al., 2018 [48], Dreesen et al., 2019 [49], Matsuoka et al., 2019 [50], Petitcollin et al., 2019 [51], Dreesen et al., 2020 [27], Bauman et al., 2020 [21], and Kantasiripitak et al., 2021 [26]) could not be evaluated because of data set incompatibility (e.g., missing covariates in our data set) or lack of reported model implementation details. The model by Grišić et al. was not included in the analysis as it was specifically focused on modeling the effects of pregnancy affecting infliximab PK [52]. In summary, models developed by Aubourg et al., 2015 [53], Buurman et al., 2015 [54], Brandse et al., 2016 [55], Edlund et al., 2017 (I–III) [43], Fasanmade et al., 2009 [23], Fasanmade et al., 2011 (adults and adults/children) [24], Passot et al., 2016 [56], Petitcollin et al., 2018 [25], and Xu et al., 2012 [57] were implemented and included in the external evaluation. Additional information on the investigated models regarding assumptions for model implementation (e.g., handling of missing units or ambiguities) are outlined in Section 1 of the Supplementary Materials.

3.3. External Evaluation Data Set

Four hundred serum infliximab concentrations from 124 patients were available in the data set. Data from 11 patients (33 infliximab concentrations total) were excluded because of insufficient information on the respective dosing regimen (e.g., unknown time of dosing). Three concentrations below the LLOQ (<1% of samples) were excluded from the external evaluation (M1 method) [58]. Moreover, 28 concentrations classified as pharmacokinetically implausible (concentrations that did not decrease over a sampling period of at least seven days within a dosing interval) were removed from the analysis. Consequently, eight patients lacked informative infliximab PK data, i.e., at least one sample with detectable infliximab concentrations, and were therefore excluded from the analysis.

As a result, a total of 336 infliximab concentrations from 105 patients with IBD, including 76 cases of CD and 29 cases of UC, were available for external evaluation (median number of infliximab samples per patient: 2; range: 1–12). Twenty-two patients had at least one positive ADA sample. In total, ADA levels above the threshold of 6.6 U/mL were measured in 49 samples. An overview of clinical and demographic patient characteristics of the external data set is presented in Table 2. Infliximab was administered to patients using various dosing regimens with a median (interquartile range (IQR)) infliximab dose of 5.5 (5.1–5.9) mg/kg and a median (IQR) dosing interval of 8.0 (7.7–8.6) weeks.

Table 1. Overview of published pharmacokinetic models for infliximab in patients with IBD.

Publication	CD/UC	Patient Cohort	No. of Patients (Samples)	Sampling Times	Base Model	Covariates on CL	Covariates on V_c	IOV	Induction/ Maintenance [1]	Inclusion of ADA+ Patients	Ref.
Ternant et al., 2008	both	adults	33 (478)	peak, trough	2-CMT	ADA	sex, weight	-	both	yes (15%)	[44]
Fasanmade et al., 2009 *	UC	adults	482 (4145)	peak, midpoint, trough	2-CMT	ADA, alb, sex	sex, weight	-	both	yes (7%)	[23]
Fasanmade et al., 2011 (a) *	CD	adults	580 (/)	peak, midpoint, trough	2-CMT	ADA, alb, IMM, weight	weight [2]	CL	both	yes (11%)	[24]
Fasanmade et al., 2011 (c)	CD	children	112 (/)	peak, midpoint, trough	2-CMT	alb, weight	weight [2]	CL	both	yes (3%)	[24]
Fasanmade et al., 2011(a/c) *	CD	both	692 (5757)	peak, midpoint, trough	2-CMT	ADA, alb, IMM, weight	weight [2]	CL	both	yes (10%)	[24]
Xu et al., 2012 *	both	both	655 [3] (/)	/	2-CMT	ADA, alb, weight [4]	weight [2]	-	/	yes (/)	[57]
Dotan et al., 2014	both	adults	54 (169)	trough	2-CMT	ADA, alb, weight [4]	weight [2]	-	both	yes (31%)	[45]
Aubourg et al., 2015 *	CD	adults	133 (/)	trough, peak	2-CMT	sex	sex, weight	-	treatment initiation	no	[53]
Buurman et al., 2015 *	both	adults	42 (188)	trough	2-CMT	ADA, period [5], sex	HBI	-	both	yes (5%)	[54]
Ternant et al., 2015	CD	adults	111 (546)	throughout dosing interval	1-CMT	FcGR3A-158V/V, hsCRP		-	maintenance	yes (2%)	[46]
Brandse et al., 2016 *	UC	adults	19 (/)	throughout dosing interval	2-CMT	ADA, alb		-	induction	yes (32%)	[55]
Passot et al., 2016 *	both	both	79 [6] (/)	trough	1-CMT	CD/UC, sex, weight	CD/UC, sex, weight	-	both	no	[56]
Brandse et al., 2017	both	adults	332 (997)	throughout dosing interval	2-CMT	ADA, alb, previous exposure, weight [4]	weight [2]	-	both	yes (23%)	[47]
Edlund et al., 2017(I-III) *,[7]	CD	adults	68 (152)	midpoint, trough	2-CMT	ADA [8], weight [4,9]	weight [2,9]	-	maintenance	yes (37%)	[43]
Kevans et al., 2018	both	adults	51 (/)	throughout dosing interval	2-CMT	ADA, alb, weight [4], time-varying CL [10]	weight [2]	-	induction	yes (11%)	[48]
Petitcollin et al., 2018 *	CD	children	20 (145)	trough	1-CMT	alb, time-varying CL/risk of immunization [11]		-	both	yes (15%)	[25]
Dreesen et al., 2019	UC	adults	204 (583)	trough	1-CMT	alb, CRP, Mayo	FFM, CS, panc.	CL	induction	yes (1%) [12]	[49]
Matsuoka et al., 2019	CD	adults	121 (832)	trough	1-CMT	ADA, alb, weight		-	maintenance	yes (26%)	[50]

244

Table 1. Cont.

Publication	CD/UC	Patient Cohort	No. of Patients (Samples)	Sampling Times	Base Model	Covariates on CL	Covariates on V_c	IOV	Induction/Maintenance [1]	Inclusion of ADA+ Patients	Ref.
Petitcollin et al., 2019	both	adults	91 (607)	trough	1-CMT	CD/UC, CRP, dose, Mayo, AZA, time-varying CL/risk of immunization [11], weight [13]	-	-	maintenance	yes (1%)	[51]
Bauman et al., 2020	both	children	135 (289)	trough	2-CMT	ADA [14], alb, ESR, weight	weight [2]	-	maintenance	yes (62%)	[21]
Dreesen et al., 2020	CD	adults	116 (1329)	midpoint, trough	2-CMT	ADA, alb, CDAI, fCal	-	-	both	yes (18%)	[27]
Grišić et al., 2020	both	pregnant	19 (172)	throughout dosing interval	1-CMT	ADA, 2nd/3rd trimester	-	-	both	yes (30%) [12,15]	[52]
Kantasiripitak et al., 2021	both	adults	104 (272)	trough	2-CMT	ADA, age, alb, CRP, FFM	-	-	induction	yes (13%)	[26]

Note: -: none; /: unknown; (a): (adults); (a/c): (adults/children); ADA: anti-drug antibodies; ADA+: anti-drug antibody positive; alb: albumin concentrations; AZA: azathioprine; (c): children; CD: Crohn's disease; CDAI: Crohn's disease activity index; CL: clearance; CMT: compartment; CRP: C-reactive protein; CS: corticosteroids; ESR: erythrocyte sedimentation rate; fCal: fecal calprotectin; FCGR3A-158V/V: Fc fragment of IgG, low affinity IIIa, receptor (CD16a) polymorphism; FFM: fat-free mass; HBI: Harvey-Bradshaw index; hsCRP: high-sensitivity C-reactive protein; IBD: inflammatory bowel disease; IMM: immunomodulators; IOV: inter-occasion variability; Mayo: Mayo score; No.: number; panc.: pancolitis; Ref.: reference; UC: ulcerative colitis; V_c: volume of central compartment; *: included in the external model performance evaluation; [1] blood sample data collected during induction and/or maintenance therapy; [2] covariate also on volume of peripheral compartment (V_p); [3] 133 more pediatric patients with other inflammatory diseases were included; [4] covariate also on intercompartmental clearance (Q); [5] induction or maintenance phase; [6] 139 more patients with other inflammatory diseases were included; [7] three similar models with different handling of the ADA covariate; [8] ADA as binary or continuous covariate; [9] allometric scaling; [10] a component of CL that varies over time independent of patient factors; [11] describing varying infliximab CL over time (independent from ADA testing); [12] percentage of ADA-positive blood samples; [13] as a covariate on the CL increase over time; [14] ADA was included as an ordinal covariate with four categories; [15] samples with infliximab concentrations ≤5 µg/mL were assessed for ADAs.

Table 2. Clinical and demographic patient characteristics.

Characteristic	Median or No.	Range	IQR
Patients, n	105		
Sex, female, n (%)	50 (48)		
Patients with CD, n (%)	76 (72)		
Patients with UC, n (%)	29 (28)		
ADA-positive patient status, n (%)	22 (21)		
IMM [1], n (%)	17 (16)		
Nonsmoker, n (%)	35 (33)		
Smoker, n (%)	41 (39)		
Past smoker, n (%)	28 (27)		
Unknown smoking status, n (%)	1 (1)		
Body weight [1] [kg]	70	47–115	59–80
Height [1] [cm]	171	155–190	165–178
Albumin [1] [g/dL]	4.35	2.53–5.08	4.12–4.54
CRP [1] [mg/dL]	0.29	0.02–7.49	0.11–0.49
HBI [1]	1	0–18	1–3
Total serum samples, n	336		
ADA-positive serum samples, n (%)	49 (15)		

Note: ADA: anti-drug antibodies; CD: Crohn's disease; CRP: C-reactive protein; HBI: Harvey–Bradshaw index; IMM: immunomodulators (including azathioprine and methotrexate); IQR: interquartile range; No.: number; UC: ulcerative colitis; [1] at the time of first drug sampling.

3.4. Predictive Model Evaluation Goodness-of-Fit Plots

The first concentration (C_{MAP}) was used for MAP estimation of EBEs, and all subsequent concentrations were predicted. Data was split into two sets of ADA-positive and ADA-negative patients. Additionally, for ADA-negative patients, predictions were stratified for different time intervals after C_{MAP} (i.e., "within 1 month", "between 1 and 6 months" and ">6 months"). For ADA-positive patients, predicted concentrations were stratified as follows: infliximab concentrations for patients that have not been tested ADA positive yet ("before ADA+"), concentrations measured within one month or at first ADA detection ("1st time ADA+ and ≤1 month"), and concentrations measured after one month of first ADA detection (">1 month of being ADA+").

Goodness-of-fit plots (Figure 1) show that model predictions of infliximab concentrations for most ADA-negative patients (turquoise symbols) matched precisely with the observed concentrations. However, predictions of concentrations of ADA-positive patients (pink symbols), especially those measured within and after one month of first ADA detection, were less accurate (turquoise symbols). Additionally, in ADA-negative patients, predictions of concentrations measured more than six months after C_{MAP} showed larger deviation from the corresponding observed concentrations compared to predictions of concentrations measured within the first six months after C_{MAP} in this study setting.

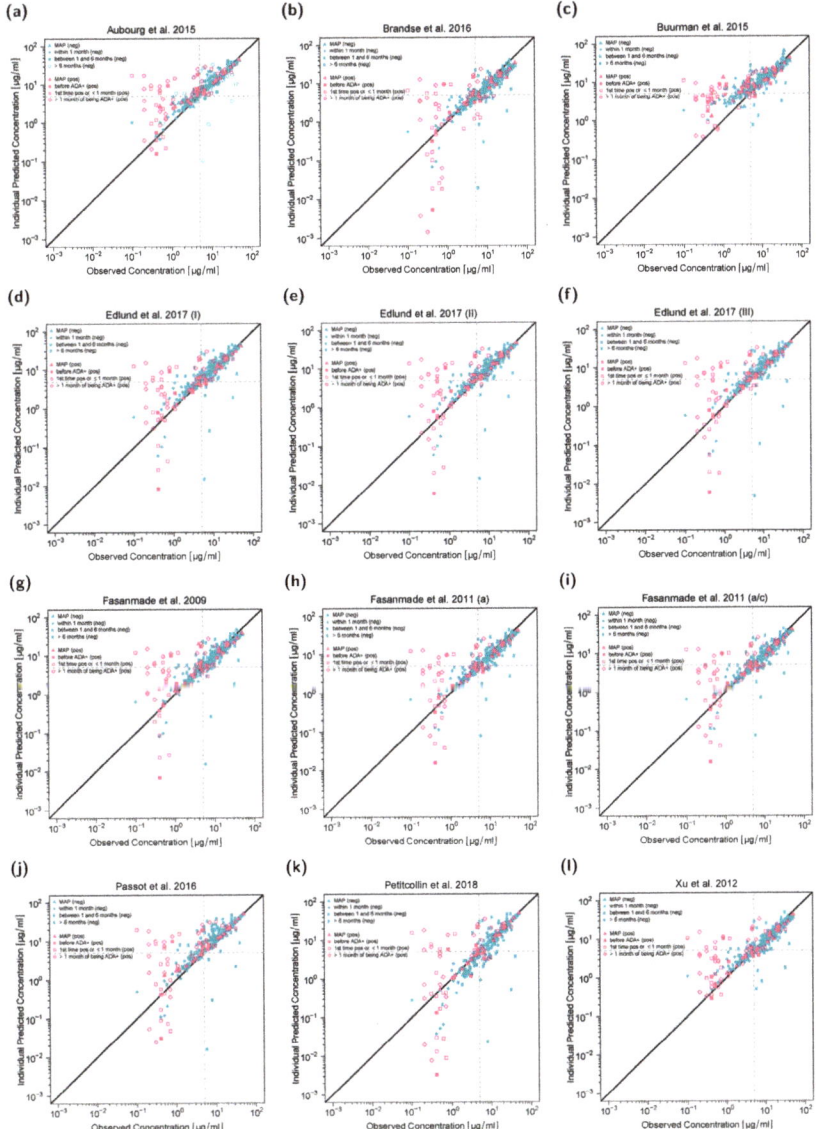

Figure 1. Individual predicted versus observed serum infliximab concentrations for twelve different population pharmacokinetic models (a–l). Concentrations of anti-drug antibody (ADA) negative patients are shown in turquoise, concentrations of ADA-positive patients in pink. Concentrations used for maximum a posteriori (MAP) estimation (C_{MAP}) are depicted as triangles, the remaining symbols depict predictions in different time intervals after C_{MAP}. Black solid lines represent the lines of identity, gray dashed lines mark the target trough concentration of 5 µg/mL. In (k), one serum concentration falls outside the plotting range but is included in the full plot depicted in the Supplementary Materials. a: adults; a/c: adults/children; (neg): ADA-negative patients; (pos): ADA-positive patients.

3.5. Accuracy and Bias of Model Predictions

ζ values represent a measure of accuracy with smaller values indicating higher accuracy, while SSPB values represent a measure of bias with values closer to zero indicating less bias. Figure 2 shows the development of ζ and SSPB values over time for all included population pharmacokinetic models in the ADA negative (Figure 2a,b) and ADA-positive (Figure 2c,d) patient subpopulations. The last category ("all pred") subsumes unstratified results for all predicted concentrations excluding C_{MAP}. The corresponding ζ values were calculated for all 12 models to be within 26–44% (median: 30%) for ADA-negative patients and 77–215% (median: 92%) for ADA-positive patients. SSPB values for all models were within −22–27% (median: 6%) for ADA-negative patients and 8–145% (median: 43%) for ADA-positive patients.

The models exhibiting the highest overall accuracy (lowest ζ) for predicted concentrations in ADA-negative patients were the two models by Fasanmade et al., 2011, both with ζ values of ~26%. Regarding bias in model predictions, four models had absolute SSPB values of ≤5% (with SSPB values for Fasanmade et al., 2009: −3%; Xu et al., 2012: −1%; and the two models from Fasanmade et al., 2011: −5%).

ζ values for predictions in ADA-negative patients increased from a median of 25% (predictions within one month of C_{MAP}) and 28% (predictions one to six months after C_{MAP}) to 54% (predictions more than six months after C_{MAP}) over time (see Figure 2a). In contrast, the median SSPB value for model predictions in ADA-negative patients did not increase over time (median (SSPB $_{< 1\ month}$): 7%, median (SSPB $_{1-6\ months}$): 8%, median (SSPB $_{> 6\ months}$): 2%; Figure 2b). All calculated ζ and SSPB values for each model are listed in Table S1 and Table S2 of the Supplementary Materials.

In ADA-positive patients, predictions of infliximab concentrations were less accurate, especially for concentrations measured within and after one month of first ADA detection (Figure 3c, median (ζ $_{1st\ time\ ADA+\ and\ \leq 1\ month}$): 97%, median (ζ $_{> 1\ month\ ADA+}$): 301%). For some models, bias (SSPB) was still low for predictions of concentrations when patients were tested ADA positive for the first time and within one month of detection (Petitcollin et al., 2018: −1%, Fasanmade et al., 2009: −2%, Fasanmade et al., 2011 (adults/children): 5%, Edlund et al., 2017 (II): 9%, and Edlund et al., 2017 (III): −9%) but was high for all models regarding concentrations measured more than one month after patients tested ADA positive for the first time (range of SSPB values: 78–344%).

ζ values for model simulations of C_{MAP} were 0–24% (median: 9%) for ADA-negative patients and 0–43% for ADA-positive patients (median: 12%). The corresponding SSPB values were −24–0% (median: −5%) for ADA-negative patients and −13–22% for ADA-positive patients (median: −4%).

The model by Edlund et al., 2017 (III) included ADA concentrations measured by HMSA (Prometheus Laboratories, San Diego, CA) as a continuous covariate on infliximab CL [43] in contrast to a binary covariate (i.e., ADA negative or ADA positive) as implemented in other evaluated models. However, since model predictions were executed with individual patient covariates imputed from time of C_{MAP}, model predictions for later time points could not benefit from continuous measurements of ADA concentrations and other time-varying covariates. In order to examine these potential benefits for the model by Edlund et al., 2017 (III), predictions were also performed with fully informed covariates for the ADA-positive subpopulation and results are depicted in Figure 2c,d (green dashed line). This led to an improvement in both model accuracy and bias, especially for concentrations measured more than one month after patients tested ADA positive for the first time (ζ: 130% vs. 206% and SSPB: 11% vs. 206%).

Predictions with fully informed time-varying covariates were also performed for all other evaluated models for both ADA-negative and ADA-positive patients, and results are shown in Tables S3 and S4, as well as in Figures S1 and S2 in the Supplementary Materials.

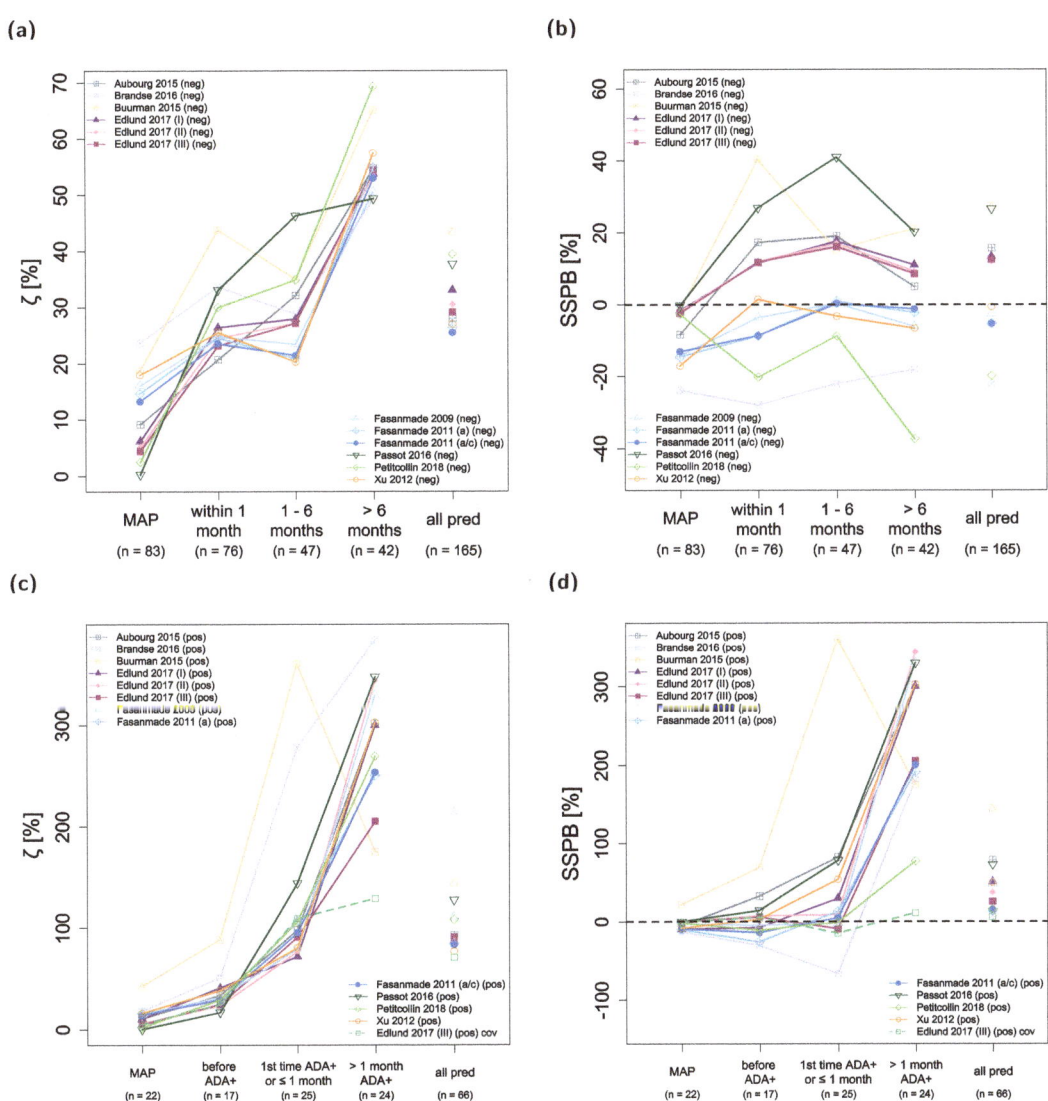

Figure 2. Model prediction accuracy (ζ, (**a,c**)) and bias (SSPB, (**b,d**)) over time. The upper panel shows results for anti-drug antibody (ADA) negative patients, the lower panel for ADA-positive patients. Numbers in parentheses refer to the number of observed concentrations in the respective time interval. "all pred" covers all predicted concentrations excluding concentrations used for maximum a posteriori (MAP) estimation (C_{MAP}) of individual pharmacokinetic parameters. Solid lines depict the results for model predictions using patient covariates determined at the time of C_{MAP}. The green dashed line shows the results for predictions with the model by Edlund et al., 2017 (III), using measured time-varying covariates. a: adults; a/c: adults/children; ADA+: anti-drug antibody positive; cov: covariates; (neg): ADA-negative patients, (pos): ADA-positive patients; pred: predictions; SSPB: symmetric signed percentage bias; ζ: median symmetric accuracy.

3.6. Predictions of "Need for Dose Escalation"

According to the American Gastroenterological Association Institute Guideline, the target trough concentration for infliximab is ≥ 5 µg/mL [13]. In total, 69 serum trough samples from the external data set exhibited infliximab concentrations ≥ 5 µg/mL (no dose escalation needed), 90 trough samples exhibited infliximab concentrations < 5 µg/mL (dose escalation needed). For serum trough samples in which ADA status was negative, 67 samples showed infliximab trough levels ≥5 µg/mL (50%) and 67 showed infliximab trough levels < 5 µg/mL (50%). In contrast, for serum trough samples in which ADA status was positive, only 2 samples showed infliximab levels ≥ 5 µg/mL (8%) and 23 showed infliximab levels < 5 µg/mL (92%).

Table 3 presents the results regarding model abilities to correctly predict the need for dose escalation in the external data set. Results were split into two groups—predictions for serum trough samples in which ADA status was negative and predictions for serum trough samples in which ADA status was positive. Models with the highest accuracy for the ADA-negative sample cohort were the models by Edlund et al., 2017 (II + III), and the models by Fasanmade et al., 2011, with 113/134 (84%) correct predictions. For the ADA-positive sample cohort, the model by Buurman et al., 2015, correctly classified 20 of 25 (80%) concentrations to be above or below the threshold of 5 µg/mL. In summary, the investigated models correctly identified the need for dose escalation (i.e., trough concentration < 5 µg/mL) in 63–89% of cases. In 4–43% of cases a dose escalation would have been recommended (predicted trough concentration < 5 µg/mL) although the measured concentration was above the target concentration.

Table 3. Predictions of "need for dose escalation" (i.e., trough concentration <5 µg/mL [13]).

Dose Escalation Needed? (C_{obs} < 5 µg/mL)	ADA Negative					ADA Positive				
	Yes (n = 67)		No (n = 67)			Yes (n = 23)		No (n = 2)		
Correctly Predicted?	Yes	No	Yes	No	Accuracy	Yes	No	Yes	No	Accuracy
Aubourg et al., 2015	48	19	63	4	82.8%	13	10	2	0	60.0%
Brandse et al., 2016	62	5	39	28	75.4%	18	5	0	2	72.0%
Buurman et al., 2015	38	29	62	5	74.6%	19	4	1	1	80.0%
Edlund et al., 2017 (I)	51	16	61	6	83.6%	16	7	2	0	72.0%
Edlund et al., 2017 (II)	50	17	63	4	84.3%	15	8	1	1	64.0%
Edlund et al., 2017 (III)	50	17	63	4	84.3%	16	7	1	1	68.0%
Fasanmade et al., 2009	54	13	58	9	83.6%	17	6	1	1	72.0%
Fasanmade et al., 2011 (a/c)	60	7	53	14	84.3%	19	4	0	2	76.0%
Fasanmade et al., 2011 (a)	60	7	53	14	84.3%	19	4	0	2	76.0%
Passot et al., 2016	44	23	64	3	80.6%	13	10	2	0	60.0%
Petitcollin et al., 2018	62	5	48	19	82.1%	15	8	0	2	60.0%
Xu et al., 2012	56	11	52	15	80.6%	18	5	1	1	76.0%

Note: a: adults; a/c: adults/children; ADA: anti-drug antibody; C_{obs}: observed trough concentration.

3.7. Prediction- and Variability-Corrected Visual Predictive Checks (pvcVPCs)

The results of pvcVPCs for each investigated population pharmacokinetic model are presented in Figure 3. The pvcVPCs showed a clear overprediction of the 95th percentile of observations for the models by Aubourg et al., 2015, Edlund et al., 2017 (II), Fasanmade et al., 2009, and Xu et al., 2012, but predictions of median infliximab concentrations were reasonable for all four models. The model by Petitcollin et al., 2018, overpredicted and the model by Brandse et al., 2016, underpredicted both the median and 95th percentile of observations. In contrast, the model by Buurman et al., 2015, overpredicted the 5th percentile while slightly underpredicting the 95th percentile. Model simulated median and 95th percentile showed high agreement with the corresponding median/percentile observed for the model by Passot et al., 2016. However, the 5th percentile was overpredicted most of the time. The remaining four models showed high congruence with a slight initial underprediction of the median observations for the two models by Fasanmade et al., 2011, and the model by Edlund et al., 2017 (III).

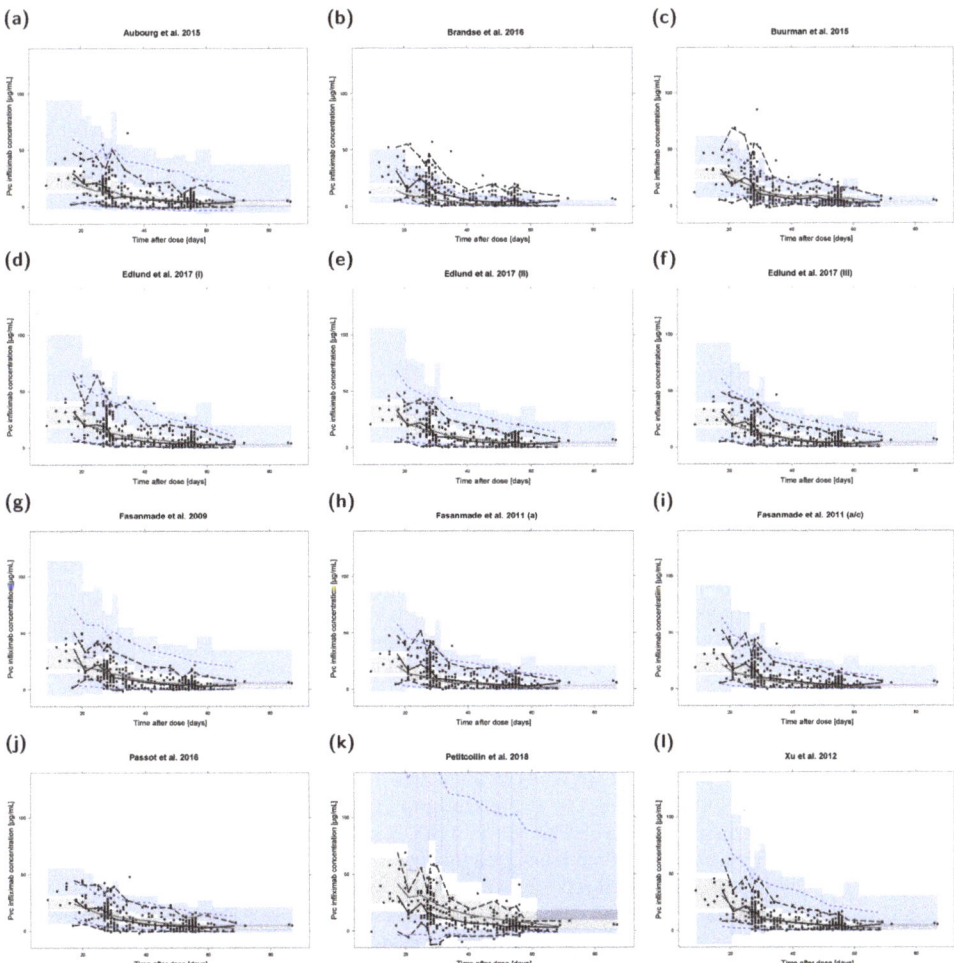

Figure 3. Prediction- and variability-corrected visual predictive checks (pvcVPCs) of serum infliximab concentrations for each investigated population pharmacokinetic model (**a–l**). Prediction- and variability-corrected observed concentrations are shown as black circles, observed medians are depicted as black solid lines, 5th and 95th data percentiles as black dashed lines. The model simulations (n = 1000 replicates) are depicted as gray solid lines (median) and blue dashed lines (5th and 95th percentiles). Colored areas represent the simulation-based 95% confidence intervals for the corresponding model-predicted median (gray areas) and 5th and 95th percentiles (blue areas). For ease of comparison, y-axis upper limits were set to 140 µg/mL. Plots with automatic y-axis limits are shown in the Supplementary Materials. a: adults; a/c: adults/children; Pvc: prediction- and variability-corrected.

4. Discussion

Several MIPD approaches have recently shown major success in supporting and optimizing dosing regimen selection for various drugs [28,59–62]. As infliximab trough concentrations exhibit high inter-individual variability and, hence, contribute to a high rate of primary and secondary non-response [9,12–14,18] and as infliximab drug exposure is a predictor of clinical response [6,10–12], dose selection for infliximab could benefit considerably from population pharmacokinetic modeling and MIPD [31,63]. Consequently, many efforts have been made to analyze infliximab PK, quantifying and explaining inter-individual variability in various population pharmacokinetic models [21,23–27,43–49,51–57].

However, for the application of population pharmacokinetic models, an extensive assessment including internal and external evaluation regarding accuracy, robustness, and predictive performance is crucial [64]. While different methods have been applied in the respective internal model evaluations, only a fraction of the models has been evaluated with an independent data set [34,65–68], and a comprehensive external evaluation for predictive model performances has not been conducted yet. External evaluation with an independent data set allows the evaluation of model performance regarding prediction and variability in patients with a clinical background similar to the internal data set and thus evaluates not only the modeling approach itself, but also other study-related factors [64].

As shown in this analysis, differences in the predictive performances of the 12 investigated models could be observed by external evaluation, and trends in the predictability of infliximab concentrations could be identified for the ADA-negative as well as the ADA-positive subpopulation when using first measured infliximab concentration for estimation of EBEs.

While in ADA-negative patients the absolute SSPB values, as a measure of model bias, did not increase for virtually all models from the predictions of concentrations within one month (SSPB median of 7%) to the predictions of concentrations after more than six months of C_{MAP} (SSPB median of 2%), model accuracy decreased noticeably for predictions of concentrations more than six months after C_{MAP} in this study setting (median ($\zeta_{< 1\ month}$): 25%, median ($\zeta_{1-6\ months}$): 28%, median ($\zeta_{> 6\ months}$): 54%). As this observation also held true for model predictions performed with time-varying covariates, yet to a lesser extent, long-term predictions should be treated carefully because of the deterioration in model accuracy.

Different analytical methods have been used to measure infliximab and ADA concentrations in the population pharmacokinetic analyses, leading to differences in immunogenicity rate [17]. While in some studies, "drug sensitive" methods (ADAs not detectable in the presence of infliximab because of analytic interferences) were used to measure ADA concentrations, "drug-tolerant" assays were applied in other investigations, yielding a much higher rate of ADA-positive patients (up to 62% compared to as low as 1%) [21,51]. Nevertheless, 18 out of 23 models that included ADA patients implemented ADA status as a covariate. The five remaining studies identified only ≤3% of patients as ADA positive or used a risk function of developing ADA. The implementation of ADA status in the majority of models highlights the importance of ADA for the PK of infliximab.

Predictions in ADA-positive patients showed much larger deviations from the corresponding observed values compared to predictions in ADA-negative patients: While prediction accuracy for concentrations before the first ADA-positive blood sample (median(ζ): 31%, range: 17–89%) were similar compared to predictions for ADA-negative patients, predictions became much less accurate as soon as ADA status turned positive (median(ζ): 97%, range 72–361%). As noted, for predictions in this analysis, individual patient covariates for times after C_{MAP} were imputed (last observation carried forward). This especially affected predictions of concentrations in patients showing changes in important covariates such as ADA status. Hence, model predictions were also performed with time-varying covariates (depicted in the Supplementary Materials). While improvements in model predictions were especially noted for concentrations in ADA-positive blood samples, predictions still exhibited ζ values of >100% for concentrations more than one month after patients tested ADA positive for the first time, albeit the inclusion of ADA status in most models.

The study by Edlund et al., 2017, aimed to tackle the challenges of predicting infliximab CL in ADA-positive patients [43]. The corresponding population pharmacokinetic model was based on the models by Fasanmade et al., 2011, and Ternant et al., 2015, with the advancement of including ADA concentrations as a continuous covariate [43]. As a result, when using time-varying covariates, the model by Edlund et al., 2017 (III), showed the highest accuracy and least bias for model predictions in ADA-positive patients for "all pred". However, the respective model predictions were still less accurate and showed a higher bias compared to predictions for the ADA-negative patient cohort. Additionally, the implemented covariates albumin and IMM in the model by Fasanmade et al., 2011, were not found to be statistically significant with the data set used for model development by Edlund et al., 2017 [43]. This may have contributed to the slightly lower accuracy and higher bias for predictions in ADA-negative patients compared to the models by Fasanmade et al., 2011.

One reason for the observed overprediction in ADA-positive patients could be due to the fact that the exact time of ADA onset is often unknown. ADA-positive patients develop ADA during a time period of unknown length before they test positive for the first time, which is supported by findings from Petitcollin and coworkers [51]. A close and regular monitoring for ADA using drug-tolerant assays as well as the development and application of models identifying predictors of ADA development [69] might help to improve predictive performances for ADA-positive patients.

For predictive performance evaluation in Bayesian forecasting, only the first measured serum infliximab concentration of each patient was used for MAP estimation of EBEs (C_{MAP}). Due to the design of the study, C_{MAP} was usually a midpoint concentration and results should be interpreted with this in mind. However, using a midpoint infliximab concentration for estimation of EBEs to predict the subsequent trough level allows potential adjustment of the current dosing interval before infliximab concentrations drop below the target concentration of 5 µg/mL.

As infliximab therapy can be adapted based on trough levels [13], model performances to correctly predict the need for dose escalation (i.e., trough concentration <5 µg/mL) were further investigated. The two examined models by Fasanmade et al., 2011, correctly identified 79 of 90 (88%) trough concentrations to be below the target trough concentration (true positive) while correctly identifying 53 of 69 (77%) trough concentrations to be above the target trough concentration (true negative). This represented the highest classification accuracy of correctly identified infliximab trough samples (132/159, 83%) in this study setting. The model by Brandse et al., 2016 [55], exhibited the highest true positive rate (89%); however, it was accompanied by a low true negative rate of 57%. The model by Passot et al., 2016 [56], showed the highest true negative rate (96%) with a low true positive rate of only 63%. While a high false negative rate yields an increased number of patients with insufficient infliximab levels and, hence, decreased drug effect, a high false positive rate corresponds to an increased number of patients with higher exposure and potentially higher rates of adverse effects (e.g., rate of infection [70]). It should be noted that these measures only reflect whether model predictions were correctly below or above the target trough concentration and do not assess how much predictions deviated from the actual measured concentration.

The investigation of factors leading to differences in model performances was outside the scope of this study, but it is worth mentioning that the vast majority of blood samples from the external data set were collected during infliximab maintenance therapy. In contrast, three examined models were developed with data only from the first 6 weeks (Brandse et al., 2016 [55]), "treatment initiation" (Aubourg et al., 2015 [53]), and the first 22 weeks of infliximab treatment (Passot et al., 2016 [56]), which might have affected prediction performance. The model by Petitcollin et al., 2018, was included in the analysis to study the performance of a model with implemented ADA risk function instead of an ADA covariate, although the model was developed with data from pediatric patients [25]. While the corresponding CL and V_d model parameters appear comparable to parameters in infliximab models developed with adult patients [25,43,46,56], the difference in patient cohorts might still explain larger deviations between predicted and measured infliximab concentrations observed in the corresponding pvcVPC and goodness-of-fit plot.

There are some limitations of this analysis, which are discussed in the following paragraphs. Since the study was based on routine therapeutic drug monitoring data, a full dosing schedule was not available for all patients. In such cases, regular dosing from the start of treatment with infliximab and from every change in dosing regimen was assumed. Moreover, sampling times as well as the included patient cohort, treatment period (induction vs. maintenance therapy), analytical methods, or dosing regimens in the external data set could have affected the results of the analysis. Hence, further evaluations with independent data sets should be conducted in future studies.

Another factor influencing the results of an analysis is the choice of quantitative measure. Here, median symmetric accuracy (ζ) and symmetric signed percentage bias (SSPB) values were computed. As illustrated by Morley et al., ζ attenuates the issues with asymmetric penalty and effects of outliers while maintaining interpretability [42]. ζ is a robust measure of accuracy minimizing the effect of the skewness of the distribution of absolute errors [42]. The SSPB estimates the central tendency of the error and can be interpreted similar to a mean percentage error (MPE) [42]. However, in contrast to the MPE, SSPB is not affected by the likely asymmetries in the distribution [42]. As illustrated throughout the analysis, different performance metrics stratified by different patient cohorts (here, ADA-negative and ADA-positive patients) can be of interest when evaluating population pharmacokinetic models in the framework of MIPD. Since different models showed strengths in different measures, we could not appraise which published model was the "best" model, as this also depends on the question of interest and was beyond the scope of this analysis.

Additionally, because of data set incompatibility (e.g., missing covariates) or the lack of reported model implementation details, only 12 of the 25 identified population pharmacokinetic models of infliximab in IBD could be evaluated. While this work already adds a comprehensive analysis to recently published evaluations of single models, an external evaluation including additional covariates (such as the erythrocyte sedimentation rate or fecal calprotectin [21,27]) would be of interest for future studies. Moreover, new modeling approaches (e.g., pharmacokinetic/pharmacodynamic models [27,49]) regarding treatment efficacy could investigate recent findings such as the relation of intestinal microbiota to anti-TNF-α treatment outcome in IBD patients [71,72]. Improvement in gut microbial dysbiosis in IBD patients has been observed during infliximab therapy [71,73], and fecal microbiota has been suggested as a response indicator of infliximab treatment [72]. Future pharmacokinetic/pharmacodynamic studies that examine therapeutic outcome could further investigate this interplay of intestinal microbiota and infliximab therapy. For this, the presented comprehensive external evaluation can also serve as guidance to adopt a suitable population pharmacokinetic model in order to explore these complex response mechanisms.

5. Conclusions

This work presents an external evaluation of the predictive performance of 12 published infliximab population pharmacokinetic models in IBD patients using an independent data set. Differences in predictive performance regarding model accuracy, model bias, and need for dose escalation have been observed for both ADA-negative and ADA-positive patients. Using the first measured infliximab concentration for MAP estimation (C_{MAP}) in a Bayesian forecasting setting, overall model accuracy decreased for predictions more than six months after C_{MAP} for ADA-negative patients, while bias did not increase. The two investigated models by Fasanmade et al., 2011, showed the highest dose escalation classification accuracy of correctly identified infliximab trough samples (83%) in this study setting. Overall, the investigated population pharmacokinetic models showed a classification accuracy of 75–84% for ADA-negative samples and of 60–80% for ADA-positive samples. The results of this predictive performance evaluation could help to guide and plan future MIPD approaches with infliximab population pharmacokinetic models to improve individual dosing strategies and prevent infliximab trough concentrations dropping below the target concentration. Yet clinical application needs to be tested and confirmed in larger, prospective clinical trials. In comparison to predictions for ADA-negative patients, model predictions of serum concentrations for ADA-positive patients showed lower accuracy and higher bias. Thus, predictions with population pharmacokinetic models remain particularly challenging for ADA-positive patients and for patients with unknown ADA status.

Supplementary Materials: The following are available online at https://www.mdpi.com/article/10.3390/pharmaceutics13091368/s1, Electronic Supplementary Materials: Additional evaluation results. Figure S1: Individual predicted versus observed serum infliximab concentrations for the population pharmacokinetic model by Petitcollin et al. 2018. Concentrations of anti-drug antibody (ADA) negative patients are shown in turquoise, concentrations of ADA positive patients in pink. Concentrations used for maximum a posteriori (MAP) estimation (CMAP) are depicted as triangles, the remaining symbols depict predictions in different time intervals after CMAP. The black solid line represents the line of identity, grey dashed lines mark the target trough concentration of 5 µg/mL. (neg): ADA negative patients; (pos): ADA positive patients, Figure S2: Model prediction accuracy (ζ, a and b) and bias (SSPB, c and d) for anti-drug antibody (ADA) negative pa-tients over time. The left panel shows ζ and SSPB values for model predictions with fixed covariates determined at the time of the first measured serum infliximab concentration of each patient (CMAP), the right panel shows ζ and SSPB val-ues for model predictions with time-varying covariates. "all pred" covers all predicted concentrations excluding CMAP. Numbers in parentheses refer to the number of observed concentrations in the respective time interval. (neg): ADA negative patients, pred: predictions; SSPB: symmetric signed percentage bias; ζ: median symmetric accuracy, Figure S3: Model prediction accuracy (ζ, a and 2b) and bias (SSPB, c and d) for anti-drug antibody (ADA) positive pa-tients over time. The left panel shows ζ and SSPB values for model predictions with fixed covariates determined at the time of the first measured serum infliximab concentration of each patient (CMAP), the right panel shows ζ and SSPB val-ues for model predictions with time-varying covariates. "all pred" covers all predicted concentrations excluding CMAP. Numbers in parentheses refer to the number of observed concentrations in the respective time interval. (pos): ADA pos-itive patients, pred: predictions; SSPB: symmetric signed percentage bias; ζ: median symmetric accuracy, Figure S4: Prediction- and variability-corrected visual predictive check (pvcVPC) of serum infliximab concentrations for the population pharmacokinetic model by Petitcollin et al. 2018. Prediction- and variability-corrected observed concen-trations are shown as black circles, observed median is depicted as black solid line, 5th and 95th data percentiles as black dashed lines. The model simulations (n = 1000 replicates) are depicted as grey solid line (median) and blue dashed lines (5th and 95th percentiles). Colored areas represent the simulation-based 95% confidence intervals for the corresponding model-predicted median (grey areas) and 5th and 95th percentiles (blue areas). Pvc: prediction- and variability-corrected, Table S1: ζ and SSPB values for model predictions with fixed covariates at time of CMAP for ADA negative patients, Table S2: ζ and SSPB values for model predictions with fixed covariates at time of CMAP for ADA positive patients, Table S3: ζ and SSPB values for model predictions with time-varying covariates for ADA negative patients, Table S4: ζ and SSPB values for model predictions with time-varying covariates for ADA positive patients.

Author Contributions: Conceptualization, C.S., L.K., U.H., F.T., W.R., M.S. and T.L.; data curation, C.S. and D.S.; formal analysis, C.S., L.K. and D.S.; funding acquisition, U.H., F.T., W.R., M.S. and T.L.; investigation, C.S., L.K., W.R. and T.L.; methodology, C.S., L.K. and D.S.; project administration, U.H., F.T., W.R., M.S. and T.L.; resources, W.R., M.S. and T.L.; software, C.S., L.K. and D.S.; supervision, U.H., F.T., W.R., M.S. and T.L.; visualization, C.S., L.K. and D.S.; writing—original draft, C.S., L.K., D.S. and T.L.; writing—review and editing, C.S., L.K., D.S., U.H., F.T., W.R., M.S. and T.L. All authors have read and agreed to the published version of the manuscript.

Funding: This research was funded by the Robert Bosch Stiftung (Stuttgart, Germany), the German Federal Ministry of Education and Research (BMBF), 031L0188D "GUIDE-IBD", and the Horizon 2020 ERACoSysMed project INSPIRATION (grant 643271).

Institutional Review Board Statement: For predictive external model evaluation, data originated from a previously published observational study that was reviewed and approved by the institutional review board of the Medical University of Vienna [35].

Informed Consent Statement: All participating patients signed an informed consent form.

Data Availability Statement: Not applicable.

Conflicts of Interest: C.S., L.K., D.S., U.H., M.S. and T.L. declare no conflicts of interest. F.T. has served as a speaker for Falk Pharma GmbH and Janssen. W.R. has served as a speaker for Abbott Laboratories, Abbvie, Aesca, Aptalis, Astellas, Centocor, Celltrion, Danone Austria, Elan, Falk Pharma GmbH, Ferring, Immundiagnostik, Mitsubishi Tanabe Pharma Corporation, MSD, Otsuka, PDL, Pharmacosmos, PLS Education, Schering-Plough, Shire, Takeda, Therakos, Vifor, Yakult. Moreover, W.R. has served as a consultant for Abbott Laboratories, Abbvie, Aesca, Algernon, Amgen, AM Pharma, AMT, AOP Orphan, Arena Pharmaceuticals, Astellas, Astra Zeneca, Avaxia, Roland Berger GmbH, Bioclinica, Biogen IDEC, Boehringer-Ingelheim, Bristol-Myers Squibb, Cellerix, Chemocentryx, Celgene, Centocor, Celltrion, Covance, Danone Austria, DSM, Elan, Eli Lilly, Ernest & Young, Falk Pharma GmbH, Ferring, Galapagos, Gatehouse Bio Inc., Genentech, Gilead, Grünenthal, ICON, Index Pharma, Inova, Intrinsic Imaging, Janssen, Johnson & Johnson, Kyowa Hakko Kirin Pharma, Lipid Therapeutics, LivaNova, Mallinckrodt, Medahead, MedImmune, Millenium, Mitsubishi Tanabe Pharma Corporation, MSD, Nash Pharmaceuticals, Nestle, Nippon Kayaku, Novartis, Ocera, OMass, Otsuka, Parexel, PDL, Periconsulting, Pharmacosmos, Philip Morris Institute, Pfizer, Procter & Gamble, Prometheus, Protagonist, Provention, Quell Therapeutics, Robarts Clinical Trial, Sandoz, Schering-Plough, Second Genome, Seres Therapeutics, Setpointmedical, Sigmoid, Sublimity, Takeda, Therakos, Theravance, Tigenix, UCB, Vifor, Zealand, Zyngenia, and 4SC. Additionally, W.R. has served as an advisory board member for Abbott Laboratories, Abbvie, Aesca, Amgen, AM Pharma, Astellas, Astra Zeneca, Avaxia, Biogen IDEC, Boehringer-Ingelheim, Bristol-Myers Squibb, Cellerix, Chemocentryx, Celgene, Centocor, Celltrion, Danone Austria, DSM, Elan, Ferring, Galapagos, Genentech, Grünenthal, Inova, Janssen, Johnson & Johnson, Kyowa Hakko Kirin Pharma, Lipid Therapeutics, MedImmune, Millenium, Mitsubishi Tanabe Pharma Corporation, MSD, Nestle, Novartis, Ocera, Otsuka, PDL, Pharmacosmos, Pfizer, Procter & Gamble, Prometheus, Sandoz, Schering-Plough, Second Genome, Setpointmedical, Takeda, Therakos, Tigenix, UCB, Zealand, Zyngenia, and 4SC, and W.R. has received research funding from Abbott Laboratories, Abbvie, Aesca, Centocor, Falk Pharma GmbH, Immundiagnostik, Janssen, MSD, Sandoz, Takeda.

References

1. European Medicines Agency Remicade—EPAR. Product Information, Annex I—Summary of Product Characteristics—EMEA/H/C/000240. 2020, pp. 1–59. Available online: https://www.ema.europa.eu/en/documents/product-information/remicade-epar-product-information_en.pdf (accessed on 25 November 2020).
2. Prescribing Information REMICADE®(Infliximab), Janssen Biotech, Inc. Available online: https://www.accessdata.fda.gov/drugsatfda_docs/label/2013/103772s5359lbl.pdf (accessed on 8 January 2021).
3. Feagan, B.G.; Choquette, D.; Ghosh, S.; Gladman, D.D.; Ho, V.; Meibohm, B.; Zou, G.; Xu, Z.; Shankar, G.; Sealey, D.C.; et al. The challenge of indication extrapolation for infliximab biosimilars. *Biologicals* **2014**, *42*, 177–183. [CrossRef]
4. Dreesen, E.; Gils, A.; Vermeire, S. Pharmacokinetic Modeling and Simulation of Biologicals in Inflammatory Bowel Disease: The Dawning of a New Era for Personalized Treatment. *Curr. Drug Targets* **2018**, *19*, 757–776. [CrossRef]
5. European Medicines Agency Remicade—EPAR. Summary for the Public, EMA/76495/2012. 2018, pp. 1–3. Available online: https://www.ema.europa.eu/en/documents/overview/remicade-epar-summary-public_en.pdf (accessed on 9 March 2020).
6. Hemperly, A.; Vande Casteele, N. Clinical Pharmacokinetics and Pharmacodynamics of Infliximab in the Treatment of Inflammatory Bowel Disease. *Clin. Pharmacokinet.* **2018**, *57*, 929–942. [CrossRef]
7. Klotz, U.; Teml, A.; Schwab, M. Clinical pharmacokinetics and use of infliximab. *Clin. Pharmacokinet.* **2007**, *46*, 645–660. [CrossRef] [PubMed]
8. Ryman, J.T.; Meibohm, B. Pharmacokinetics of Monoclonal Antibodies. *CPT Pharmacomet. Syst. Pharmacol.* **2017**, *6*, 576–588. [CrossRef]
9. Buhl, S.; Dorn-Rasmussen, M.; Brynskov, J.; Ainsworth, M.A.; Bendtzen, K.; Klausen, P.H.; Bolstad, N.; Warren, D.J.; Steenholdt, C. Therapeutic thresholds and mechanisms for primary non-response to infliximab in inflammatory bowel disease. *Scand. J. Gastroenterol.* **2020**, *55*, 884–890. [CrossRef] [PubMed]
10. Lee, L.Y.W.; Sanderson, J.D.; Irving, P.M. Anti-infliximab antibodies in inflammatory bowel disease. *Eur. J. Gastroenterol. Hepatol.* **2012**, *24*, 1078–1085. [CrossRef]
11. Seow, C.H.; Newman, A.; Irwin, S.P.; Steinhart, A.H.; Silverberg, M.S.; Greenberg, G.R. Trough serum infliximab: A predictive factor of clinical outcome for infliximab treatment in acute ulcerative colitis. *Gut* **2010**, *59*, 49–54. [CrossRef] [PubMed]
12. Maser, E.A.; Villela, R.; Silverberg, M.S.; Greenberg, G.R. Association of trough serum infliximab to clinical outcome after scheduled maintenance treatment for Crohn's disease. *Clin. Gastroenterol. Hepatol.* **2006**, *4*, 1248–1254. [CrossRef]
13. Feuerstein, J.D.; Nguyen, G.C.; Kupfer, S.S.; Falck-Ytter, Y.; Singh, S.; Gerson, L.; Hirano, I.; Rubenstein, J.H.; Smalley, W.E.; Stollman, N.; et al. American Gastroenterological Association Institute Guideline on Therapeutic Drug Monitoring in Inflammatory Bowel Disease. *Gastroenterology* **2017**, *153*, 827–834. [CrossRef]
14. Santacana, E.; Rodríguez-Alonso, L.; Padullés, A.; Guardiola, J.; Bas, J.; Rodríguez-Moranta, F.; Serra, K.; Morandeira, F.; Colom, H.; Padullés, N. Predictors of Infliximab Trough Concentrations in Inflammatory Bowel Disease Patients Using a Repeated-Measures Design. *Ther. Drug Monit.* **2020**, *42*, 102–110. [CrossRef]

15. Papamichael, K.; Gils, A.; Rutgeerts, P.; Levesque, B.G.; Vermeire, S.; Sandborn, W.J.; Vande Casteele, N. Role for therapeutic drug monitoring during induction therapy with TNF antagonists in IBD: Evolution in the definition and management of primary nonresponse. *Inflamm. Bowel Dis.* **2015**, *21*, 182–197. [CrossRef]
16. Gisbert, J.P.; Panés, J. Loss of response and requirement of infliximab dose intensification in Crohn's disease: A review. *Am. J. Gastroenterol.* **2009**, *104*, 760–767. [CrossRef]
17. Chirmule, N.; Jawa, V.; Meibohm, B. Immunogenicity to therapeutic proteins: Impact on PK/PD and efficacy. *AAPS J.* **2012**, *14*, 296–302. [CrossRef] [PubMed]
18. Roda, G.; Jharap, B.; Neeraj, N.; Colombel, J.F. Loss of Response to Anti-TNFs: Definition, Epidemiology, and Management. *Clin. Transl. Gastroenterol.* **2016**, *7*, e135. [CrossRef]
19. Mould, D.R.; Dubinsky, M.C. Dashboard systems: Pharmacokinetic/pharmacodynamic mediated dose optimization for monoclonal antibodies. *J. Clin. Pharmacol.* **2015**, *55*, S51–S59. [CrossRef]
20. Wojciechowski, J.; Upton, R.N.; Mould, D.R.; Wiese, M.D.; Foster, D.J.R. Infliximab Maintenance Dosing in Inflammatory Bowel Disease: An Example for In Silico Assessment of Adaptive Dosing Strategies. *AAPS J.* **2017**, *19*, 1136–1147. [CrossRef]
21. Bauman, L.E.; Xiong, Y.; Mizuno, T.; Minar, P.; Fukuda, T.; Dong, M.; Rosen, M.J.; Vinks, A.A. Improved Population Pharmacokinetic Model for Predicting Optimized Infliximab Exposure in Pediatric Inflammatory Bowel Disease. *Inflamm. Bowel Dis.* **2020**, *26*, 429–439. [CrossRef] [PubMed]
22. Vande Casteele, N.; Ferrante, M.; Van Assche, G.; Ballet, V.; Compernolle, G.; Van Steen, K.; Simoens, S.; Rutgeerts, P.; Gils, A.; Vermeire, S. Trough concentrations of infliximab guide dosing for patients with inflammatory bowel disease. *Gastroenterology* **2015**, *148*, 1320–1329.e3. [CrossRef]
23. Fasanmade, A.A.; Adedokun, O.J.; Ford, J.; Hernandez, D.; Johanns, J.; Hu, C.; Davis, H.M.; Zhou, H. Population pharmacokinetic analysis of infliximab in patients with ulcerative colitis. *Eur. J. Clin. Pharmacol.* **2009**, *65*, 1211–1228. [CrossRef]
24. Fasanmade, A.A.; Adedokun, O.J.; Blank, M.; Zhou, H.; Davis, H.M. Pharmacokinetic Properties of Infliximab in Children and Adults with Crohn's Disease: A Retrospective Analysis of Data from 2 Phase III Clinical Trials. *Clin. Ther.* **2011**, *33*, 946–964. [CrossRef]
25. Petitcollin, A.; Leuret, O.; Tron, C.; Lemaitre, F.; Verdier, M.C.; Paintaud, G.; Bouguen, G.; Willot, S.; Bellissant, E.; Ternant, D. Modeling Immunization to Infliximab in Children with Crohn's Disease Using Population Pharmacokinetics: A Pilot Study. *Inflamm. Bowel Dis.* **2018**, *24*, 1745–1754. [CrossRef]
26. Kantasiripitak, W.; Verstockt, B.; Alsoud, D.; Lobatón, T.; Thomas, D.; Gils, A.; Vermeire, S.; Ferrante, M.; Dreesen, E. The effect of aging on infliximab exposure and response in patients with inflammatory bowel diseases. *Br. J. Clin. Pharmacol.* **2021**, 1–14. [CrossRef]
27. Dreesen, E.; Berends, S.; Laharie, D.; D'Haens, G.; Vermeire, S.; Gils, A.; Mathôt, R. Modelling of the relationship between infliximab exposure, faecal calprotectin and endoscopic remission in patients with Crohn's disease. *Br. J. Clin. Pharmacol.* **2020**, 1–13. [CrossRef]
28. Darwich, A.S.; Ogungbenro, K.; Vinks, A.A.; Powell, J.R.; Reny, J.-L.; Marsousi, N.; Daali, Y.; Fairman, D.; Cook, J.; Lesko, L.J.; et al. Why Has Model-Informed Precision Dosing Not Yet Become Common Clinical Reality? Lessons From the Past and a Roadmap for the Future. *Clin. Pharmacol. Ther.* **2017**, *101*, 646–656. [CrossRef]
29. Gonzalez, D.; Rao, G.G.; Bailey, S.C.; Brouwer, K.L.R.; Cao, Y.; Crona, D.J.; Kashuba, A.D.M.; Lee, C.R.; Morbitzer, K.; Patterson, J.H.; et al. Precision Dosing: Public Health Need, Proposed Framework, and Anticipated Impact. *Clin. Transl. Sci.* **2017**, *10*, 443–454. [CrossRef]
30. Santacana Juncosa, E.; Rodríguez-Alonso, L.; Padullés Zamora, A.; Guardiola, J.; Rodríguez-Moranta, F.; Serra Nilsson, K.; Bas Minguet, J.; Morandeira Rego, F.; Colom Codina, H.; Padullés Zamora, N. Bayes-based dosing of infliximab in inflammatory bowel diseases: Short-term efficacy. *Br. J. Clin. Pharmacol.* **2021**, *87*, 494–505. [CrossRef]
31. Strik, A.S.; Löwenberg, M.; Mould, D.R.; Berends, S.E.; Ponsioen, C.I.; van den Brande, J.M.H.; Jansen, J.M.; Hoekman, D.R.; Brandse, J.F.; Duijvestein, M.; et al. Efficacy of dashboard driven dosing of infliximab in inflammatory bowel disease patients; a randomized controlled trial. *Scand. J. Gastroenterol.* **2021**, *56*, 145–154. [CrossRef]
32. Buclin, T.; Gotta, V.; Fuchs, A.; Widmer, N.; Aronson, J. Monitoring drug therapy. *Br. J. Clin. Pharmacol.* **2012**, *73*, 917–923. [CrossRef] [PubMed]
33. Frymoyer, A.; Piester, T.L.; Park, K.T. Infliximab Dosing Strategies and Predicted Trough Exposure in Children With Crohn Disease. *J. Pediatr. Gastroenterol. Nutr.* **2016**, *62*, 723–727. [CrossRef]
34. Frymoyer, A.; Hoekman, D.R.; Piester, T.L.; de Meij, T.G.; Hummel, T.Z.; Benninga, M.A.; Kindermann, A.; Park, K.T. Application of Population Pharmacokinetic Modeling for Individualized Infliximab Dosing Strategies in Crohn Disease. *J. Pediatr. Gastroenterol. Nutr.* **2017**, *65*, 639–645. [CrossRef]
35. Eser, A.; Primas, C.; Reinisch, S.; Vogelsang, H.; Novacek, G.; Mould, D.R.; Reinisch, W. Prediction of Individual Serum Infliximab Concentrations in Inflammatory Bowel Disease by a Bayesian Dashboard System. *J. Clin. Pharmacol.* **2018**, *58*, 790–802. [CrossRef] [PubMed]
36. IDKmonitor® Infliximab Drug Level ELISA, Immundiagnostik AG. Available online: http://www.immundiagnostik.com/fileadmin/pdf/IDKmonitor_Infliximab_K9655.pdf (accessed on 20 January 2021).
37. Prometheus Therapeutics & Diagnostics Prometheus Anser IFX Monohraph. Available online: www.anserifx.com/PDF/AnserIFX-Monograph.pdf (accessed on 8 January 2021).
38. Wang, S.L.; Ohrmund, L.; Hauenstein, S.; Salbato, J.; Reddy, R.; Monk, P.; Lockton, S.; Ling, N.; Singh, S. Development and validation of a homogeneous mobility shift assay for the measurement of infliximab and antibodies-to-infliximab levels in patient serum. *J. Immunol. Methods* **2012**, *382*, 177–188. [CrossRef]

39. Lindbom, L.; Ribbing, J.; Jonsson, E.N. Perl-speaks-NONMEM (PsN)—A Perl module for NONMEM related programming. *Comput. Methods Programs Biomed.* **2004**, *75*, 85–94. [CrossRef]
40. Lindbom, L.; Pihlgren, P.; Jonsson, N. PsN-Toolkit—A collection of computer intensive statistical methods for non-linear mixed effect modeling using NONMEM. *Comput. Methods Programs Biomed.* **2005**, *79*, 241–257. [CrossRef]
41. Abrantes, J.A.; Jönsson, S.; Karlsson, M.O.; Nielsen, E.I. Handling interoccasion variability in model-based dose individualization using therapeutic drug monitoring data. *Br. J. Clin. Pharmacol.* **2019**, *85*, 1326–1336. [CrossRef]
42. Morley, S.K.; Brito, T.V.; Welling, D.T. Measures of Model Performance Based On the Log Accuracy Ratio. *Sp. Weather* **2018**, *16*, 69–88. [CrossRef]
43. Edlund, H.; Steenholdt, C.; Ainsworth, M.A.; Goebgen, E.; Brynskov, J.; Thomsen, O.; Huisinga, W.; Kloft, C. Magnitude of Increased Infliximab Clearance Imposed by Anti-infliximab Antibodies in Crohn's Disease Is Determined by Their Concentration. *AAPS J.* **2017**, *19*, 223–233. [CrossRef]
44. Ternant, D.; Aubourg, A.; Magdelaine-Beuzelin, C.; Degenne, D.; Watier, H.; Picon, L.; Paintaud, G. Infliximab Pharmacokinetics in Inflammatory Bowel Disease Patients. *Ther. Drug Monit.* **2008**, *30*, 523–529. [CrossRef]
45. Dotan, I.; Ron, Y.; Yanai, H.; Becker, S.; Fishman, S.; Yahav, L.; Ben Yehoyada, M.; Mould, D.R. Patient Factors That Increase Infliximab Clearance and Shorten Half-life in Inflammatory Bowel Disease. *Inflamm. Bowel Dis.* **2014**, *20*, 2247–2259. [CrossRef]
46. Ternant, D.; Berkane, Z.; Picon, L.; Gouilleux-Gruart, V.; Colombel, J.F.; Allez, M.; Louis, E.; Paintaud, G. Assessment of the Influence of Inflammation and FCGR3A Genotype on Infliximab Pharmacokinetics and Time to Relapse in Patients with Crohn's Disease. *Clin. Pharmacokinet.* **2015**, *54*, 551–562. [CrossRef]
47. Brandse, J.F.; Mould, D.; Smeekes, O.; Ashruf, Y.; Kuin, S.; Strik, A.; van den Brink, G.R.; D'Haens, G.R. A Real-life Population Pharmacokinetic Study Reveals Factors Associated with Clearance and Immunogenicity of Infliximab in Inflammatory Bowel Disease. *Inflamm. Bowel Dis.* **2017**, *23*, 650–660. [CrossRef]
48. Kevans, D.; Murthy, S.; Mould, D.R.; Silverberg, M.S. Accelerated clearance of infliximab is associated with treatment failure in patients with corticosteroid-refractory acute ulcerative colitis. *J. Crohn's Colitis* **2018**, *12*, 662–669. [CrossRef]
49. Dreesen, E.; Faelens, R.; Van Assche, G.; Ferrante, M.; Vermeire, S.; Gils, A.; Bouillon, T. Optimising infliximab induction dosing for patients with ulcerative colitis. *Br. J. Clin. Pharmacol.* **2019**, *85*, 782–795. [CrossRef]
50. Matsuoka, K.; Hamada, S.; Shimizu, M.; Nanki, K.; Mizuno, S.; Kiyohara, H.; Arai, M.; Sugimoto, S.; Iwao, Y.; Ogata, H.; et al. Factors contributing to the systemic clearance of infliximab with long-term administration in Japanese patients with Crohn's disease: Analysis using population pharmacokinetics. *Int. J. Clin. Pharmacol. Ther.* **2020**, *58*, 89–102. [CrossRef]
51. Petitcollin, A.; Brochard, C.; Siproudhis, L.; Tron, C.; Verdier, M.C.; Lemaitre, F.; Lucidarme, C.; Bouguen, G.; Bellissant, É. Pharmacokinetic Parameters of Infliximab Influence the Rate of Relapse After De-Escalation in Adults With Inflammatory Bowel Diseases. *Clin. Pharmacol. Ther.* **2019**, *106*, 605–615. [CrossRef]
52. Grišić, A.M.; Dorn-Rasmussen, M.; Ungar, B.; Brynskov, J.; Ilvemark, J.F.K.F.; Bolstad, N.; Warren, D.J.; Ainsworth, M.A.; Huisinga, W.; Ben-Horin, S.; et al. Infliximab clearance decreases in the second and third trimesters of pregnancy in inflammatory bowel disease. *United Eur. Gastroenterol. J.* **2020**, *9*, 91–101. [CrossRef]
53. Aubourg, A.; Picon, L.; Lecomte, T.; Bejan-Angoulvant, T.; Paintaud, G.; Ternant, D. A robust estimation of infliximab pharmacokinetic parameters in Crohn's disease. *Eur. J. Clin. Pharmacol.* **2015**, *71*, 1541–1542. [CrossRef]
54. Buurman, D.J.; Maurer, J.M.; Keizer, R.J.; Kosterink, J.G.W.; Dijkstra, G. Population pharmacokinetics of infliximab in patients with inflammatory bowel disease: Potential implications for dosing in clinical practice. *Aliment. Pharmacol. Ther.* **2015**, *42*, 529–539. [CrossRef]
55. Brandse, J.F.; Mathôt, R.A.; van der Kleij, D.; Rispens, T.; Ashruf, Y.; Jansen, J.M.; Rietdijk, S.; Löwenberg, M.; Ponsioen, C.Y.; Singh, S.; et al. Pharmacokinetic Features and Presence of Antidrug Antibodies Associate With Response to Infliximab Induction Therapy in Patients With Moderate to Severe Ulcerative Colitis. *Clin. Gastroenterol. Hepatol.* **2016**, *14*, 251–258.e2. [CrossRef]
56. Passot, C.; Mulleman, D.; Bejan-Angoulvant, T.; Aubourg, A.; Willot, S.; Lecomte, T.; Picon, L.; Goupille, P.; Paintaud, G.; Ternant, D. The underlying inflammatory chronic disease influences infliximab pharmacokinetics. *MAbs* **2016**, *8*, 1407–1416. [CrossRef]
57. Xu, Z.; Mould, D.R.; Hu, C.; Ford, J.; Keen, M.; Davis, H.M.; Zhou, H. Population pharmacokinetic analysis of infliximab in pediatrics using integrated data from six clinical trials. *Clin. Pharmacol. Drug Dev.* **2012**, *1*, 203.
58. Xu, X.S.; Dunne, A.; Kimko, H.; Nandy, P.; Vermeulen, A. Impact of low percentage of data below the quantification limit on parameter estimates of pharmacokinetic models. *J. Pharmacokinet. Pharmacodyn.* **2011**, *38*, 423–432. [CrossRef]
59. Janssen, E.J.H.; Välitalo, P.A.J.; Allegaert, K.; de Cock, R.F.W.; Simons, S.H.P.; Sherwin, C.M.T.; Mouton, J.W.; van den Anker, J.N.; Knibbe, C.A.J. Towards Rational Dosing Algorithms for Vancomycin in Neonates and Infants Based on Population Pharmacokinetic Modeling. *Antimicrob. Agents Chemother.* **2016**, *60*, 1013–1021. [CrossRef]
60. Smits, A.; De Cock, R.F.W.; Allegaert, K.; Vanhaesebrouck, S.; Danhof, M.; Knibbe, C.A.J. Prospective Evaluation of a Model-Based Dosing Regimen for Amikacin in Preterm and Term Neonates in Clinical Practice. *Antimicrob. Agents Chemother.* **2015**, *59*, 6344–6351. [CrossRef]
61. Neely, M.; Philippe, M.; Rushing, T.; Fu, X.; van Guilder, M.; Bayard, D.; Schumitzky, A.; Bleyzac, N.; Goutelle, S. Accurately Achieving Target Busulfan Exposure in Children and Adolescents With Very Limited Sampling and the BestDose Software. *Ther. Drug Monit.* **2016**, *38*, 332–342. [CrossRef] [PubMed]
62. Krekels, E.H.J.; Tibboel, D.; de Wildt, S.N.; Ceelie, I.; Dahan, A.; van Dijk, M.; Danhof, M.; Knibbe, C.A.J. Evidence-Based Morphine Dosing for Postoperative Neonates and Infants. *Clin. Pharmacokinet.* **2014**, *53*, 553–563. [CrossRef] [PubMed]

63. Darwich, A.S.; Polasek, T.M.; Aronson, J.K.; Ogungbenro, K.; Wright, D.F.B.; Achour, B.; Reny, J.-L.; Daali, Y.; Eiermann, B.; Cook, J.; et al. Model-Informed Precision Dosing: Background, Requirements, Validation, Implementation, and Forward Trajectory of Individualizing Drug Therapy. *Annu. Rev. Pharmacol. Toxicol.* **2021**, *61*, 225–245. [CrossRef]
64. Zhao, W.; Kaguelidou, F.; Biran, V.; Zhang, D.; Allegaert, K.; Capparelli, E.V.; Holford, N.; Kimura, T.; Lo, Y.; Peris, J.; et al. External evaluation of population pharmacokinetic models of vancomycin in neonates: The transferability of published models to different clinical settings. *Br. J. Clin. Pharmacol.* **2013**, *75*, 1068–1080. [CrossRef] [PubMed]
65. Santacana, E.; Rodríguez-Alonso, L.; Padullés, A.; Guardiola, J.; Rodríguez-Moranta, F.; Serra, K.; Bas, J.; Morandeira, F.; Colom, H.; Padullés, N. External Evaluation Of Population Pharmacokinetic Models Of Infliximab In Inflammatory Bowel Disease Patients. *Ther. Drug Monit.* **2017**, *40*, 120–129. [CrossRef]
66. Santacana Juncosa, E.; Padullés Zamora, A.; Colom Codina, H.; Rodríguez Alonso, L.; Guardiola Capo, J.; Bas Minguet, J.; Padullés Zamora, N. Contribution of infliximab population pharmacokinetic model for dose optimization in ulcerative colitis patients. *Rev. Esp. Enferm. Dig.* **2016**, *108*, 104–105. [CrossRef]
67. Candel, M.G.; Gascón Cánovas, J.J.; Espín, R.G.; Nicolás de Prado, I.; Redondo, L.R.; Sanz, E.U.; Navalón, C.I. Usefulness of population pharmacokinetics to optimize the dosage regimen of infliximab in inflammatory bowel disease patients. *Rev. Esp. Enfermedades Dig.* **2020**, *112*, 590–597. [CrossRef]
68. Dave, M.B.; Dherai, A.J.; Desai, D.C.; Mould, D.R.; Ashavaid, T.F. Optimization of infliximab therapy in inflammatory bowel disease using a dashboard approach—An Indian experience. *Eur. J. Clin. Pharmacol.* **2021**, *77*, 55–62. [CrossRef]
69. Eser, A.; Reinisch, W.; Schreiber, S.; Ahmad, T.; Boulos, S.; Mould, D.R. Increased Induction Infliximab Clearance Predicts Early Antidrug Antibody Detection. *J. Clin. Pharmacol.* **2020**, *61*, 224–233. [CrossRef]
70. Landemaine, A.; Petitcollin, A.; Brochard, C.; Miard, C.; Dewitte, M.; Le Balc'h, E.; Grainville, T.; Bellissant, E.; Siproudhis, L.; Bouguen, G. Cumulative Exposure to Infliximab, But Not Trough Concentrations, Correlates With Rate of Infection. *Clin. Gastroenterol. Hepatol.* **2021**, *19*, 288–295.e4. [CrossRef]
71. Magnusson, M.K.; Strid, H.; Sapnara, M.; Lasson, A.; Bajor, A.; Ung, K.; Öhman, L. Anti-TNF Therapy Response in Patients with Ulcerative Colitis Is Associated with Colonic Antimicrobial Peptide Expression and Microbiota Composition. *J. Crohn's Colitis* **2016**, *10*, 943–952. [CrossRef]
72. Seong, G.; Kim, N.; Joung, J.; Kim, E.R.; Chang, D.K.; Chun, J.; Hong, S.N.; Kim, Y.-H. Changes in the Intestinal Microbiota of Patients with Inflammatory Bowel Disease with Clinical Remission during an 8-Week Infliximab Infusion Cycle. *Microorganisms* **2020**, *8*, 874. [CrossRef]
73. Wang, Y.; Gao, X.; Ghozlane, A.; Hu, H.; Li, X.; Xiao, Y.; Li, D.; Yu, G.; Zhang, T. Characteristics of Faecal Microbiota in Paediatric Crohn's Disease and Their Dynamic Changes During Infliximab Therapy. *J. Crohn's Colitis* **2018**, *12*, 337–346. [CrossRef]

Article

Evaluation of the Predictive Performance of Population Pharmacokinetic Models of Adalimumab in Patients with Inflammatory Bowel Disease

Silvia Marquez-Megias [1,†], Amelia Ramon-Lopez [1,2,*,†], Patricio Más-Serrano [1,2,3], Marcos Diaz-Gonzalez [2,3], Maria Remedios Candela-Boix [4] and Ricardo Nalda-Molina [1,2]

1. School of Pharmacy, Miguel Hernández University, 03550 San Juan de Alicante, Spain; silvia.marquez@goumh.umh.es (S.M.-M.); mas_pat@gva.es (P.M.-S.); jnalda@umh.es (R.N.-M.)
2. Alicante Institute for Health and Biomedical Research (ISABIAL-FISABIO Foundation), 03010 Alicante, Spain; diaz_marcosgon@gva.es
3. Clinical Pharmacokinetics Unit, Pharmacy Department, Alicante University General Hospital, 03010 Alicante, Spain
4. Virgen de la Salud General Hospital of Elda, 03600 Elda, Spain; candela_marboi@gva.es
* Correspondence: aramon@umh.es
† These authors contributed equally to this work.

Abstract: Adalimumab is a monoclonal antibody used for inflammatory bowel disease. Due to its considerably variable pharmacokinetics, the loss of response and the development of anti-antibodies, it is highly recommended to use a model-informed precision dosing approach. The aim of this study is to evaluate the predictive performance of different population-pharmacokinetic models of adalimumab for inflammatory bowel disease to determine the pharmacokinetic model(s) that best suit our population to use in the clinical routine. A retrospective observational study with 134 patients was conducted at the General University Hospital of Alicante between 2014 and 2019. Model adequacy of each model was evaluated by the distribution of the individual pharmacokinetic parameters and the NPDE plots whereas predictive performance was assessed by calculating bias and precision. Moreover, stochastic simulations were performed to optimize the maintenance doses in the clinical protocols, to reach the target of 8 mg/L in at least 75% of the population. Two population-pharmacokinetic models were selected out of the six found in the literature which performed better in terms of adequacy and predictive performance. The stochastic simulations suggested the benefits of increasing the maintenance dose in protocol to reach the 8 mg/L target.

Keywords: pharmacokinetics; drug monitoring; adalimumab; inflammatory bowel diseases; Crohn's disease; colitis; ulcerative

1. Introduction

Crohn's disease (CD) and ulcerative colitis (UC) are chronic inflammatory bowel diseases (IBD) characterized by the intermittent destructive inflammation of the intestinal tract associated with significant morbidity, high burden of hospitalization and a severe impact on the quality of life of patients. There are several pharmacological alternatives available, including corticosteroids, immunosuppressive agents (methotrexate or azathioprine) and monoclonal antibodies that have shown clinical response in the treatment of these diseases [1–3].

Adalimumab is a human monoclonal antibody that binds specifically to the tumor necrosis factor (TNF) and neutralizes its biological function, decreasing the process of inflammation. Adalimumab is effective for induction and maintenance of remission in patients with moderate-to-severe IBD older than 6 years who fail with corticosteroids, immunosuppressive agents or other biologic therapy [4–6].

Several published studies of adalimumab have shed light on the clinical relevance of individualized dosing. Historically, the empiric approach to adapt the adalimumab dosage consists of intensifying the treatment in patients with loss of response and later, if this fails, switching to another biological treatment. In the last decade, several studies have shown that some patients can experience a loss of response to adalimumab or can develop antibodies against adalimumab (AAA) after long periods of subtherapeutic drug levels [7–14]. However, most of the time, the serum concentration guide dosing was done through algorithms [15,16].

In this line, Model-Informed Precision Dosing (MIPD) is the approach based on the use of population PK (PopPK) models and prospective Bayesian approach to increase the homogeneity in the drug exposure in patients in order to improve outcomes of treatments by achieving the optimal balance between efficacy and toxicity for each individual patient [17]. IBD patients could benefit from dose optimization because adalimumab has highly variable pharmacokinetics (PK) [16,18].

Recently, a multicenter retrospective study showed that the potential importance of early monitoring levels of adalimumab and MIPD approach can prevent immunogenicity and achieve better long-term outcomes in terms of IBD-related surgery or hospitalization, lower risk of developing AAA or serious infusion reactions and also it proved to be more cost-effective in comparison to empirical and/or reactive dose optimization program dose escalation [19]. However, the selection of the appropriate PopPK model is fundamental to apply MIPD, especially when there are multiple models in the literature in patients with IBD. The structural model is defined, in most of them, as one-compartment model with linear kinetics in the absorption and elimination processes, although the value of the PopPK parameters, and the covariates included in the model, vary significantly. Therefore, the aim of this study is to evaluate the predictive performance of PopPK models of adalimumab found in literature, in patients with IBD to determine the pharmacokinetic model(s) best suited for our population to subsequently use it in the clinical setting using MIPD.

2. Materials and Methods

2.1. Literature Search

A systematic literature search was conducted of databases in the field of Health Sciences: MEDLINE (via PubMed), Embase and Scopus. To define the search terms, the Medical Subject Headings (MeSH), a thesaurus developed by the U.S. National Library of Medicine, was used. The MeSH descriptors "Chron Disease", "Colitis, Ulcerative", "adalimumab" and "pharmacokinetics" were considered suitable. Likewise, these terms, "inflammatory bowel diseases" and "pharmacokinetics" were used to query the databases using the title and abstract field (Title/Abstract). The search was performed from the first available date until May 2021 according to the characteristics of each database. Additionally, a manual search for population models was conducted by inspecting the bibliographies of relevant journal articles to minimize the number of unrecovered papers by the review.

The following search was used in Pubmed, and it was adapted to the other databases: ((((("Inflammatory Bowel Diseases"[Mesh]) OR (Inflammatory Bowel Diseases[Title/Abstract])) OR (((Crohn Disease[Title/Abstract]) OR (Crohn's Disease[Title/Abstract])) OR ("Crohn Disease"[Mesh]))) OR ((ulcerative colitis[Title/Abstract]) OR ("Colitis, Ulcerative"[Mesh]))) AND ((Adalimumab[Title/Abstract]) OR ("Adalimumab"[Mesh]))) AND ((Pharmacokinetics[Title/Abstract]) OR ("Pharmacokinetics"[Mesh])).

The inclusion criteria were the following: original articles published in peer-reviewed journals, articles that describe a novel population pharmacokinetic model and pertinent works with the available complete text, which must be written in English or Spanish. Additionally, the full text of the document should be accessible and only one version of each document was included. The following were the exclusion criteria: articles that included different diseases to CD or UC and studies developed in animal models.

The following information was extracted from the articles: patient characteristics, model structure, typical PopPK parameters, inter-individual variability (IIV), residual variability (RV) and covariates.

2.2. Study Design

A retrospective observational study was conducted at the General University Hospital of Alicante, performed on patients diagnosed with IBD undergoing treatment with adalimumab and who followed a dose optimization program developed between 2014 and 2019.

2.3. Patients and Data Collection

Trough serum concentrations (TSC) were collected from patients diagnosed with moderate or severe IBD treated with adalimumab in General University Hospital of Alicante, Spain. The following inclusion criteria were applied: participants had to be diagnosed with IBD, treated with adalimumab, and there had to be at least two adalimumab TSC in their medical history. Exclusion criteria included patients treated with other monoclonal antibodies different to adalimumab like infliximab, vedolizumab and ustekinumab and subjects who were diagnosed with other autoimmune diseases different to IBD such as rheumatoid arthritis, psoriasis and ankylosing spondylitis.

Relevant data were collected from the medical records and included age, sex, height, body weight, lean body weight (LBW), body mass index (BMI), AAA status and AAA serum concentration, dose of adalimumab, adalimumab serum concentration, serum albumin levels, serum C-reactive protein (CRP) levels, fecal calprotectin (FCP), type of disease, use of concomitant immunomodulators and time of the event recorded. Missing values of continuous covariates were imputed by their expected mean values. Data were excluded from the analysis if there was uncertainty about any relevant information such as the time of dosing or the time of drug concentration measurement and the loss to follow-up during their treatment.

Serum adalimumab concentrations and AAA were measured using an enzyme-linked immunosorbent assay (LISA TRACKER Duo Drug + ADAb from TheraDiag®) with a limit of quantification established to be 0.1 mg/L. Patients were considered as positive for AAA if titers were above 10 mg/L on at least one occasion.

2.4. Evaluation of Model Adequacy

The first step in the evaluation of the different PopPk models found in the literature was the evaluation of the model adequacy by analyzing and comparing how the different PopPK models describe the studied population using all the available TSC in the dataset (full dataset). Models that show the greater systematic bias in the Empirical Bayesian estimate (EBEs) of the PK parameters, or in the Normalised Prediction Distribution Errors (NPDE) [20,21] will be discarded. Only the models that described properly our population will be used to evaluate the predictive performance later.

Therefore, the distribution of the EBEs of the PK parameters for each of the PopPk models was calculated after performing a post-hoc analysis using the full dataset. Then, this distribution would be compared with the theoretical distribution of these PK parameters according to each of the PopPK models.

On the other hand, any trends observed in the NPDE plots (e.g., cone-shaped graph) might indicate model misspecifications and inferior model adequacy.

2.5. Evaluation of Predictive Performance

The evaluation of predictive performance was only performed in those models which best describe the studied population, according to the evaluation of the model adequacy.

To evaluate the predictive performance, the individual predictions of the last TSC were estimated for each patient, using the EBEs. These last TSC concentrations, named "last observed TSC", were left out and not used to calculate the EBEs. To evaluate the predictive

performance, the bias and the precision were calculated with the last observed TSC by comparing them with their individual predictions calculated by each of the PK models. The predictive performance of the patients was evaluated considering two different scenarios;
Scenario 1: The EBES were calculated from the previous TSC obtained from each patient 2
Scenario 2: The EBES were calculated from the two previous TSC of each patient.

The mean prediction error (MPE, Equation (1)) and root mean square prediction error (RMSPE, Equation (2)) were calculated for bias and precision, respectively.

$$\text{MPE} = \frac{\sum(\hat{Y} - Y)}{n} \quad (1)$$

$$\text{RMSPE} = \sqrt{\frac{\sum(\hat{Y} - Y)^2}{n}} \quad (2)$$

In both equations Y-hat represents the model-predicted adalimumab concentration, Y represents the observed adalimumab concentration, and n is the number of observations.

A bootstrap of the data was performed to compare the statistical significance of the differences between bias and precision among the selected models.

2.6. Clinical Impact

Stochastic simulations were performed to optimize the initial maintenance doses in the clinical protocols, in order to acquire the target TSC in at least 75% of the population. The dosage regimens that were simulated were 40 and 80 mg administered subcutaneously every week or every other week. The target TSC that were considered were 8 mg/L for clinical remission [18,22].

2.7. Software

The PopPK models found in the literature were implemented in NONMEM® version 7.4 software package [23]. The posterior statistical analysis and graphics were performed using R software v4.0.3 [24], implemented in R-studio v1.3.1093 [25].

2.8. Ethical Considerations

2.8.1. Ethics Approval

All studies were conducted in accordance with principles for human experimentation as defined in the Declaration of Helsinki and were approved by the Human Investigational Review Board of each study center.

2.8.2. Consent

The need for written consent was waived because of the retrospective nature of the study.

3. Results

3.1. Literature Search

A total of 211 publications 72, 52 and 87 from PubMed, Embase and Scopus, respectively, from 2003 to 2021, were found and collected in the search of databases using the keywords mentioned in the methods section. After removing duplicate articles and applying the inclusion and exclusion criteria, six PopPK models [26–31] were selected. The models were numbered from 1 to 6 and are referred to as M1 to M6. All selected PopPK models were one-compartment models. Four of them included only trough levels of adalimumab (M2, M3, M4 and M5) whereas the others (M1 and M6) derived from complete profiles of serum concentrations of adalimumab. Five of the six models were developed using NONMEM® software, while one model (M2) was developed using Monolix® software. Further information can be found in Table 1.

Table 1. Summary of specifications of selected models.

Model No.	Study	No. of Patients (Total No. of Samples)	Parameter Values and Covariate Relationships Included	IIV (CV)	Residual Variability
M1	FDA, 2008	646 adult patients (NA)	$CL^*/F\,(L/h) = 0.0127$ $V/F\,(L) = 9.39 + 0.126 \cdot (WT - 72))$ $ka\,(1/h) = 0.027$ FIX	IIV-CL/F: 16.4% IIV-V/F: 35.1%	Prop = 31.6%
M2	Ternant D et al., 2015	65 adult CD patients (341)	$CL/F\,(L/h) = 0.0175 \cdot (1 + 4.5 \cdot AAA)$ $V/F\,(L) = 13.5$ $ka\,(1/h) = 0.00625$ $CL/F\,(L/h) =$	IIV-CL/F: 65% IIV-V/F: 48%	Add = 1.8 mg/L Prop = 16%
M3	Sharma S et al., 2015	189 pediatric CD patients (852)	$0.0117 \cdot (1 + 1.08 \cdot AAA) \cdot (WT/45.2)^{0.48}$ $V/F\,(L) = 4.75 \cdot (WT/45.2)^{0.904}$ $ka\,(1/h) = 0.00833$ $CL/F\,(L/h) =$	IIV-CL/F: 21.1%	Add = 1.9 mg/L Prop = 7.1%
M4	Berends SE et al., 2018	96 adult CD patients (181)	$0.0133 \cdot (1 + 3.14 \cdot AAA) \cdot (1 + 0.4 \cdot DOSING)$ $V/F\,(L) = 4.07$ $ka\,(1/h) = 0.00833$ FIX $CL/F\,(L/h) =$	IIV-CL/F: 49.1%	Add = 1.02 mg/L Prop = 9%
M5	Vande Castelee et al., 2019	28 adult CD patients (185)	$0.01375 \cdot (1 + 1.59 \cdot AAA) \cdot (LBW/47.8)^{1.97}$ $V/F\,(L) = 7.8$ $ka\,(1/h) = 0.0143$ $CL/F\,(L/h) = 0.0157 \cdot (BMI/23.7)^{1.11}$	IIV-CL/F: 32.6% IIV-V/F: 35.6% IIV-ka: 103.9%	Prop = −16.6%
M6	Sánchez-Hernández et al., 2020	104 adult IBD patients (303)	$(1 + 1.20 \cdot UDASC) \cdot (1 + 0.24 \cdot PEN) \cdot (FCP/74)^{0.064}$ $V/F\,(L) = 11.2$ $ka\,(1/h) = 0.00625$ FIX	IIV-CL/F: 23.2%	Prop = 21.7%

IIV: inter-individual variability; CV: coefficient of variation; CD: Crohn's disease; IBD: Inflammatory Bowel Disease; WT: weight; AAA: antibodies against adalimumab; DOSING: adalimumab dosing regimen (0: every other week, 1: every week); UDASC: unexplained decline in adalimumab serum concentrations (0: NO, 1: YES); PEN: administration pen device during maintenance phase (0:40 mg, 1:80 mg); FCP: fecal calprotectin; add:additive error; prop: proportional error; NA: not available. The M numbers represent the selected models.

Typical values for adalimumab apparent clearance (CL/F) in the studies ranged from 11.7 to 17.5 mL/h, with the lowest value being reported in studies performed with pediatric population (M3). The typical apparent volume of distribution (V/F) ranged from 4.07 to 13.5 L. The absorption rate constant (ka) was estimated in three models and fixed in the others. All models estimated the IIV (coefficient of variation [CV], in percent) associated with adalimumab CL/F, with values ranging from 16.4% to 65%. Three models (M1, M2 and M5) estimated the IIV of V/F ranged from 35.1% to 48%. The summary of the characteristics of each study is listed in Table 2.

3.2. Patients

The dataset included 134 IBD patients in treatment with adalimumab with at least two TC. Baseline demographics, disease characteristics and missing values for the different covariates of the patient population are listed in Table 3. 75% of the patients are below 57 years old and 75 kg. Approximately 85% of the patients were diagnosed as CD and 8% of them developed AAA.

82 patients were treated subcutaneously with 160/80 mg and 18 with 80/40 mg at weeks 0/2 as an induction phase. For the rest, the information regarding the induction phase was not available in their medical histories. Following this phase, as a maintenance phase, all patients were treated with 40 mg of adalimumab every other week. A total of 398 TSC in the maintenance phase were available for the analysis, where 25.4% of these concentrations were over 8 mg/L, 46.3% between 3 and 8 mg/L and 28.3% below 3 mg/L in the first measure. AAA were detected in 11 patients. 73 patients were on a concomitant immunomodulator (azathioprine, 6 mercaptopurine, methotrexate or prednisone).

The dosage regimen was increased to 40 mg every 10 days or 40 mg every week, on 31 and 70 dose adjustments, respectively. Similarly, the dosage regimen was increased to 80 mg every other week or 80 mg every week, on 7 and 11 dose adjustments, respectively. On the other hand, on 7 dose adjustments, the dosage regimen was decreased to 40 mg every 3 weeks, at any time during their treatment. In 36 patients the dosage regimen was maintained at 40 mg every other week.

3.3. Evaluation of Model Adequacy

The distribution of the individual CL/F obtained in the post-hoc analysis compared with their theoretical distribution is represented in Figure 1. The distribution of the individual V/F was not performed because half of the models (M3, M4 and M6) did not include IIV in the V/F. The QQ-plot of the NPDE and their distribution versus time are depicted in Figure 2.

In M2 and M4, the 20% and 80% percentiles of the EBE of CL/F are close to the 95% confidence interval of the 20% and 80% percentiles of the simulated distribution of CL/F for these models. Moreover, the NPDE performed better in these models. Hence, M2 and M4 were the models that best described the studied population, with less bias and better NPDE performance. Therefore, the predictive performance would be evaluated in these models.

3.4. Evaluation of Predictive Performance

Figure 3 shows the predictive performance for M2 and M4 represented as the IRES vs. the model-based prediction of the last observed TSC. Both models behave similarly, with a limited bias and a similar dispersion of the IRES. Table 4 also shows the bias and precision for M2 and M4 and their confidence interval. M2 and M4 are statistically better ($p < 0.05$) than the other models in terms of bias and precision in both scenarios (data not shown).

Table 2. Summary of patient characteristics of selected models.

Model No.	Age (yr)	Weight (kg)	Disease (cd/uc)	Sex (m/f)	AAA Positive (%)	Albumin (g/dL)	Dosage Regimen	Measured Adalimumab Concentration	Measured AAA
M1	NA	NA	NA	NA	NA	NA	- Induction phase: 160/80 mg or 80/40 at weeks 0/2 - Maintenance phase: 40 every other week	ELISA	ELISA
M2	37 (17–61)	68 (43–109)	100/0	17/48	9 (13.8%)	NA	- Induction phase: 160/80 mg or 80/40 at weeks 0/2 - Maintenance phase: 40 mg every other week	ELISA	Double-antigen ELISA

M3	13.6 (6–17)	45.2 (18–119)	100/0	105/84	83 (43.9%)	4.0 (2.4–5.3)	- Induction phase:
							  ○ ≥40 kg: 160/80 mg at weeks 0/2
							  ○ <40 kg: 80/40 at weeks 0/2
							- Maintenance phase:
							  ○ ≥40 kg: 40 or 20 mg every other week
							  ○ <40 kg: 20 or 10 mg every other week
								Double-antigen ELISA	Bridging ELISA

M4	38 (32–44)	65 (58–76)	100/0	35/96	17 (18%)	4.3 (4.05–4.5)	- Maintenance phase: 40 mg every week or every other week	TNF ELISA	Antigen-binding test
M5	37 (30–49)	66 (55–73)	100/0	13/28	5 (17.9%)	3.99 (3.6–4.4)	- Induction phase: 160/80 mg at weeks 0/2 - Maintenance phase: 40 mg every other week	In-house developed TNF-coated ELISA	In-house developed drug resistant AAA assay
M6	43 (32–56)	68 (56–80)	84/20	58/46	0	4.5 (4.3–4.7)	- Induction phase: 160/80 mg at weeks 0/2 - Maintenance phase: dose adjustment according to TDM	ELISA	ELISA

CD: Crohn's disease; UC: ulcerative colitis; AAA: antibodies against adalimumab; NA = not available. The M numbers represent the models described in Table 1.

Table 3. Summary of characteristics of included patients.

Characteristics	Count (%)/ Median (Percentile 25th–75th)	Missings, n (%)
Patients	134	0
Age (yr)	45 (34–57)	0
Sex, male, n (%)	70 (52.2%)	0
Weight (kg)	66 (58–75)	1 (0.75%)
Body mass index (kg/m^2)	23.85 (20.52–27.36)	10 (7.46%)
Lean Body Weight (kg)	46.84 (42.60–52.10)	10 (7.46%)
Albumin (g/dL)	3.84 (3.53–4.12)	5 (3.73%)
CRP (mg/dL)	0.64 (0.25–2.1)	37 (27.61%)
FCP (mg/kg)	487 (217.11–884.68)	37 (27.61%)
IBD type, CD, n (%)	115 (85.8%)	0
Concomitant immunomodulator, n (%)		
Aminosalicylate	7 (5.2%)	0
Methotrexate	10 (7.5%)	0
Azathioprine	53 (39.6%)	0
6-Mercaptopurine	6 (4.5%)	0
Corticosteroids	16 (11.9%)	0
Combined	14 (10.4%)	0
Adalimumab serum samples	398	0
Adalimumab serum concentrations (mg/L)	6.75 (4.58–8.65)	0
AAA serum concentrations (mg/L)	29 (4.53–76.30)	0
AAA positive, n (%)	11 (8%)	0

CRP: C-reactive protein; FCP: fecal calprotectin; IBD: inflammatory bowel disease; CD: Crohn's disease; AAA: antibodies against adalimumab.

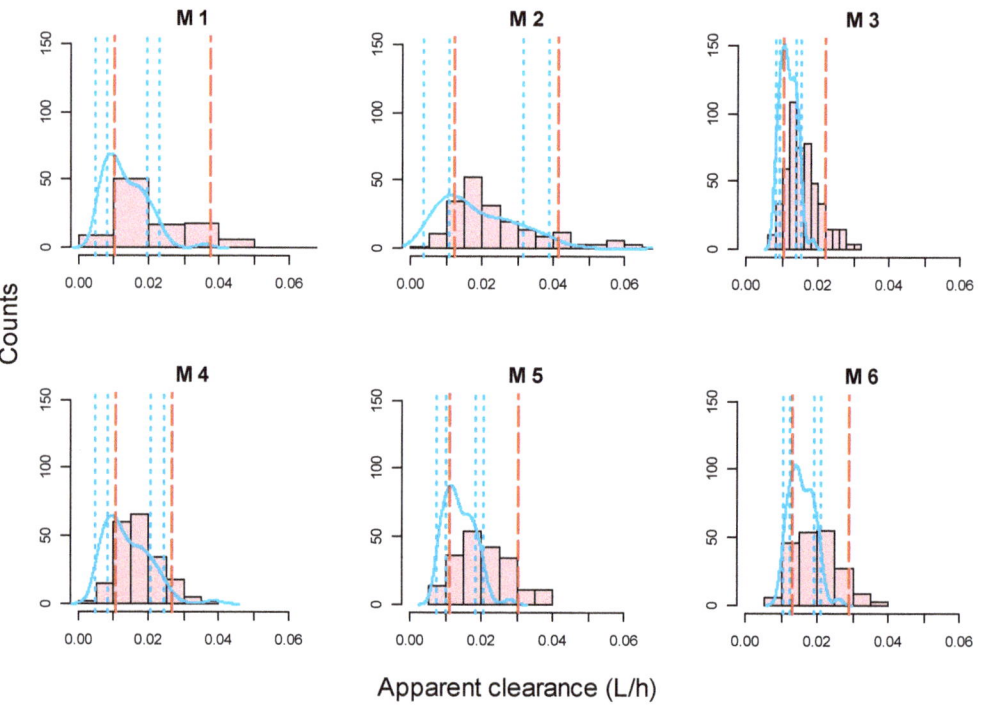

Figure 1. Histograms of EBEs for CL/F. Red dashed line; 20th and 80th percentile of EBEs CL/F; blue solid line represents the density of the simulated CL/F; blue dotted line, 95% confidence interval (CI) for the 20th and 80th percentiles of simulated CL/F. The M numbers represent the models described in Table 1.

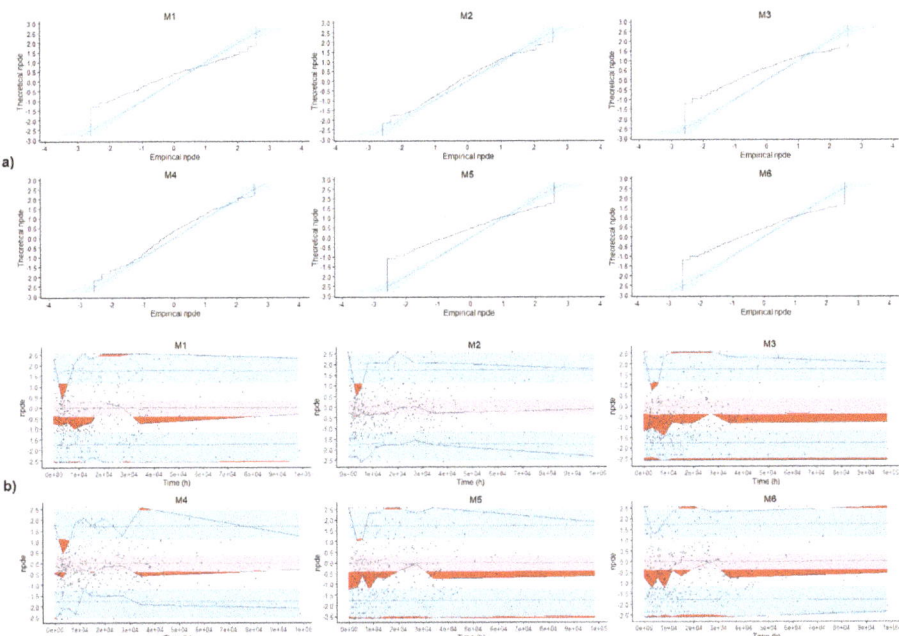

Figure 2. NPDE for each model. (a) Quantile-quantile plot of the npde versus the corresponding quantiles of a normal distribution. (b) Plot of npde versus time. Solid horizontal lines are the lines corresponding to 0, 5% and 95% critical values; gray solid lines, prediction intervals; blue-shaded area, 90% confidence interval (CI) of the 5% and 95% critical values; pink-shaded area, 90% CI of 0; red-shaded area, outliers of the bounds of the CI. The M numbers represent the models described in Table 1.

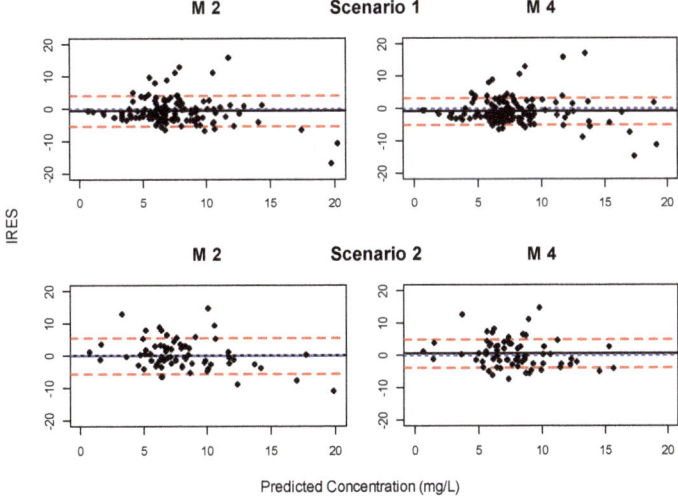

Figure 3. Individual residual (IRES) versus the individual predicted concentrations for M2 and M4 in Scenario 1 and Scenario 2. The mean IRES (black solid line) represents the bias of each model; red dashed line, 5th and 95th percentile for IRES; blue dotted line to highlight the line corresponding to 0. The M numbers represent the models described in Table 1.

Table 4. Values of bias and precision with its 95% confidence interval for each model in both scenarios.

Model	Scenario 1		Scenario 2	
	Bias	Precision	Bias	Precision
M2	−0.59 (−1.37:0.19)	4.61 (3.55:5.67)	0.012 (−1.27:1.29)	5.43 (3.81:7.06)
M4	−0.91 (−1.62:−0.19)	4.30 (3.47:5.12)	0.52 (−0.52:1.56)	4.43 (3.49:5.37)

The M numbers represent the models described in Table 1.

3.5. Clinical Impact

The results of the stochastic simulations of different dosage regimens using M2 and M4 are summarized in Figure 4. None of the dosage regimens could reach the desired target (TSC > 8 mg/mL) in at least 75% of the population that developed AAA. Similarly, 40 mg every other week was insufficient to reach the target for at least 75% of the population without AAA, although it is the standard dose recommended by protocol. 40 mg every week or 80 mg every week or every other week are enough to reach the target in at least 75% of the population. Interestingly, according to M2, the plasma concentration profiles of 40 mg every week or 80 mg every other week are very similar, which is not the case in M4.

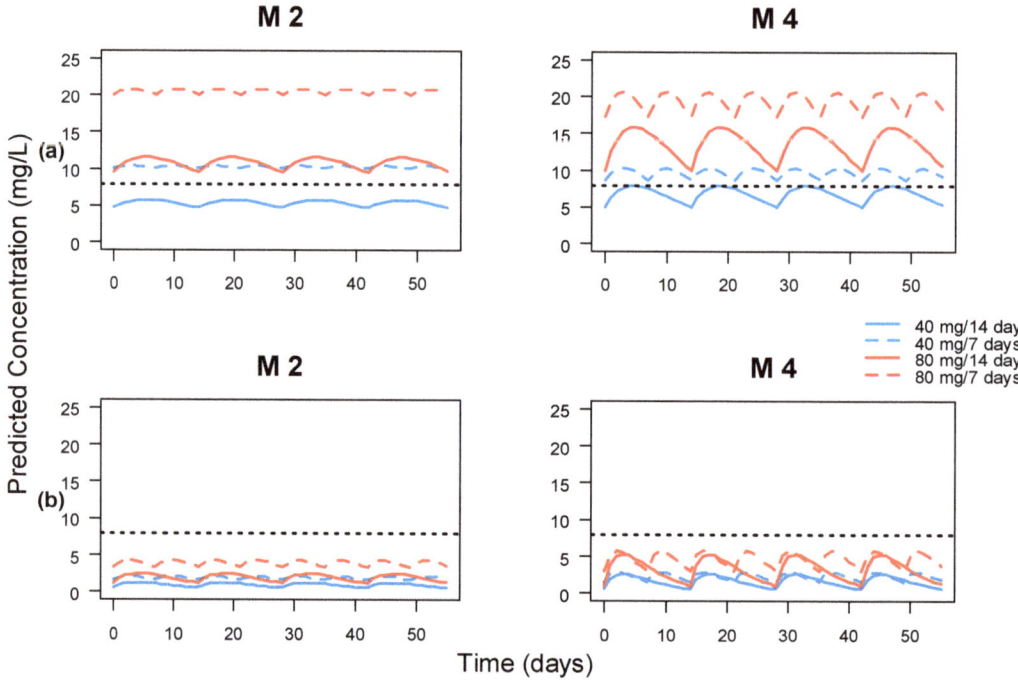

Figure 4. Stochastic simulation of the 25th percentile of serum concentrations over time for M2 and M4. Black dotted line was drawn to highlight the line corresponding to 8 mg/L. (**a**) Serum concentrations of patients without AAA. (**b**) Serum concentrations of patients with AAA. The M numbers represent the models described in Table 1.

4. Discussion

The MDPI applied in the clinical routine commonly makes use of PopPK models found in literature, given the lack of data available to develop in-house models in most of the hospitals. However, these models must be validated in the target population. An important aspect to validate is the predictive performance of the models, in similar conditions to the clinical routine. Many validations published in the literature do not really validate the predictive performance, but rather evaluate the model adequacy to the data. In the present work, the predictive performance was done with TSC that has not been used to calculate the EBEs, mimicking the real-world scenario. To our knowledge, this is the first validation and comparison of the PopPK models of adalimumab in the literature for their use in clinical routine. Six PopPK models for adalimumab were found in the literature for CD and/or UC patients, with similar structure (one-compartment model), although the covariates included differ among them. The PopPK models included patients with both induction and maintenance treatment, and only one was performed with data from pediatric population.

The model adequacy showed that M2 and M4 performed better than the rest. However, the mean individual CL/F obtained in all six PopPK models after the Bayesian post-hoc estimation (Figure 1) is somehow higher than the expected mean CL/F. One possible explanation for this systematic trend is that the mean albumin value of our population is slightly lower than the referenced in the models found in literature, which indicates a worse disease control. There are several studies that demonstrate the correlation between low levels of albumin and an increase in the clearance of other similar drugs like infliximab [32,33].

Consequently, four out of the six models were discarded due to the significant bias in the distribution of the NPDE as well as the EBEs of the PopPK parameters, therefore, the models M2 and M4 were the candidates to evaluate the predictive performance. The predictive performance of both models performed reasonably well, with a bias less than −0.91, which is less than 13% of the trough target (8 mg/L). The bootstrap analysis of the predictive performance showed no statistical difference between both models, so, with the available data, both models could be considered as equally good for the clinical routine purposes. AAA is considered the covariate with the highest impact in the pharmacokinetic parameters, according to the results of the stochastic simulations.

According to the drug label, the recommended maintenance dose after the induction phase is 40 mg every other week [5]. This scheme results in a mean steady-state TSC of approximately 7 mg/L in Crohn's disease patients, which agrees with the mean steady-state TSC observed in our population (7.3 mg/L). So far, the exposure target is highly dependent on the therapeutic objective (clinical, endoscopic, biochemical or histologic remission) and whether patients are diagnosed with CD or UC [34]. A recent study showed that patients with concentrations <8.3 mg/L had more risk to develop AAA by week 12 and experienced less clinical benefit from dose escalation due to a loss of response [22]. Another study indicates that 8–12 mg/L TSC of adalimumab are required to achieve mucosal healing in 80–90% of IBD patients [18]. According to the stochastic simulations performed with M2 and M4 and considering a target TSC over 8 mg/mL, the recommended maintenance regimen dosage that should be included in the protocols is 40 mg every week or 80 mg every other week, in order to reach the target in, at least, 75% of the population. These recommendations are in line with the MDPI interventions in our population, where 75% of the patients needed a dose increase to reach the 8 mg/mL target.

The limitation of this study relies on its retrospective design, where patients were selected for MDPI based on the clinical decision of the physician, which implies a bias in the severity of the disease, reflected in the mean albumin values of our population. A prospective study in which patients were included for MDPI in a structured way regardless of the clinical situation of the patients should be carried out to avoid selection bias and validate these results in a wider population.

In summary, two of the PopPK models found in the literature were found to be better than the others in terms of model adequacy and predictive performance. However, the EBEs of the individual CL/F were found biased when compared with the population mean values in the models. That suggested the need to update the model with the available data. On the other hand, the stochastic simulations performed with these models suggested the benefits of increasing the maintenance dose in protocol to reach the 8 mg/L target.

Author Contributions: Conceptualization, R.N.-M., A.R.-L. and P.M.-S.; data curation, R.N.-M., P.M.-S., M.D.-G. and M.R.C.-B.; formal analysis, S.M.-M. and A.R.-L.; investigation, S.M.-M. and A.R.-L.; methodology, S.M.-M., A.R.-L., R.N.-M.; supervision, R.N.-M.; writing—original draft, S.M.-M. and A.R.-L.; writing—review and editing, R.N.-M., P.M.-S., M.D.-G and M.R.C.-B. All authors have read and agreed to the published version of the manuscript.

Funding: This research was funded by a research grant offered by the Miguel Hernandez University. Reference number [PAR-00385/2021].

Institutional Review Board Statement: The study was conducted according to the guidelines of the Declaration of Helsinki and approved by the Institutional Review Board (or Ethics Committee) of Alicante University General Hospital.

Informed Consent Statement: Patient consent was waived due to the retrospective nature of the study.

Data Availability Statement: The datasets used and/or analyzed during the current study are available from the corresponding author on reasonable request.

Acknowledgments: The authors thank Gastroenterology Department of the Alicante University General Hospital for the support in the treatment clinical approach.

Conflicts of Interest: The authors declare no conflict of interest.

References

1. Gomollón, F.; Dignass, A.; Annese, V.; Tilg, H.; Van Assche, G.; Lindsay, J.O.; Peyrin-Biroulet, L.; Cullen, G.J.; Daperno, M.; Kucharzik, T.; et al. 3rd European Evidence-based Consensus on the diagnosis and management of Crohn's disease 2016: Part 1: Diagnosis and medical management. *J. Crohn's Colitis* **2017**, *11*, 3–25. [CrossRef]
2. Baumgart, D.C.; Sandborn, W.J. Inflammatory bowel disease: Clinical aspects and established and evolving therapies. *Lancet* **2007**, *369*, 1641–1657. [CrossRef]
3. Bernstein, C.N.; Eliakim, A.; Fedail, S.; Fried, M.; Gearry, R.; Goh, K.; Hamid, S.; Khan, A.G.; Khalif, I.; Ng, S.C.; et al. World Gastroenterology Organisation Global Guidelines inflammatory bowel disease. *J. Clin. Gastroenterol.* **2016**, *50*, 803–818. [CrossRef]
4. Fakhoury, M.; Negrulj, R.; Mooranian, A.; Al-Salami, H. Inflammatory bowel disease: Clinical aspects and treatments. *J. Inflamm. Res.* **2014**, *7*, 113–120. [CrossRef]
5. European Medicines Agency (EMA). HUMIRA: Summary of Product Characteristics. *EMA.* 2021. Available online: https://www.ema.europa.eu/en/documents/product-information/humira-epar-product-information_en.pdf (accessed on 11 August 2021).
6. Cohen, L.B.; Nanau, R.M.; Delzor, F.; Neuman, M.G. Biologic therapies in inflammatory bowel disease. *Transl. Res.* **2014**, *163*, 533–556. [CrossRef] [PubMed]
7. Roda, G.; Jharap, B.; Neeraj, N.; Colombel, J.F. Loss of response to anti-TNFs: Definition, epidemiology, and management. *Clin. Transl. Gastroenterol.* **2016**, *7*, e135. [CrossRef] [PubMed]
8. Ma, C.; Huang, V.; Fedorak, D.K.; Kroeker, K.I.; Dieleman, L.A.; Halloran, B.P.; Fedorak, R.N. Adalimumab dose escalation is effective for managing secondary loss of response in Crohn's disease. *Aliment. Pharmacol. Ther.* **2014**, *40*, 1044–1055. [CrossRef]
9. Yanai, H.; Lichtenstein, L.; Assa, A.; Mazor, Y.; Weiss, B.; Levine, A.; Ron, Y.; Kopylov, U.; Bujanover, Y.; Rosenbach, Y.; et al. Levels of drug and antidrug antibodies are associated with outcome of interventions after loss of response to infliximab or adalimumab. *Clin. Gastroenterol. Hepatol.* **2015**, *13*, 522–530. [CrossRef]
10. Vande Casteele, N.; Gils, A. Pharmacokinetics of anti-TNF monoclonal antibodies in inflammatory bowel disease: Adding value to current practice. *J. Clin. Pharmacol.* **2015**, *55*, 39–50. [CrossRef]
11. Lopetuso, L.R.; Gerardi, V.; Papa, V.; Scaldaferri, F.; Rapaccini, G.L.; Antonio Gasbarrini, A.; Papa, A. Can we predict the efficacy of anti-TNF-α agents? *Int. J. Mol. Sci.* **2017**, *18*, 1973. [CrossRef]
12. Ding, N.S.; Hart, A.; De Cruz, P. Systematic review: Predicting and optimising response to anti-TNF therapy in Crohn's disease—algorithm for practical management. *Aliment. Pharmacol. Ther.* **2016**, *43*, 30–51. [CrossRef] [PubMed]
13. Papamichael, K.; Gils, A.; Rutgeerts, P.; Levesque, B.G.; Vermeire, S.; Sandborn, W.J.; Vande Casteele, N. Role for therapeutic drug monitoring during induction therapy with TNF antagonists in IBD: Evolution in the definition and management of primary nonresponse. *Inflamm. Bowel Dis.* **2015**, *21*, 182–197. [CrossRef]
14. Papamichael, K.; Vande Casteele, N.; Ferrante, M.; Gils, A.; Cheifetzl, A.S. Therapeutic drug monitoring during induction of antitumor necrosis factor therapy in inflammatory bowel disease: Defining a therapeutic drug window. *Inflamm. Bowel Dis.* **2017**, *23*, 1510–1515. [CrossRef]
15. Papamichael, K.; Vogelzang, E.H.; Lambert, J.; Wolbink, G.; Cheifetz, A.S. Therapeutic drug monitoring with biologic agents in immune mediated inflammatory diseases. *Expert Rev. Clin. Immunol.* **2019**, *15*, 837–848. [CrossRef] [PubMed]
16. Papamichael, K.; Cheifetz, A.S.; Melmed, G.Y.; Irving, P.M.; Vande Casteele, N.; Kozuch, P.L.; Raffals, L.E.; Baidoo, L.; Bressler, B.; Devlin, S.M.; et al. Appropriate Therapeutic Drug Monitoring of Biologic Agents for Patients With Inflammatory Bowel Diseases. *Clin. Gastroenterol. Hepatol.* **2019**, *17*, 1655–1668. [CrossRef]

17. Darwich, A.S.; Ogungbenro, K.; Vinks, A.A.; Powell, J.R.; Reny, J.L.; Marsousi, N.; Daali, Y.; Fairman, D.; Cook, J.; Lesko, L.J.; et al. Why has model-informed precision dosing not yet become common clinical reality? Lessons from the past and a roadmap for the future. *Clin. Pharmacol. Ther.* **2017**, *101*, 646–656. [CrossRef] [PubMed]
18. Ungar, B.; Levy, I.; Yavne, Y.; Yavzori, M.; Picard, O.; Fudim, E.; Loebstein, R.; Chowers, Y.; Eliakim, R.; Kopylov, U.; et al. Optimizing anti-TNFα therapy: Serum levels of infliximab and adalimumab associate with mucosal healing in patients with inflammatory bowel diseases. *Clin. Gastroenterol. Hepatol.* **2015**, *14*, 550–557. [CrossRef]
19. Papamichael, K.; Juncadella, A.; Wong, D.; Rakowsky, S.; Sattler, L.A.; Campbell, J.P.; Vaughn, B.P.; Cheifetz, A.S. Proactive therapeutic drug monitoring of adalimumab is associated with better long-term outcomes compared to standard of care in patients with inflammatory bowel disease. *J. Crohn's Colitis* **2019**, *13*, 976–981. [CrossRef] [PubMed]
20. Brendel, K.; Comets, E.; Laffont, C.; Laveille, C.; Mentre, F. Metrics for external model evaluation with an application to the population pharmacokinetics of gliclazide. *Pharm. Res.* **2006**, *23*, 2036–2049. [CrossRef] [PubMed]
21. Brendel, K.; Comets, E.; Laffont, C.; Laveille, C.; Mentre, F. Evaluation of different tests based on observations for external model evaluation of population analyses. *J. Pharmacokinet. Pharmacodyn.* **2010**, *37*, 49–65. [CrossRef] [PubMed]
22. Verstockt, B.; Moors, G.; Bian, S.; Van Stappen, T.; Van Assche, G.; Vermeire, S.; Gils, A.; Ferrante, M. Influence of early adalimumab serum levels on immunogenicity and long-term outcome of anti-TNF naive Crohn's disease patients: The usefulness of rapid testing. *Aliment. Pharmacol. Ther.* **2018**, *48*, 731–739. [CrossRef]
23. Beal, S.L.; Sheiner, L.B.; Boeckmann, A.J.; Bauer, R.J. *NONMEM 7.4.0 Users Guides. (1989–2013)*; ICON Development Solutions: Hanover, MD, USA, 2021; Available online: https://iconplc.com/innovation/nonmem/ (accessed on 10 May 2021).
24. R Core Team. *R: A Language and Environment for Statistical Computing*; R Foundation for Statistical Computing: Vienna, Austria, 2021; Available online: http://www.R-project.org/ (accessed on 10 May 2021).
25. RStudio. *RStudio: Integrated Development Environment for R*; RStudio: Boston, MA, USA, 2021; Available online: http://www.rstudio.org/ (accessed on 10 May 2021).
26. Food and Drug Administration (FDA). HUMIRA: Clinical Pharmacology and Biopharmaceutics Review(s). *FDA*. 2008. Available online: https://www.accessdata.fda.gov/drugsatfda_docs/bla/2007/125057_S0089.pdf (accessed on 11 August 2021).
27. Ternant, D.; Karmiris, K.; Vermeire, S.; Desvignes, C.; Azzopardi, N.; Bejan-Angoulvant, T.; van Assche, G.; Paintaud, G. Pharmacokinetics of adalimumab in Crohn's disease. *Eur. J. Clin. Pharmacol.* **2015**, *71*, 1155–1157. [CrossRef] [PubMed]
28. Sharma, S.; Eckert, D.; Hyams, J.S.; Mensing, S.; Thakkar, R.B.; Robinson, A.M.; Rosh, J.R.; Ruemmele, F.M.; Awni, W.M. Pharmacokinetics and exposure-efficacy relationship of adalimumab in pediatric patients with moderate to severe Crohn's disease: Results from a randomized, multicenter, phase-3 study Pharmacokinetics and exposure-efficacy relationship of adalimumab in pediatric patients with moderate to severe Crohn's disease: Results from a randomized, multicenter, phase-3 study. *Inflamm. Bowel Dis.* **2015**, *21*, 783–792. [CrossRef]
29. Berends, S.E.; Strik, A.S.; Van Selm, J.C.; Löwenberg, M.; Ponsioen, C.Y.; D'Haens, G.R.; Mathôt, R.A. Explaining interpatient variability in adalimumab pharmacokinetics in patients with Crohn's disease. *Ther. Drug Monit.* **2018**, *40*, 202–211. [CrossRef]
30. Vande Casteele, N.; Baert, F.; Bian, S.; Dreesen, E.; Compernolle, G.; Van Assche, G.; Ferrante, M.; Vermeire, S.; Gils, A. Subcutaneous absorption contributes to observed interindividual variability in adalimumab serum concentrations in Crohn's disease: A prospective multicentre study. *J. Crohn's Colitis* **2019**, *27*, 1248–1256. [CrossRef] [PubMed]
31. Sánchez-Hernández, J.G.; Pérez-Blanco, J.S.; Rebollo, N.; Muñoz, F.; Prieto, V.; Calvo, M.V. Biomarkers of disease activity and other factors as predictors of adalimumab pharmacokinetics in inflammatory bowel disease. *Eur. J. Pharm. Sci.* **2020**, *150*, 105369. [CrossRef] [PubMed]
32. Hemperly, A.; Vande Casteele, N. Clinical Pharmacokinetics and Pharmacodynamics of Infliximab in the Treatment of Inflammatory Bowel Disease. *Clin. Pharmacokinet.* **2018**, *57*, 929–942. [CrossRef]
33. Brandse, J.F.; Mould, D.; Smeekes, O.; Ashruf, Y.; Kuin, S.; Strik, A.; van den Brink, G.R.; D'Haens, G.R. A Real-life Population Pharmacokinetic Study Reveals Factors Associated with Clearance and Immunogenicity of Infliximab in Inflammatory Bowel Disease. *Inflamm. Bowel Dis.* **2017**, *23*, 650–660. [CrossRef]
34. Juncadella, A.; Papamichael, K.; Vaughn, B.P.; Cheifetz, A.S. Maintenance adalimumab concentrations are associated with biochemical, endoscopic, and histologic remission in inflammatory bowel disease. *Dig. Dis. Sci.* **2018**, *63*, 3067–3073. [CrossRef]

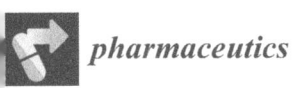

Article

No Time Dependence of Ciprofloxacin Pharmacokinetics in Critically Ill Adults: Comparison of Individual and Population Analyses

Martin Šíma [1,*], Danica Michaličková [1], Pavel Ryšánek [1,*], Petra Cihlářová [2], Martin Kuchař [2], Daniela Lžičařová [3], Jan Beroušek [4], Jan Miroslav Hartinger [1], Tomáš Vymazal [4] and Ondřej Slanař [1]

[1] Department of Pharmacology, First Faculty of Medicine, Charles University and General University Hospital in Prague, 128 00 Prague, Czech Republic; danica.michalickova@lf1.cuni.cz (D.M.); jan.hartinger@vfn.cz (J.M.H.); ondrej.slanar@lf1.cuni.cz (O.S.)

[2] Forensic Laboratory of Biologically Active Substances, Department of Chemistry of Natural Compounds, University of Chemistry and Technology Prague, 166 28 Prague, Czech Republic; Petra.Cihlarova@vscht.cz (P.C.); Martin.Kuchar@vscht.cz (M.K.)

[3] Department of Medical Microbiology, Second Faculty of Medicine, Charles University in Prague and Motol University Hospital, 150 06 Prague, Czech Republic; Daniela.lzicarova@lfmotol.cuni.cz

[4] Department of Anesthesiology and ICM, Second Faculty of Medicine, Charles University in Prague and Motol University Hospital, 150 06 Prague, Czech Republic; jan.berousek@fnmotol.cz (J.B.); tomas.vymazal@fnmotol.cz (T.V.)

* Correspondence: martin.sima@lf1.cuni.cz (M.Š.); pavel.rysanek@lf1.cuni.cz (P.R.)

Abstract: The aim of this prospective PK study was to evaluate the pharmacokinetics of ciprofloxacin dosed within the first 36 h (early phase) and after 3 days of treatment (delayed phase) using individual and population PK analysis. The secondary aim of the study was to evaluate possible dosing implications of the observed PK differences between early and delayed phases to achieve a PK/PD target for ciprofloxacin of $AUC_{24}/MIC \geq 125$. Blood concentrations of ciprofloxacin (1 and 4 h after dose and trough) were monitored in critically ill adults in the early and delayed phases of the treatment. Individual and population PK analyses were performed. Complete concentration-time profiles in the early phase, delayed phase, and both phases were obtained from 29, 15, and 14 patients, respectively. No systematic changes in ciprofloxacin PK parameters between the early and delayed phases were observed, although variability was higher at the early phase. Both individual and population analyses provided similar results. Simulations showed that after standard dosing, it is practically impossible to reach the recommended ciprofloxacin PK/PD target (AUC/MIC ≥ 125) for pathogens with MIC ≥ 0.5 mg/L. A dosing nomogram utilizing patients' creatinine clearance and MIC values was constructed. Both individual and population analyses provided similar results. Therapeutic drug monitoring should be implemented to safeguard the optimal ciprofloxacin exposure.

Keywords: ciprofloxacin; pharmacokinetics; covariates; dosing; NONMEM; renal function

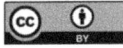

1. Introduction

Antibiotic treatment is commonly used to eradicate bacterial infections in critically ill patients admitted to the intensive care unit. Ciprofloxacin is a wide-spectrum antibiotic that is commonly prescribed for various infections either in monotherapy or in combination with other antibiotics [1]. Its bactericidal action is distinguished by an activity primarily against Gram-negative aerobic bacteria, of which *Pseudomonas aeruginosa* and *Enterobacterales* are the most clinically important [2]. Specific pharmacokinetic/pharmacodynamic (PK/PD) target for ciprofloxacin is defined as the ratio of the 24 h area under the concentration-time curve (AUC_{24}) over the minimum inhibitory concentration (MIC), where the MIC is determined as the lowest concentration of an antibiotic that prevents visible growth of bacteria in vitro [3]. Generally, attaining the PK/PD target of $AUC_{24}/MIC \geq 125$ should be predictive of sufficient anti-infective treatment. Nonetheless, $AUC_{24}/MIC \geq 125$ is usually not attained in critically ill patients treated with the standard recommended doses of ciprofloxacin (200–1500 mg/day), as shown in previous studies [4–6].

Both population and individual PK analyses are well-established and recognized types of PK explorations with distinct features that may lead to the preference for one procedure over another. In a population PK analysis performed using non-linear mixed-effects modeling (NLME), data of all patients included in the study are analyzed at the same time, providing estimates of population parameter values and inter- and intra-individual variability [7]. There are several advantages of the population PK analysis, such as the possibility to analyze sparse and unbalanced data, identification and quantification of predictive covariates, and ability to distinguish between inter- and intra-individual variability, or residual unexplained variability [7]. On the other hand, individual PK explorations are generally conducted to describe PK parameters and determine the most prominent factors with the highest potential to affect drug exposures. Although this individual approach leaves many possible sources of variability unexplored, the most important ones are generally better captured in a limited-sample-size population, provided a sufficient number of samples is obtained.

There is a high heterogeneity in the group of critically ill patients regarding the patients' age, comorbidities, disease severity, pathogens and loci of infections [4,8]. Various pathophysiological factors in these patients usually lead to alteration of PK of the drugs. Altered PK of a drug may result in an inadequate exposure, causing insufficient bacterial eradication, an increased risk of antibiotic resistance, and surplus morbidity and mortality [9]. Therefore, detailed understanding of the PK of an individual antibiotic drug is necessary for its dosing optimization. Volume of distribution (Vd) can be increased due to the reduced protein binding, systemic inflammatory response syndrome (SIRS), and capillary leak [10]. Additionally, the elimination rate can be impaired or augmented, depending on the clinical condition of the patient [10]. SIRS can downregulate CYP enzymes, and this may lead to reduced clearance (CL) of drugs cleared by these enzymes [10]. On the other hand, CL of an antibiotic can be enhanced in sepsis, burn injury, or by concomitant use of inotropic agents [10].

Our hypothesis was that there might be a context-sensitive pharmacokinetic profile of ciprofloxacin as a result of complex instability of factors affecting ciprofloxacin PK in critically ill patients at the beginning of treatment, compared to likely more-stabilized conditions after 3 days of treatment.

The aim of this prospective study was therefore to evaluate the pharmacokinetics of ciprofloxacin dosed within first 36 h (early phase) and after 3 days of treatment (delayed phase). The secondary aim of the study was to evaluate possible dosing implications of the observed PK differences between the early and delayed phases to achieve a PK/PD target for ciprofloxacin of $AUC_{24}/MIC \geq 125$.

2. Materials and Methods

2.1. Study Design

This was a prospective, open-label (laboratory-blinded) pharmacokinetic study in adult patients treated with intravenous ciprofloxacin admitted to the Department of Anesthesiology and Intensive Care Medicine, Second Faculty of Medicine, Charles University in Prague, and Motol University Hospital between February 2019 and June 2020. The study was approved by the local Ethics Committee under No. EK 1492/18 on 2 January 2019 and was conducted in compliance with the Declaration of Helsinki. Written informed consent was obtained from all subjects before undertaking any study-related procedures. The study was registered in EudraCT under No. 2019-003732-24.

Ciprofloxacin was administered according to the standard clinical care in 30 min intravenous infusions of 400 or 600 mg every 8 or 12 h. The choice of dosing regimen was at the discretion of the clinician. Blood samples for the PK analysis were taken at 1, 4, and 7.5 or 11.5 h following completion of the infusion (the last sample was taken as a trough, depending on the dosing interval). This concentration-time profile was collected twice during the therapy—at the early phase (within 36 h after initiation of ciprofloxacin dosing) and at the delayed phase (72–96 h after initiation of ciprofloxacin dosing). Patients from whom at least one complete concentration-time profile was not collected were excluded from the study. Blood samples (5 mL) were collected via cannula into serum collecting tubes without clot activator and immediately placed in the cold. Samples were then centrifuged at $4500 \times g$ for 10 min at 4 °C, and serum aliquots were stored at -80 °C until analysis.

The following demographic, laboratory, and clinical features of patients were recorded as a potential covariates of ciprofloxacin pharmacokinetics: sex, age, body weight, height, smoking status, total bilirubin, serum creatinine, fluid balance, and co-medication with norepinephrine and furosemide. All clinical and laboratory parameters were determined separately on each sampling day. Hence, actual values were used for PK analysis both in the early and delayed phase.

Creatinine clearance (CL_{CR}) was measured using serum creatinine (enzymatic assay) and 24 h urine output. CL_{CR} was calculated using the traditional equation $CL_{CR} = U_{CR} \times V/S_{CR}$, where U_{CR} is urine creatinine level (µmol/L), V is the urinary flow rate (mL/s), and S_{CR} is the serum level of creatinine (µmol/L) [11].

Glomerular filtration rate was also estimated using Chronic Kidney Disease Epidemiology Collaboration (CKD-EPI), Modification of Diet in Renal Disease (MDRD), Cockroft–Gault (C-G), and revised Lund–Malmö (L-M) formulas [12–15].

For each patient, body surface area (BSA) according to the DuBois formula and lean body mass (LBM) according to the Boer formula were calculated [16,17].

2.2. Bioanalytical Assay

Acetonitrile (ACN) and methanol (MeOH) (all LC-MS grade) were obtained from Honeywell (Charlotte, NC, USA). Ammonium acetate, formic acid, and ammonia solution 25% (all LC-MS grade) were supplied by Fluka (Buchs, Switzerland). Ultra-pure water was produced by a Smart2Pure system (Thermo Fisher Scientific, Waltham, MA, USA). Charcoal-stripped fetal bovine serum and ciprofloxacin ($\geq$98%) were purchased from Sigma-Aldrich (Saint Louis, MO, USA), and internal standard ciprofloxacin-d8 (IS) from TRC (Totonto, ON, Canada). Standard stock solutions were prepared in water/acetic acid (60/40 v/v) at a concentration of 1 mg/mL and stored at -20 °C.

For serum samples, protein precipitation was used. Several procedures and reagents were tested; e.g., ACN, ACN/MeOH, and ACN/formic acid mixtures in several ratios. For the final procedure, 10 µL of IS solution (5 µg/mL) was added to 100 µL of serum and vortexed. Then, 200 µL of ice-cold mixture of ACN with 0.1% of formic acid was added and vortexed for 5 min. The procedure was repeated with another 200 uL of ACN/formic acid. The mixture was centrifuged at $13,000 \times g$ for 15 min, then 400 µL of the supernatant was evaporated and reconstituted in 500 µL of 10% methanol. All samples were prepared in triplicate.

The same procedure was used for the calibration curve; 100 µL of stripped bovine serum was spiked with ciprofloxacin standard solution to construct a calibration curve with the final range of 0.1–750 ng/mL.

For the UHPLC-MS/MS analysis, an Agilent 1290 Infinity UHPLC system coupled with an Agilent 6460 Triple quadrupole mass spectrometer (Agilent Technologies, Inc., Santa Clara, CA, USA) was used. Chromatographic separation was performed on a Kinetex EVO C18 column (2.1 × 50 mm; 1.7 µm) equipped with a guard column (both Phenomenex, Torrance, CA, USA). The mobile phases for gradient elution were ammonium acetate in water (0.5 mM) with ammonia solution, pH adjusted to 10.5 (A) and methanol (B). The flow rate was 0.45 mL/min and column temperature 30 °C. Gradient elution was carried out as follows: 0 min, 90:10 (A:B); 2 min, 60:40; 3.5 min, 0:100; 4.5 min, 0:100; 4.7 min, 90:10; 6.5 min, 90:10.

The MS/MS apparatus was operated in positive mode. The applied conditions of the electrospray ion source were: drying gas temperature 300 °C; drying gas flow 13 L/min; sheath gas temperature 350 °C; sheath gas flow 11 L/min; nebulizer pressure 40 psi; nozzle voltage 0 V; capillary voltage 2500 V. Multiple reaction monitoring (MRM) mode was used for the detection. Two transitions of m/z were used: 332.14 → 314.1 and 231 for ciprofloxacin and 340.19 → 322.2 and 235 for ciprofloxacin-d8.

An Agilent Mass Hunter (Agilent Technologies, Inc., Santa Clara, CA, USA) was used for data acquisition and quantification of samples.

2.3. Primary PK Analysis

Individual ciprofloxacin pharmacokinetic parameters—Vd, CL, and elimination half-life ($t_{1/2}$)—were calculated in a one-compartmental pharmacokinetic model with first-order elimination kinetics based on individual demographic and clinical data and observed ciprofloxacin serum levels using MWPharm^{++} software version 1.8.2 (MediWare, Prague, Czech Republic). The ciprofloxacin PK data derived from Drusano et al. was used for an a priori estimation of the concentration-time profile in each patient [18]. These estimated PK profile curves were a posteriori individualized to maximize fitting with observed concentration points in each patient. The fitting was performed using Bayesian method separately for both the early and delayed phase concentrations set. The goodness of fit was expressed using weighted sum of squares and root mean square values.

Subsequently, a Mann–Whitney U-test and linear regression model were used to evaluate the relationships between ciprofloxacin individual PK parameters with categorical and continuous variables, respectively. PK parameters and measured CL_{CR} obtained from early and delayed concentration-time profiles were compared using a Mann–Whitney U-test (for this analysis, only patients with both complete phase profiles were included). GraphPad Prism software version 8.2.1 (GraphPad Inc., La Jolla, CA, USA) was used for all comparisons, and p-levels < 0.05 were considered as statistically significant.

2.4. Population PK Analysis

Population PK analysis was performed using NONMEM version 7.3.0 (ICON Development Solutions, Ellicott City, MD, USA) and PsN v3.4.2 [19,20] both running under Pirana 2.9.0 [21]. Modeling was carried out using the first-order conditional estimation method with interaction (FOCE-I). R 3.3.2 was used for the visualization of the data and model diagnostics.

Model development was performed in three steps:

(1) Development of structural and statistical model

For the structural model, one- and two-compartment models were tested to describe the distribution of ciprofloxacin. First-order clearance of ciprofloxacin was assumed. Log-normally distributed inter-individual variability terms with estimated variance were tested on each PK parameter. As change in the clinical status of the patients between the early phase and delayed phase of ciprofloxacin treatment was expected, inter-occasional variability was also tested. Proportional, additive, and combination error models were tested for the residual error model.

(2) Covariate analysis

The following variables were tested as covariates (characteristics predictive of inter-individual variability):

- Body weight, height, LBM, BSA, serum level of bilirubin, CL_{CR}, age, daily fluid balance, and doses of concomitantly used drugs (noradrenalin and furosemide) were tested as continuous covariates;
- Smoking status (smoker/non-smoker), concomitant therapy with continuous veno-venous hemodialysis—CVVHD (on CVVHD/off CVVHD) and sex were tested as categorical covariates.

A stepwise covariate modeling procedure was performed. Continuous covariates were tested in linear and power functions. Categorical covariates were tested by estimating the parameter value for one category as a fraction of the parameter value for the other category. For model selection, a decrease in objective function value (OFV) of more than 3.84 points between nested models ($p < 0.01$) was considered statistically significant, assuming a χ^2 distribution. Additional criteria for model selection were relative standard error (RSE) of the estimates of structural model parameters <30%, physiological plausibility of the obtained parameter values, and absence of bias in goodness-of-fit (GOF) plots.

(3) Validation of the final model

To evaluate the stability of the model, a bootstrap analysis was performed. In this procedure, 1000 replicates of the original data were generated, and the parameter estimates for each of the 1000 samples were re-estimated by NONMEM in the final model. The median and 95% confidence intervals (CI) obtained for each parameter estimated for bootstrap samples were compared with the estimates in the final model. The predictive properties of the structural and statistical model were validated using normalized prediction distribution errors (NPDEs). For this, the dataset was simulated 1000 times, after which the observed concentrations were compared to the range of simulated values using the NPDE package developed for R [22]. Additionally, a visual predictive check (VPC) was performed to evaluate the predictive accuracy of the final model [23]. For this, 1000 replicates of the original dataset were simulated using the final model parameter estimates, and the simulated distribution was compared with that from the observed data. The 95% CIs for the 10th, 50th, and 90th percentiles of the simulations were calculated from all replicates and presented graphically.

Monte Carlo Simulations

Monte Carlo simulations ($n = 1000$) were performed to assess the probability of target attainment (PTA) of the PK/PD target for ciprofloxacin (AUC/MIC ratio > 125) for various MICs (0.0625 to 1 mg/L). Standard dosing regimens consisting of 400 mg b.i.d. and t.i.d were simulated for different levels of CL_{CR} (0.5, 1, 1.5 mL/s). Dosing regimen was regarded to be successful if the PTA was >100%.

3. Results

3.1. Study Population

There were 35 patients enrolled in the study. Five patients were excluded due to deviations in sampling times or missing samples. Complete concentration-time profile in the early phase, delayed phase, and both phases was obtained from 29, 15, and 14 patients, respectively. The main reasons for not completing both study phases were discontinuation of ciprofloxacin therapy, patient transfer from the intensive care unit, or significant deviations from sampling schedule. Demographic, laboratory, and clinical characteristics of patients are summarized in Table 1. The most frequent indications for ciprofloxacin use were acute exacerbations of chronic obstructive pulmonary disease, lower respiratory tract infections, and soft tissue infections. Among patients included in the PK analysis ($n = 30$), only one subject received CVVHD support, and none were treated with extracorporeal membrane oxygenation. Ciprofloxacin dose ranged from 800 mg/day (400 mg every 12 h) to 1200 mg/day (400 mg every 8 h or 600 mg every 12 h). In total, 132 ciprofloxacin serum concentrations were included in the analysis.

Table 1. Demographic, laboratory, and clinical characteristics of patients ($n = 30$).

Characteristics	Early Phase ($n = 29$)	Delayed Phase ($n = 15$)
Sex (M/F)	21/8	11/4
Age (years)	58 (35–85)	57 (35–85)
Body weight (kg)	90 (56–140)	90 (58–130)
Height (cm)	175 (150–196)	175 (160–190)
BSA (m^2)	2.09 (1.60–2.65)	2.09 (1.60–2.45)
LBM (kg)	63 (44–81)	63 (44–76)
Smoking status (Y/N/NA)	15/6/8	9/3/3
CL$_{CR}$ (mL/s)	1.16 (0.12–3.32)	1.36 (0.66–2.49)
CKD-EPI (mL/s)	1.60 (0.16–2.98)	1.24 (0.76–2.37)
MDRD (mL/s)	1.70 (0.18–4.26)	1.99 (0.94–4.95)
C–G (mL/s)	1.77 (0.25–4.96)	2.10 (0.72–5.31)
L–M (mL/s)	1.45 (0.20–2.81)	1.76 (0.82–2.95)
Total bilirubin (μmol/L)	11.3 (3.5–90.3)	11.0 (4.4–46.4)
Fluid balance (mL/day)	−490 (−4000–4300)	−500 (−3502–1900)
Norepinephrine (mg/day)	17 (0–61)	5 (0–60)
Furosemide (mg/day)	5 (0–320)	19 (0–148)

Data are presented as median (range). BSA—body surface area; LBM—lean body mass; CL$_{CR}$—measured creatinine clearance; M—men; W—women; Y—yes; N—no; NA—not available; CKD-EPI—Chronic Kidney Disease Epidemiology Collaboration; MDRD—Modification of Diet in Renal Disease; C–G—Cockroft–Gault; and L–M—revised Lund–Malmö equations for estimation of glomerular filtration rate.

3.2. Primary PK Analysis

Individual pharmacokinetic parameters of ciprofloxacin are summarized in Table 2. Median (interquartile range) weighted sum of squares and root mean square values were 7.43 (2.60–10.98) and 0.96 (0.91–0.98), respectively. We observed medium to high inter-individual variability of PK parameters normalized per kg of body weight demonstrated by coefficients of variation of 46%, 74%, and 37% for Vd, CL, and t$_{1/2}$, respectively (early-phase group). On the contrary, there were no significant differences either in ciprofloxacin PK parameters or in measured CL$_{CR}$ between the early and delayed phases (p-values of 0.2798, 0.6673, 0.7088, and 0.5189 for body-weight-normalized Vd, CL, t$_{1/2}$, and CL$_{CR}$, respectively).

Table 2. Individual pharmacokinetic parameters of ciprofloxacin.

PK Parameter	Early Phase ($n = 29$)	Delayed Phase ($n = 15$)
Vd (L)	136.9 (76.6–322.6)	158.3 (98.0–386.6)
Vd (L/kg)	1.73 (0.76–3.83)	1.98 (0.75–4.55)
CL (L/h)	18.59 (8.13–74.94)	20.57 (6.20–74.63)
CL (L/h/kg)	0.209 (0.068–0.906)	0.291 (0.107–0.878)
t$_{1/2}$ (h)	5.6 (2.3–11.7)	4.7 (2.8–11.6)

Data are presented as median (range). Vd—volume of distribution; CL—clearance; t$_{1/2}$—elimination half-life.

Both ciprofloxacin Vd and CL were significantly and positively related with CL$_{CR}$ ($p = 0.0009$ and $p < 0.0001$, respectively) and negatively related with age ($p < 0.0001$ for both Vd and CL). Since CL$_{CR}$ significantly decreased with increasing age ($p < 0.0001$), we assumed that the real independent variable was only CL$_{CR}$. Measured CL$_{CR}$ was the most predictive of the ciprofloxacin CL ($r^2 = 0.6275$), but estimated glomerular filtration rates according to various formulas were also significantly related to ciprofloxacin CL (r^2 of 0.4342, 0.4301, 0.4088, and 0.3701 according to CKD-EPI, L–M, MDRD, and C–G equation, respectively). The weakest predictive performance for estimating of ciprofloxacin CL was observed in serum creatinine level ($r^2 = 0.1717$). These relations are presented in Figure S1. Ciprofloxacin CL was also negatively related to the daily dose of norepinephrine ($p = 0.0249$), but analogically, since the dose of norepinephrine was associated with CL$_{CR}$ ($p = 0.0060$), we assumed that the only dependent variable and the real covariate was CL$_{CR}$. Both ciprofloxacin Vd and CL were also positively related with height ($p = 0.0263$ and

$p = 0.0240$, respectively). PK of ciprofloxacin was neither related to body weight nor to any derived body-size descriptors such as BSA and LBM. We also observed no relationships with smoking status, serum level of bilirubin, fluid balance, or daily dose of furosemide. There were no differences in the ciprofloxacin PK between the sexes.

Based on the strongest observed relationship (ciprofloxacin CL = 18.54 × CL_{CR} + 3.261; $r^2 = 0.6275$) and the well-known equation (AUC = dose/CL), we constructed a nomogram (Figure 1) representing the relation between patient CL_{CR}, MIC for pathogen, and ciprofloxacin PK/PD target attainment (AUC_{24}/MIC ratio of 125) at the usual ciprofloxacin dosage (800 or 1200 mg/day).

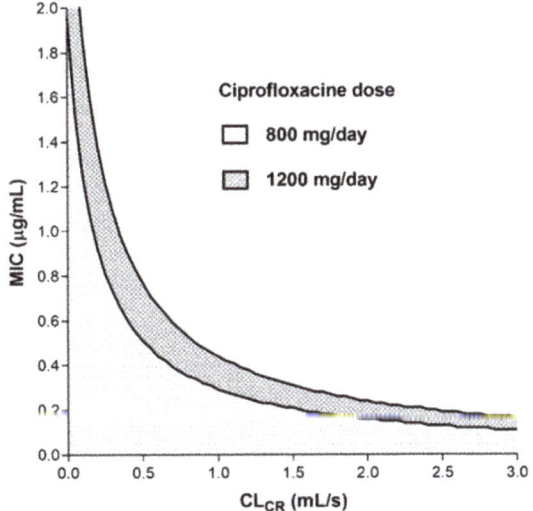

Figure 1. Nomogram representing the relation between patient creatinine clearance (CL_{CR}), minimum inhibitory concentration for the pathogen (MIC), and ciprofloxacin PK/PD target attainment (AUC_{24}/MIC ratio of 125) at the usual ciprofloxacin dosage (800 or 1200 mg/day). The white area of the graph corresponds to renal clearance and MIC values, for which the standard dosing could not achieve the PK/PD target.

3.3. Population PK Analysis

Observed ciprofloxacin plasma concentrations were best described by a one-compartment model with log-normally distributed intra-individual variability on CL and Vd. A combination residual error model provided the best description of residual variability. Interoccasion variability tested as a third level of random effects was not found to be significant.

Inclusion of CL_{CR} in a linear relationship as a covariate on CL resulted in a statistically significant improvement of the model fit ($p < 0.001$). Inclusion of this covariate in the model led to a decrease in inter-individual variability of CL from 71.6% (basic model without covariates) to 44.9% (final model). None of the other covariates were statistically significant.

The final parameter estimates are presented in Table 3. In the final model, for a typical individual with CL_{CR} of 1.25 mL/s, CL and Vd were 21.5 L/h and 143 L (34%), respectively.

Table 3. Parameter estimates of the final model for ciprofloxacin in critically ill patients.

Parameter (Units)	Final Model (RSE %)	Bootstrap Method (95% CI)
Fixed effects		
CL (L/h) = $CL_p + \theta CL_{CR} \times (CL_{CR}/1.25)$		
CL_p (L/h)	5.4 (28%)	5.33 (2.21–8.50)
θCL_{CR}	16.1 (16%)	16 (11.3–21.8)
Vd (L) = Vd_p		
Vd_p (L)	143 (9%)	142 (112–168)
Inter-individual variability		
CL (%)	44.9% (3%)	43.6% (34.9–52.4)
Vd (%)	34.8% (17%)	43.6% (34.9–52.4)
Residual variability		
Additive (%)	0.981 (34%)	1.05 (0.6–2.1)
Proportional (%)	4.78 (26%)	4.5 (2.3–7.5)

RSE—relative standard error of the estimate; CL—clearance; CL_p—population clearance value; CL_{CR}—creatinine clearance; θCL_{CR}—increase in CL per L/s CL_{CR}; Vd—volume of distribution; Vd_p—population volume of distribution value.

The precision of the estimated structural parameter values was acceptable, with RSE values below 30%. The basic GOF plots in Figure 2 indicate that the final model could describe the data accurately, as the predicted population and predicted individual concentrations were described without bias. All median parameter values in the bootstrap procedure were within 10% of the values obtained in the final model fit, indicating that the model was robust.

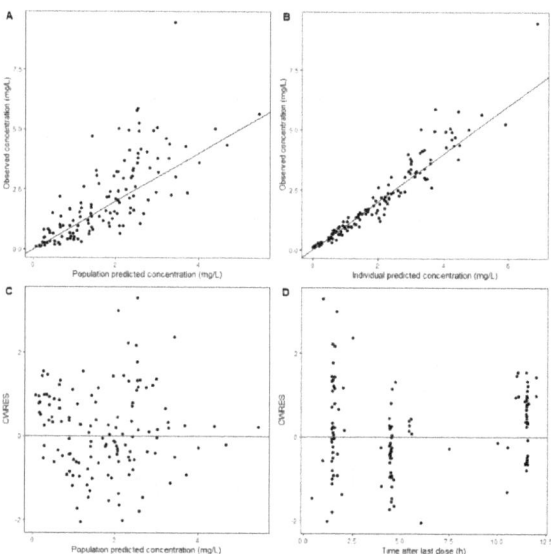

Figure 2. Goodness-of-fit plots for the final model for ciprofloxacin concentrations in critically ill patients. (**A**) Population-predicted ciprofloxacin concentrations vs. observed ciprofloxacin concentrations. (**B**) Individual-predicted ciprofloxacin concentrations vs. observed ciprofloxacin concentrations. (**C**) Conditional weighted residuals (CWRES) vs. population-predicted ciprofloxacin concentrations. (**D**) Conditional weighted residuals (CWRES) vs. time after last dose.

The distribution of the NPDEs obtained with the model for the dataset had a mean of 0.039 (SE = 0.087) and variance of 1 (SE = 0.12). Neither of these values were significantly different from the expected values of 0 ($p = 1$) and 1 ($p = 1$), respectively (Figure 3). This indicates that predictions regarding the structural model and the variability in the data were accurate. Adequate performance of the final model was confirmed with the VPC analysis (Figure S2). However, the VPC showed that the median of the observed concentrations did not fall into the CI of median prediction (red shaded area); therefore, caution should be taken when using this model for extrapolation to early time points after dosing.

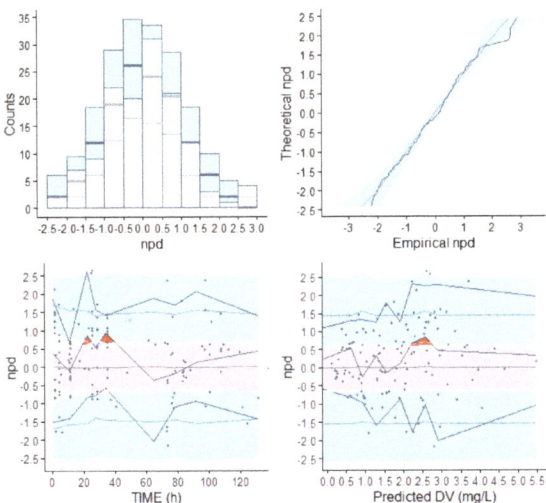

Figure 3. Visual output of the normalized prediction distribution error (NPDE) analysis. Shown at the top are the QQ plot and histogram of the NPDEs in the overall dataset. The red dotted line and blue shaded areas show the expected trends and 95% confidence intervals of these trends, while the dark blue lines and bars show the observed NPDE distributions. At the bottom, the individual NPDE values for each observation are plotted versus time and versus the predicted concentrations with the symbols. The solid lines in the bottom graphs indicate the mean (red) and the 95% percentiles (blue) of the NPDEs, and the shaded areas are the simulated 95% confidence intervals of the NPDE median (red) and 95% percentiles (blue), while the dotted red and blue lines show the expected values for the median and 95% percentiles.

Monte Carlo Simulations

Figure 4 shows the PTA values for different dosing regimens (400 mg b.i.d. and t.i.d.) of ciprofloxacin for various MIC values (0.0625–1 mg/L) for patients with different values of CL_{CR} (0.5, 1, 1.5 mL/s). Dosing regimen including 400 mg b.i.d. (Figure 4A) was sufficient for MICs $\leq$ 0.125 mg/L, but was insufficient for MICs $\geq$ 0.25 mg/L, except for impaired renal function (CL_{CR} = 0.5 mL/s). Dosing regimen consisting of ciprofloxacin t.i.d. (Figure 4B) enabled PTA > 100% for MIC $\leq$ 0.25 mg/L. No approved dosing regimen achieved sufficient PTA for MICs $\geq$ 0.5 mg/L.

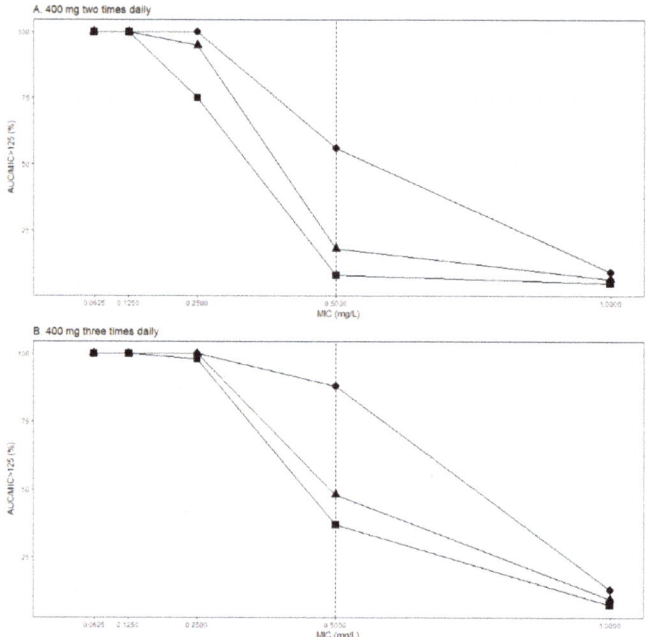

Figure 4. Monte Carlo simulations for ciprofloxacin PTA (AUC/MIC > 125) at different creatinine clearance (CL_{CR}) values. (**A**) 400 mg two times daily and (**B**) 400 mg three times daily.

4. Discussion

Variability in the clinical status of the patients between the early phase and delayed phase of ciprofloxacin treatment was expected, therefore inter-occasion variability was tested. However, no significant differences of ciprofloxacin PK parameters between the early and delayed phases of treatment was observed. Similarly, inter-occasion variability tested as a third level of random effects in the population PK analysis, and it was not significant. Since shifts in body fluid have been implicated as a major cause of alteration in distribution [24], it can be assumed that especially Vd of hydrophilic drugs may be altered. Ciprofloxacin is lipophilic, and as such it is likely to be less susceptible to changes in distribution during critical illness; however, our study could not precisely describe the distribution phase. Substantial changes in functional of eliminating organs resulting in significant variability of a drug CL are also common in critically ill patients [24]. In our study population, we consistently observed higher spread (both increase and decrease) of renal-function status in the early phase in comparison with the delayed phase. However, median CL_{CR} values were without statistically significant difference ($p = 0.5189$) in both phases, and thus no significant difference in ciprofloxacin CL between the early and delayed phase was also noted.

In a recent position paper, individualized antibiotic dosing was unambiguously recommended for aminoglycosides, glycopeptides, beta-lactams, and linezolid, while for ciprofloxacin (fluoroquinolones), the therapeutic drug monitoring was neither recommended nor discouraged [25]. The nomogram based on individual PK analysis (Figure 1) shows that at standard dosage (800–1200 mg/day), it was practically impossible to reach the recommended ciprofloxacin PK/PD target (AUC/MIC $\geq$ 125) when the MIC $\geq$ 0.5 mg/L (except for patients with moderate to severe renal impairment). This observation was consistent with ciprofloxacin-resistance breakpoint value of 0.5 mg/L stated by the European Committee on Antimicrobial Susceptibility Testing (EUCAST). On the other hand, the ciprofloxacin PK/PD target should be reached at standard dosing when the MIC is less than

0.25 mg/L (except in patients with augmented renal clearance), which fully corresponds with the EUCAST-sensitivity breakpoint value for ciprofloxacin. However, it is evident from the nomogram that in patients with augmented renal clearance, even a ciprofloxacin dose of 1200 mg/day may not be effective, and on the contrary, commonly used doses may lead to overexposure in patients with renal impairment.

Monte Carlo simulations were performed to assess PTA of the ciprofloxacin PK/PD target (AUC/MIC $\geq$ 125). Dosing regimen including 400 mg b.i.d. was sufficient for MICs $\leq$ 0.125 mg/L but was insufficient for MICs $\geq$ 0.25 mg/L, except for patients with impaired renal function (CL_{CR} = 0.5 mL/s). Additionally, a dosing regimen consisting of ciprofloxacin 400 mg t.i.d. enabled PTA > 100% for MICs $\leq$ 0.25 mg/L. Finally, no dosing regimen achieved sufficient PTA for MICs $\geq$ 0.5 mg/L. Similar results were obtained in the previous studies conducted in critically ill patients [4,26]. Roberts et al. showed that for a directed therapy against *P. aeruginosa* (MIC value of 0.5 mg/L), a dose of 600 mg t.i.d. would be needed to achieve an adequate PTA in patients with septic shock [26]. Although simulations show daily doses > 1200 mg would be required for optimal exposure of ciprofloxacin for MICs $\geq$ 0.5 mg/L, it is important to note that these dosing regimens have never been prospectively and externally validated. Higher doses increase risk of unwanted effects, which may go undiscovered in critically ill patients who are predisposed to similar adverse effects due to co-medication or their underlying illness. Relatively high incidence of both augmented renal clearance and impaired renal function status among critically ill patients support the clinically reasonable approach to implement therapeutic drug monitoring of fluoroquinolones to safeguard efficacious and safe antimicrobial treatment in this vulnerable patient population.

We can distinguish between the individual and population approaches to perform PK analyses. Advantages and disadvantages of these approaches or their suitability for specific situation are often discussed, but there is a lack of direct comparison of these methods on the same dataset [27]. Population approach offers significant advantages with respect to comprehensive PK exploration and drug-dosing posology in the population, while the individual approach is superior in terms of the routine clinical care of an individual patient. We analyzed data from our study using both individual and population PK approaches. The median values of ciprofloxacin PK parameters from individual analysis were almost the same as Vd and CL values for a typical individual in the final population model. CL_{CR} also proved to be the main independent covariate of ciprofloxacin CL in both analyses. In individual analysis CL_{CR} was also associated with ciprofloxacin Vd. This observation can be explained by fluid retention in patients with impaired renal function resulting in a relative decrease in distribution space for lipophilic agents such as ciprofloxacin. Relation of PK parameters with body size is common, but body weight is usually the strongest covariate, especially in lipophilic drugs [28]. Since we observed only a weak relationship with height in the individual PK analysis and the other body size descriptors were without significance, it might be considered as a chance finding.

We also compared glomerular filtration rate (measured CL_{CR}) with multiple estimation equations (CKD-EPI, L–M, C–G, and MDRD) and simple serum creatinine level as determinants of ciprofloxacin CL. As expected, the best predictive performance was shown for measured CL_{CR} (r^2 = 0.6275). The CKD-EPI or L–M showed numerically better performance in comparison with MDRD, C–G, or simple serum creatinine level, which was in accordance with previous observations in other renally excreted antibiotic agents [29,30]. The MDRD formula is applicable primarily in chronic kidney disease subjects. The C–G equation includes body weight, which can lead to a distortion in under- or overweight patients. This may be the reason for the worse performance of glomerular filtration rate calculated by the MDRD or C–G formulas when used in a heterogeneous population. However, estimation of glomerular filtration rate by means of any equation may be reliable only in patients with a stable renal function. Therefore, measurement of CL_{CR} is considered the "gold standard" in the routine care of patients with unstable renal functions, and estimation methods will likely not be used in the patient population included in our study.

For the individual PK analysis, we used a two-stage method, in the first stage of which the values of the PK parameters in each patient were calculated. Although we used mean (SD) from Drusano et al. as a Bayesian prior [18], the PK parameters were adapted as random variables via a large number of iterations to achieve maximum fitting of the simulated PK profile with the true observed concentration points in each individual. The fitting was very tight, as evidenced by the goodness-of-fit values. In the second stage, the individual PK parameters were associated with patient characteristics using regression models (continuous variables) or column statistics (categorical variables). The values of PK parameters obtained from this analysis corresponded well with data from other ciprofloxacin individual PK studies [31–34].

Although a direct comparison of findings between population PK studies using a NLME approach is difficult due to differences in parameterization and covariate relationships, it is possible to make comparisons between parameter values for typical individuals. So far, two studies using NLME modeling to describe PK ciprofloxacin in critically ill patients have been published [4,26]. One of these studies (Roberts et al.) was conducted in patients with sepsis [26]. To allow comparison of PK parameters, we calculated parameter values for the typical individual from our study with CL_{CR} of 1.25 mL/s using the provided equations in the corresponding publications. The estimated values of CL in this study for a typical individual (21.5 L/h) were similar to the values reported in the previous studies (25 L/h according to Abdulla et al. [4], and 15 L/h according to Roberts et al. [26]). Moreover, Roberts et al. [26] found CL_{CR} to be a significant covariate for CL, and this relationship was described as a power function. In our study, this relationship was found to be linear. On the other hand, Abdulla et al. [4] found no significant covariates for CL. Regarding Vd, we found no predictive covariates, similarly to Abdulla et al. [4]. Conversely, Roberts et al. [26] reported body weight to be a predictive covariate for central Vd.

The studies by Abdulla et al. [4] and Roberts et al. [26] found the two-compartment model to provide the best description of ciprofloxacin disposition, whereas we selected a one-compartment model. These differences can be explained by a relatively sparse blood sampling at early time points after onset of treatment with ciprofloxacin in the current study, therefore caution should be taken when using this model for extrapolation to early time points after dosing. This was also confirmed by the VPC, as the median of the observed concentrations did not fall into the CI of the median prediction in the early time points after the first dose of ciprofloxacin.

5. Conclusions

In conclusion, we described PK of ciprofloxacin using both individual and population approaches and obtained similar results. We observed no changes in ciprofloxacin PK parameters between the early and delayed phases of treatment. CL_{CR} (as a marker of functional renal status) was identified as a significant covariate of ciprofloxacin PK. Standard dosing regimens might be insufficient for achieving the optimal therapeutic target, therefore therapeutic drug monitoring should be implemented to increase the probability of optimal ciprofloxacin exposure and to avoid unnecessary high concentrations.

Supplementary Materials: The following are available online at https://www.mdpi.com/article/10.3390/pharmaceutics13081156/s1, Figure S1: Relationships of ciprofloxacin clearance (CL_{CIP}) with creatinine serum concentrations, with measured creatinine clearance (CL_{CR}), and with glomerular filtration rate estimations according to Chronic Kidney Disease Epidemiology Collaboration (CKD-EPI), Modification of Diet in Renal Disease (MDRD), Cockroft-Gault (C-G), and revised Lund-Malmö (L-M) equations, Figure S2: Visual predictive check of the final model. Black dots—observations, black dashed lines—80%-interval and median of the observations, red shaded area—95%-confidence interval (CI) of the median prediction, blue shaded area—95%-CI of the 10 and 90th prediction interval.

Author Contributions: Conceptualization, M.Š. and O.S.; methodology, M.Š., P.C., and D.M.; validation, P.C. and M.K.; formal analysis, D.M., P.R., J.M.H., and M.Š.; investigation, M.Š., D.M., P.R., D.L., J.B., and J.M.H.; resources, P.R., D.L., and J.B.; data curation, P.R., D.L., and J.B.; writing—original draft preparation, M.Š., D.M., and P.C.; writing—review and editing, T.V. and O.S.; visualization,

M.Š.; supervision, M.Š., M.K., T.V., and O.S.; project administration, M.Š.; funding acquisition, O.S. All authors have read and agreed to the published version of the manuscript.

Funding: This research is funded by the Ministry of Education, Youth, and Sports (Czech Republic), Inter-Excellence (Action), under Grant No. LTAUSA-19049, by the Charles University projects PROGRES Q25/LF1 and SVV 260523, and by the specific university research under Grant No. A1_FPBT_2021_002.

Institutional Review Board Statement: The study was conducted according to the guidelines of the Declaration of Helsinki, and approved by the Ethics Committee of Motol University Hospital under No. EK 1492/18 on 2 January 2019.

Informed Consent Statement: Written informed consent was obtained from all subjects involved in the study.

Data Availability Statement: The data that support the findings of this study are available from the corresponding author upon reasonable request.

Acknowledgments: P.R. wishes to acknowledge the support provided by the Pharmaceutical Applied Research Centre (The Parc) for his scientific work.

Conflicts of Interest: The authors declare no conflict of interest.

References

1. Dalhoff, A. Global Fluoroquinolone Resistance Epidemiology and Implictions for Clinical use. *Interdiscip. Perspect. Infect Dis.* **2012**, *2012*. [CrossRef] [PubMed]
2. Cruciani, M.; Bassetti, D. The Fluoroquinolones as Treatment for Infections Caused by Gram-positive Bacteria. *J. Antimicrob. Chemother.* **1994**, *33*, 403–417. [CrossRef] [PubMed]
3. Mouton, J.W.; Muller, A.E.; Canton, R.; Giske, C.G.; Kahlmeter, G.; Turnidge, J. MIC-based Dose Adjustment: Facts and Fables. *J. Antimicrob. Chemother.* **2018**, *73*, 564–568. [CrossRef]
4. Abdulla, A.; Rogouti, O.; Hunfeld, N.G.; Endeman, H.; Dijkstra, A.; van Gelder, T.; Muller, A.E.; de Winter, B.C.; Koch, B.C. Population Pharmacokinetics and Target Attainment of Ciprofloxacin in Critically Ill Patients. *Eur. J. Clin. Pharmacol.* **2020**, *76*, 957–967. [CrossRef] [PubMed]
5. Khachman, D.; Conil, J.-M.; Georges, B.; Saivin, S.; Houin, G.; Toutain, P.-L.; Laffont, C.M. Optimizing Ciprofloxacin Dosing in Intensive Care Unit Patients through the Use of Population Pharmacokinetic–pharmacodynamic Analysis and Monte Carlo Simulations. *J. Antimicrob. Chemother.* **2011**, *66*, 1798–1809. [CrossRef]
6. Van Zanten, A.R.; Polderman, K.H.; van Geijlswijk, I.M.; van der Meer, G.Y.; Schouten, M.A.; Girbes, A.R. Ciprofloxacin Pharmacokinetics in Critically Ill Patients: A Prospective Cohort Study. *J. Crit. Care* **2008**, *23*, 422–430. [CrossRef] [PubMed]
7. De Cock, R.F.; Piana, C.; Krekels, E.H.; Danhof, M.; Allegaert, K.; Knibbe, C.A. The Role of Population PK-PD Modelling in Paediatric Clinical Research. *Eur. J. Clin. Pharmacol.* **2011**, *67*, 5–16. [CrossRef]
8. Leligdowicz, A.; Matthay, M.A. Heterogeneity in Sepsis: New Biological Evidence with Clinical Applications. *Crit. Care* **2019**, *23*, 1–8. [CrossRef] [PubMed]
9. Roberts, J.A.; Paul, S.K.; Akova, M.; Bassetti, M.; De Waele, J.J.; Dimopoulos, G.; Kaukonen, K.-M.; Koulenti, D.; Martin, C.; Montravers, P. DALI: Defining Antibiotic Levels in Intensive Care Unit Patients: Are Current β-Lactam Antibiotic Doses Sufficient for Critically Ill Patients? *Clin. Infect. Dis.* **2014**, *58*, 1072–1083. [CrossRef]
10. Blot, S.I.; Pea, F.; Lipman, J. The Effect of Pathophysiology on Pharmacokinetics in The Critically Ill Patient—Concepts Appraised by the Example of Antimicrobial Agents. *Adv. Drug Deliv. Rev.* **2014**, *77*, 3–11. [CrossRef]
11. Traynor, J.; Mactier, R.; Geddes, C.C.; Fox, J.G. How to Measure Renal Function in Clinical Practice. *BMJ* **2006**, *333*, 733–737. [CrossRef]
12. Cockcroft, D.W.; Gault, M.H. Prediction of Creatinine Clearance from Serum Creatinine. *Nephron* **1976**, *16*, 31–41. [CrossRef] [PubMed]
13. Levey, A.S.; Stevens, L.A.; Schmid, C.H.; Zhang, Y.L.; Castro, A.F.; Feldman, H.I., III; Kusek, J.W.; Eggers, P.; Van Lente, F.; Greene, T.; et al. A New Equation to Estimate Glomerular Filtration Rate. *Ann. Intern. Med.* **2009**, *150*, 604–612. [CrossRef] [PubMed]
14. Levey, A.S.; Bosch, J.P.; Lewis, J.B.; Greene, T.; Rogers, N.; Roth, D. A More Accurate Method to Estimate Glomerular Filtration Rate from Serum Creatinine: A New Prediction Equation. Modification of Diet in Renal Disease Study Group. *Ann. Intern. Med.* **1999**, *130*, 461–470. [CrossRef] [PubMed]
15. Nyman, U.; Grubb, A.; Larsson, A.; Hansson, L.O.; Flodin, M.; Nordin, G.; Lindstrom, V.; Bjork, J. The Revised Lund-Malmo GFR Estimating Equation Outperforms MDRD and CKD-EPI Across GFR, Age and BMI Intervals in a Large Swedish Population. *Clin. Chem. Lab. Med.* **2014**, *52*, 815–824. [CrossRef] [PubMed]
16. Dubois, D.; Dubois, E.F. Nutrition Metabolism Classic–A Formula to Estimate the Approximate Surface-Area If Height and Weight Be Known (Reprinted from Archives Internal Medicine, Vol 17, Pg 863, 1916). *Nutrition* **1989**, *5*, 303–313.

17. Boer, P. Estimated Lean Body Mass as an Index for Normalization of Body Fluid Volumes in Humans. *Am. J. Physiol.* **1984**, *247*, F632–F636. [CrossRef] [PubMed]
18. Drusano, G.L.; Weir, M.; Forrest, A.; Plaisance, K.; Emm, T.; Standiford, H.C. Pharmacokinetics of Intravenously Administered Ciprofloxacin in Patients with Various Degrees of Renal Function. *Antimicrob. Agents Chemother.* **1987**, *31*, 860–864. [CrossRef] [PubMed]
19. Lindbom, L.; Pihlgren, P.; Jonsson, E.N. PsN-Toolkit–A Collection of Computer Intensive Statistical Methods for Non-Linear Mixed Effect Modeling using NONMEM. *Comput. Methods Programs Biomed.* **2005**, *79*, 241–257. [CrossRef] [PubMed]
20. Lindbom, L.; Ribbing, J.; Jonsson, E.N. Perl-speaks-NONMEM (PsN)–A Perl Module for NONMEM Related Programming. *Comput. Methods Programs Biomed.* **2004**, *75*, 85–94. [CrossRef]
21. Keizer, R.J.; van Benten, M.; Beijnen, J.H.; Schellens, J.H.; Huitema, A.D. Pirana and PCluster: A Modeling Environment and Cluster Infrastructure for NONMEM. *Comput. Methods Programs Biomed.* **2011**, *101*, 72–79. [CrossRef] [PubMed]
22. Comets, E.; Brendel, K.; Mentré, F. Computing Normalised Prediction Distribution Errors to Evaluate Nonlinear Mixed-effect Models: The Npde Add-on Package for R. *Comput. Methods Programs Biomed.* **2008**, *90*, 154–166. [CrossRef] [PubMed]
23. Byon, W.; Smith, M.K.; Chan, P.; Tortorici, M.A.; Riley, S.; Dai, H.; Dong, J.; Ruiz-Garcia, A.; Sweeney, K.; Cronenberger, C. Establishing Best Practices and Guidance in Population Modeling: An Experience with an Internal Population Pharmacokinetic Analysis Guidance. *CPT Pharmacomet. Syst. Pharmacol.* **2013**, *2*, e51. [CrossRef]
24. Boucher, B.A.; Wood, G.C.; Swanson, J.M. Pharmacokinetic Changes in Critical Illness. *Crit. Care Clin.* **2006**, *22*, 255–271. [CrossRef] [PubMed]
25. Abdul-Aziz, M.H.; Alffenaar, J.C.; Bassetti, M.; Bracht, H.; Dimopoulos, G.; Marriott, D.; Neely, M.N.; Paiva, J.A.; Pea, F.; Sjovall, F.; et al. Antimicrobial Therapeutic Drug Monitoring in Critically Ill Adult Patients: A Position Paper. *Intensive Care Med.* **2020**, *46*, 1127–1153. [CrossRef] [PubMed]
26. Roberts, J.A.; Alobaid, A.S.; Wallis, S.C.; Perner, A.; Lipman, J.; Sjövall, F. Defining Optimal Dosing of Ciprofloxacin in Patients with Septic Shock. *J. Antimicrob. Chemother.* **2019**, *74*, 1662–1669. [CrossRef]
27. De Velde, F.; Mouton, J.W.; de Winter, B.C.M.; van Gelder, T.; Koch, B.C.P. Clinical Applications of Population Pharmacokinetic Models of Antibiotics: Challenges and Perspectives. *Pharmacol Res* **2018**, *134*, 280–288. [CrossRef]
28. Alobaid, A.S.; Hites, M.; Lipman, J.; Taccone, F.S.; Roberts, J.A. Effect of Obesity on The Pharmacokinetics of Antimicrobials in Critically Ill Patients: A Structured Review. *Int. J. Antimicrob. Agents* **2016**, *47*, 259–268. [CrossRef] [PubMed]
29. Sima, M.; Hartinger, J.; Cikankova, T.; Slanar, O. Estimation of Once-daily Amikacin Dose in Critically Ill Adults. *J. Chemother.* **2018**, *30*, 37–43. [CrossRef]
30. Sima, M.; Hartinger, J.; Stenglova Netikova, I.; Slanar, O. Creatinine Clearance Estimations for Vancomycin Maintenance Dose Adjustments. *Am. J. Ther.* **2018**, *25*, e602–e604. [CrossRef] [PubMed]
31. Fabre, D.; Bressolle, F.; Gomeni, R.; Arich, C.; Lemesle, F.; Beziau, H.; Galtier, M. Steady-state Pharmacokinetics of Ciprofloxacin in Plasma from Patients with Nosocomial Pneumonia: Penetration of The Bronchial Mucosa. *Antimicrob. Agents Chemother.* **1991**, *35*, 2521–2525. [CrossRef] [PubMed]
32. Gasser, T.C.; Ebert, S.C.; Graversen, P.H.; Madsen, P.O. Ciprofloxacin Pharmacokinetics in Patients with Normal and Impaired Renal Function. *Antimicrob. Agents Chemother.* **1987**, *31*, 709–712. [CrossRef] [PubMed]
33. Webb, D.B.; Roberts, D.E.; Williams, J.D.; Asscher, A.W. Pharmacokinetics of Ciprofloxacin in Healthy Volunteers and Patients with Impaired Kidney Function. *J. Antimicrob. Chemother.* **1986**, *18*, 83–87. [CrossRef] [PubMed]
34. Wingender, W.; Graefe, K.H.; Gau, W.; Forster, D.; Beermann, D.; Schacht, P. Pharmacokinetics of Ciprofloxacin After Oral and Intravenous Administration in Healthy Volunteers. *Eur. J. Clin. Microbiol.* **1984**, *3*, 355–359. [CrossRef] [PubMed]

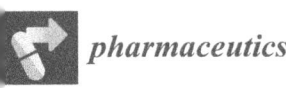

Review

Review of Pharmacokinetics and Pharmacogenetics in Atypical Long-Acting Injectable Antipsychotics

Francisco José Toja-Camba [1,2,†], Nerea Gesto-Antelo [3,†], Olalla Maroñas [3,†], Eduardo Echarri Arrieta [4], Irene Zarra-Ferro [2,4], Miguel González-Barcia [2,4], Enrique Bandín-Vilar [2,4], Victor Mangas Sanjuan [2,5,6], Fernando Facal [7,8], Manuel Arrojo Romero [7], Angel Carracedo [3,9,10,*], Cristina Mondelo-García [2,4,*] and Anxo Fernández-Ferreiro [2,4,*]

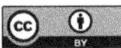

Citation: Toja-Camba, F.J.; Gesto-Antelo, N.; Maroñas, O.; Echarri Arrieta, E.; Zarra-Ferro, I.; González-Barcia, M.; Bandín-Vilar, E.; Mangas Sanjuan, V.; Facal, F.; Arrojo Romero, M.; et al. Review of Pharmacokinetics and Pharmacogenetics in Atypical Long-Acting Injectable Antipsychotics. *Pharmaceutics* **2021**, *13*, 935. https://doi.org/10.3390/pharmaceutics13070935

Academic Editors: Jonás Samuel Pérez-Blanco, José Martínez Lanao and Aristeidis Dokoumetzidis

Received: 30 April 2021
Accepted: 21 June 2021
Published: 23 June 2021

Publisher's Note: MDPI stays neutral with regard to jurisdictional claims in published maps and institutional affiliations.

Copyright: © 2021 by the authors. Licensee MDPI, Basel, Switzerland. This article is an open access article distributed under the terms and conditions of the Creative Commons Attribution (CC BY) license (https://creativecommons.org/licenses/by/4.0/).

1. Pharmacy Department, University Clinical Hospital of Ourense (SERGAS), Ramón Puga 52, 32005 Ourense, Spain; kikotoja@gmail.com
2. Clinical Pharmacology Group, Institute of Health Research (IDIS), Travesía da Choupana s/n, 15706 Santiago de Compostela, Spain; irene.zarra.ferro@sergas.es (I.Z.-F.); miguel.gonzalez.barcia@sergas.es (M.G.-B.); enriquebandinvilar@gmail.com (E.B.-V.); victor.mangas@uv.es (V.M.S.)
3. Genomic Medicine Group, CIMUS, University of Santiago de Compostela, 15782 Santiago de Compostela, Spain; nerea.gesto@rai.usc.es (N.G.-A.); olalla.maronas@hotmail.com (O.M.)
4. Pharmacy Department, University Clinical Hospital of Santiago de Compostela (SERGAS), 15706 Santiago de Compostela, Spain; eduardo.echarri.arrieta@sergas.es
5. Department of Pharmacy and Pharmaceutical Technology and Parasitology, University of Valencia, 46100 Valencia, Spain
6. Interuniversity Research Institute for Molecular Recognition and Technological Development, Polytechnic University of Valencia-University of Valencia, 46100 Valencia, Spain
7. Psychiatry Department, University Clinical Hospital of Santiago de Compostela (SERGAS), Travesía da Choupana s/n, 15706 Santiago de Compostela, Spain; ferfacal92@hotmail.com (F.F.); Manuel.Arrojo.Romero@sergas.es (M.A.R.)
8. Institute of Health Research (IDIS), Travesía da Choupana s/n, 15706 Santiago de Compostela, Spain
9. Genomic Medicine Group, Biomedical Research Center of Rare Diseases (CIBERER), University of Santiago de Compostela, 15782 Santiago de Compostela, Spain
10. Galician Foundation of Genomic Medicine, Foundation of Health Research Institute of Santiago de Compostela (FIDIS), SERGAS, 15706 Santiago de Compostela, Spain
* Correspondence: angel.carracedo@usc.es (A.C.); crismondelo1@gmail.com (C.M.-G.); anxordes@gmail.com (A.F.-F.)
† These authors contributed equally to this work.

Abstract: Over the last two decades, pharmacogenetics and pharmacokinetics have been increasingly used in clinical practice in Psychiatry due to the high variability regarding response and side effects of antipsychotic drugs. Specifically, long-acting injectable (LAI) antipsychotics have different pharmacokinetic profile than oral formulations due to their sustained release characteristics. In addition, most of these drugs are metabolized by *CYP2D6*, whose interindividual genetic variability results in different metabolizer status and, consequently, into different plasma concentrations of the drugs. In this context, there is consistent evidence which supports the use of therapeutic drug monitoring (TDM) along with pharmacogenetic tests to improve safety and efficacy of antipsychotic pharmacotherapy. This comprehensive review aims to compile all the available pharmacokinetic and pharmacogenetic data regarding the three major LAI atypical antipsychotics: risperidone, paliperidone and aripiprazole. On the one hand, CYP2D6 metabolizer status influences the pharmacokinetics of LAI aripiprazole, but this relation remains a matter of debate for LAI risperidone and LAI paliperidone. On the other hand, developed population pharmacokinetic (popPK) models showed the influence of body weight or administration site on the pharmacokinetics of these LAI antipsychotics. The combination of pharmacogenetics and pharmacokinetics (including popPK models) leads to a personalized antipsychotic therapy. In this sense, the optimization of these treatments improves the benefit–risk balance and, consequently, patients' quality of life.

Keywords: population pharmacokinetic models; pharmacogenetics; LAI; risperidone; paliperidone; aripiprazole; CYP2D6; antipsychotics

1. Introduction

Schizophrenia is a severe mental disorder that is presented clinically heterogeneously in patients. It is estimated that approximately 0.7–1% of the world population suffer from this condition, currently affecting 24–25 million people worldwide according to data from the World Health Organization [1–3]. Mainly, it causes disorder of behavior, thoughts, perception and emotions. The core features are positive symptoms (delusions, hallucinations and disorganized speech), negative symptoms (such as abulia, anhedonia and social withdrawal), cognitive impairment (mainly in speed of mental processing, working memory and executive functions) and affective symptoms (i.e., anxiety and depression) [4]. There are well-defined instruments such as the Brief Psychiatric Rating Scale (BPRS), the Scale for the Assessment of Positive Symptoms (SAPS), the Scale for the Assessment of Negative Symptoms (SANS) or the Positive and Negative Symptoms Scale (PANSS) to measure these positive and negative symptoms as well as general psychopathology. In clinical studies, reductions in these scales have been used to define treatment response [5]. There are several theories that try to explain the pathophysiology of this complex and highly polygenic disease, including brain structure defects or neurochemical alterations [6]. Recently Genome Wide Association Studies have supported some of those classic neurochemical hypotheses such as the dopaminergic and glutamatergic from a genetic perspective [7]. Nowadays, the pharmacological treatment of schizophrenia is based on antipsychotics, a family of drugs which are classified into two separate groups: first generation or typical (i.e., haloperidol, chlorpromazine) and second generation or atypical (i.e., risperidone, paliperidone, aripiprazole). Both of them present affinity toward D2 receptors and reduce positive symptoms. Atypical antipsychotics form a heterogenous group of drugs with regard to their different receptor affinity. In addition to D2 receptor affinity, they have other pharmacological actions involving different signaling pathways such as serotoninergic receptors (5-HT$_{2A}$,5-HT$_{1A}$ and 5-HT$_{2C}$) that could be the main cause of their safer profile compared to typical antipsychotics [8].

The effectivity of these drugs is far from expected. Treatment resistance requires dose optimization that is based on a trial-and-error method caused by the current inability to predict response to treatment; this added to severe and frequent adverse events are commonly the reasons that lead the patients to discontinue antipsychotic therapies. The main handicap of oral antipsychotics formulations is adherence. Many factors have influence on non-adherence such as forgetting doses of medication, adverse events during therapy and poor insight that condition drug intake. According to various studies, which define adherence as taking medication at least 75% of the time, non-adherence is around 50% of treated patients [9,10]. This problem has been partially solved since typical long-acting injectable (LAI) antipsychotics were released. Later, arrival of atypical LAI antipsychotics introduced an improvement in the safety profile of these drugs, which are administered at long intervals of time (from 2 weeks to 3 months). At this point, the tandem of pharmacogenetics and pharmacokinetics plays a key role, and personalized prescription of antipsychotics improves the safety and efficacy of pharmacotherapy. Combining pharmacogenetics with therapeutic drug monitoring (TDM) of LAI antipsychotics would be a great tool to predict and anticipate patient response in order to achieve mental wellness and minimize side effects. Furthermore, population pharmacokinetic (popPK) models should be considered as a useful tool to understand the relationship between patient characteristics and drug exposure.

Among all over the genes involved in pharmacokinetics of drugs, the *Cytocrome P450* family is, by far, the most important in terms of interindividual variability. Most of drugs that are commonly used in psychiatry are *CYP2D6*-dependent [11,12], an enzyme encoded from a highly polymorphic gene. Nowadays, there are already 145 alleles described for CYP2D6. These alleles can have different functions, frequency and clinical impact on metabolism across different populations [13–15]. Depending on allele combination, it is possible to differentiate the following metabolizer status [16–21]: extensive or normal metabolizer (EM/NM): their metabolic pathway is not altered; poor metabolizers (PM): the activity enzyme is significantly reduced or absent; intermediate metabolizer (IM): those who can metabolize substances in lower ratios compared to an EM but better than a PM. Rapid or ultrarrapid metabolizer (UM): enzymatic hyperactivity compared to EM. Those attracting more interest are PM, IM and UM due to their risk of developing adverse reactions or lack of efficacy in clinical practice [22–24], so currently development in this area of knowledge holds great promise for reducing time between diagnosis and seeking an effective treatment. Lastly, a mismatch has been observed between the genotype-based prediction of *CYP450*-mediated drug metabolism and the true capacity of an individual to metabolize drugs (phenotype) due to non-genetic factors, which is called phenoconversion [25].

Compared to classical pharmacokinetics, where several samples at different time points are collected from a patient to estimate their individual pharmacokinetic parameters (clearance, distribution volume, half-life, etc.), population pharmacokinetics (popPK) analyzes the pooled data available of several patients in order to estimate pharmacokinetic parameter values and their variance, identify covariates and study the random effects (parameter variance which cannot be explained by covariates). All this information implemented in a mathematical model (popPK models) plus Bayesian computational methods allows us to estimate our patients' individual pK parameters, which can be a very helpful tool to individualize dosing and optimize the treatment efficacy and safety.

The three major prescribed LAI-antipsychotics are risperidone, paliperidone and aripiprazole, while LAI-olanzapine prescription has been decreasing over time [26]. Our aim is to comprehensively review all the available literature about these three major prescribed LAI-antipsychotics pharmacogenetics and pharmacokinetics, including the existing popPK models as a crucial tool for predicting drug exposure, focusing on risperidone, paliperidone and aripiprazole.

2. Long-Acting Risperidone

Risperidone is an atypical antipsychotic derived from benzisoxazole with potent D2 and 5-HT2 receptor antagonism. LAI risperidone is an aqueous suspension of microspheres formed by a glycolic and lactic acid degradable matrix where risperidone is encapsulated [27]. More recently, a new formulation of once-monthly subcutaneous LAI risperidone has been approved by the FDA in which risperidone is suspended in ATRIGEL®, a polymer that solidifies in contact with tissues [28,29].

2.1. Pharmacokinetics

Considering the physicochemical properties of polymers of risperidone, a reduced release occurs a few days after injection (around 1% of the dose administered) followed by a lag time of 3 weeks and then a significant release is observed in weeks 4–6 [27,30]. Due to this lag phase, oral supplementation should be given in the first three weeks of treatment. Metabolism of risperidone goes through hydroxylation and N-dealkylation processes in which CY2D6 plays a predominant role in the formation of 9-OH-risperidone (9-OH-R), main active and "equipotent" metabolite [31]. Product monograph states that the half-life ($t_{1/2}$) of risperidone plus 9-OH-R is 3–6 days [32] and the steady-state is reached after the fourth injection and maintained for 4–5 weeks after the last injection [30]. As well as $t_{1/2}$, steady-states were determined by inspection of the concentration–time curve and not by the rule of the five $t_{1/2}$. As Lee et al. [33] point out, this can cause an underestimation of the time when the steady state is reached and can lead to an increase in dosage and an accumulation of the drug.

More recently, a new formulation of once-monthly subcutaneous LAI risperidone has been approved by the FDA, in which risperidone is suspended in ATRIGEL®, a polymer that solidifies in contact with tissues, providing a sustained release. Risperidone ATRIGEL® does not need oral supplementation due to its characteristic pharmacokinetic profile. After subcutaneous injection, a first peak appears 4–6 h post-dose followed by a second one 10–14 days after. Steady state is reached by the end of the second injection and the apparent half-life ranges between 8 and 9 days [28,29].

With regard to the therapeutic range of reference, the German working group for neuropsychopharmacology and pharmacopsychiatry (AGNP) Consensus Guidelines for Therapeutic Drug Monitoring established between 20 and 60 ng/mL for risperidone plus 9-OH-R [34]. This range is derived exclusively from orally given risperidone studies, extrapolating this range to patients treated with long-acting formulations, which has not yet been extensively studied. Two different studies used this AGNP range [35,36] but the other two studies differ and propose other ranges for LAI risperidone [37,38]. De Leon et al. [39] proposed an updated therapeutic range (20–30 ng/mL) for LAI risperidone as a consequence of the prolonged absorption of LAI formulations and the reduction in the administration frequency, which leads to less oscillations at steady-state conditions. Despite this, until new data about LAI risperidone are available, the AGNP therapeutic reference range is the most recommended [40].

2.2. Pharmacogenetics

2.2.1. Efficacy

Polymorphisms in the *CYP2D6* gene could affect plasma concentrations of risperidone plus 9-OH-R (active moiety) although the product monograph reflects that concentration of the active moiety is the same in PM individuals as in other phenotypes [32]. Therefore, adjusting the dose to the patient's phenotype is not necessary but many published studies differ on this point. It is suggested that *CYP2D6* metabolizer status cause differences in active moiety exposure and consequently in efficacy and tolerability, but there are still controversies (Table 1).

Table 1. Studies between *CYP2D6* phenotype and relation with active moiety exposure.

Study	LAI/Oral	n	Race	Age (Median)	Male/Female	CYP2D6 Phenotypes	Outcome
Vermeulen A et al. [41]	Oral	407	NR	38	267/140	PM/IM/NM	Irrelevant
Scordo MG et al. [42]	Oral	37	Caucasians	41	30/7	PM/IM/NM/UM	Irrelevant
Cho HY et al. [43]	Oral	24	Asian	24.6	NR	PM/NM	Irrelevant
Hendset, M et al. [35]	LAI	90	Caucasians	38	53/37	PM/IM/NM/UM	Relevant (higher plasma exposure for IM and PM)
Llerena A et al. [44]	Oral	35	Caucasians	43	NR	PM/IM/NM/UM	Irrelevant
Choong, E et al. [45]	LAI	42	Caucasian (76%)	35	30/12	PM/IM/NM/UM	Relevant (higher plasma exposure for IM and PM and lower for UM)
Leon, J. D et al. [46]	Oral	277	Caucasian (78%)	43.7	150/127	PM/IM/NM/UM	Relevant (higher plasma exposure for PM)
Jovanović, N et al. [47]	Oral	83	Caucasians	30.3	17/66	PM/NM/IM	Irrelevant

Table 1. Cont.

Study	LAI/Oral	n	Race	Age (Median)	Male/Female	CYP2D6 Phenotypes	Outcome
Jukic, M et al. [48]	Oral	725	Caucasians	42.8	355/370	PM/IM/NM/UM	Relevant (higher plasma exposure for IM and PM and lower for UM)
Locatelli, I et al. [49]	LAI	50	Caucasian	30	39/11	PM/IM/NM/UM	Irrelevant
Vandenberghe, F et al. [50]	Oral	150	Caucasian (81%)	39	82/68	PM/IM/NM/UM	Relevant (higher plasma exposure for PM)
Gunes, A et al. [51]	Oral	46	Caucasian	45	35/11	PM/NM/PM	Relevant (higher plasma exposure for PM)

Classified in relevant (significant association between CYP2D6 phenotype and active moiety exposure) or irrelevant (no significative association between CYP2D6 phenotype and active moiety exposure or incorrect assignment of CYP2D6 genotype due to missing copy number variation analysis). Abbreviations: PM, Poor Metabolizer; IM, Intermediate Metabolizer; NM, Normal Metabolizer; UM, Ultra Metabolizer; NR: Not reported. Those studies that do not analyze the number of copies of the gene have been classified as irrelevant. Among those classified as relevant, it is important to highlight that they should be taken as a guideline, taking into account that the main limitation is the high heterogeneity that exists between the different methods of analysis used, as well as the polymorphisms explored in the determination of the phenotype of CYP2D6.

A recent meta-analysis of 15 studies involving 2125 patients taking oral risperidone concluded that *CYP2D6* activity is associated with increased exposure of both risperidone and active moiety. Risperidone steady-state plasma concentration was 2.35-fold higher in IM and 6.20-fold higher in PM, while active moiety concentration was 1.18-fold higher in IM and 1.44-fold higher in PM [52].

Furthermore, some studies suggest that PM are associated with a greater number of adverse events and treatment discontinuation which decreases clinical efficacy [53,54]. In addition, some popPK models based on oral regimens of risperidone showed large differences in CL/F depending on *CYP2D6* phenotype. Mean CL/F values reported by Feng et al. were 65.4, 36 and 12.5 L/h for EM, IM and PM, respectively [55]. The popPK model developed by Sherwin et al. [56] obtained mean values of CL/F for EM, IM and PM patients of 37.4, 29.2 and 9.38 L/h, respectively. Similar differences in CL/F between PM (three-fold lower) and EM individuals were reported by Thyssen et al. [57] in a study including pediatric and adult patients. More recently, a popPK model based on oral regimen of risperidone showed that a reduced activity of *CYP2D6* (PM) could increase up to a 106% steady-state plasma concentration and up to a 53% higher Cmax compared with NM, so dose adjustment may be necessary [58].

Nevertheless, LAI antipsychotics exhibit large differences compared to oral formulations in terms of their PK profile due to their slow and sustained absorption. To our knowledge, only a popPK LAI model of the risperidone ATRIGEL® formulation has been published, which found body mass index and dose as covariates of absorption rate constants and risperidone and 9-OH-R distribution volumes, respectively. In contrast, *CYP2D6* polymorphisms were not statistically significant to any structural popPK parameter [59], which might be explained by the unbalanced and reduced number of patients recruited.

It is possible to obtain approximated information about *CYP2D6* activity using quantitative methods by the following ratios. On the one hand, the R/9-OH-R ratio (relates risperidone and 9-OH-R plasma concentrations) values <1 are normal plasma ratios that indicate normal *CYP2D6* activity (UM, NM, IM) while a value >1 indicates a lack of activity (PM) or the presence of a strong inhibitor [39,60,61]. On the other hand, total risperidone C/D ratio is a measure of drug clearance that relates the concentration of the active moiety with the dose of risperidone. The normal value for oral risperidone and for LAI formulation is approximately around 7 ng/mL per mg/day and patients with ratios >14 ng/mL per mg/day are expected to be *CYP2D6* PM [40,60]. Previous procedures could be an alternative for psychiatrists and could be a possibility for clinicians who do not have access to genotype *CYP2D6*, but it is important to take into account that these methods would only be useful when *CYP2D6* constitutes the main pathway of metabolization. It is important to take into account that the *CYP2D6* allele combination in a patient is an invariable condition; once analyzed it will not change. Thus, analyzing polymorphisms in *CYP2D6* by pharmacogenetics can be useful to select the most appropriate drugs for a patient, avoiding adverse effects or lack of efficacy concerning its *CYP2D6* metabolizer status. As a result, individualized treatment selection would become easier for prescribers.

Therefore, it seems clear that genetic variations in *CYP2D6* have an impact on plasma concentrations of risperidone, but there are controversies when it comes to relating it to the efficacy of the treatment and clinical outcome. A study of 136 patients diagnosed with schizophrenia and evaluating clinical improvement using the Positive and Negative Syndrome Scale (PANSS) did not showed association between *CYP2D6* activity variations and clinical outcome [61]. Along the same line another study of 83 drug-naïve patients experiencing a first episode of psychosis did not match the clear relation between *CYP2D6* genetic variations and clinical improvement [47]. On the contrary, another study of 76 patients with schizophrenia evaluated changes on total PANSS and *CYP2D6* polymorphism founding correlation between PMs and better response to risperidone treatment. Only three patients were classified as PMs but the power of the study was enough to establish an association with PANSS improvement. [62]. Likewise, Jukic et al. recently identified a higher incidence of therapeutic failure (discontinuation or switch to another antipsychotic) in PMs [48]. These pharmacogenetic studies are based on oral risperidone administration and not all of them had been conducted in patients with schizophrenia.

2.2.2. Safety

Antipsychotics can cause hyperprolactinemia by blocking dopaminergic receptors at the tuberoinfundibular system [63]. Risperidone was reported to have a high prevalence of hyperprolactinemia among all atypical antipsychotics [64,65]. Association between *CYP2D6* and hyperprolactinemia was described in a observational study of 47 children and adolescents with autism spectrum disorder in a long-term treatment with risperidone; the number of patients with hyperprolactinemia was 100% (2/2) for PM, 47% (8/17) for IM, 48% (12/25) for NM and 0% (0/2) for UM [66]. Sex influence in hyperprolactinemia incidence has been studied, observing a higher incidence in female than in males, a study of Schoretsanitis et al. [67] involving 111 patients (61 males and 49 females) evaluates association between *CYP2D6* activity, risperidone levels and sex finding a significant association across them. Another cause of reduced patient compliance is weight gain produced by risperidone, relation between genetic polymorphisms and this adverse drug reaction is still under study. Some studies like the one performed by Lane et al. found significant association between *CYP2D6×10* allele (PM) and weight gain but data about this relation up-to-date are limited [68].

Extrapyramidal Symptoms (EPS) are the most evaluated adverse effects with *CYP2D6* in a large number of studies. Nevertheless, it is not clear the impact of *CYP2D6* variations on EPS from risperidone. Several studies showed no significant difference between these two variables and only a few find some correlation. Adverse effects were also examined in a study of 70 healthy volunteers, several genes and respective polymorphisms were associated with adverse effects (*CYP2C9*, *NAT2*, *DRD2*, *CYP2C19*) but no relation was found between *CYP2D6* polymorphisms and EPS [69]. De Leon et al. [53] showed this association in 73 patients with moderate to severe EPS and 81 patients that discontinued risperidone due to EPS. *CYP2D6* PM phenotype was associated with the first group (OR = 3.4; CI = 1.5–8.0, p = 0.004) and with the second group. (OR = 6; CI = 1.4–25.4, p = 0.02). Another recent study evaluated 22 patients and the Drug-induced Extrapyramidal Symptoms Scale (DIEPSS) score; they observed that DIEPSS score was significantly higher in the IM group (7) than in the EM group (15) [70]. A summary of LAI-risperidone pharmacokinetic and pharmacogenetic characteristics is available in Table 2.

Table 2. Summary of PK/PG characteristics of LAI-Risperidone.

Drug	Main Active Metabolite	Therapeutic Reference Range	Metabolism	TDM Recommendation (33)	Mean PK Values	Genetic Test Recommendation (94)
LAI-Risperidone microespheres	9-OH-Risperidone	20–60 ng/mL	CYP2D6/CYP3A4	2	T_{max}: 28 days T_{ss}: 8 weeks $T_{1/2}$: 3–6 days	Informative
LAI-Risperidone ATRIGEL®	9-OH-Risperidone	20–60 ng/mL	CYP2D6/CYP3A4	2	Double T_{max}: 4–6 h and 10–14 days T_{ss}: 8 weeks $T_{1/2}$: 8–9 days	Informative

Abbreviations: T_{max}, time to maximum concentration after administration; T_{ss}, time to reach steady state; $t_{1/2}$, apparent half-life of elimination. TDM Levels of recommendation: 1: Strongly recommended; 2: Recommended; 3: Useful; 4: Potentially useful (33). Genetic test; informative: the label contains information stating that a particular gene affects or does not effect drug efficacy, not clinically significant.

3. Long-Acting Paliperidone

Paliperidone (9-OH-Risperidone) is the primary active metabolite of risperidone. This long-acting drug is formulated as a palmitate ester of paliperidone in an aqueous suspension of nanocrystals resulting in a sustained release profile [71,72]. This technology confers an increased solubility, absorption and bioavailability [73]. Monthly formulation (PP1M) was approved by the FDA in 2009 and trimestral formulation (PP3M) in 2015, a semi-annual formulation is currently being developed [74]. For developing PP3M, the manufacturer used a PP1M population-pharmacokinetic model and avoid phase II study [75]. The main difference between PP1M and PP3M is that this last one has an increased particle size what allows its longer sustained release [76].

3.1. Pharmacokinetics

Paliperidone palmitate is slowly dissolved at the injection site after the intramuscular, deltoid or gluteal, administration and then rapidly hydrolyzed. Peak plasma concentration is achieved 13 days after injection while steady-state conditions last nearly 8 months. The apparent half-life ranges between 25 and 49 days. In contrast to risperidone, paliperidone is not extensively metabolized in the liver and nearly half of the dose is excreted unchanged in urine, so dose reduction is recommended in patients with mild renal impairment [71]. LAI Paliperidone treatment is not recommended in patients with moderate to severe renal impairment.

A popPK model of LAI PP1M statistically identified BMI, creatinine clearance, injection site (deltoid vs. gluteal), injection volume and needle length as statistical covariates, demonstrating that administration procedure and the site of injection play a key role on PP1M pharmacokinetic profile [77]. The summary of product characteristics recommends a first deltoid injection of 234 mg of paliperidone palmitate followed by a second deltoid injection of 156 mg one week later [71]. Different studies evaluated therapeutical equivalence of deltoid versus gluteal injection sites. While some authors stated that differences between deltoid and gluteal injection are not clinically relevant [78], Yin et al. reported that it can compromise maintenance treatment [79]. A case report observed that absorption rate after gluteal injection decreased in obese patients due to subcutaneous fat [80]. According to this, another study estimates that time to reach steady-state differs by 4 weeks between deltoid (38w) and gluteal (42w) injection [81]. It seems that deltoid injection provides better absorption so it should be chosen instead of the gluteal zone whenever is possible, especially in obese patients.

On the other hand, PP3M is approved for use in patients previously treated with PP1M formulation for at least 4 months with a dose 3.5 times higher than the previous PP1M dosage. PP3M has a larger particle size compared to PP1M, which allows for longer sustained release and administration every 3 months. Peak plasma concentrations are achieved 30–33 days after administration while consecution of steady-state lasts nearly 15 months. Apparent half-life ranges from 84 to 95 days (deltoid administration) versus 118 to 139 days (gluteal administration). This difference in half-life of PP3M depending on site of injection could be due to flip-flop kinetics that occur on these long-acting formulations. According to Schoretsanitis et al., urgent real-world half-life studies are needed in steady-state conditions to clarify dose-dependent half-lives on dose and influence of injection site [40]. The most relevant parameters of the popPK models of PP1M and PP3M are summarized in Table 3.

Table 3. Population pharmacokinetic models of paliperidone palmitate.

Author	Formulation	Model	Covariates	Parameters Values	Equations
Samtani et al. [77]	LAI-PP1M	- One-compartment model with first-order elimination - Dual and sequential input absorption: rapid zero order followed by first-order absorption after a lag time. - Flip-flop kinetics due to dissolution rate limited absorption.	- SEX, AGE, IVOL and INJS on Ka - CLCR on CL - BMI and SEX on Vd	KA: 0.488 h^{-1} CL: 4.95 L/h VD: 391 L	$CL = 4.95 \times \left(\frac{CLCR}{110.6}\right)^{0.376}$ $V = SEX \times 391 \times \left(\frac{BMI}{26.8}\right)^{0.889}$ SEX = 1 for males SEX = 0.726 for females
Magnusson et al. [82]	LAI-PP3M	- One-compartment model with first-order elimination - Dual and sequential input absorption processes: rapid zero absorption followed by first-order absorption.	- IVOL on Ka - INJS and SEX on Ka$_{max}$ - CLCR on CL - BMI on Vd	KA: not available. CL/F: 3.84 L/h VD/F: 1960 L	$CL = 3.84 \times \left(\frac{CLCR}{115}\right)^{0.316}$ $V = 1960 \times \left(\frac{BMI}{26.15}\right)^{1.18}$

Abbreviations: LAI: long-acting injectable. PP1M: once-monthly paliperidone palmitate. PP3M: once every 3 months paliperidone palmitate. IVOL: injection volume. INJS: injection site. BMI: body mass index. NDLL: needle length. KA: first-order absorption rate constant. Ka$_{max}$: maximum absorption rate. CL: clearance. VD: apparent volume of distribution. CL/F: clearance relative to bioavailability (in the absence of intravenous administration). VD/F: apparent volume of distribution relative to bioavailability (in the absence of intravenous administration).

With regard to the reference range, AGNP consensus guidelines established the paliperidone palmitate reference range between 20 and 60 ng/mL, but this range is again an extrapolation from oral paliperidone studies and discordance exists. A study of non-steady-state patients revealed that 45% of them were under the AGNP range [83]; on the other hand, two different studies agreed with the AGNP therapeutic range [84,85].

3.2. Pharmacogenetics

Metabolism and elimination information provided by the manufacturer are based on a study of five healthy male subjects given a 1 mg single dose of ^{14}C-paliperidone oral solution; 59% of the dose was excreted unchanged in urine. They identified four metabolic pathways but none of them metabolized more than 6.5% of the dose. Three subjects were classified as EM and two were classified as PM for *CYP2D6* using the dextrometorphan metabolic ratio. No differences in the overall plasma pharmacokinetics were observed between EM and PM. A total of 80% of the administered radioactivity was recovered in urine and 11% in the feces [86]. The small sample size (n = 5) of the study and the fact of oral administration instead of injectable does not make it possible to draw definitive conclusions with a sufficient level of evidence. Another study including 31 patients treated with paliperidone (Oral: 9 LAI: 22) did not find a statistical difference in either for the C/D ratios between different *CYP2D6* phenotypes (4 PM, 3 IM, 22 EM, 2 UM) [87]. A summary of LAI-paliperidone pharmacokinetic and pharmacogenetic characteristics is available in Table 4.

Table 4. Summary of PK/PG characteristics of LAI-Paliperidone.

Drug	Main Active Metabolite	Therapeutic Reference Range	Metabolism	TDM Recommendation (33)	Mean PK Values	Genetic Test Recommendation (94)
LAI-Paliperidone PP1M	-	20–60 ng/mL	60% excreted unmetabolized/ CYP2D6/CYP3A4 In vitro	2	T_{max}: 13 days T_{ss}: 8–9 months $T_{1/2}$: 25–49 days	Informative
LAI-Paliperidone PP3M	-	2–60 ng/mL	60% excreted unmetabolized/ CYP2D6/CYP3A4 In vitro	2	T_{max}: 30–33 days T_{ss}: 15 months $T_{1/2}$: 84–95 days (deltoid) 118–139 days (gluteal)	Informative

Abbreviations: T_{max}, time to maximum concentration after administration; T_{ss}, time to reach steady state; $t_{1/2}$, apparent half-life of elimination. TDM Levels of recommendation: 1: Strongly recommended; 2: Recommended; 3: Useful; 4: Potentially useful (33). Genetic test; informative: label contains information stating that a particular gene affects or does not affect drug efficacy, not clinically significant.

With these data it is expected that co-treatment with cytochrome inducers does not play any role in metabolism of paliperidone; however, a study performed by Yasui-Furukori et al. [88] in steady-state conditions observed that paliperidone concentrations decrease nearly 48% when carbamazepine, a potent CYP3A4 inductor, was administered concomitantly. Due to the lack of evidence regarding the influence of CYP2D6 polymorphisms in paliperidone plasma concentrations (Table 5), it is not expected that it could be associated with a higher risk of adverse effects.

Table 5. Studies between CYP2D6 phenotype and the relation with paliperidone plasma exposure.

STUDY	Oral/LAI	n	Race	Age (Median)	Male/Female	CYP2D6 Phenotypes	Outcome
Vermeir et al. [86]	Oral	5	Caucasian	51	5/0	PM/NM *	Irrelevant
Lisbeth et al. [87]	Oral/LAI	31	Caucasian	35	22/9	PM/IM/EM/UM	Irrelevant
Berwaerts et al. [89]	Oral	60	Caucasian (75%)	NR	60/0	NM/UM	Irrelevant (Coadministration with paroxetine)

Irrelevant outcome (no significative association between CYP2D6 phenotype and paliperidone plasma exposure or incorrect assignment of CYP2D6 genotype due to missing copy number variation analysis). Abbreviations: PM, Poor Metabolizer; IM, Intermediate Metabolizer; NM, Normal Metabolizer; UM, Ultra Metabolizer; NR: Not reported. * Phenotyped using the dextromethorphan metabolic ratio.

4. Long-Acting Aripiprazole

Aripiprazole was the first antipsychotic to have partial agonist effects at D2 receptors. This property, plus D3 and 5-HT1A partial agonism and 5-HT2A receptor antagonism translates, into a reduction in negative, positive and cognitive symptoms of schizophrenia, minimizing the risk of some adverse effects compared with other atypical antipsychotics.

4.1. Pharmacokinetics

The aripiprazole once monthly (AOM) long-acting injectable is the monohydrate polymorphic form of aripiprazole [90]; currently, doses of 400 mg and 300 mg are approved for induction (along with 14 days of oral supplementation) and maintenance therapy of schizophrenia. Recently, an induction start of two injections of 400 mg has been approved, avoiding the need for oral supplementation for 14 days [90]. Due to low solubility, AOM absorption into the systemic circulation is slow and prolonged after intramuscular injection. Peak plasma concentration is reached after 4 days in deltoid injection versus 5–7 days in gluteal injection, in steady-state conditions. The mean apparent half-life is 29.9 days for

300 mg and 46.5 days for 400 mg; steady-state concentrations are achieved by the fourth injection for both sites of injection according to the manufacturer [90,91].

Systemic metabolism is carried out mainly by liver biotransformation, mediated by *CYP3A4* and *CYP2D6*, yielding to its main active metabolite dehydro-aripiprazole [92]. Dehydro-aripiprazole is also a ligand at the D2 receptor and has similar pharmacological properties to the original compound [93]. At steady state, this metabolite represents up to 40% of plasma drug concentration [94]. Therefore, both compounds are thought to contribute to the antipsychotic effects. As well as risperidone and paliperidone, aripiprazole and dehydro-aripiprazole are substrates of P-gp [95]. In this case, to our knowledge no literature is available about binding affinity to P-gp of aripiprazole and dehydro-aripiprazole.

Recently, the new lauroxil LAI aripiprazole formulation has been approved. After intramuscular injection, aripiprazole lauroxil slowly dissolves and it is then hydrolyzed to aripiprazole. Peak plasma concentrations are achieved 41 days post-dose, while the steady-state is reached after 4 months. Supplementation with oral aripiprazole is needed 21 days after first administration. A 1-day regimen composed of 30 mg oral aripiprazole plus an intramuscular 675 mg nanocrystalline aripiprazole has also been approved. Aripiprazole lauroxil can be after administrated every 4, 6 or 8 weeks depending on the dose.

Therapeutic reference range based on oral formulation studies were reported between 100 and 350 ng/mL for aripiprazole and 150 and 500 ng/mL for the active moiety (aripiprazole plus dehydro-aripiprazole) [34]. AOM 400 mg provided sustained mean plasma concentrations comparable to those achieved by oral aripiprazole, 10–30 mg/day at steady-state. These data were evaluated in a 24-week, open-label, phase I study conducted in 41 patients with schizophrenia, receiving oral supplementation with 10 mg of aripiprazole for the first 14 days following the initial injection [91,96]. Pharmacokinetic data about AOM are to date limited; no third-party studies with PK analysis are available.

A study performed by the manufacturer comparing deltoid and gluteal administration verified that exposure was similar between the two injection sites but absorption rate and C_{max} were higher in the deltoid group; it seems that, as in other LAI antipsychotics, deltoid administration is a better injection site [96].

Most relevant parameters of the popPK models of aripiprazole lauroxil are summarized in Table 6, which simultaneously modeled aripiprazole and dehydro-aripriprazole observations. Surprisingly, factors related with its administration (needle length or injection volume) were not statistically significant covariates in LAI-aripiprazole lauroxil pharmacokinetics, in contrast to PP1M and PP3M findings. CYP2D6 and total weight significantly affected LAI-aripiprazole pharmacokinetics.

Table 6. Population pharmacokinetic model of LAI aripiprazole.

Author	Formulation	Model	Covariates	Parameters Values	Equations
Hard et al. [97]	Aripiprazole lauroxil	- 2-compartment model with sequential zero-order absorption followed by a first-order process - Zero-order conversion of aripiprazole lauroxil to aripiprazole	- CYP2D6 PM on CL - Total weight on Vd	KA: 0.574 h^{-1} CL/F: 0.767 L/H (PM) vs. 2.02 L/h (non-PM) VD/F: 2122 L	CL equation not reported $VD = 268 \times \left(\frac{WT}{70}\right)$

Abbreviations: KA: first-order absorption rate constant. CL/F: clearance relative to bioavailability (in the absence of intravenous administration). VD/F: apparent volume of distribution relative to bioavailability (in the absence of intravenous administration).

4.2. Pharmacogenetics

The FDA recommends dose adjustment for aripiprazole in patients who are known *CYP2D6* PMs and AOM product monograph recommends an adjusted dose of 300 mg for this group of patients [90]. According to these data, C/D ratios observed in 62-patient study treated with oral aripiprazole indicated that PMs typically need 30–40% lower doses to achieve similar serum concentrations as NMs [98]. As aripiprazole and dehydro-aripiprazole are regarded as equipotent [93], Suzuki et al. [99] in a study of 89 healthy patients demonstrated that subjects with any or reduced functional alleles (×5 and ×10) for *CYP2D6* had higher C/D ratios of the active moiety of the two compounds than those without the alleles. In a recent retrospective cohort study including pharmacokinetic data of 890 patients it was found that aripiprazole active moiety exposure increased 1.6 times and 1.4 times for PMs and IMs, respectively [48]. All these data and those of other studies are available in Table 7, showing the necessary dose adjustment in PMs.

Table 7. Studies between *CYP2D6* phenotype and the relation with aripiprazole plasma exposure.

Study	Oral/LAI	n	Race	Age (Median)	Male/Female	CYP2D6 Phenotypes	Outcome
Suzuki et al. [99]	Oral	89	Asian	38	46/43	IM/NM/UM	Relevant (higher plasma exposure for IM and PM)
Suzuki et al. [100]	Oral	63	Asian	NR	36/33	PM/IM	Relevant (For ×10 allele)
Hendset et al. [54]	Oral	266	Caucasian	33	NR	IM/NM	Irrelevant
Hendset et al. [98]	Oral	62	Caucasian	31	29/33	PM/NM	Relevant (higher plasma exposure for PM)
Belmonte et al.* [101]	Oral	148	Caucasian	26	85/63	PM/IM/NM/UM	Relevant (higher plasma exposure for PM and IM)
Tveito et al. [102]	Oral/LAI	635 (469/166)	Caucasian	40	294/341	PM/IM/NM/UM	Relevant (higher plasma exposure for PM and IM)
Jukic et al. [48]	Oral	890	Caucasian	37	400/490	PM/IM/NM/UM	Relevant (higher plasma exposure for PM and IM)
Lisbeth et al. [87]	Oral/Lai	18 (17/1)	Caucasian	36	11/7	PM/IM/NM/UM	Relevant (higher plasma exposure for PM)
van der Weide et al. [103]	Oral	130	Caucasian	NR	NR	PM/IM/NM/UM	Irrelevant
Azuma et al.** [104]	Oral	27	Asian	NR	NR	IM/NM	Relevant (Coadministration with CYP2D6 inhibitors)
Kubo et al.** [105]	Oral	20	Asian	24	20/0	IM/NM	Irrelevant

Classified in relevant (significative association between CYP2D6 phenotype and active moiety exposure) or irrelevant (no significative association between CYP2D6 phenotype and active moiety exposure or incorrect assignment of CYP2D6 genotype due to missing copy number variation analysis). Abbreviations: PM, Poor Metabolizer; IM, Intermediate Metabolizer; NM, Normal Metabolizer; UM, Ultra Metabolizer; NR: Not reported. * Those studies which do not analyze the number of copies of the gene have been classified as irrelevant. Among those classified as relevant, it is important to highlight that it should be taken as a guideline, taking into account that the main limitation is the high heterogeneity that exists between the different methods of analysis used, as well as the polymorphisms explored in the determination of the phenotype of CYP2D6. ** Single-dose study.

Current FDA recommendation only takes into account dose adjustment in *CYP2D6* PMs, but available studies show that dose reduction should also be carried out in *CYP2D6* IMs. In this sense, Tveito et al. [102] established that IM phenotype increases aripiprazole plasma concentration by 50% and active moiety concentration by 40%, both compared to NM. Further pharmacogenetic studies must be carried out in order to confirm this effect on plasma exposure, which could entail updating the product information regarding this group of patients. Among all the studies, only a few of them were performed with AOM, in which substantial influence of *CYP2D6* phenotype on serum concentrations was observed too, as in oral formulations [102].

Aripiprazole is generally well tolerated due to its good safety profile concerning extrapyramidal reactions which are less common than in the other atypical antipsychotics, except for akathisia [106,107]. Hendset et al. [98] observed that *CYP2D6*-defective alleles patients were associated with more potent adverse effects. In addition, a case–control study with eight patients suggested that IM and PM *CYP2D6* status are more frequently associated with extrapyramidal reactions [108]. Another study found that PM and IM were associated with higher incidence of nausea/vomiting due to higher plasma concentrations of aripiprazole in these subjects [101]. A summary of LAI-aripiprazole pharmacokinetic and pharmacogenetic characteristics is available in Table 8.

Table 8. Summary of PK/PG characteristics of LAI-Aripiprazole.

Drug	Main Active Metabolite	Therapeutic Reference Range	Metabolism	TDM Recommendation (33)	Mean PK Values	Genetic test Recommendation (94)
LAI-Aripiprazole Monohydrate	Dehydro-aripiprazole	100–350 ng/Ml Active moiety: 150–500 ng/mL	CYP2D6/CYP3A4	2	T_{max}: 4–7 days T_{ss}: 4 months $T_{1/2}$ 400 mg: 46.5 days 300 mg: 29.9 days	Actionable
LAI-Aripiprazole Lauroxil	Dehydro-aripiprazole	100–350 ng/mL Active moiety: 150–500 ng/mL	CYP2D6/CYP3A4	2	T_{max}: 41 days T_{ss}: 4 months $T_{1/2}$: 53.9–57.2 days	Actionable

Abbreviations: T_{max}, time to maximum concentration after administration; T_{ss}, time to reach steady state; $t_{1/2}$, apparent half-life of elimination. TDM Levels of recommendation: 1: Strongly recommended; 2: Recommended; 3: Useful; 4: Potentially useful (33). Genetic test; Informative: this label contains information stating that a particular gene affects or does not affect drug efficacy, not clinically significant; Actionable: this label may contain information about changes in efficacy due to gene variants.

Only a few of the summarized studies are developed using LAI formulations of antipsychotics; there is an urgent need for independent and real-world LAI antipsychotics TDM studies to clarify pharmacokinetic data such as the half-life and therapeutic reference range.

5. Pharmacokinetics/Pharmacogenetics Implementation

Pharmacogenetics can also contribute to understand antipsychotics behavior in the organism, and this information can be totally complemented with pharmacokinetics data of LAI. The use of pharmacogenetics on treatment optimization is exemplified in different case reports [109–111]. Moreover, nowadays there are multiple initiatives that are already translating pharmacogenetics into clinical care around the world. To cite several examples, there is the Electronic Medical Records and Genomics (eMERGE-PGx) and St. Jude Children's Research Hospital that are using pharmacogenetic analysis to guide treatment in patients; both initiatives are from the United States [112,113]. In Europe, the Ubiquitous Pharmacogenomics project (U-PGx) can be found, with seven countries taking part, one of them Spain [114]. In our country, there are already hospitals incorporating pharmacogenetics into health services [115]. There is also a Pharmacogenomic Society, the Spanish Society of Pharmacogenetics and Pharmacogenomics (SEFF), which is actively working on promoting pharmacogenetics knowledge and developing guidelines for healthcare professionals [116].

Viability of pharmacogenetics testing in psychiatry has been observed. Five years ago, two different studies were performed where physicians were asked about pharmacogenetics in psychiatry practice. Around 95% of the physicians believe that this can help them and their patients in decision-making [117] and 80–85% think that pharmacogenetics will become a standard practice in the future [117,118], which is currently a reality as aforementioned [119]. Curiously, in 2012 Mas et al. [120] studied *CYP2D6* polymorphisms in 151 patients treated with risperidone and realized that PMs received the lowest doses and UM the higher doses, without physicians knowing patients' metabolic status. However, a preventive pharmacogenetics test would resolve the casuistry with better cost-effectiveness for the health care system and the patient versus traditional prescribing methods [121].

As we have mentioned, schizophrenia implies a great economic cost for health care systems, families and society. A study performed in patients with psychiatric conditions taking drugs not recommended based on genetic information showed that they have 69% more total health care visits, 67% more medical visits and three times more medical absence days compared to patients taking drugs recommended based on their genotypes [122]. Another study associated *CYP2D6* PMs and UMs to longer hospital stay duration compared to EMs [123]. In 2013, Herbild et al. [124] demonstrated cost-effectiveness of preemptive *CYP2D6* or *CYP2C19* genotyping in patients with schizophrenia. TDM and preemptive genotyping of patients could reduce the time spent seeking the right antipsychotic drug and dose, minimizing hospital stay and visits, preventing adverse drug reactions and reducing associated costs. To all of these expenses must be added the expensive treatment with LAI, so studies focused on therapies with this group of drugs are needed to assess the cost–benefit ratio of preemptive *CYP2D6* genotyping.

6. Unsolved Questions and Future Directions

According to the LAI risperidone product monograph, 9-OH-R has similar pharmacological activity to risperidone [32]; however, oral paliperidone has been approved with twice the daily dose of risperidone. Accordingly, de Leon et al. [60,125] suggest that risperidone is twice as potent as paliperidone. In this sense, brain imaging studies showed that lower doses of risperidone cause a similar percentage of binding to higher doses of paliperidone [126,127]. This could be explained by the high affinity of paliperidone to P-gp, minimizing blood–brain barrier (BBB) penetration.

The correlations between plasma and brain concentration for risperidone and 9-OH-R have been studied by Aravagiri et al. [128] in rats documenting differences in the distribution of both compounds in the brain, showing plasma/brain ratios of 6.7 for risperidone and 32.9 for 9-OH-R. These differences could be explained by two different factors: first, affinity of risperidone and 9-OH-R for P-glycoprotein (P-gp) in BBB. Wang et al. [129] conducted a study in abcb1a/b knockout mouse model dysfunctional in P-gp. Data showed that the ratio of plasma to brain of 9-OH-R was 2.4-fold higher than that for risperidone. This could mean that 9-OH-R presents a higher affinity for P-gp than risperidone and it could explain the greater toxicity of risperidone than 9-0H-R [60]; second, hydroxylation of risperidone to 9-OH-R makes it more hydrophilic, decreasing the ability to cross the BBB.

A preliminary assessment has demonstrated the prediction performance of D2/3 receptor occupancy a priori to optimize the dosing regimen based on risperidone blood concentrations. Accordingly, a 65–80% D2/3 receptor occupancy is associated with maximal effectiveness, minimal risk of adverse events and reduced risk of relapse in patients receiving supra-therapeutic doses [130]. Similar D2/3 receptor occupancy was also reported by Shin et al. after aripiprazole administration, demonstrating the improvement of the cognitive function in a small sample size of patients with schizophrenia [131]. Therefore, predictive popPK models are encouraged to better characterize the PK properties of LAI antipsychotics and identify the sources of inter-individual variability in order to establish a PK/PD framework able to assess D2/3 receptor occupancy. The mathematical framework would allow the evaluation of dosing strategies in special sub-groups of patients, which will help to achieve an optimal efficacy/safety balance.

7. Conclusions

Atypical LAI have resulted in a great increase in safety compared with the previously available typical LAI. However, limited evidence has restricted the proper characterization of their pharmacokinetic properties, specifically regarding LAI of risperidone, paliperidone and aripiprazole. The role of CYP2D6 has been demonstrated on the PK of LAI aripriprazole, although it remains uncertain for LAI risperidone and LAI paliperidone. In spite of that fact, the developed popPK models showed common aspects regarding the influence of body weight, administration site and needle characteristics on the pharmacokinetic behavior of these drugs. However, the reduced number of patients enrolled, the prolonged drug half-life and the limited number of clinical studies available may limit the identification of covariates and pharmacogenetic effects that would help to explain the large inter-individual differences concerning drug exposure. Pharmacogenetic analysis should be considered with caution because the CYP2D6 polymorphisms analyzed in each study are different. Assuming that all the polymorphisms that were not analyzed are wild-type allele; consequently, exceedance of NM would be obtained. The CYP2D6 gene is a complex gene, which presents duplications, deletions and even non-functional hybrids and, therefore, requires a more exhaustive approach to be able to determine the relationship between kinetics and genetics. Additional evaluations, including continuous PK endpoints, are encouraged to provide a more comprehensive characterization of the PK/PD properties of LAI in order to guide the individual dose selection.

Funding: This project was partially supported by Fundación Española de Farmacia Hospitalaria "Convocatoria de ayudas de proyectos para grupos de trabajo de la SEFH 2021-2022", Plan Galego de Saude Mental (SERGAS) and Axencia Galega Innovación (Grupos de Potencial Crecimiento IN607B2020/11). Bandín-Vilar E.: Mondelo-García C. and Fernández-Ferreiro A. are grateful to the Carlos III Health Institute for financing their personnel contracts: CM20/00135, JR20/00026 and JR18/00014.

Institutional Review Board Statement: Not applicable.

Informed Consent Statement: Not applicable.

Data Availability Statement: Not applicable.

Conflicts of Interest: The authors declare no conflict of interest.

References

1. Saha, S.; Chant, D.; Welham, J.; McGrath, J. A Systematic Review of the Prevalence of Schizophrenia. *PLoS Med.* **2005**, *2*, e141. [CrossRef]
2. Organización Mundial de Salud. *Informe Sobre la Salud en el Mundo 2001: Salud Mental: Nuevos Conocimientos, Nuevas Esperanzas*; OMS: Genebra, Switzerland, 2001; ISBN 978-92-4-356201-8.
3. Tandon, R.; Keshavan, M.S.; Nasrallah, H.A. Schizophrenia, "Just the Facts" What We Know in 2008. 2. Epidemiology and Etiology. *Schizophr Res.* **2008**, *102*, 1–18. [CrossRef]
4. American Psychiatric Association. *Diagnostic and Statistical Manual of Mental Disorders*, 5th ed.; American Psychiatric Association: Washington, DC, USA, 2013; ISBN 978-0-89042-555-8.
5. Kay, S.R.; Fiszbein, A.; Opler, L.A. The Positive and Negative Syndrome Scale (PANSS) for Schizophrenia. *Schizophr Bull.* **1987**, *13*, 261–276. [CrossRef] [PubMed]
6. Combs, D.R.; Mueser, K.T. Schizophrenia and Severe Mental Illness. In *Treatments for Psychological Problems and Syndromes*; McKay, D., Abramowitz, J.S., Storch, E.A., Eds.; John Wiley & Sons, Ltd: Chichester, UK, 2017; pp. 188–201. ISBN 978-1-118-87714-2.
7. Schizophrenia Working Group of the Psychiatric Genomics Consortium Biological Insights from 108 Schizophrenia-Associated Genetic Loci. *Nature* **2014**, *511*, 421–427. [CrossRef] [PubMed]
8. Flórez, J. *Farmacología Humana*; Elsevier Masson: Barcelona, Spain, 2012; ISBN 978-84-458-1861-9.
9. Nosé, M.; Barbui, C.; Tansella, M. How Often Do Patients with Psychosis Fail to Adhere to Treatment Programmes? A Systematic Review. *Psychol Med.* **2003**, *33*, 1149–1160. [CrossRef]
10. Haddad, P.M.; Brain, C.; Scott, J. Nonadherence with Antipsychotic Medication in Schizophrenia: Challenges and Management Strategies. *Patient Relat Outcome Meas* **2014**, *5*, 43–62. [CrossRef]
11. FDA. *Table of Pharmacogenomic Biomarkers in Drug Labeling*; FDA: White Oak, MD, USA, 2020.
12. Hicks, J.K.; Bishop, J.R.; Sangkuhl, K.; Müller, D.J.; Ji, Y.; Leckband, S.G.; Leeder, J.S.; Graham, R.L.; Chiulli, D.L.; LLerena, A.; et al. Clinical Pharmacogenetics Implementation Consortium (CPIC) Guideline for CYP2D6 and CYP2C19 Genotypes and Dosing of Selective Serotonin Reuptake Inhibitors. *Clin. Pharmacol. Ther.* **2015**, *98*, 127–134. [CrossRef]
13. Daly, A.K.; Brockmöller, J.; Broly, F.; Eichelbaum, M.; Evans, W.E.; Gonzalez, F.J.; Huang, J.D.; Idle, J.R.; Ingelman-Sundberg, M.; Ishizaki, T.; et al. Nomenclature for Human CYP2D6 Alleles. *Pharmacogenetics* **1996**, *6*, 193–201. [CrossRef]
14. Sistonen, J.; Sajantila, A.; Lao, O.; Corander, J.; Barbujani, G.; Fuselli, S. CYP2D6 Worldwide Genetic Variation Shows High Frequency of Altered Activity Variants and No Continental Structure. *Pharm. Genom.* **2007**, *17*, 93–101. [CrossRef] [PubMed]
15. Friedrich, D.C.; Genro, J.P.; Sortica, V.A.; Suarez-Kurtz, G.; de Moraes, M.E.; Pena, S.D.J.; dos Santos, A.K.R.; Romano-Silva, M.A.; Hutz, M.H. Distribution of CYP2D6 Alleles and Phenotypes in the Brazilian Population. *PLoS ONE* **2014**, *9*, e110691. [CrossRef]

16. Caudle, K.E.; Sangkuhl, K.; Whirl-Carrillo, M.; Swen, J.J.; Haidar, C.E.; Klein, T.E.; Gammal, R.S.; Relling, M.V.; Scott, S.A.; Hertz, D.L.; et al. StandardizingCYP *2D6* Genotype to Phenotype Translation: Consensus Recommendations from the Clinical Pharmacogenetics Implementation Consortium and Dutch Pharmacogenetics Working Group. *Clin. Transl. Sci.* **2020**, *13*, 116–124. [CrossRef] [PubMed]
17. Sachse, C.; Brockmöller, J.; Bauer, S.; Roots, I. Cytochrome P450 2D6 Variants in a Caucasian Population: Allele Frequencies and Phenotypic Consequences. *Am. J. Hum. Genet.* **1997**, *60*, 284–295.
18. Marez, D.; Legrand, M.; Sabbagh, N.; Lo Guidice, J.M.; Spire, C.; Lafitte, J.J.; Meyer, U.A.; Broly, F. Polymorphism of the Cytochrome P450 CYP2D6 Gene in a European Population: Characterization of 48 Mutations and 53 Alleles, Their Frequencies and Evolution. *Pharmacogenetics* **1997**, *7*, 193–202. [CrossRef] [PubMed]
19. Bradford, L.D. CYP2D6 Allele Frequency in European Caucasians, Asians, Africans and Their Descendants. *Pharmacogenomics* **2002**, *3*, 229–243. [CrossRef]
20. Ji, L.; Pan, S.; Marti-Jaun, J.; Hänseler, E.; Rentsch, K.; Hersberger, M. Single-Step Assays to Analyze CYP2D6 Gene Polymorphisms in Asians: Allele Frequencies and a Novel *14B Allele in Mainland Chinese. *Clin. Chem.* **2002**, *48*, 983–988. [CrossRef]
21. Johansson, I.; Lundqvist, E.; Bertilsson, L.; Dahl, M.L.; Sjöqvist, F.; Ingelman-Sundberg, M. Inherited Amplification of an Active Gene in the Cytochrome P450 CYP2D Locus as a Cause of Ultrarapid Metabolism of Debrisoquine. *Proc. Natl. Acad. Sci. USA* **1993**, *90*, 11825–11829. [CrossRef]
22. Müller, D.J.; Kekin, I.; Kao, A.C.C.; Brandl, E.J. Towards the Implementation of CYP2D6 and CYP2C19 Genotypes in Clinical Practice: Update and Report from a Pharmacogenetic Service Clinic. *Int Rev. Psychiatry* **2013**, *25*, 554–571. [CrossRef] [PubMed]
23. Laika, B.; Leucht, S.; Heres, S.; Steimer, W. Intermediate Metabolizer: Increased Side Effects in Psychoactive Drug Therapy. The Key to Cost-Effectiveness of Pretreatment CYP2D6 Screening? *Pharm. J.* **2009**, *9*, 395–403. [CrossRef]
24. Dagostino, C.; Allegri, M.; Napolioni, V.; D'Agnelli, S.; Bignami, E.; Mutti, A.; van Schaik, R.H. CYP2D6 Genotype Can Help to Predict Effectiveness and Safety during Opioid Treatment for Chronic Low Back Pain: Results from a Retrospective Study in an Italian Cohort. *Pharmgenomics Pers. Med.* **2018**, *11*, 179–191. [CrossRef]
25. Klomp, S.D.; Manson, M.L.; Guchelaar, H.-J.; Swen, J.J. Phenoconversion of Cytochrome P450 Metabolism: A Systematic Review. *J. Clin. Med.* **2020**, *9*, 2890. [CrossRef]
26. Patel, R.; Chesney, E.; Taylor, M.; Taylor, D.; McGuire, P. Is Paliperidone Palmitate More Effective than Other Long-Acting Injectable Antipsychotics? *Psychol. Med.* **2018**, *48*, 1616–1623. [CrossRef]
27. Ramstack, M.; Grandolfi, G.P.; Mannaert, E.; D'Hoore, P.; Lasser, R.A. Long-Acting Risperidone: Prolonged-Release Injectable Delivery of Risperidone Using Medisorbo Microsphere Technology. *Schizophr. Res.* **2003**, *60*, 314. [CrossRef]
28. Karas, A.; Burdge, G.; Rey, J.A. PerserisTM: A New and Long-Acting, Atypical Antipsychotic Drug-Delivery System. *Pharm. Ther.* **2019**, *44*, 460–466.
29. Nasser, A.F.; Henderson, D.C.; Fava, M.; Fudala, P.J.; Twumasi-Ankrah, P.; Kouassi, A.; Heidbreder, C. Efficacy, Safety, and Tolerability of RBP-7000 Once-Monthly Risperidone for the Treatment of Acute Schizophrenia: An 8-Week, Randomized, Double-Blind, Placebo-Controlled, Multicenter Phase 3 Study. *J. Clin. Psychopharmacol.* **2016**, *36*, 130–140. [CrossRef] [PubMed]
30. Gefvert, O.; Eriksson, B.; Persson, P.; Helldin, L.; Björner, A.; Mannaert, E.; Remmerie, B.; Eerdekens, M.; Nyberg, S. Pharmacokinetics and D2 Receptor Occupancy of Long-Acting Injectable Risperidone (Risperdal Consta^{TM}) in Patients with Schizophrenia. *Int J. Neuropsychopharmacol* **2005**, *8*, 27–36. [CrossRef] [PubMed]
31. Fang, J.; Bourin, M.; Baker, G.B. Metabolism of Risperidone to 9-Hydroxyrisperidone by Human Cytochromes P450 2D6 and 3A4. *Naunyn Schmiedebergs Arch. Pharm.* **1999**, *359*, 147–151. [CrossRef] [PubMed]
32. AEMPS Ficha Técnica Risperdal Consta®. Available online: https://cima.aemps.es/cima/pdfs/es/ft/65213/FT_65213.pdf (accessed on 15 January 2021).
33. Lee, L.H.N.; Choi, C.; Collier, A.C.; Barr, A.M.; Honer, W.G.; Procyshyn, R.M. The Pharmacokinetics of Second-Generation Long-Acting Injectable Antipsychotics: Limitations of Monograph Values. *CNS Drugs* **2015**, *29*, 975–983. [CrossRef] [PubMed]
34. Hiemke, C.; Bergemann, N.; Clement, H.W.; Conca, A.; Deckert, J.; Domschke, K.; Eckermann, G.; Egberts, K.; Gerlach, M.; Greiner, C.; et al. Consensus Guidelines for Therapeutic Drug Monitoring in Neuropsychopharmacology: Update 2017. *Pharmacopsychiatry* **2018**, *51*, 9–62. [CrossRef]
35. Hendset, M.; Molden, E.; Refsum, H.; Hermann, M. Impact of CYP2D6 Genotype on Steady-State Serum Concentrations of Risperidone and 9-Hydroxyrisperidone in Patients Using Long-Acting Injectable Risperidone. *J. Clin. Psychopharmacol.* **2009**, *29*, 537–541. [CrossRef] [PubMed]
36. Remington, G.; Mamo, D.; Labelle, A.; Reiss, J.; Shammi, C.; Mannaert, E.; Mann, S.; Kapur, S. A PET Study Evaluating Dopamine D2 Receptor Occupancy for Long-Acting Injectable Risperidone. *Am. J. Psychiatry* **2006**, *163*, 396–401. [CrossRef]
37. Ganoci, L.; Lovrić, M.; Živković, M.; Šagud, M.; Klarica Domjanović, I.; Božina, N. The Role Of Cyp2d6, Cyp3a4/5, And Abcb1 Polymorphisms In Patients Using Long-Acting Injectable Risperidone. *Clin. Ther.* **2016**, *38*, e10–e11. [CrossRef]
38. Nesvåg, R.; Tanum, L. Therapeutic Drug Monitoring of Patients on Risperidone Depot. *Nord. J. Psychiatry* **2005**, *59*, 51–55. [CrossRef]
39. de Leon, J. Personalizing Dosing of Risperidone, Paliperidone and Clozapine Using Therapeutic Drug Monitoring and Pharmacogenetics. *Neuropharmacology* **2020**, *168*, 107656. [CrossRef]
40. Schoretsanitis, G.; Spina, E.; Hiemke, C.; de Leon, J. A Systematic Review and Combined Analysis of Therapeutic Drug Monitoring Studies for Long-Acting Risperidone. *Expert Rev. Clin. Pharmacol.* **2017**, *10*, 965–981. [CrossRef]

41. Vermeulen, A.; Piotrovsky, V.; Ludwig, E.A. Population Pharmacokinetics of Risperidone and 9-Hydroxyrisperidone in Patients with Acute Episodes Associated with Bipolar I Disorder. *J. Pharm. Pharm.* **2007**, *34*, 183–206. [CrossRef] [PubMed]
42. Scordo, M.G.; Spina, E.; Facciolà, G.; Avenoso, A.; Johansson, I.; Dahl, M.L. Cytochrome P450 2D6 Genotype and Steady State Plasma Levels of Risperidone and 9-Hydroxyrisperidone. *Psychopharmacology* **1999**, *147*, 300–305. [CrossRef]
43. Cho, H.-Y.; Lee, Y.-B. Pharmacokinetics and Bioequivalence Evaluation of Risperidone in Healthy Male Subjects with Different CYP2D6 Genotypes. *Arch. Pharm Res.* **2006**, *29*, 525–533. [CrossRef] [PubMed]
44. Llerena, A.; Berecz, R.; Dorado, P.; de la Rubia, A. QTc Interval, CYP2D6 and CYP2C9 Genotypes and Risperidone Plasma Concentrations. *J. Psychopharmacol.* **2004**, *18*, 189–193. [CrossRef]
45. Choong, E.; Polari, A.; Kamdem, R.H.; Gervasoni, N.; Spisla, C.; Sirot, E.J.; Bickel, G.G.; Bondolfi, G.; Conus, P.; Eap, C.B. Pharmacogenetic Study on Risperidone Long-Acting Injection: Influence of Cytochrome P450 2D6 and Pregnane X Receptor on Risperidone Exposure and Drug-Induced Side-Effects. *J. Clin. Psychopharmacol.* **2013**, *33*, 289–298. [CrossRef]
46. De Leon, J.; Susce, M.T.; Pan, R.-M.; Wedlund, P.J.; Orrego, M.L.; Diaz, F.J. A Study of Genetic (CYP2D6 and ABCB1) and Environmental (Drug Inhibitors and Inducers) Variables That May Influence Plasma Risperidone Levels. *Pharmacopsychiatry* **2007**, *40*, 93–102. [CrossRef] [PubMed]
47. Jovanović, N.; Božina, N.; Lovrić, M.; Medved, V.; Jakovljević, M.; Peleš, A.M. The Role of CYP2D6 and ABCB1 Pharmacogenetics in Drug-Naïve Patients with First-Episode Schizophrenia Treated with Risperidone. *Eur. J. Clin. Pharm.* **2010**, *66*, 1109–1117. [CrossRef]
48. Jukic, M.M.; Smith, R.L.; Haslemo, T.; Molden, E.; Ingelman-Sundberg, M. Effect of CYP2D6 Genotype on Exposure and Efficacy of Risperidone and Aripiprazole: A Retrospective, Cohort Study. *Lancet Psychiatry* **2019**, *6*, 418–426. [CrossRef]
49. Locatelli, I.; Kastelic, M.; Koprivšek, J.; Kores-Plesničar, B.; Mrhar, A.; Dolžan, V.; Grabnar, I. A Population Pharmacokinetic Evaluation of the Influence of CYP2D6 Genotype on Risperidone Metabolism in Patients with Acute Episode of Schizophrenia. *Eur. J. Pharm. Sci.* **2010**, *41*, 289–298. [CrossRef] [PubMed]
50. Vandenberghe, F.; Guidi, M.; Choong, E.; von Gunten, A.; Conus, P.; Csajka, C.; Eap, C.B. Genetics-Based Population Pharmacokinetics and Pharmacodynamics of Risperidone in a Psychiatric Cohort. *Clin. Pharm.* **2015**, *54*, 1259–1272. [CrossRef] [PubMed]
51. Gunes, A.; Spina, E.; Dahl, M.-L.; Scordo, M.G. ABCB1 Polymorphisms Influence Steady-State Plasma Levels of 9-Hydroxyrisperidone and Risperidone Active Moiety. *Ther. Drug Monit.* **2008**, *30*, 628–633. [CrossRef] [PubMed]
52. Zhang, T.; Brown, S.J.; Shan, Y.; Lee, A.M.; Allen, J.D.; Eum, S.; de Leon, J.; Bishop, J.R. CYP2D6 Genetic Polymorphisms and Risperidone Pharmacokinetics: A Systematic Review and Meta-Analysis. *Pharmacotherapy* **2020**, *40*, 632–647. [CrossRef] [PubMed]
53. de Leon, J.; Susce, M.T.; Pan, R.-M.; Fairchild, M.; Koch, W.H.; Wedlund, P.J. The CYP2D6 Poor Metabolizer Phenotype May Be Associated with Risperidone Adverse Drug Reactions and Discontinuation. *J. Clin. Psychiatry* **2005**, *66*, 15–27. [CrossRef]
54. Hendset, M.; Molden, E.; Knape, M.; Hermann, M. Serum Concentrations of Risperidone and Aripiprazole in Subgroups Encoding CYP2D6 Intermediate Metabolizer Phenotype. *Ther. Drug Monit* **2014**, *36*, 80–85. [CrossRef]
55. Feng, Y.; Pollock, B.G.; Coley, K.; Marder, S.; Miller, D.; Kirshner, M.; Aravagiri, M.; Schneider, L.; Bies, R.R. Population Pharmacokinetic Analysis for Risperidone Using Highly Sparse Sampling Measurements from the CATIE Study. *Br. J. Clin. Pharmacol.* **2008**, *66*, 629–639. [CrossRef]
56. Sherwin, C.M.T.; Saldaña, S.N.; Bies, R.R.; Aman, M.G.; Vinks, A.A. Population Pharmacokinetic Modeling of Risperidone and 9-Hydroxyrisperidone to Estimate CYP2D6 Subpopulations in Children and Adolescents. *Ther. Drug Monit.* **2012**, *34*, 535–544. [CrossRef]
57. Thyssen, A.; Vermeulen, A.; Fuseau, E.; Fabre, M.-A.; Mannaert, E. Population Pharmacokinetics of Oral Risperidone in Children, Adolescents and Adults with Psychiatric Disorders. *Clin. Pharm.* **2010**, *49*, 465–478. [CrossRef]
58. Kneller, L.A.; Abad-Santos, F.; Hempel, G. Physiologically Based Pharmacokinetic Modelling to Describe the Pharmacokinetics of Risperidone and 9-Hydroxyrisperidone According to Cytochrome P450 2D6 Phenotypes. *Clin. Pharm.* **2020**, *59*, 51–65. [CrossRef] [PubMed]
59. Gomeni, R.; Heidbreder, C.; Fudala, P.J.; Nasser, A.F. A Model-Based Approach to Characterize the Population Pharmacokinetics and the Relationship between the Pharmacokinetic and Safety Profiles of RBP-7000, a New, Long-Acting, Sustained-Released Formulation of Risperidone. *J. Clin. Pharmacol.* **2013**, *53*, 1010–1019. [CrossRef]
60. de Leon, J.; Sandson, N.B.; Cozza, K.L. A Preliminary Attempt to Personalize Risperidone Dosing Using Drug–Drug Interactions and Genetics: Part I. *Psychosomatics* **2008**, *49*, 258–270. [CrossRef]
61. Kakihara, S.; Yoshimura, R.; Shinkai, K.; Matsumoto, C.; Goto, M.; Kaji, K.; Yamada, Y.; Ueda, N.; Ohmori, O.; Nakamura, J. Prediction of Response to Risperidone Treatment with Respect to Plasma Concencentrations of Risperidone, Catecholamine Metabolites, and Polymorphism of Cytochrome P450 2D6. *Int. Clin. Psychopharmacol.* **2005**, *20*, 71–78. [CrossRef]
62. Almoguera, B.; Riveiro-Alvarez, R.; Lopez-Castroman, J.; Dorado, P.; Vaquero-Lorenzo, C.; Fernandez-Piqueras, J.; LLerena, A.; Abad-Santos, F.; Baca-García, E.; Dal-Ré, R.; et al. CYP2D6 Poor Metabolizer Status Might Be Associated with Better Response to Risperidone Treatment. *Pharm. Genom.* **2013**, *23*, 627–630. [CrossRef] [PubMed]
63. Petty, R. Prolactin and Antipsychotic Medications: Mechanism of Action. *Schizophr. Res.* **1999**, *35*, S67–S73. [CrossRef]
64. Turrone, P.; Kapur, S.; Seeman, M.V.; Flint, A.J. Elevation of Prolactin Levels by Atypical Antipsychotics. *AJP* **2002**, *159*, 133–135. [CrossRef] [PubMed]

65. Madhusoodanan, S.; Parida, S.; Jimenez, C. Hyperprolactinemia Associated with Psychotropics-a Review. *Hum. Psychopharmacol. Clin. Exp.* **2010**, *25*, 281–297. [CrossRef]
66. Roke, Y.; van Harten, P.N.; Franke, B.; Galesloot, T.E.; Boot, A.M.; Buitelaar, J.K. The Effect of the Taq1A Variant in the Dopamine D$_2$ Receptor Gene and Common CYP2D6 Alleles on Prolactin Levels in Risperidone-Treated Boys. *Pharm. Genom.* **2013**, *23*, 487–493. [CrossRef]
67. Schoretsanitis, G.; de Leon, J.; Diaz, F.J. Prolactin Levels: Sex Differences in the Effects of Risperidone, 9-Hydroxyrisperidone Levels, CYP2D6 and ABCB1 Variants. *Pharmacogenomics* **2018**, *19*, 815–823. [CrossRef]
68. Lane, H.-Y.; Liu, Y.-C.; Huang, C.-L.; Chang, Y.-C.; Wu, P.-L.; Lu, C.-T.; Chang, W.-H. Risperidone-Related Weight Gain: Genetic and Nongenetic Predictors. *J. Clin. Psychopharmacol.* **2006**, *26*, 128–134. [CrossRef] [PubMed]
69. Cabaleiro, T.; Ochoa, D.; López-Rodríguez, R.; Román, M.; Novalbos, J.; Ayuso, C.; Abad-Santos, F. Effect of Polymorphisms on the Pharmacokinetics, Pharmacodynamics, and Safety of Risperidone in Healthy Volunteers. *Hum. Psychopharmacol.* **2014**, *29*, 459–469. [CrossRef] [PubMed]
70. Ito, T.; Yamamoto, K.; Ohsawa, F.; Otsuka, I.; Hishimoto, A.; Sora, I.; Hirai, M.; Yano, I. Association of CYP2D6 Polymorphisms and Extrapyramidal Symptoms in Schizophrenia Patients Receiving Risperidone: A Retrospective Study. *J. Pharm. Health Care Sci.* **2018**, *4*, 28. [CrossRef]
71. AEMPS Ficha Técnica Xeplion®. Available online: https://cima.aemps.es/cima/pdfs/ft/11672002/FT_11672002.pdf (accessed on 29 January 2021).
72. Chue, P.; Chue, J. A Review of Paliperidone Palmitate. *Expert Rev. Neurother.* **2012**, *12*, 1383–1397. [CrossRef]
73. Muller, R.H.; Keck, C.M. Challenges and Solutions for the Delivery of Biotech Drugs—a Review of Drug Nanocrystal Technology and Lipid Nanoparticles. *J. Biotechnol.* **2004**, *113*, 151–170. [CrossRef] [PubMed]
74. Janssen Pharmaceuticals. A Study of Paliperidone Palmitate 6-Month Formulation (NCT03345342). Available online: https://Clinicaltrials.Gov/Ct2/Show/Study/NCT03345342 (accessed on 7 May 2018).
75. Samtani, M.N.; Nandy, P.; Ravenstijn, P.; Remmerie, B.; Vermeulen, A.; Russu, A.; D'hoore, P.; Baum, E.Z.; Savitz, A.; Gopal, S.; et al. Prospective Dose Selection and Acceleration of Paliperidone Palmitate 3-Month Formulation Development Using a Pharmacometric Bridging Strategy. *Br. J. Clin. Pharmacol.* **2016**, *82*, 1364–1370. [CrossRef]
76. Ravenstijn, P.; Remmerie, B.; Savitz, A.; Samtani, M.N.; Nuamah, I.; Chang, C.-T.; De Meulder, M.; Hough, D.; Gopal, S. Pharmacokinetics, Safety, and Tolerability of Paliperidone Palmitate 3-Month Formulation in Patients with Schizophrenia: A Phase 1, Single Dose, Randomized, Open-Label Study. *J. Clin. Pharmacol.* **2016**, *56*, 330–339. [CrossRef] [PubMed]
77. Samtani, M.N.; Vermeulen, A.; Stuyckens, K. Population Pharmacokinetics of Intramuscular Paliperidone Palmitate in Patients with Schizophrenia: A Novel Once-Monthly, Long-Acting Formulation of an Atypical Antipsychotic. *Clin. Pharm.* **2009**, *48*, 585–600. [CrossRef]
78. Ravenstijn, P.; Samtani, M.; Russu, A.; Hough, D.; Gopal, S. Paliperidone Palmitate Long-Acting Injectable Given Intramuscularly in the Deltoid Versus the Gluteal Muscle: Are They Therapeutically Equivalent? *J. Clin. Psychopharmacol.* **2016**, *36*, 744–745. [CrossRef] [PubMed]
79. Yin, J.; Collier, A.C.; Barr, A.M.; Honer, W.G.; Procyshyn, R.M. Paliperidone Palmitate Long-Acting Injectable Given Intramuscularly in the Deltoid Versus the Gluteal Muscle: Are They Therapeutically Equivalent? *J. Clin. Psychopharmacol.* **2015**, *35*, 447–449. [CrossRef]
80. Helland, A.; Syrstad, V.E.G.; Spigset, O. Prolonged Elimination of Paliperidone after Administration of Paliperidone Palmitate Depot Injections. *J. Clin. Psychopharmacol.* **2015**, *35*, 95–96. [CrossRef]
81. Coppola, D.; Liu, Y.; Gopal, S.; Remmerie, B.; Samtani, M.N.; Hough, D.W.; Nuamah, I.; Sulaiman, A.; Pandina, G. A One-Year Prospective Study of the Safety, Tolerability and Pharmacokinetics of the Highest Available Dose of Paliperidone Palmitate in Patients with Schizophrenia. *BMC Psychiatry* **2012**, *12*, 26. [CrossRef]
82. Magnusson, M.O.; Samtani, M.N.; Plan, E.L.; Jonsson, E.N.; Rossenu, S.; Vermeulen, A.; Russu, A. Population Pharmacokinetics of a Novel Once-Every 3 Months Intramuscular Formulation of Paliperidone Palmitate in Patients with Schizophrenia. *Clin. Pharm.* **2017**, *56*, 421–433. [CrossRef] [PubMed]
83. Helland, A.; Spigset, O. Serum Concentrations of Paliperidone After Administration of the Long-Acting Injectable Formulation. *Ther. Drug Monit.* **2017**, *39*, 659–662. [CrossRef] [PubMed]
84. Boumba, V.A.; Petrikis, P.; Patteet, L.; Baou, M.; Rallis, G.; Metsios, A.; Karampas, A.; Maudens, K.; Mavreas, V. A Pilot Study of Plasma Antipsychotic Drugs Concentrations of First Episode Patients with Psychosis From Epirus—Greece. *CPSP* **2019**, *8*, 123–129. [CrossRef]
85. Nazirizadeh, Y.; Vogel, F.; Bader, W.; Haen, E.; Pfuhlmann, B.; Gründer, G.; Paulzen, M.; Schwarz, M.; Zernig, G.; Hiemke, C. Serum Concentrations of Paliperidone versus Risperidone and Clinical Effects. *Eur. J. Clin. Pharmacol.* **2010**, *66*, 797–803. [CrossRef]
86. Vermeir, M.; Naessens, I.; Remmerie, B.; Mannens, G.; Hendrickx, J.; Sterkens, P.; Talluri, K.; Boom, S.; Eerdekens, M.; van Osselaer, N.; et al. Absorption, Metabolism, and Excretion of Paliperidone, a New Monoaminergic Antagonist, in Humans. *Drug Metab. Dispos.* **2008**, *36*, 769–779. [CrossRef]
87. Lisbeth, P.; Vincent, H.; Kristof, M.; Bernard, S.; Manuel, M.; Hugo, N. Genotype and Co-Medication Dependent CYP2D6 Metabolic Activity: Effects on Serum Concentrations of Aripiprazole, Haloperidol, Risperidone, Paliperidone and Zuclopenthixol. *Eur J. Clin. Pharmacol.* **2016**, *72*, 175–184. [CrossRef]

88. Yasui-Furukori, N.; Kubo, K.; Ishioka, M.; Tsuchimine, S.; Inoue, Y. Interaction between Paliperidone and Carbamazepine. *Ther. Drug Monit.* **2013**, *35*, 649–652. [CrossRef]
89. Berwaerts, J.; Cleton, A.; Herben, V.; van de Vliet, I.; Chang, I.; van Hoek, P.; Eerdekens, M. The Effects of Paroxetine on the Pharmacokinetics of Paliperidone Extended-Release Tablets. *Pharmacopsychiatry* **2009**, *42*, 158–163. [CrossRef]
90. AEMPS Ficha Técnica Abilify Maintena®. Available online: https://cima.aemps.es/cima/pdfs/es/ft/113882002/FT_113882002.pdf (accessed on 21 January 2021).
91. Mallikaarjun, S.; Kane, J.M.; Bricmont, P.; McQuade, R.; Carson, W.; Sanchez, R.; Forbes, R.A.; Fleischhacker, W.W. Pharmacokinetics, Tolerability and Safety of Aripiprazole Once-Monthly in Adult Schizophrenia: An Open-Label, Parallel-Arm, Multiple-Dose Study. *Schizophr Res.* **2013**, *150*, 281–288. [CrossRef] [PubMed]
92. Silvio Caccia N-Dealkylation of Arylpiperazine Derivatives: Disposition and Metabolism of the 1-Aryl-Piperazines Formed. *CDM* **2007**, *8*, 612–622. [CrossRef] [PubMed]
93. Tadori, Y.; Forbes, R.A.; McQuade, R.D.; Kikuchi, T. In Vitro Pharmacology of Aripiprazole, Its Metabolite and Experimental Dopamine Partial Agonists at Human Dopamine D2 and D3 Receptors. *Eur. J. Pharmacol.* **2011**, *668*, 355–365. [CrossRef]
94. Swainston Harrison, T.; Perry, C.M. Aripiprazole: A Review of Its Use in Schizophrenia and Schizoaffective Disorder. *Drugs* **2004**, *64*, 1715–1736. [CrossRef]
95. Kirschbaum, K.M.; Uhr, M.; Holthoewer, D.; Namendorf, C.; Pietrzik, C.; Hiemke, C.; Schmitt, U. Pharmacokinetics of Acute and Sub-Chronic Aripiprazole in P-Glycoprotein Deficient Mice. *Neuropharmacology* **2010**, *59*, 474–479. [CrossRef] [PubMed]
96. Raoufinia, A.; Peters-Strickland, T.; Nylander, A.-G.; Baker, R.A.; Eramo, A.; Jin, N.; Bricmont, P.; Repella, J.; McQuade, R.D.; Hertel, P.; et al. Aripiprazole Once-Monthly 400 Mg: Comparison of Pharmacokinetics, Tolerability, and Safety of Deltoid Versus Gluteal Administration. *Int. J. Neuropsychopharmacol.* **2017**, *20*, 295–304. [CrossRef]
97. Hard, M.L.; Mills, R.J.; Sadler, B.M.; Turncliff, R.Z.; Citrome, L. Aripiprazole Lauroxil: Pharmacokinetic Profile of This Long-Acting Injectable Antipsychotic in Persons With Schizophrenia. *J. Clin. Psychopharmacol.* **2017**, *37*, 289–295. [CrossRef]
98. Hendset, M.; Hermann, M.; Lunde, H.; Refsum, H.; Molden, E. Impact of the CYP2D6 Genotype on Steady-State Serum Concentrations of Aripiprazole and Dehydroaripiprazole. *Eur. J. Clin. Pharmacol.* **2007**, *63*, 1147–1151. [CrossRef]
99. Suzuki, T.; Mihara, K.; Nakamura, A.; Kagawa, S.; Nagai, G.; Nemoto, K.; Kondo, T. Effects of Genetic Polymorphisms of CYP2D6, CYP3A5, and ABCB1 on the Steady-State Plasma Concentrations of Aripiprazole and Its Active Metabolite, Dehydroaripiprazole, in Japanese Patients with Schizophrenia. *Ther. Drug Monit.* **2014**, *36*, 651–655. [CrossRef]
100. Suzuki, T.; Mihara, K.; Nakamura, A.; Nagai, G.; Kagawa, S.; Nemoto, K.; Ohta, I.; Arakaki, H.; Uno, T.; Kondo, T. Effects of the CYP2D6*10 Allele on the Steady-State Plasma Concentrations of Aripiprazole and Its Active Metabolite, Dehydroaripiprazole, in Japanese Patients with Schizophrenia. *Ther. Drug Monit.* **2011**, *33*, 21–24. [CrossRef] [PubMed]
101. Belmonte, C.; Ochoa, D.; Román, M.; Saiz-Rodríguez, M.; Wojnicz, A.; Gómez-Sánchez, C.I.; Martín-Vílchez, S.; Abad-Santos, F. Influence of CYP2D6, CYP3A4, CYP3A5 and ABCB1 Polymorphisms on Pharmacokinetics and Safety of Aripiprazole in Healthy Volunteers. *Basic Clin. Pharm. Toxicol.* **2018**, *122*, 596–605. [CrossRef] [PubMed]
102. Tveito, M.; Molden, E.; Høiseth, G.; Correll, C.U.; Smith, R.L. Impact of Age and CYP2D6 Genetics on Exposure of Aripiprazole and Dehydroaripiprazole in Patients Using Long-Acting Injectable versus Oral Formulation: Relevance of Poor and Intermediate Metabolizer Status. *Eur. J. Clin. Pharmacol.* **2020**, *76*, 41–49. [CrossRef]
103. van der Weide, K.; van der Weide, J. The Influence of the CYP3A4*22 Polymorphism and CYP2D6 Polymorphisms on Serum Concentrations of Aripiprazole, Haloperidol, Pimozide, and Risperidone in Psychiatric Patients. *J. Clin. Psychopharmacol.* **2015**, *35*, 228–236. [CrossRef]
104. Azuma, J.; Hasunuma, T.; Kubo, M.; Miyatake, M.; Koue, T.; Higashi, K.; Fujiwara, T.; Kitahara, S.; Katano, T.; Hara, S. The Relationship between Clinical Pharmacokinetics of Aripiprazole and CYP2D6 Genetic Polymorphism: Effects of CYP Enzyme Inhibition by Coadministration of Paroxetine or Fluvoxamine. *Eur J. Clin. Pharmacol.* **2012**, *68*, 29–37. [CrossRef]
105. Kubo, M.; Koue, T.; Maune, H.; Fukuda, T.; Azuma, J. Pharmacokinetics of Aripiprazole, a New Antipsychotic, Following Oral Dosing in Healthy Adult Japanese Volunteers: Influence of CYP2D6 Polymorphism. *Drug Metab Pharm.* **2007**, *22*, 358–366. [CrossRef]
106. Kane, J.M.; Carson, W.H.; Saha, A.R.; McQuade, R.D.; Ingenito, G.G.; Zimbroff, D.L.; Ali, M.W. Efficacy and Safety of Aripiprazole and Haloperidol versus Placebo in Patients with Schizophrenia and Schizoaffective Disorder. *J. Clin. Psychiatry* **2002**, *63*, 763–771. [CrossRef]
107. Potkin, S.G.; Saha, A.R.; Kujawa, M.J.; Carson, W.H.; Ali, M.; Stock, E.; Stringfellow, J.; Ingenito, G.; Marder, S.R. Aripiprazole, an Antipsychotic with a Novel Mechanism of Action, and Risperidone vs Placebo in Patients with Schizophrenia and Schizoaffective Disorder. *Arch. Gen. Psychiatry* **2003**, *60*, 681–690. [CrossRef]
108. Subuh Surja, A.A.; Reynolds, K.K.; Linder, M.W.; El-Mallakh, R.S. Pharmacogenetic Testing of *CYP2D6* in Patients with Aripiprazole-Related Extrapyramidal Symptoms: A Case–Control Study. *Pers. Med.* **2008**, *5*, 361–365. [CrossRef]
109. Sangüesa, E.; Cirujeda, C.; Concha, J.; Padilla, P.P.; Ribate, M.P.; García, C.B. Implementation of Pharmacogenetics in a Clozapine Treatment Resistant Patient: A Case Report. *Pharmacogenomics* **2019**, *20*, 871–877. [CrossRef]
110. Franco-Martin, M.A.; Sans, F.; García-Berrocal, B.; Blanco, C.; Llanes-Alvarez, C.; Isidoro-García, M. Usefulness of Pharmacogenetic Analysis in Psychiatric Clinical Practice: A Case Report. *Clin. Psychopharmacol. Neurosci.* **2018**, *16*, 349–357. [CrossRef]
111. Smith, T.; Sharp, S.; Manzardo, A.M.; Butler, M.G. Pharmacogenetics Informed Decision Making in Adolescent Psychiatric Treatment: A Clinical Case Report. *Int. J. Mol. Sci.* **2015**, *16*, 4416–4428. [CrossRef]

112. Gottesman, O.; Kuivaniemi, H.; Tromp, G.; Faucett, W.A.; Li, R.; Manolio, T.A.; Sanderson, S.C.; Kannry, J.; Zinberg, R.; Basford, M.A.; et al. The Electronic Medical Records and Genomics (EMERGE) Network: Past, Present, and Future. *Genet. Med.* **2013**, *15*, 761–771. [CrossRef] [PubMed]
113. Hoffman, J.M.; Haidar, C.E.; Wilkinson, M.R.; Crews, K.R.; Baker, D.K.; Kornegay, N.M.; Yang, W.; Pui, C.-H.; Reiss, U.M.; Gaur, A.H.; et al. PG4KDS: A Model for the Clinical Implementation of Pre-Emptive Pharmacogenetics. *Am. J. Med. Genet.* **2014**, *166*, 45–55. [CrossRef]
114. Blagec, K.; Koopmann, R.; Crommentuijn van Rhenen, M.; Holsappel, I.; van der Wouden, C.H.; Konta, L.; Xu, H.; Steinberger, D.; Just, E.; Swen, J.J.; et al. Implementing Pharmacogenomics Decision Support across Seven European Countries: The Ubiquitous Pharmacogenomics (U-PGx) Project. *J. Am. Med Inform. Assoc.* **2018**, *25*, 893–898. [CrossRef] [PubMed]
115. Borobia, A.M.; Dapia, I.; Tong, H.Y.; Arias, P.; Muñoz, M.; Tenorio, J.; Hernández, R.; García García, I.; Gordo, G.; Ramírez, E.; et al. Clinical Implementation of Pharmacogenetic Testing in a Hospital of the Spanish National Health System: Strategy and Experience Over 3 Years: Clinical Implementation of Pharmacogenetic Testing. *Clin. Transl. Sci.* **2018**, *11*, 189–199. [CrossRef]
116. Quiénes Somos. Available online: http://www.seff.es/ (accessed on 23 January 2021).
117. Thompson, C.; Steven, P. Hamilton; Catriona Hippman Psychiatrist Attitudes towards Pharmacogenetic Testing, Direct-to-Consumer Genetic Testing, and Integrating Genetic Counseling into Psychiatric Patient Care. *Psychiatry Res.* **2015**, *226*, 68–72. [CrossRef]
118. Walden, L.M.; Brandl, E.J.; Changasi, A.; Sturgess, J.E.; Soibel, A.; Notario, J.F.D.; Cheema, S.; Braganza, N.; Marshe, V.S.; Freeman, N.; et al. Physicians' Opinions Following Pharmacogenetic Testing for Psychotropic Medication. *Psychiatry Res.* **2015**, *229*, 913–918. [CrossRef] [PubMed]
119. Fundación Instituto Roche. *Medicina Personalizada de Precisión En España: Mapa de Comunidades*; Fundación Instituto Roche: Madrid, Spain, 2019.
120. Mas, S.; Gassò, P.; Alvarez, S.; Parellada, E.; Bernardo, M.; Lafuente, A. Intuitive Pharmacogenetics: Spontaneous Risperidone Dosage Is Related to CYP2D6, CYP3A5 and ABCB1 Genotypes. *Pharm. J.* **2012**, *12*, 255–259. [CrossRef]
121. Verbelen, M.; Weale, M.E.; Lewis, C.M. Cost-Effectiveness of Pharmacogenetic-Guided Treatment: Are We There Yet? *Pharm. J.* **2017**, *17*, 395–402. [CrossRef]
122. Winner, J.; Allen, J.D.; Altar, C.A.; Spahic-Mihajlovic, A. Psychiatric Pharmacogenomics Predicts Health Resource Utilization of Outpatients with Anxiety and Depression. *Transl. Psychiatry* **2013**, *3*, e242. [CrossRef]
123. Kurylev, A.A.; Brodyansky, V.M.; Andreev, B.V.; Kibitov, A.O.; Limankin, O.V.; Mosolov, S.N. The Combined Effect of CYP2D6 and DRD2 Taq1A Polymorphisms on the Antipsychotics Daily Doses and Hospital Stay Duration in Schizophrenia Inpatients (Observational Naturalistic Study). *Psychiatr. Danub* **2018**, *30*, 157–163. [CrossRef]
124. Herbild, L.; Andersen, S.E.; Werge, T.; Rasmussen, H.B.; Jürgens, G. Does Pharmacogenetic Testing for CYP450 2D6 and 2C19 among Patients with Diagnoses within the Schizophrenic Spectrum Reduce Treatment Costs? *Basic Clin. Pharmacol. Toxicol.* **2013**, *113*, 266–272. [CrossRef]
125. de Leon, J.; Wynn, G.; Sandson, N.B. The Pharmacokinetics of Paliperidone versus Risperidone. *Psychosomatics* **2010**, *51*, 80–88. [CrossRef]
126. Arakawa, R.; Ito, H.; Takano, A.; Takahashi, H.; Morimoto, T.; Sassa, T.; Ohta, K.; Kato, M.; Okubo, Y.; Suhara, T. Dose-Finding Study of Paliperidone ER Based on Striatal and Extrastriatal Dopamine D2 Receptor Occupancy in Patients with Schizophrenia. *Psychopharmacology* **2008**, *197*, 229–235. [CrossRef]
127. Kapur, S.; Remington, G.; Zipursky, R.B.; Wilson, A.A.; Houle, S. The D2 Dopamine Receptor Occupancy of Risperidone and Its Relationship to Extrapyramidal Symptoms: A PET Study. *Life Sci.* **1995**, *57*, PL103–PL107. [CrossRef]
128. Aravagiri, M.; Marder, S. Brain, Plasma and Tissue Pharmacokinetics of Risperidone and 9-Hydroxyrisperidone after Separate Oral Administration to Rats. *Psychopharmacology* **2002**, *159*, 424–431. [CrossRef]
129. Wang, J.-S.; Ruan, Y.; Taylor, R.M.; Donovan, J.L.; Markowitz, J.S.; DeVane, C.L. The Brain Entry of Risperidone and 9-Hydroxyrisperidone Is Greatly Limited by P-Glycoprotein. *Int. J. Neuropsychopharm.* **2004**, *7*, 415–419. [CrossRef]
130. Nakajima, S.; Uchida, H.; Bies, R.R.; Caravaggio, F.; Suzuki, T.; Plitman, E.; Mar, W.; Gerretsen, P.; Pollock, B.G.; Mulsant, B.H.; et al. Dopamine D2/3 Receptor Occupancy Following Dose Reduction Is Predictable With Minimal Plasma Antipsychotic Concentrations: An Open-Label Clinical Trial. *Schizophr Bull.* **2016**, *42*, 212–219. [CrossRef]
131. Shin, S.; Kim, S.; Seo, S.; Lee, J.S.; Howes, O.D.; Kim, E.; Kwon, J.S. The Relationship between Dopamine Receptor Blockade and Cognitive Performance in Schizophrenia: A [11C]-Raclopride PET Study with Aripiprazole. *Transl. Psychiatry* **2018**, *8*, 87. [CrossRef] [PubMed]

www.ingramcontent.com/pod-product-compliance
Lightning Source LLC
LaVergne TN
LVHW070050120526
838202LV00102B/2011

MDPI
St. Alban-Anlage 66
4052 Basel
Switzerland
Tel. +41 61 683 77 34
Fax +41 61 302 89 18
www.mdpi.com

Pharmaceutics Editorial Office
E-mail: pharmaceutics@mdpi.com
www.mdpi.com/journal/pharmaceutics

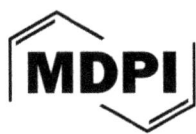